Surgical Decision-Making

Rifat Latifi
Editor

Surgical Decision-Making

Evidence and Beyond

Second Edition

Springer

Editor
Rifat Latifi
Department of Surgery
The University of Arizona
Tucson, AZ, USA

ISBN 978-3-031-67390-0 ISBN 978-3-031-67391-7 (eBook)
https://doi.org/10.1007/978-3-031-67391-7

This Springer imprint is published by the registered company Springer Nature Switzerland AG
The registered company address is: Gewerbestrasse 11, 6330 Cham, Switzerland

December 22, 2024

Tucson AZ USA

In loving memory of, and my deep appreciation for, Dr. Rao Ivatury's invaluable mentorship and unwavering support throughout my career, I dedicate this book to his enduring legacy and profound impact on surgery and trauma care worldwide.

May his wisdom, compassion, humility, and dedication continue to inspire future generations of surgeons, and his memory forever be a guiding light in the field of trauma and acute care surgery.

Foreword

For decades, various urban legends have remarked about the ability (or lack of ability) of surgeons to make rapid decisions based on little data, to then reflect upon these decisions, and to learn from their successes and their mistakes. Surgical decision-making always starts with the ability to make correct diagnoses regarding a patient's illness and then to decide if an intervention is indicated either alone or as part of a continuum of care, including medical therapies. Medicine is truly a team "sport," but, fundamentally, each patient deserves to have an individual (captain model): to provide an overall view, to bring together consultants from many fields when necessary, and to present fully the pros and cons of the decided intervention, the risks and potential complications of such intervention, and the consequences of nonintervention to the patient for his/her decision as to what they wish done. Underlying this process of surgeon–patient interaction and decision-making is the requirement for up-to-date clinical knowledge regarding best practices, clinical knowledge, and judgment.

The evolution of surgical clinical knowledge has not always proceeded in a stepwise fashion. Historically, surgeons learned from each other by apprenticeship through observing operations and inpatient/outpatient perioperative care. More experienced surgeons would travel long distances to learn new techniques that were being introduced by another master surgeon. This method evolved into the publication of an individual surgeon's results in treating a variety of surgical problems in patients, presenting such results in a professional public forum, and defending his/her various surgical approaches. Surgical societies and organizations were formed to exchange ideas. This was an attempt to improve surgical decision-making from the eighteenth through the twentieth centuries. With time, it became apparent that greater knowledge could be obtained by understanding how "an institution" handled certain patients with different diagnoses and how the patients' outcomes varied based upon their comorbidities and the surgical decisions made before, during, and after operations. These retrospective studies taught us "associations" but not causations.

Later, institutions with large clinical volumes created their own prospective databases from which multiple questions could be answered when the clinical volumes were large enough to provide some statistical validity. Interspersed over time have been prospective, randomized, clinical trials in which surgical therapies were instituted based upon randomization of the patients, and certain predetermined outcomes were then measured. All of these types of studies taken together provide a base of clinical knowledge that assist the decision-making process.

Yet, each patient is an individual with different genetic and environmental backgrounds, ages, genders, comorbidities, socioeconomic and cultural circumstances, and goals for their lives. In addition, the disease processes patients encounter have different durations, severities, prognoses, and potential outcomes. Taken together, the complexities of human diseases in patients make physician decision-making difficult despite knowledge of basic sciences and current best practice guidelines. This book, written and edited by Dr. Latifi and others, provides an important and timely resource for surgical decision-making because it defines and recognizes the many internal and external factors that influence certain surgical decisions for better or worse.

Several points made in this book deserve emphasis. While each operation should have a surgeon's standard approach, many factors that occur during an operation may alter that approach, requiring surgeon flexibility in techniques used and goals to be obtained. Recognizing that each operation is comprised of a team, we agree with Dr. Latifi that the surgeon's leadership ability and his/her ability to communicate effectively the tasks at hand to other members of the team are critical to a successful operation. As described by Dr. Latifi in Chap. 1, managing resources (including time); directing, training, and supporting others; and coping with pressure are some of the critical components of the surgeon's leadership ability. It is that ability that usually determines the patient's successful outcome.

This book nicely outlines the generic components of the surgeon's leadership and decision-making abilities and the factors that influence them. It also defines difficult clinical situations—from sepsis and trauma to elective or urgent operations for a variety of pathologic conditions—and provides guidance based on the best current clinical evidence. An expert surgical leader combines such guidance with focused training, proper communication for team members, avoidance of intraoperative distractions, and a proper mental state. These attributes lead to optimal surgical decision-making, which leads to optimal patient outcomes.

Hamden, NJ, USA Maureen D. Moore
Philadelphia, PA, USA John M. Daly (Deceased)

Preface

In the ever-evolving landscape of medicine, the practice of surgery stands as one of the most challenging and dynamic fields. The stakes are high, as every surgical decision made can profoundly impact patient outcomes, and these decisions become increasingly complicated in a rapidly changing world, where patient demographics are changing like never before. As societal values shift and technological advancements unfold, the practice of surgery is required to adapt, necessitating a profound understanding of both clinical nuances and ethical considerations. This book, a compilation of invaluable insights and experiences from leading voices in the surgical community, seeks to navigate the intricacies of surgical decision-making that have become increasingly relevant in today's healthcare environment.

The journey through this text begins with an examination of the legacy imbued in surgical decision-making. We began by paying homage to the foundational philosophies championed by our mentors, including Professor Rao Ivatury, who dedicated his life to the fields of trauma surgery and surgical education. His renowned commitment to excellence, compassion, and humility serves as a guiding light for current and future surgeons. It calls upon us to reflect not only on the decisions we make but also on the underlying motives driving those decisions. Professor Ivatury's insights remind us that the practice of surgery is not simply a technical endeavor but a profound moral responsibility that must be approached with care and contemplation.

As you delve deeper into the chapters of this second edition of this book, you will encounter the stark realities of the contemporary challenges in acute care surgery. The rapid advancement of technology in the form of artificial intelligence (AI) presents both new opportunities and ethical dilemmas in surgical planning. While there is excitement and much expectation for AI, there is still much to be discovered and it is unknown at the present time. What is well known is the fact that increasingly, surgeons must navigate complex algorithms and data analytics in their decision-making processes, raising questions about the balance of human intuition and machine-generated recommendations. Equally pressing is the exploration of the critical factors influencing the surgeon's state of mind. The mental and emotional health of surgeons, which directly impacts their decision-making capabilities and patient interactions, is addressed with the seriousness it deserves.

The parallels drawn between pilots and surgeons serve to highlight the high-stakes nature of our profession. Just as pilots must hone their skills to react in unpredictable environments, surgeons are faced with rapidly changing clinical scenarios that demand sharp acuity and preparedness. This comparative analysis effectively emphasizes the layered complexities involved in ensuring patient safety and optimal recovery outcomes, drawing on established practices in aviation that may offer valuable lessons for surgical professionals.

This book does not shy away from confronting and discussing difficult discussions surrounding surgical burnout, an issue that is increasingly recognized as a crisis in the medical community. This chapter explores the emotional toll that the demands of surgical practice can exact on individuals, providing insights into coping mechanisms and organizational strategies that can foster support for those on the front lines of patient care. Moreover, it addresses the pivotal moments when a surgeon must consider whether to continue operating or transition to different roles. The real conversations about when it is appropriate to step back from the operating room underscore the importance of self-awareness and the ethical responsibility to prioritize patient welfare amid personal challenges.

Each chapter showcases contributions from a diverse range of experts, combining contemporary research findings, case studies, and heuristic knowledge that reflect the myriads of scenarios surgeons encounter daily. From tackling complex medical issues such as managing polytrauma patients to navigating ethical dilemmas in challenging oncological cases, this text offers an expansive and nuanced overview of decision-making processes across a multitude of intricate surgical contexts. It emphasizes the need for continuing education and interdisciplinary collaboration to remain informed and adaptable to the multifaceted challenges faced by modern surgeons.

Ultimately, I hope this volume will serve not only as a valuable resource for surgeons at all levels but also as a call to action for a new paradigm of surgical decision-making—one that embraces adaptability, compassion, and ethical foresight in equal measure. The complexities of modern medicine demand that we don't simply rely on established protocols; rather, we must be inspired to think critically, explore alternative approaches, and engage in dialogue that challenges the status quo. As you turn the pages, you are invited to reflect upon our shared commitment to the art and science of surgery, a profession that continually demands the best of us and inspires the profound responsibility of keeping human lives at its core.

While the editor of each book is the driving force behind this compilation, it is the individual chapter authors who embody the dedication and pioneering spirit that characterizes the surgeon's journey. Collectively these authors' visionary leadership and commitment to surgical education shine through in the rich tapestry of perspectives compiled in this book. May this collection of wisdom, reflection, and inquiry ignite critical discussions and inspire the next generation of surgeons to navigate the complexities of their craft with courage, wisdom, and integrity.

Tucson, AZ, USA Rifat Latifi
September 22, 2024

Prologue to First Edition

Complex surgical procedures carry significant risks and complications. Despite the most conscientious preoperative preparations, surprising events may still occur. If the operation takes an unplanned turn, the surgeon has to make difficult decisions. An absolute must is continuous awareness of the patient's physiologic status—including fluid status, urine output, use of blood and blood products, bleeding, current medications (such as vasopressors), and biochemical endpoints of resuscitation. Even when the operation is going well, the biochemical profile of the patient may not be optimal or even satisfactory, which may directly affect the outcome. In addition, the surgeon must recognize his/her own physiologic status; if tired, for example, cutting corners and making major errors are much more likely. In this book, we address these and other elements that are important for the intraoperative decision-making process. How do we as surgeons make intraoperative decisions under what can be inauspicious conditions? That question has not been answered appropriately in the literature. When a patient is dying in our hands from bleeding that we cannot control, when irreversible metabolic shock does not respond to anything that we do, when new problems emerge out of the blue, when things go alarmingly wrong: In such dire moments during a carefully planned operation, how do we decide what to do next and how should we overcome our own fear? Many of us make decisions that later on we cannot explain, that we cannot say why we did things a certain way. Usually these are decisions made on the basis of a "gut feeling," or "intuition," or the "gray hair effect," among other attributes. Yet, the anatomy of such decisions is of great importance to all surgeons and to those who work with surgeons. In this book, we will review theoretical as well as any objective data that we as surgeons use to make intraoperative decisions. The decision we make, often with very limited amount of information, will decide between someone living or dying. How do we make decisions in split seconds to take someone to the operating room now as opposed to a bit later? How do we decide to operate on a dying patient without a CT scan and no laboratory data, just based on the fact that he or she is in shock, just to find liters of blood in the abdomen, a torn vena cava, liver, spleen, or some major blood vessel?

When the patient is dying in the operation room, everyone panics, but the surgeon reaches in the open abdomen and compresses the aorta between his/her fingers, in order to let the team catch up. Is there a molecular explanation for this? Non-surgeons have created and put forth many theories and hypotheses in the literature. But our collective firsthand experience as surgeons' points to a combination of factors contributing to our intraoperative decision-making process. These factors include education, clinical know-how, mentoring, and the creativity and excellence that come with long practice and with strict discipline.

The aim of this book is to evaluate the current literature on the subject and to explore what is known and, more importantly, what is not known about this process. Frankly, while the surgeon may be considered the "captain of the ship," there are many aspects of the surgical process that have recently received major public interest, and these aspects are not in the hands of surgeons at all. Involvement of these other disciplines—mainly administration, regulations, insurance, and government—has become a priority in many cases. Often, we forget that surgery is both a science and an art, and surgeons are the conductors of a symphony that truly needs to run perfectly. There are other differences between surgeons and the physicians in many other clinical disciplines. While I was a medical student at the University of Prishtina, Kosova, Professor of Surgery, Dr. Gazmend Shaqiri would tell me and others: "When a patient dies in a medical ward, he or she dies from the disease; however, when the patient dies in surgical ward, the patient dies from the surgery, or more importantly, from the decisions made by the surgeon." This may be a decision by the surgeon to operate or not to operate. While surgical procedures are far more complex than one individual's decisions during surgery, there are elements to this small surgical microcosm that add additional pressure on the surgeon and how he or she copes with this decision. Over the years, I have been reminded often of the consequences of making a decision, both wrong and right.

When I started this book, I thought it would be a single-author book, somewhat of a real rarity these days. However, as the months were passing by and the project was not being completed, I saw the real reason why: I really wanted to have other opinions on the matter.

I am hoping this book will serve as a good reference or even inspiration for others to explore the subject further. I did not and do not envision this as a book of algorithms and strict protocols although in a few chapters such suggestions have been made. I wanted myself and the other chapter authors to go a bit "beyond" the surgical decision-making process and inside the surgeon as being. I wanted to see if we can explore what makes the surgeon's brain and heart "buzz" and continue to work nonstop for many hours.

While at Yale University, before the regulation of working hours for residents, one of my vascular attendings and I operated basically nonstop from Friday morning until Sunday afternoon, with a few "power naps" between cases. I thought I was doing "fine" until I went to start my car. Now that the adrenaline was gone, I could not even drive myself home. I was completely exhausted and could not keep my eyes open. I had to call my wife Drita to come pick me up and take me home. How was I able to go on for so long while we were operating and yet I could not drive myself the 10 miles home? The anatomy and the physiology of the surgeon are addressed in Chaps. 1 and 2. We cannot forget that we are not super creatures, despite what everyone may think of us; we are all just human.

Have you ever seen a surgeon emotionally "naked," burnt out, exhausted, disillusioned, and simply tired of everything? Even worse, most of us do not talk about the matter until it becomes a real problem. Not a pretty picture by any means. At this point, you may be thinking of friends and colleagues who committed suicide or were on the brink of doing so. Drug and alcohol abuse, difficulties with personal relationships, multiple divorces, or simply becoming obese and not caring for oneself are not uncommon among surgeons. We are just human, and yet, like many other professions, we still have to get up and go to work and make some incredible decisions that will affect our patients and their families and, of course, us, and we have to live with those decisions.

I hope this book will explain some of those decisions and how we make them, but, most importantly, how we live with the decisions we make and how we improve constantly.

Valhalla, NY, USA
Spring 2016

Rifat Latifi

Prologue to Second Edition

Since the publications of the first edition of this book, there have been significant advancements in surgical decision-making that surgeons have embraced and developed. Here are some noteworthy developments:

1. **Minimally Invasive Surgery (MIS)**: Over the past decade, MIS techniques have expanded to numerous surgical specialties, including general surgery, urology, gynecology, and orthopedics. These procedures involve smaller incisions, specialized instruments, and often the use of laparoscopes or endoscopes for visualization. Benefits include reduced damage to surrounding tissues, less postoperative pain, shorter hospital stays, and faster recovery times for patients. Surgeons now have a broader range of minimally invasive options to consider when planning surgeries.
2. **Robotic-Assisted Surgery**: Robotic surgical systems, such as the da Vinci Surgical System, have made significant strides in the last decade. These systems offer enhanced visualization, improved dexterity, and tremor reduction for surgeons. The robotic arms mimic the surgeon's movements while scaling them down, providing precise control during complex operations. Surgeons have embraced robotic assistance for procedures like prostatectomies, hysterectomies, and colorectal surgeries, resulting in potentially decreased blood loss, shorter hospital stays, and improved patient outcomes.
3. **Decision Support Systems (DSS):** Technological advancements and the advent of electronic health records have paved the way for digital DSS in surgery. These systems leverage algorithms, data analytics, and artificial intelligence to analyze patient-specific information and provide evidence-based recommendations. DSS can assist surgeons in preoperative planning, predicting surgical outcomes, selecting treatment options, and assessing risks. By integrating clinical data and evidence-based guidelines, DSS programs help surgeons make well-informed decisions tailored to individual patients.
4. **Personalized Medicine**: Genomic research and molecular profiling have enabled personalized surgical approaches. Genetic testing can identify specific genetic markers or mutations that influence a patient's response to surgery, anesthesia, or drug therapies. This knowledge can guide surgical decision-making by identifying patients who might benefit from particular procedures, predicting the likelihood of complications, optimizing drug selection, or identifying potential risks. Personalized medicine

allows surgeons to customize treatment plans to individual patients, improving outcomes and reducing risks.

5. **Enhanced Imaging Modalities**: Advanced imaging technologies have had a profound impact on surgical decision-making. Magnetic resonance imaging (MRI), computed tomography (CT), and intraoperative ultrasound provide surgeons with detailed anatomical information, facilitating precise surgical planning and execution. These modalities help identify vital structures, vessels, and tumor margins, reducing the risk of complications and enabling more accurate and minimally invasive procedures. Additionally, intraoperative imaging systems provide real-time feedback, enabling surgeons to adapt their strategies during surgery.
6. **Risk Stratification Models**: Predictive models and risk stratification tools have emerged to estimate surgical risks and outcomes. These models use patient characteristics, clinical data, comorbidities, and sometimes genetic information to predict the probability of complications, length of hospital stay, or mortality rates. Surgeons can utilize this information to discuss risks and benefits with patients, set realistic expectations, and adapt surgical plans or interventions accordingly. Risk stratification models aid in shared decision-making, allowing patients to make informed choices about their surgical options.
7. **Multidisciplinary Approach**: Collaboration among multiple healthcare professionals has become integral to surgical decision-making. Surgeons now work closely with radiologists, pathologists, anesthesiologists, and other specialists to ensure comprehensive patient evaluation and optimize treatment plans. This multidisciplinary approach enables a holistic assessment of patients, incorporating expertise from various domains to develop the most appropriate surgical strategies. Collaborative discussions and input from different perspectives enhance surgical decision-making and contribute to improved patient outcomes.

These advancements collectively pave the way for more precise, individualized, and optimal surgical decision-making, improving patient outcomes and quality of care. Ongoing research, innovations in artificial intelligence, and further advancements in technology will likely continue to shape and refine surgical decision-making approaches in the coming years.

But let's get down to what really matters. While the new technological advances are very important, in the center of all the above advances is the surgeon and what constitute the decision-making. Despite the most conscientious preoperative preparations, surprising events may still occur. If the operation takes an unplanned turn, the surgeon has to make difficult decisions. Depending on the procedure, continuous knowledge and awareness of the patient's physiologic status—including fluid status, urine output, use of blood and blood products, bleeding, current medications (such as vasopressors), and biochemical endpoints of resuscitation, frailty index and how the patients look and feel, are cornerstone of surgical decision-making. Even when the operation is going well, the biochemical profile of the patient may not be optimal, or even satisfactory, which may directly affect the outcome. In addition, the surgeon must recognize his or her own physiologic status; if tired, for example, cutting corners and making major errors are much more likely. In my recent complex release of adhesion in patient with complete mechanical bowel obstruction from adhesions (grade 3 and 4), I noticed oozing from the raw surfaces. When I asked the anesthesia team, what was the patient's temperature, I was told 35.5 °C. He became cold and coagulopathic after 3 h of intense lysis of adhesions. I decided to stop the procedure, pack his abdomen, and performed a temporary abdominal closure. The next day, after resuscitation and warming him up, I worked on him for three more hours and he recovered fine. The decision was a result of observation and communication. In order to assist in surgical decision-making, and reduce errors and bias, among others, we suggest the use of artificial intelligence (AI) models that are continuously fed real-time data from electronic health records through mobile devices. By streamlining the data collection process and leveraging AI algorithms, the authors suggest that this approach may improve the accuracy and efficiency of surgical decision-making. However, implementing this approach successfully would require overcoming certain obstacles. These include standardizing the data, ensuring the interpretability of AI models, implementing and monitoring the system carefully, addressing ethical concerns related to algorithm bias, being accountable for errors, and maintaining the importance of bedside assessments and human intuition in the decision-making process (Debas 2002). Irrespective of how helpful, and fast AI can potentially be, the missing link between AI and the patient will be trust and bond between the patient and the surgeon that needs to be established and maintained. This bond and trust between the patient and the surgeon is most important element and can only be established with a "hand shake", a straight look in the eye of the patient, detailed explanations, even the regrets when we have, happiness when things go well, and sadness seen on the surgeon's face when things do not go as planned, or when there is not much that he or she can do. These are the most difficult conversations that we surgeons have with patients and their families. AI cannot do that. It can summarize the literature quickly, so it will be useful for some of us who are not up to date on every clinical issue.

In this book, as in the first edition, we address these and other elements that are important for the perioperative decision-making process. For the majority of elective surgeries, the general checklist for surgery that includes some common steps and considerations include the preoperative evaluation, anesthesia consultation, preoperative instructions for the patient, surgical consent and discussion, preoperative preparation, preoperative medications and precautions, and time-out before the procedure starts, suffices, and it is designed to reduce surgical errors.

But, the question that has not been answered yet is, how do we as surgeons make intraoperative decisions? When a patient is dying in our hands from bleeding that we cannot control, when irreversible metabolic shock does not respond to anything that we do, when new problems emerge out of the blue, when things go alarmingly wrong—in such dire moments during a carefully planned operation, how do we decide what to do next, and how should we overcome our own fears? Many of us make decisions that later on we cannot explain why we did things a certain way. Usually these are decisions made on the basis of a "gut feeling," or "intuition," or the "gray hair effect," among other attributes. Yet, the anatomy of such decisions is of great importance to all surgeons, patients, and those who work with surgeons. In this book, we will review theoretical as well as any objective data that we as surgeons use to make perioperative decisions. The decision we make, often with very limited amount of information, will decide between someone living or dying. How do we make decisions in split seconds to take someone to the operating room now, as opposed to, let's say "a bit later"? How do we decide to operate on a dying patient, without a CT scan, no laboratory data, just based on the fact that he or she is in shock, just to find liters of blood in the abdomen, a torn vena cava, grade 4–5 liver injury, spleen, or some major blood vessel?

When the patient is dying in the operating room from massive bleeding, everyone panics, but the surgeon reaches in the open abdomen and compresses the aorta between his or her fingers, or puts a clamp on to let the anesthesia team catch up. Personally, when things get "tight," I lower my voice and give deliberate commands. Is there a molecular explanation for this? Our collective firsthand experience as surgeons' points to a combination of factors contributing to our intraoperative decision-making process, including education, clinical know-how, mentoring, and the creativity and excellence that come with long practice and with strict discipline.

Frankly, while the surgeon is the "captain of the ship," there are many aspects of the surgical process that have recently received major public interest, which are not in the hands of surgeons at all. Involvement of administration, regulations by varies agencies, insurance, and governmental involvement, may affect how surgeons make potential decisions. Recently, my decision to use a certain medical product was questioned by administration. Direct interference in my surgical decision making. The majority of private and independent surgical groups are no longer private, and no longer independent. They have been swallowed by the corporate world.

Prof Haile Debas, on his presidential address titled "Surgery: A Noble Profession in a Changing World" given to the American Surgical Association, called surgery noble and quoted Webster's Third New International Dictionary that defines the word *noble as*: (1) possessing outstanding qualities such as eminence, dignity; (2) having power of transmitting by inheritance; (3) indicating superiority or commanding excellence of mind, character, or high ideals or morals. Further, Prof Debas continued: "These three attributes befit the profession of surgery. Over centuries, the surgical profession has set the standards of ethical and humane practice. Surgeons have made magnificent contributions in education, clinical care, and science. Their landmark accomplishments in surgical science and innovations in operative technique have revolutionized surgical care, saved countless lives, and significantly improved longevity and the quality of human life. Generations of surgeons have developed their craft and passed it on to succeeding generations, as they have to me and to each one of you, to take into the future."

Practice of surgery has changed significantly and dramatically, and surgeons have become a replaceable workforce of major corporations, and worse we have become "shift doctors" managed by several VPs in expensive suites that often have just come out of MBA schools and have no clue how surgery or department of surgery is run. Furthermore, as Prof Debas writes in the above-cited paper: "Financial control and control of access to healthcare were taken over by HMOs and insurance companies. As for-profit medicine proliferated, the health of our patients has come to be treated as a commodity traded daily on Wall Street. History will record that the medical profession was sidelined and watched haplessly as MBAs and business executives defined the fate of healthcare." He calls these effects of HMO "deplorable."

While director and chairman of a major medical center and academic department, I witnessed senior academic surgeons, deans, and other major academicians being "walked out" of the hospital or their offices without any cause or explanation. They wanted to "move in a new direction." The academic surgeons and surgery itself once the "crème de la crème" of the hospital have become under major corporate attacks in the last 2 to 3 decades. Unfortunately, this is not happening only in America. However, this hijacking of the surgical world by the corporate world should not cloud our thoughts and our surgical decisions, and we should make the best decision possible for every single patient that we evaluate and care for, by being trained well, being ready to care for every surgical disease. Surgeons as true leaders, should own the care of the patient, lead the multidisciplinary and complex care with passion, love, and respect for everyone, and these affect people's lives, save lives, and prevent morbidity.

The consequences may be because the surgeon decided to operate, or when the surgeon makes a decision not to operate, or not to operate in a timely fashion. As my former Professor of Surgery, Gazmend Shaqiri, a true (general, vascular, cardiothoracic) surgeon used to tell us students at the University of Prishtina, Kosova, "When a patient dies in a medical ward, he or she dies from the disease; however, when the patient dies in surgical ward, the patient dies from the surgery, or more importantly, of the decisions made by the surgeon."

Every surgical decision that we make as surgeons may have consequences, and regrets that have been reported in about 1 in 7 surgical patients (Loftus et al. 2020), both patient related and procedure related. Yet, despite this surgery was, and remains, the best clinical discipline, and represents both a science and art, and surgeons are the conductors of a symphony that truly needs to play perfectly. There are other somewhat more silent consequences of surgical decision-making.

In a study of almost 8 million patients, analyzed from the National Inpatient Sample data base, we found that delaying the operation and not performing in the optimal time was the most common cause of mortality (Smiley and Latifi n.d). While we were unable to discern why the decision to operate was delayed, the decision to operate or not is the surgeon's, and it is the decision not to operate that had major consequences. While surgical procedures are far more complex than one individual's decisions during surgery, there are elements to this small surgical microcosm that add additional pressure on the surgeon and how he or she copes with this decision. Over the years, I have been reminded often of the consequences of making a decision, both wrong and right.

I am hoping this book will serve as a good reference, or even inspiration, for others to explore the subject further and remind yourself what I teach everyone who listens—that "surgery is easy, the decision is not." I did not and do not envision this as a book of a bunch of algorithms both from some great books on the subject, or created by AI, whose computers are major polluters of our environment, to create strict protocols, although in a couple of chapters such suggestions have been made. I wanted this book to go a bit "beyond" the glory of being a surgeon and at the soul of the surgical decision-making process, and inside the surgeon being, under his or her skin. I wanted to explore what makes the surgeon's brain and heart "buzz," and continue to work nonstop for many hours. While at Yale University, before the regulation of working hours for residents, one of my vascular attendings and I operated basically nonstop from Friday morning until Sunday afternoon, with few "power naps" in the PACU or noisy operating room lounge between cases. When we finished Sunday afternoon, I thought I was doing "fine" until I went to start my car. Now that adrenaline was gone, I could not even drive myself home. I was completely exhausted and could not keep my eyes open. I had to call my wife Drita to come pick me up and take me home. How was I able to go on for so long while we were operating and yet I could not drive myself home the 10 miles to Hamden?

The anatomy and the physiology of the surgeon are addressed in Chaps. 1 and 2. We cannot forget that we are not super creatures, despite what everyone may think of us; we are all just humans, like all others except we are leaders who really care.

Have you ever seen a surgeon emotionally "naked," helpless, lonely, exhausted, disillusioned, and simply tired of everything? Even worse, most of us do not talk about the matter until it becomes real problem. Not a pretty picture by all means. At this point, you may be thinking of friends and colleagues who committed suicide or were on the brink of doing so. Drug and alcohol abuse, difficulties with personal relations, multiple divorces, or simply becoming obese and not caring for oneself are not uncommon among us surgeons. We are just humans, and yet, like many other professions, we still have to get up and go to work and make some incredible decisions that will affect our patients and their families, and of course us, that we have to live with those decisions. Hopefully, this book will explain some of those decisions, and how we make them, but most importantly how we live with the decisions we make and how we improve constantly.

Further Reading

Debas, Haile T. MD. Surgery: A Noble Profession in a Changing World. Annals of Surgery 236(3):p 263–269, September 2002

Loftus TJ, Tighe PJ, Filiberto AC, Efron PA, Brakenridge SC, Mohr AM, Rashidi P, Upchurch GR Jr, Bihorac A. Artificial Intelligence and Surgical Decision-making. JAMA Surg. 2020 Feb 1;155(2):148–158. https://doi.

org/10.1001/jamasurg.2019.4917. PMID: 31825465; PMCID: PMC7286802.

Abbas Smiley, Rifat Latifi. The Role of Delayed Operation in Hospital Mortality in Emergency General Surgery Admissions: A 10-year Study of 6,805,380 Patients. Unpublished data.

Wilson A, Ronnekleiv-Kelly SM, Pawlik TM. Regret in Surgical Decision Making: A Systematic Review of Patient and Physician Perspectives. World J Surg. 2017 Jun;41(6):1454–1465. https://doi.org/10.1007/s00268-017-3895-9. PMID: 28243695.

Rifat Latifi

Contents

Editor and Contributors

About the Editor

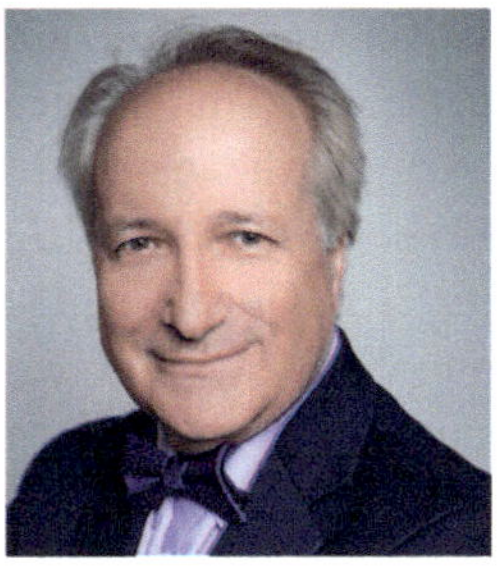

Rifat Latifi MD, FACS, FICS, FKCS, is currently a general surgeon at Tucson Medical Center in Arizona and a Professor of Surgery at the University of Arizona. He has held prestigious positions, including serving as the immediate past Minister of Health of the Republic of Kosova and as the former Chairman and Professor of Surgery at New York Medical College, School of Medicine. Additionally, he has served as the Director of the Department of Surgery at Westchester Medical Center Health Network in Valhalla, New York, and as the Medical Director of the Trauma Center in Doha, Qatar.

Dr. Latifi is a Fellow of the American College of Surgeons (ACS), Fellow of the International College of Surgeons (ICS), and a Fellow and founding President of the Kosova College of Surgeons (KCS).

Throughout his prolific academic career, Dr. Latifi has authored and co-authored near 350 peer-reviewed articles and more than 150 book chapters. He has published 20 books covering a range of surgical topics, including nutrition support, telemedicine, geriatrics, surgical decision-making, and reoperative surgery with complex abdominal wall reconstruction. Some of his latest book publications include titles such as:

1. *Telemedicine, Telehealth, and Telepresence: Principles, Strategies, Applications, and New Directions* (Springer Nature, 2020)

2. *Emergency General Surgery in Geriatrics* (Springer Nature, 2020)

3. *Surgical Decision-Making in Geriatrics: A Comprehensive Multidisciplinary Approach* (Springer Nature, 2020)

4. *The Modern Hospital: Patient-Centered, Disease-Based, Research-Oriented, Technology Driven* (Springer Nature, 2019)

5. *Surgery of Complex Abdominal Wall Defects: Practical Approaches* (2nd ed.) (Springer, 2017)

6. *Surgical Decision-Making: Beyond the Evidence* (Springer, 2016)

7. *Technological Advances in Surgery, Trauma, and Critical Care* (Springer, 2015)

In addition to his academic pursuits, Dr. Latifi is the Founder and President of the International Virtual e-Hospital Foundation, a non-profit organization that has created pioneering telemedicine programs in various countries, including Kosova, Albania, Cabo Verde, and Vietnam. Dr. Latifi established the first teletrauma and telepresence program in Arizona, known as the Southern Arizona Telemedicine and Telepresence (SATT) program, in 2004, and used telemedicine for the first time to support the long-distance swimmer, Martin Strel, while he swam the entire Amazon River in 2007.

For his outstanding contributions to telemedicine and sustainable surgical volunteerism globally, Dr. Latifi was honored with the 2015 American College of Surgeons (ACS)/Pfizer International Surgical Volunteerism award and "The 21st Century Achievement Award for Health." Over the past few years, he has been dedicated to establishing and advancing the Kosova College of Surgeons and its initiatives, including overseeing the publication of the *Kosova Journal of Surgery* as its Editor-in-Chief, while establishing telemedicine in post-conflict countries and other developing countries. Most recently he was awarded "Life-time Achieving" award for his contribution and global impact with telemedicine program by Global Digital Summit, Mumbai, India.

Contributors

Mentor Ahmeti Department of Surgery, University of North Dakota School of Medicine and Health Science, Grand Forks, ND, USA

Department of Trauma and Acute Care Surgery, Sanford Medical Center Fargo, Fargo, ND, USA

Edward S. Anderson Physician Assistant Studies, Misericordia University, Dallas, PA, USA

Emeritus of Surgery, Yale University Medical School, New Haven, CT, USA

Sateesh Babu Vascular Section of the Department of Surgery, Westchester Medical Center, Valhalla, NY, USA

New York Medical College, Valhalla, NY, USA

Zsolt J. Balogh Department of Traumatology, Division of Surgery, John Hunter Hospital & University of Newcastle, Newcastle, NSW, Australia

Gary A. Bass Division of Traumatology, Surgical Critical Care and Emergency Surgery, Department of Surgery, Perelman School of Medicine, University of Pennsylvania, Philadelphia, PA, USA

European Society for Trauma and Emergency Surgery, Vienna, Austria

Genna Beattie Clinical Fellow (PGY-9), Trauma & Acute Care Surgery, University of California San Francisco, San Francisco, CA, USA

Ryan Bendl New York Medical College, Westchester Medical Center, Valhalla, NY, USA

Sai Krishna Bhogadi Division of Trauma, Critical Care, Burns, and Emergency Surgery, Department of Surgery, University of Arizona, Tucson, AZ, USA

Heepeel Chang Westchester Medical Center, Valhalla, NY, USA

Beatriz Chumbinho Hepato-Biliary-Pancreatic and Transplantation Centre, Curry Cabral Hospital/Local Health Unit of São José, and NOVA Medical School, Lisbon, Portugal

James Clarke Westchester Medical Center, Valhalla, NY, USA

Christina Colosimo Division of Trauma, Critical Care, Burns, and Emergency Surgery, Department of Surgery, University of Arizona, Tucson, AZ, USA

Pedro Custódio Hepato-Biliary-Pancreatic and Transplantation Centre, Curry Cabral Hospital/Local Health Unit of São José, and NOVA Medical School, Lisbon, Portugal

Stanley J. Dudrick Surgery, The Commonwealth Medical College, Scranton, PA, USA

Anthony Duncan Department of Surgery, University of North Dakota School of Medicine and Health Science, Grand Forks, ND, USA

Kurt Alois Ebeleseder Department of Dental Medicine and Oral Health, Division of Restorative Dentistry, Periodontology and Prosthodontics, Medical University of Graz, Graz, Austria

Alberto R. Ferreres School of Medical Sciences, University of Buenos Aires, Buenos Aires, Argentina

Hospital de Clínicas "José de San Martín" University of Buenos Aires, Buenos Aires, Argentina

University of Washington, Seattle, WA, USA

J. Esteban Foianini Surgeon and Medical Director, Clinica Foianini, Santa Cruz, Bolivia

Joseph Fulton Vascular Section of the Department of Surgery, Westchester Medical Center, Valhalla, NY, USA

New York Medical College, Valhalla, NY, USA

Jonathan Giannone Department of Surgery, Westchester Medical Center, Valhalla, NY, USA

Arun Goyal Vascular Section of the Department of Surgery, Westchester Medical Center, Valhalla, NY, USA

New York Medical College, Valhalla, NY, USA

J. M. Guido Department of Surgery, University of South Dakota Sanford School of Medicine, Sioux Falls, SD, USA

Diane N. Haddad Division of Traumatology, Surgical Critical Care and Emergency Surgery, Department of Surgery, Perelman School of Medicine, University of Pennsylvania, Philadelphia, PA, USA

Stephanie Y. Hung Department of Surgery, University of South Dakota Sanford School of Medicine, Sioux Falls, SD, USA

Ergest Isak Department of Surgery, University of North Dakota School of Medicine and Health Science, Grand Forks, ND, USA

Daniel Jo Department of Surgery, Westchester Medical Center, Valhalla, NY, USA

Bellal Joseph Division of Trauma, Critical Care, Burns, and Emergency Surgery, Department of Surgery, University of Arizona, Tucson, AZ, USA

Rondi Kauffmann Division of Surgical Oncology and Endocrine Surgery, Vanderbilt University Medical Center, Nashville, TN, USA

Ashutosh Kaul Department of Surgery, Westchester Medical Center, Valhalla, NY, USA

Geeta Kekre Department of Pediatric Surgery, Ruby Hall Clinic, Pune, India

Tricia Kim Department of Surgery, Westchester Medical Center, Valhalla, NY, USA

Kate L. King Department of Traumatology, Division of Surgery, John Hunter Hospital & University of Newcastle, Newcastle, NSW, Australia

Lumnije Kqiku Department of Dental Medicine and Oral Health, Division of Restorative Dentistry, Periodontology and Prosthodontics, Medical University of Graz, Graz, Austria

Kshama Kulkarni Department of Pediatric Surgery, Surya Hospital, Pune, India

Igor A. Laskowski Vascular Section of the Department of Surgery, Westchester Medical Center, Valhalla, NY, USA

New York Medical College, Valhalla, NY, USA

Rifat Latifi Department of Surgery, The University of Arizona, Tucson, AZ, USA

Tucson Medical Center, Department of Surgery, Tucson, AZ, USA

Hugo Pinto Marques Hepato-Biliary-Pancreatic and Transplantation Centre, Curry Cabral Hospital/Local Health Unit of São José, and NOVA Medical School, Lisbon, Portugal

Terence O'Keeffe Division of Trauma/Surgical Critical Care/General Surgery, Department of Surgery, Augusta University, Augusta, GA, USA

Ruben Peralta Department of Surgery, Trauma Surgery Section, Hamad General Hospital, Doha, Qatar

Universidad Nacional Pedro Henriquez Urena, Santo Domingo, Dominican Republic

Ruben Peralta Department of Surgery, Trauma Surgery Section, Hamad General Hospital, Doha, Qatar

Universidad Nacional Pedro Henriquez Urena, Santo Domingo, Dominican Republic

B. S. Ratta Department of Pediatric Surgery, Ruby Hall Clinic, Pune, India

Trista Rosing Abrazo Health Network General Surgery Residency, Phoenix, AZ, USA

Cameron Schlegel Division of Surgical Oncology and Endocrine Surgery, Vanderbilt University Medical Center, Nashville, TN, USA

Abbas Smiley Department of Surgery, University of Arizona, Tucson, AZ, USA

Mafalda Sobral Hepato-Biliary-Pancreatic and Transplantation Centre, Curry Cabral Hospital/Local Health Unit of São José, and NOVA Medical School, Lisbon, Portugal

Erin Switzer Division of Trauma/Surgical Critical Care/General Surgery, Department of Surgery, Augusta University, Augusta, GA, USA

Thav Thambi-Pillai Department of Surgery, University of South Dakota Sanford School of Medicine, Sioux Falls, SD, USA

Ryan S. Ting St George & Sutherland Clinical School, University of New South Wales, Sydney, NSW, Australia

Hassan Turaihi Department of Surgery, University of South Dakota Sanford School of Medicine, Sioux Falls, SD, USA

Dhananjay Vaze Department of Pediatric Surgery, DY Patil Medical College, Pune, India

Daniel Ventarola Vascular Section of the Department of Surgery, Westchester Medical Center, Valhalla, NY, USA

New York Medical College, Valhalla, NY, USA

Part I

Changing World and the Legacy of Surgical Decision-Making

1 Surgical Decision-Making and the Changing World

Rifat Latifi and Abbas Smiley

During their professional lifetimes, surgeons must make many decisions, virtually daily, often continually, mostly "on the spot," sometimes "life or death," and almost always critically important to the optimal care, outcomes, and well-being of their patients. These decisions are based primarily on the cumulative knowledge, experience, judgment, and wisdom gained throughout years of education, training, mentoring, conferences, consultations, study, and introspection; coupled with dedication, motivation, persistence, resilience, integrity, equanimity, core values, ethics, and courage; along with a wide variety of additional, often unique, virtues which comprise the individual essence and character of each of the multitude of surgeons throughout the world.

Stanley J. Dudrick, MD, FACS- Chap. 26 in this book

Introduction

Significant advancements have been made in surgical decision-making that surgeons have embraced and further developed since the publication of the first edition of this book. Major noteworthy developments include large scale advances in robotic assisted surgery in most major and community hospitals in the USA and applied to every surgical discipline. In addition, the advent of electronic health records have increased support systems, genomic research and molecular profiling have enabled personalized surgical approaches, and advanced imaging technologies and target cell immunotherapy for cancer and other diseases in daily practice have had a profound impact on surgical decision-making. Finally all these advancements combined collectively have helped in more precise, individualized, and optimal surgical decision-making, improving patient outcomes and quality of care. In summary the following is noteworthy:

1. **Minimally Invasive Surgery (MIS)**: Over the past decade, MIS techniques have expanded to numerous surgical specialties, including general surgery, urology, gynecology, and orthopedics. These procedures involve smaller incisions, specialized instruments, and often the use of laparoscopes or endoscopes for visualization. Benefits include reduced damage to surrounding tissues, less postoperative pain, shorter hospital stays, and faster recovery times for patients. Surgeons now have a broader range of minimally invasive options to consider when planning surgeries.
2. **Robotic-assisted Surgery**: Robotic surgical systems, such as the da Vinci Surgical System, have made significant strides in the last decade. These systems offer enhanced visual-

R. Latifi (✉)
Department of Surgery, The University of Arizona, Tucson, AZ, USA

Tucson Medical Center, Department of Surgery, Tucson, AZ, USA
e-mail: Latifi@surgery.arizona.edu

A. Smiley
Department of Surgery, University of Arizona, Tucson, AZ, USA

R. Latifi (ed.), *Surgical Decision-Making*, https://doi.org/10.1007/978-3-031-67391-7_1

ization, improved dexterity, and tremor reduction for surgeons. The robotic arms mimic the surgeon's movements while scaling them down, providing precise control during complex operations. Surgeons have embraced robotic assistance for procedures in every clinical surgical discipline from neurosurgeries to like prostatectomies, hysterectomies, and colorectal surgeries, hepatobiliary surgery, and endocrine surgery, resulting in potentially decreased blood loss, shorter hospital stays, and improved patient outcomes.

3. **Decision Support Systems (DSS):** Technological advancements and the advent of electronic health records have paved the way for digital decision support systems in surgery. These systems leverage algorithms, data analytics, and artificial intelligence to analyze patient-specific information and provide evidence-based recommendations. DSS can assist surgeons in preoperative planning, predicting surgical outcomes, selecting treatment options, and assessing risks. By integrating clinical data and evidence-based guidelines, DSS programs help surgeons make well-informed decisions tailored to individual patients.
4. **Personalized Medicine**: Genomic research and molecular profiling have enabled personalized surgical approaches. Genetic testing can identify specific genetic markers or mutations that influence a patient's response to surgery, anesthesia, or drug therapies. This knowledge can guide surgical decision-making by identifying patients who might benefit from particular procedures, predicting the likelihood of complications, optimizing drug selection, or identifying potential risks. Personalized medicine allows surgeons to customize treatment plans to individual patients, improving outcomes and reducing risks.
5. **Enhanced Imaging Modalities**: Advanced imaging technologies have had a profound impact on surgical decision-making. Magnetic resonance imaging (MRI), computed tomography (CT), and intraoperative ultrasound provide surgeons with detailed anatomical information, facilitating precise surgical planning and execution. These modalities help identify vital structures, vessels, and tumor margins, reducing the risk of complications and enabling more accurate and minimally invasive procedures. Additionally, intraoperative imaging systems provide real-time feedback, enabling surgeons to adapt their strategies during surgery.
6. **Risk Stratification Models**: Predictive models and risk stratification tools have emerged to estimate surgical risks and outcomes. These models use patient characteristics, clinical data, comorbidities, and sometimes genetic information to predict the probability of complications, length of hospital stay, or mortality rates. Surgeons can utilize this information to discuss risks and benefits with patients, set realistic expectations, and adapt surgical plans or interventions accordingly. Risk stratification models aid in shared decision-making, allowing patients to make informed choices about their surgical options.
7. **Multidisciplinary Approach**: Collaboration among multiple healthcare professionals has become integral to surgical decision-making. Surgeons now work closely with radiologists, pathologists, anesthesiologists, and other specialists to ensure comprehensive patient evaluation and optimize treatment plans. This multidisciplinary approach enables a holistic assessment of patients, incorporating expertise from various domains to develop the most appropriate surgical strategies. Collaborative discussions and input from different perspectives enhance surgical decision-making and contribute to improved patient outcomes.

These advancements collectively pave the way for more precise, individualized, and optimal surgical decision-making, improving patient outcomes and quality of care [1–4]. Ongoing research, innovations in artificial intelligence, and further advancements in technology will likely continue to shape and refine surgical decision-making approaches in the coming years.

But let's get down to what really matters. Yet, in the center of all the above advances is the surgeon and what constitutes decision-making, since every surgical procedure potentially carries significant risks and complications. Despite the most conscientious preoperative preparations, surprising events may still occur. If the operation takes an unplanned turn, the surgeon has to make difficult decisions. Depending on the procedure, but an absolute must, continuous awareness of the patient's physiologic status—including fluid status, urine output, use of blood and blood products, bleeding, current medications (such as vasopressors), and biochemical endpoints of resuscitation, frailty index, and how the patients look and feel, are the cornerstone of surgical decision-making. Even when the operation is going well, the biochemical profile of the patient may not be optimal, or even satisfactory, which may directly affect the outcome. In addition, the surgeon must recognize his or her own physiologic status; if tired, for example, cutting corners and making major errors are much more likely. In my recent complex release of adhesion in a patient with complete mechanical bowel obstruction from adhesions (grade 3 and 4), I noticed oozing from the raw surfaces. When I asked the anesthesia team, what was the patient's temperature, I was told 35.5^{0}C. He became cold and coagulopathic after three hours of intense lysis of adhesions. I decided to stop the procedure, pack his abdomen and performed a temporary abdominal closure. Next day, after resuscitation and warming him up, I worked on him for three more hours and now he is recovering fine. The decision was a result of intense observation and communication.

Most recently, in order to assist in surgical decision-making and reduce errors and bias, among others, it has been suggested [3] the use of artificial intelligence models that are continuously fed real-time data from electronic health records through mobile devices. By streamlining the data collection process and leveraging AI algorithms, the authors suggest that this approach may improve the accuracy and efficiency of surgical decision-making. However, implementing this approach successfully would require overcoming certain obstacles. These include standardizing the data, ensuring the interpretability of AI models, implementing and monitoring the system carefully, addressing ethical concerns related to algorithm bias, being accountable for errors, and maintaining the importance of bedside assessments and human intuition in the decision-making process [1]. Irrespective of how helpful and crisp and fast, can AI be helpful, or potentially be helpful, the missing link between AI and the patient will be trust and bond between the patient and surgeon that needs to be established and maintained. This bond and trust can only be established with a handshake, looking straight in the eye of the patient, with detailed explanations or even regrets when we have, happiness when things go well, and sadness on the surgeon's face, when things do not go as planned, or when there is not much that he/she can do. These are the most difficult conversations that we surgeons have with patients and their families. Artificial intelligence cannot do that. It can summarize the literature quickly, so it will be useful, for some of us who are not up to date on every clinical issue.

In this book, as in the first edition, we address these and other elements that are important for the perioperative decision-making process. For the majority of elective surgeries, the general checklist for surgery that includes some common steps and considerations include the preoperative evaluation, anesthesia consultation, preoperative instructions for the patient, surgical consent and discussion, preoperative preparation, preoperative medications and precautions, and time-out before the procedure starts, suffices, and it is designed to reduce surgical errors.

The question that has not been answered yet, is how do we as surgeons make intraoperative decisions? When a patient is dying in our hands from bleeding that we cannot control, when irreversible metabolic shock does not respond to anything that we do, when new problems emerge out of the blue, when things go alarmingly wrong—in such dire moments during a carefully planned operation, how do we decide what to do next, and how should we overcome our own fears? Many of us make decisions that later on we cannot explain why we did things a certain way. Usually these are decisions made on the basis of a "gut feeling," or "intuition," or the "gray hair effect," among other attributes. Yet, the anatomy of such decisions is of great importance to all surgeons, patients, and those who work with surgeons. In this book, we will review theoretical as well as any objective data that we as surgeons use to make perioperative decisions. The decisions we make, often with very limited information, will decide between someone living or dying. How do we make decisions in split seconds to take someone to the operating room now, as opposed to, let's say "a bit later"? How do we decide to operate on a dying patient, without a CT scan, no laboratory data, just based on the fact that he or she is in shock, just to find liters of blood in the abdomen, a torn vena cava, grade 4-5 liver injury, spleen, or some major blood vessel?

When the patient is dying in the operating room from massive bleeding, everyone panics, but the surgeon reaches in the open abdomen and compresses the aorta between his or her fingers, or puts a clamp on to let the anesthesia team catch up. Personally, when things get "tight," I lower my voice and give deliberate commands. Is there a molecular explanation for this? Our collective firsthand experience as surgeons' points to a combination of factors contributing to our intraoperative decision-making process, including education, clinical know-how, mentoring, and the creativity and excellence that come with long practice and with strict discipline.

Frankly, while the surgeon is the "captain of the ship," there are many aspects of the surgical process that have recently received major public interest, which are not in the hands of surgeons at all. Involvement of other disciplines, mainly administration, regulations, insurance and governmental involvement, has taken many of these priorities, and even prevent surgeons from taking potential decisions. The majority of private and independent surgical groups, are no longer private, and no longer independent. They have been swallowed by the corporate world.

Prof Haile Debas, on his presidential address [1] titled "Surgery: A Noble Profession in a Changing World" given to American Surgical Association called surgery noble and quoted Webster's Third New International Dictionary that defines the word *noble as*:" (1) possessing outstanding qualities such as eminence, dignity; (2) having power of transmitting by inheritance; (3) indicating superiority or commanding excellence of mind, character, or high ideals or morals. Further, Prof Debas continues: "*These three attributes befit the profession of surgery. Over centuries, the surgical profession has set the standards of ethical and humane practice. Surgeons have made magnificent contributions in education, clinical care, and science. Their landmark accomplishments in surgical science and innovations in operative technique have revolutionized surgical care, saved countless lives, and significantly improved longevity and the quality of human life. Generations of surgeons have developed their craft and passed it on to succeeding generations, as they have to me and to each one of you, to take into the future.*"

Practice of surgery has changed significantly and dramatically; surgeons have become a replaceable workforce for major corporations, and worse we have become "shift doctors" managed by several VPs in expensive suits who often have just come out of MBA school, and have no clue how surgery or the department of surgery is run. Furthermore, As Prof Debas writes in the above cited paper: "*Financial control and control of access to healthcare were taken over by HMOs and insurance companies. As for-profit medicine proliferated, the health of our patients has come to be treated as a commodity traded daily on Wall Street. History will record that the medical profession was sidelined and watched haplessly as MBAs and business executives defined the fate of healthcare.* He calls these effects of HMO *"deplorable"*."

While director and chairman of a major medical center and academic department, I witnessed senior academic surgeons, deans, and others major academicians being "walked out" of the hospital or their offices without any cause or explanation. They wanted to "move in a new direction." The academic surgeons and surgery itself once the "crème de la crème" of the hospital, have come under major corporate attacks in the last 2-3 decades. Unfortunately, this is not happening only in America. However, this hijacking of the surgical world by the corporate world should not cloud our thoughts, our surgical decisions, and we should make the best decision possible for every single patient that we evaluate and care for, by being trained well, being ready to care for every surgical disease. Surgeons should act like true leaders, own the care of the patient, lead the multidisciplinary and complex care with passion, love, and respect for everyone and those who directly affect people's lives, save lives, and prevent morbidity.

The consequences may be because the surgeon decided to operate, or when the surgeon makes a decision not to operate, or not to operate in a timely fashion. As my former Professor of surgery, Gazmend Shaqiri, a true (general, vascular, cardiothoracic) surgeon used to tell us students at the University of Prishtina, Kosova, "When a patient dies in a medical ward, he or she dies from the disease; however, when the patient dies in the surgical ward, the patient dies from the surgery, or more importantly, of the decisions made by the surgeon."

Every surgical decision that we make as surgeons may have consequences, and regrets that have been reported in about 1 in 7 surgical patients [2], both patient- and procedure-related. Yet, despite this gloomy outlook, surgery was and remains the best clinical discipline, and represents both a science and an art, and surgeons are the conductors of a symphony that truly needs to run perfectly. There are other somewhat more silent consequences of surgical decision-makings. How artificial intelligence will affect surgical decision making in the future it is not clear [3].

In a study of almost seven million patients, analyzed from the National Inpatient Sample database, we found that delaying the operation and not performing in the optimal time was the most common cause of mortality [4]. While we were unable to discern why the decision to operate was delayed, the decision to operate or not is the surgeon's and this decision not to operate had major consequences. While surgical procedures are far more complex than one individual's decisions during surgery, there are elements to this small surgical microcosm that add additional pressure on the surgeon and how he or she copes with this decision. Over the years, I have been reminded often of the consequences of making a decision, both wrong and right.

I am hoping this book will serve as a good reference or even inspiration for others to explore the subject further and remind yourself what I teach everyone who listens that "*surgery is easy, the decision is not.*" I did not and do not envision this as book of a bunch of algorithms both from some great books on the subject, or created by AI, whose computers are major polluter of our environment, to create strict protocols, although in a couple of chapters such suggestions have been made. I wanted this book to go a bit "beyond" the glory of being a surgeon and at the soul of the surgical decision-making process, and inside the surgeon being under his or her skin. I wanted to explore what makes the surgeon's brain and heart "buzz," and continue to work nonstop for many hours. While at Yale University, before the regulation of working hours for residents, one of my vascular attending and I operated basically non-stop from Friday morning until Sunday afternoon, with few "power naps" in the PACU or noisy operating room lounge between cases. When we finished Sunday afternoon, I thought I was doing "fine" until I went to start my car. Now that adrenaline was gone, I could not even drive myself home. I was completely exhausted, and could not keep my eyes open. I had to call my wife Drita to come pick me up and take me home. How was I able to go on for so long while we were operating and yet, I could not drive myself home the ten miles to Hamden?

The anatomy and the physiology of the surgeon are addressed in Chaps. 1 and 2. We cannot forget that we are not super creatures, despite what everyone may think of us; we are all just humans, like all others except we are leaders who really care.

Have you ever seen a surgeon emotionally "naked," helpless, lonely, exhausted, disillusioned and, simply tired of everything? Even worse, most of us do not talk about the matter until it becomes a real problem. Not a pretty picture by all means. At this point, you may be thinking of friends and colleagues who committed suicide or were on the brink of doing so. Drug and alcohol abuse, difficulties with personal relations, multiple divorces, or simply becoming obese and not caring for oneself are not uncommon among us surgeons. We are just humans, and yet like many other professions, we still have to get up and go to work, and make some incredible decisions, that will affect our patients and their families, and of course us, that we have to live with those decisions. Hopefully, this book will explain some of those decisions, and how we make them, but most importantly how we live with the decisions we make, and how we improve constantly.

References

1. Debas HT. Surgery: a noble profession in a changing world. Annals of Surgery. 236(3):263–9.
2. Wilson A, Ronnekleiv-Kelly SM, Pawlik TM. Regret in surgical decision making: a systematic review of patient and physician perspectives. World J Surg. 2017;41(6):1454–65. https://doi.org/10.1007/s00268-017-3895-9.
3. Loftus TJ, Tighe PJ, Filiberto AC, Efron PA, Brakenridge SC, Mohr AM, Rashidi P, Upchurch GR Jr, Bihorac A. Artificial intelligence and surgical decision-making. JAMA Surg. 2020;155(2):148–58. https://doi.org/10.1001/jamasurg.2019.4917. PMID: 31825465; PMCID: PMC7286802.
4. Smiley A., Latifi R.. The role of delayed operation in hospital mortality in emergency general surgery admissions: a 10-year study of 6,805,380 Patients. Unpublished data.

2 Professor Rao Ivatury: A Legacy of Surgical Decision-Making in Trauma Surgery, Excellence, Compassion, and Humility

Rifat Latifi

Throughout his illustrious career, Dr. Rao R. Ivatury

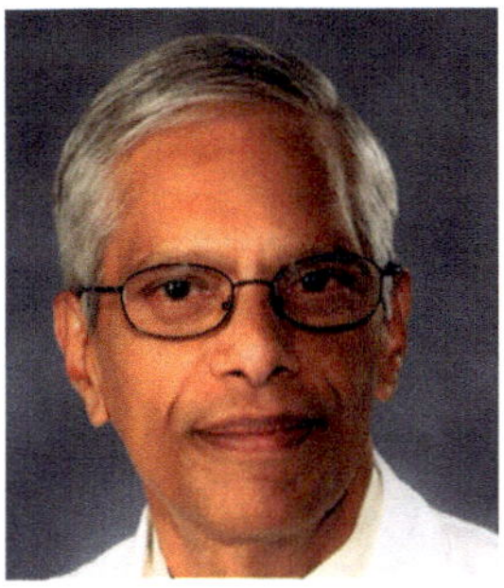

revolutionized penetrating trauma with his groundbreaking advancements and unwavering commitment to patient care.

R. Latifi (✉)
Department of Surgery, The University of Arizona, Tucson, AZ, USA

Tucson Medical Center, Department of Surgery, Tucson, AZ, USA
e-mail: Latifi@surgery.arizona.edu

R. Latifi (ed.), *Surgical Decision-Making*, https://doi.org/10.1007/978-3-031-67391-7_2

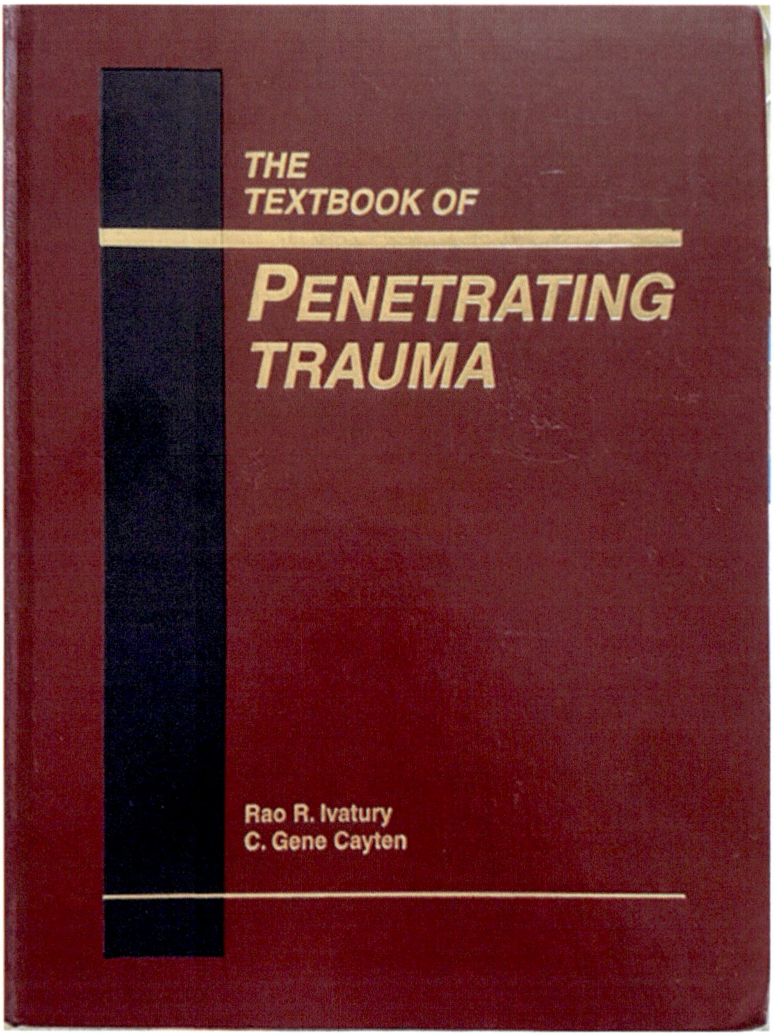

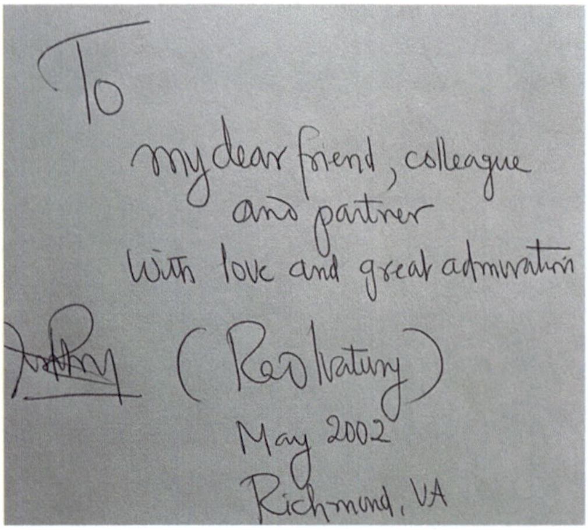

His *Textbook of Penetrating Trauma* has been a bible of management of trauma surgery since it came out in 1996. (Photo of the book that I have on my desk and consult often to this day with his autograph and dedication to me.) In addition, the book *Operative Techniques for Severe Liver Injury* (2014) became a new model of management of liver trauma.

His expertise and dedication were unmatched, earning him immense respect and admiration from colleagues, patients, and the medical community at large in all continents of the world. Dr. Ivatury's legacy extends far beyond his professional accomplishments; he was known for his exceptional human character and humility, touching the lives of all who had the privilege of knowing him. His compassionate bedside manner, genuine empathy, and tireless advocacy for patient well-being set him apart as a truly remarkable individual. His surgical decision making was impeccable, always calm and collected, and always got ahead of death.

The loss of Dr. Ivatury is deeply felt by the trauma community worldwide, as his contributions have had a lasting impact on the field of emergency medicine. His innovative approaches to trauma care have saved countless lives and inspired future generations of medical professionals. Dr. Ivatury's absence leaves a void that will be difficult to fill, and his memory will continue to be cherished by all of us who were fortunate enough to have crossed paths with this exceptional healer and visionary in the world of trauma medicine. He taught surgical decision making without making noise about it. He simply did it.

I met Dr. Ivatury or Iva as we fondly called him in June 1996 as a third-year General Surgery resident at Yale University Hospital, in New Haven, CT. That day, my Chairman, Dr. Ronald C Merrell, called me to his office to inform me that I needed to vacate my spot as the incoming fourth year resident to make room for another resident, Dr. Robert Knox, from the closing Bridgeport hospital residency program. Though unexpected, for me and for Dr. Merrell, he had arranged for me to join Professor Irvin Modlin's laboratory at the VA Hospital, West Haven, CT few weeks later.

Coincidentally, on that Friday evening, one of the surgical critical care fellows informed me that Dr. Ivatury was giving a talk in New Haven and asked me to join him and go to that program. That evening, I met Dr. Ivatury, presented him with a copy of my book, *Surgical Nutrition: Strategies in Critically Ill Patients,* and told him that I am interested in a surgical critical care fellowship and sought his advice, since I have done 5 years of research before joining the residency. He invited me to an interview the following Monday and to meet some of other faculty. Following an interview with Dr. Ivatury and his partner Dr. John Porter that Monday in June 1996, I was offered a fellowship in Surgical Critical Care at Lincoln Hospital in the Bronx, which due to Dr. Rao Ivatury was known as the Mecca of trauma surgery. And, thus, I entered the orbit of Rao Ivatury.

This meeting with Dr. Ivatury was one of the most important encounters, similar to the one when I met Dr. Stanley Dudrick (see chapter 23) in my life and career. I had been too busy operating and was enjoying being a third-year resident and had not thought of a fellowship until then. However, after this fateful meeting with Dr. Merrell, I made the pivotal decision to pursue surgical critical care fellowship, and eventually become a trauma surgeon, a choice that would shape my future professional trajectory for years to come. This encounter with Dr. Ivatury was truly transformative and set me on a path that I am eternally grateful for. Daily trips by car or train (most of the time) to southern Bronx were memorable. I listen to books on tapes, or read books on trauma and critical care.

Finishing a fellowship in Surgical Critical Care was the best way to prepare for the next two final chief years of my residency. Gaining competency in trauma and critical care is the most important way to really join the last few years of surgical residency. Walking (or running) in a trauma room without any hesitation or fear of what you will find is an amazing and liberating feeling for a novice surgeon. Training in the Lincoln Bronx, the country's most premier trauma center of those times, was a special treat and real destiny.

Following graduation from residency in July 1999, I joined both Dr. Ivatury and Dr. Merrell at Virginia Commonwealth University (VCU). Both had taken on new roles, with Dr. Merrell as the chairman of the department of surgery, and Dr. Ivatury as the chief of trauma. I became a close confidant and partner of Dr. Ivatury during my time at VCU, forming a strong bond with him. Dr. Merrell, whom I had met during my time with Dr. Dudrick in Houston, Texas, at the Herman Hospital, the University of Texas, and who had become chairman of the department of Surgery at Yale University, invited me to leave

Cleveland Clinic in Cleveland Ohio on December 6, 1993, where I was a categorical resident, and join Yale surgical residency program as a second year.

The transition from Yale to VCU marked a significant chapter in my career and solidified my relationship with Dr. Ivatury, further shaping my journey as a trauma and acute care surgeon. As the title of this essay, Dr. Rao Ivatury was an excellent and true master trauma and general surgeon, outstanding author, editor, and researcher, all the while maintaining compassion and humility, under whose quiet mentorship, I and many others who were lucky to work with him developed and grew as a trauma surgeon.

While working together or being friends with Dr. Ivatury, after I moved to Arizona to work with John Porter, I recall another significant moment that played a pivotal role in shaping further my destiny and professional journey. Dr. Merrell, a true pioneer in telemedicine, influenced my interest in utilizing telemedicine and technology for rebuilding post-war countries. This newfound passion led me to delve into this field further, when Dr. Merrell sent me to Toulouse in early 2000 for a telemedicine meeting. Subsequently, Dr. Merrell asked me to present him at the G8 Meeting in Berlin on May 4–5, 2000. My presentation titled *The Anatomy of War and Destruction of Kosovo: The Alumni's View on Reconstruction of Health in Kosovo*, showcased the vision for leveraging telemedicine to aid in the reconstruction and improvement of healthcare services in Kosova. This presentation marked a significant milestone in my involvement with telemedicine and the advancement of healthcare initiatives in post-war regions like Kosova. It was in Berlin that I presented the idea to create the Telemedicine Project of Kosova and the International Virtual e-Hospital Network concept. Despite Dr. Merrell's global leadership in telemedicine, there were no opportunities to establish trauma telemedicine in Virginia at that time. I shared with Dr. Ivatury my plans to relocate to Tucson, Arizona, where Iva's former partner John Porter was working, in January 2003. However, due to my commitment to oversee the building of the telemedicine center and program in Prishtina starting in September 2002, I needed to leave, but still had to come back monthly to take calls at VCU and to meet my financial obligations. Dr. Ivatury approved both decisions but expressed his hope that I would prioritize assisting my country, Kosova, before anything else.

Dr. Ivatury's love and passion for helping underserved individuals in the Bronx and developing countries around the world were truly immense. His unwavering commitment to supporting those in need, whether in local communities or on a global scale, resonated deeply with all of us who knew him. His approval for me to travel the world, building telemedicine and trauma programs in various countries, was the best testament to his belief in the power of education, innovation, and compassion to make a positive impact on healthcare systems and those they serve. Dr. Ivatury's endorsement of my endeavors underscored his legacy of generosity, mentorship, and dedication to improving healthcare access for all. Our bond remained steadfast over the years, and Dr. Ivatury graciously accepted to become an Honorary Fellow of the Kosova College of Surgeons in 2021. Unfortunately, due to declining health, he was unable to travel to Kosovo and witness the progress we had made since the war. Our last conversation on the phone took place after the passing of his wife, Laila. I will deeply miss him, as will the world of trauma, which will feel the absence of his expertise and guidance, his compassion and humility. However, his written works will continue to educate and inspire generations to come. Dr. Ivatury's legacy, wisdom, and compassion will forever be cherished and remembered through his writings and the lives he touched in profound ways.

Conclusion

Surgical decision-making is taught in a number of ways. Much of what I have done over the years and surgical decision that I made in trauma, I learned from Professor Rao Ivatury. He was master surgeon, a renowned trauma and critical care educator who has dedicated his career to improving patient outcomes in emergency and trauma care. Dr. Ivatury has made significant contributions to the field through his research, teaching, and clinical practice, particularly in the areas of abdominal trauma, sepsis, and emergency medical response. He has held leadership positions at multiple medical institutions and is considered a leading expert in the field of trauma surgery. Dr. Ivatury's work has had a lasting impact on the field of emergency medicine and he continues to be a driving force in advancing the care of critically ill and injured patients.

In addition to his professional achievements, Rao Ivatury, MD was known and will be remembered for his exceptional human character and humble demeanor. He was and continues to be highly regarded by colleagues, patients, and students for his compassion, integrity, and dedication to providing high-quality care. Despite his significant accomplishments in the field of trauma surgery, Dr. Ivatury remained approachable and down-to-earth, always putting the needs of his patients first. His humble nature and genuine concern for others have earned him the respect and admiration of those who have had the privilege of working with him. Dr. Ivatury's combination of medical expertise and genuine kindness make him a truly exceptional physician and mentor.

3 Surgical Decision-Making: More Questions than Answers?

Rifat Latifi and Abbas Smiley

Introduction

How do we surgeons make decisions under what can be inauspicious conditions is not entirely clear. One would think and hope that we have streamlined this process clearly by now since such decisions are made countless times daily across the world. Dissecting the anatomy of this process is of great importance to all surgeons and those who work with surgeons. Most importantly, however, is the question, do patients understand entirely the thought process of their surgeon and how is this incorporated into the consent for the operation? Many of us make decisions for which later we may not have solid reason why we did it. Usually, these are decisions made on the basis of "a gut feeling" or "intuition" or the "gray hair effect" among other "techniques." The surgical decision-making process is complex, demanding the integration of evidence, inference, and the experience, but often times it goes beyond the evidence and it becomes a matter of creativity and intuition [1]. How do we surgeons make decisions under what can be inauspicious conditions is not entirely clear. As conductors of the operation, or this most complex surgical symphony, we are cognizant of the intricacies of each decision and complexity. Yet, despite the enormous implication of the surgical decision-making process (SDMP) on surgical outcomes, the subject has not received adequate attention [1]. Furthermore, while evidence based is for the most part the standard of care and the modus operandi for most of us surgeons, the question "how do we surgeons make intraoperative decisions?" has not been answered and is often not understood by even co-surgeons, residents, or other assistants. Or perhaps, irrespective of the fact that we make decisions, most of the times on evidence based, and/or intuition, often we surgeons have difficulty in describing exactly how we came to specific decisions during surgery. The question is why we do not talk more about it? Are we simply too busy clinically, day in and day out, and do not have time to study and dissect our own decisions? Or, do we simply think that is the way we do, our mentors did it before us, we do, and we teach the youngsters the same procedure or the same elements of the surgical procedure. How to perform an evaluation of the surgical decision while gaining a better understanding of a seemingly gut-level process, which helps surgeons combat the external factors experienced

The authors has no financial or proprietary interest in the subject matter or materials discussed in the manuscript.

R. Latifi (✉)
Department of Surgery, The University of Arizona, Tucson, AZ, USA

Tucson Medical Center, Department of Surgery, Tucson, AZ, USA
e-mail: Latifi@surgery.arizona.edu

A. Smiley
Department of Surgery, University of Arizona, Tucson, AZ, USA

R. Latifi (ed.), *Surgical Decision-Making*, https://doi.org/10.1007/978-3-031-67391-7_3

before and during surgery, is wholly another subject altogether. Clearly, there are many factors that affect decision-making for surgeons before and during operations. These factors are experience and training, previous personal outcomes, the physiologic state of the surgeon, the harmony of teamwork, external factors at work, and the surgeon's ability to adapt quickly to a changing environment, are the main ones. The aim of this chapter is to set the stage for the entire book on this complex and very important process, which if done properly and timely may prevent, minimize, or avoid altogether serious intraoperative and postoperative complications. The recent developments in artificial intelligence (AI) and super computers will undoubtedly add more interesting discussions to the role of AI in surgical decision-making. As of now, there is no doubt that surgical decision-making is both a science and an art, and involves intuition. Theories on naturalistic and complex problem-solving methods have attempted to explain the decision-making processes of high-risk professionals. However, these theories often lump surgeons together with other professionals, such as pilots and nuclear plant scientists, whose decisions require exceptional accuracy, and creativity [1]. It is customary in the literature to compare pilots, surgeons, and some other high-demanding professions, and figure out how do they all make decisions when in a difficult situation.

Later in this book, in a separate chapter, I will delve into a comparison between the surgeons and the pilots, highlighting common elements in their daily routines, such as the use of checklists before commencing procedures, but in this introductory chapter, I will set the stage for further discussion. While both professions involve continuous vigilant monitoring, crisis prevention, and resolution when it occurs, pilots rely on standardized checklists during emergencies, whereas surgeons heavily depend on their experience, training, and intuition, and decide based on patient's physiology at hand. Unlike pilots, surgeons face the challenge of making critical decisions independently, even though they operate within a team. Pilots, on the other hand have been assisted and or directed by computers, and in recent years, advanced super computers, which control, just about everything that aircraft should do or not do, and there is not much that pilots can change on their own. The inability of pilots to take over the computer software brought down two Boeing Max 737 with catastrophic consequences [2]. Moreover, the unmanned aircrafts (airplanes, drones, and other flying machines with extraordinary precision) have become very common, both in peace and more so in conflicts, and may render pilots unnecessary, although they are still controlled by someone somewhere in this planet of ours. Humans control a number of sophisticated unmanned aircraft in other planets as well. What will be the role of artificial intelligence and computer programming in the airline industry in the future, remains to be seen.

The Complexity of Surgical Decision-Making

Several factors contribute to the complexity of surgical decision-making, distinguishing it from other highly demanding professions and underscoring its unique challenges.

Challenges in Standardization

While the aviation industry has successfully implemented a stepwise checklist model for pilots, the surgical field lacks a direct equivalent. Unlike the standardized steps universally followed by pilots in aviation, surgeons encounter difficulties in standardizing their decision-making processes. Although the WHO Surgical Safety Checklist was created to enhance teamwork, communication, reduce errors, and adverse events in surgery, it does not directly address the intricacies of intraoperative surgical decision-making and the dynamic environment of the operating room.

While certain operations adhere strictly to standardized steps, most surgical procedures involve flexible intra-operative steps. Even routine operations like cholecystectomy vary in instrument usage and technique (open, laparoscopic or robotic) among individual surgeons. This individualized approach hinders the creation of a reliable, reproducible, and easy-to-follow step-wise surgical model, making standardization difficult, even in the face of evidence of preferred practice [3].

Although general safety standards exist, surgical steps lack subtle rules, allowing surgeons considerable discretion. A four-grade classification of intraoperative difficulties, reflecting the diverse challenges surgeons encounter has been proposed [3], but it is not universally adopted. If we concede that we will not be able to standardize every thought of the surgeon, or every move in the operating room, is there a way that we can clean up the process of surgical decision-making from all external factors and make it dynamic, yet consistent. If we could achieve this consistency, trainees anywhere in the world can have access to a consistent model every time they do the given procedure. What will constitute " consistency" is another matter to be discussed and defined, altogether. Will all the surgeons around the world act like robots and behave as creatures with no "brain and emotional input"? Obviously, the practicality of such an attempt will certainly be an impossible mission. Yet, such models are being examined and created, practiced and reported. The fact is that we surgeons have simply not written enough to explain how we have arrived at a particular decision intraoperatively. The reasons for this are multifactorial as well, but the current ways of reporting data on our outcomes including very sophisticated statistical analyses do not permit such reporting, and thus there is a huge void of literature describing surgical decision-making processes. Just try to write a paper where you describe your thoughts, and see if it will be published in any peer reviewed journal.

Individualization in Surgical Procedures

The individualization of surgical approaches stems from various factors, including training, education, institutional practices, geography (location), and institutional culture and memory. At the Mayo, Cleveland, and other major clinics around the world, changes are slow. The memory and the culture prevail.

Even for routine surgeries, such as intestinal anastomosis, variations exist in techniques, whether stapler or hand-sewn [4, 5, 6, 7]. First, there are a number of variations on stapler techniques, and certainly a number of variations on the hand-sewn technique: single layer, double layer, silk, vicryl, PDS, and other suturing materials are all used. Even when we narrow the discussion to one type of suture, for example silk suture, one surgeon may use only 2.0 silk, while another surgeon never uses 2.0, but instead uses 3.0 silk; the differences on outcomes are so minute, but each individual surgeon would have a strong opinion on why he or she uses their preferred type of sutures. Because it not easy to explain these individual preferences, it comes back to the surgeons' education and training, technology available to the surgeon, institutional tradition, region, and finally, the culture of the surgeon and the patient that is being operated on. These simple variations, underscore the challenge of creating standardized surgical models.

Intraoperative Decision-Making

The intraoperative decision-making process is complex and can be difficult. It draws on the factors that we outlined above, but few factors such as leadership ability, mental state, physiology, and creativity, as well as objective data from the patient's physiology and anatomy. Flexibility and an open-minded approach, along with a respect for sound surgical principles, are most important. The physiology of both the patient and the surgeon is imperative. Still, most difficult intraoperative decisions, as mention above, are made "on the fly" and are hard to theorize, quantify, categorize or explain. Additional work, especially from and on surgeons themselves, is needed to delineate further how we make life-changing intraoperative decisions.

The construct of situational awareness can be applied to these "gut feeling" evaluations. How situational awareness and decision-making is affected by factors such as sleep deprivation, alcohol, or other substance consumption and other lifestyle habits is most important in understanding the decision-making process.

Leadership, Creativity, and Surgical Decision-Making

Apart from the technical aspects, a surgeon's leadership ability, often overlooked, proves crucial in navigating complex and unexpected intraoperative challenges. Managing adroitly crises by applying technical skills, clearly delegating tasks, and communicating effectively can significantly impact outcomes. Intraoperative decision-making involves monitoring, assessing situations, taking appropriate actions, and reevaluating patient responses [8, 9], While surgeon may have a lot of data to consider, eventually he or she has to rely on their own experience and knowledge, their grasp of the patient's clinical information, and occasionally on their assistants' help. A dynamic stepwise model of the surgeons' intraoperative decision-making process involves monitoring and reassessing the situation, taking appropriate actions, and reevaluating the patients' response. This dynamic model encompasses intuition, recognized as "recognition-primed decision-making," analytical ability, and creativity [10]. The surgeons' mental states play a vital role, as evidenced by studies monitoring cardiac arrhythmia and emotional levels during different stages of surgery [11]. In this study, surgeons were monitored using EEC, while opening the wound during the operation process, and while closing the skin immediately after the operation. From the ECG recordings, indices reflecting cardiac arrhythmia and emotional levels were calculated. The authors concluded that the process of decision-making during the vital stages of operations causes a fall in the coefficient of heart rate variability, the variance of R-R intervals, and the variability range of R-R intervals. During all the stages of surgery studied, and immediately after the operation, an increase in tonus of the sympathetic nervous system occurs in surgeons, indicating a rise in emotional level [11]. Factors such as task visualization, communication, and mental models have also been identified as critical in surgical decision-making [12, 13]. Creativity in complex surgical procedures is a key element in shaping surgical practices and challenging established norms [14]. While adhering to sound surgical principles, surgeons must remain open-minded and flexible to adapt to new intraoperative challenges. Nowhere is that model more applicable than in complex reoperative surgical procedures, which are often associated with an array of unanticipated problems [14]. In the author's opinion, an important non-technical component that has not received sufficient attention is the surgeon's leadership ability.

Influence of Technology on Decision-Making

The evolution of technology has significantly influenced the peri- and intraoperative decision-making process by using technological tools and modifying decisions accordingly [15]. One has to review the progress made only within the last few decades, from all open surgery, to laparoscopically, to endovascularly and robotically assisted, just basically every surgical procedure, to see the real effect of technological advances. The availability of technology shapes surgical practices, particularly artificial intelligence, as evidenced by the historical development of surgical advancements. However, the increasing reliance on technology prompts contemplation of a future where surgical decisions might be guided by advanced systems, possibly surpassing human capabilities.

Summary: From all the elements associated with the entire continuum of complex surgical process, for us as surgeons, surgery itself is and should be the easiest one. Deciding what to do, and more often what not to do, is more complex, more demanding, more tasking, and requires more thinking and planning from the surgeon and the surgical team than the procedure itself. Because there are no minor or simple surgical interventions, surgical decision-making is complex in every procedure, in every patient, and all the time. Each complex surgical procedure carries significant risks and complications, whether performed alone or in combination, if every detail is not executed exactly. Surgery is a symphony where everyone plays their notes based on the script and are led from the conductor. Yet, there is a difference between the emergency surgery that is required to save someone's life or relieve the pain and suffering and elective surgery. Even more different is the surgical decision in prophylactic surgery [16].

Consequences of Surgical Decision-Making

Sometimes not all that we do goes as smoothly as planned, and not every operation is successful. In the past, surgeons have been known to use the saying: "*The surgery was successful, but the patient died.*" While this is not uttered as often today, sometimes everything during the operation did go as we had wished, but the patient does not recuperate, develops one or more major complications, or worse the patient dies. Even when things do go well, the patient may still need to undergo a subsequent procedure, another exposure to anesthesia, endure a longer hospital stay, and experience a number of unforeseen issues. The cost of surgical errors is massive, and probably cannot be quantified realistically, as many of the errors go unnoticed, and often outcomes are "assigned" to the patient's disease or at best to "opportunity for improvement."

It's important to note that the exact costs can vary widely depending on the severity of the mistake, the resulting harm to the patient, and the specific circumstances surrounding the incident. Healthcare systems continually strive to improve safety measures to minimize the occurrence of surgical mistakes and mitigate their associated costs. One only need to consider the impact of potential complications to appreciate that no surgery should be dismissed as minor or merely routine. Does surgical decision-making contribute to postoperative complications?

The Factors Affecting Intraoperative Decisions

As a medical student, a surgical resident, and as a young faculty, I was fascinated by the surgical decision-making and how surgeons came up with them. Often time, for the same disease process and the same diagnosis, my professors would have different approaches and often different or alternative decisions altogether. The first edition of this book was the result of this interest. Recently, I have expanded the surgical decision-making to the geriatric population, as the fastest growing group of world population decisions in a number of situations [17].

Distracting Factors on Perioperative Surgical Decision-Making and Disruption of Surgical Symphony

The most important factors in surgical decision-making that have not attracted enough attention are those that we surgeons encounter in the preoperative phase. These factors, and I call them distracting, may have a profound effect on outcomes. Such perioperative factors could be the state of the patient's physiology and age (often we act differently in young patients compared to elderly ones), comorbidities or lack of other diseases, staff or family members of the staff (do we act differently when a patient is a doctor or nurse or a family member of the healthcare provider who we know or not), patient is famous or a well-known persona (we all have received those phone calls from people that know someone popular and wishes to have the best surgeon to take out the gallbladder or fix the hernia), your own experience with the patient and the family in the past and other factors. How many times, we have dealt with such factors in our practice and when things did not go as well as we wanted. In Kaizen conferences, we the surgeons bring these factors up in our conversation: "The family wanted everything on 92 years old grandpa" who in everyone's opinion, upon hearing the story, felt he had no chance of making it; or more common, "this is not a mortality from the operation"; " family withdrew care" after the procedure, which we should not have done to begin with. A wife of one my high-ranking bosses in one of the institutions that I worked for in the past, and who had severe mechanical small bowel obstruction from previous surgeries, insisted that I manage her non-operatively. I made it clear that she needs an operation. I was glad she allowed me to operate on her. Clearly, I resisted to distraction, and did not succumb to this external factor. A delay in the operation and she would have had gangrene of a large segment of the small bowel.

What the crew of this ship, named "The Operating Theater," does and does not do will have profound consequences. A team of surgeons, nurses, an anesthesiologist, scrub technicians, a radiologist, and scheduling personnel, are all led by the surgeon to execute a surgical procedure affecting the patient's life, and the lives of their family, friends, and their community. Everyone expects that this orchestrated set of tasks will be executed like a perfectly coordinated symphony. After all, this is a hospital with highly-trained professionals. Other distracting factors are the operating team composition, such as the anesthesiologist, your scrub nurse or tech, the equipment that is missing or does not work. Each and every one of these factors affects the outcomes of surgery, and most people have not studied them. We need to.

Each individual surgeon will differ on what they identify as a potential stressor, but those commonly reported include laparoscopic (versus robotic) surgery, procedural complexity, distractions, and lack of time [18]. Observational studies indicated that movement and case-irrelevant conversations were the most frequently occurring distractions, but equipment and procedural distractions were the most severe [19]. While distractions in particular may lead to an increase in surgical errors, because tasks that require more concentration tend to be more stressful, it has been shown that deliberate practice and minimization of intermittent auditory distractions can help a surgeon to better multitask during a procedure [19, 20]. Surgical trainees undergo extensive medical training that prepares them to form a cognitive representation for comparison that stimulates arousal, alertness, and focused attention. Brain structures involved when confronting a stressor are the hippocampus (involved in retention and memory), the amygdala (emotional stimuli processing), and the prefrontal cortex (part of the executive function control). Psychological stressors, such as performing complex surgery, will activate regions such as the amygdala which promotes the memory of salient but not neutral information. For example, when faced with a surgical procedure, a surgeon may recall key complex procedures more accurately than procedures that are not as pressing or salient. Can one extract a memory that has been stored somewhere in the brain, under stress?

This is a fluid and dynamic process [9, 21], encompassing components such as intuition (also known as "recognition-primed decision-making" analytical ability), flexibility, and creativity [22]. This model is particularly important in complex reoperative surgical procedures, which are often associated with an array of unanticipated or unrecognized problems preoperatively. While performing, a take-down ileostomy and end-colostomy (serving as mucus fistula, as described in medical record) a few years ago, I found a couple of surprises that complicated the operation greatly. First, instead of ileostomy, patient actually had a jejunostomy (mid small bowel stoma) and this explained why he could not gain weight since he was operated three years ago in another hospital. Second, there was an unrecognized small bowel to end-colostomy fistula, requiring resection (20 cm from ligament of Trietz). And third, he required a colo-colonic anastomosis. In all, I spent about six hours dissecting and freeing his intestines from severe adhesions, and performed three anastomoses, plus complex abdominal wall reconstruction, as he had a known large abdominal defect requiring posterior component separation. To make the proper decision, it is essential to be continuously aware of the patient's physiologic status—including fluid status, urine output, use of blood and blood products, bleeding, use of medications used by anesthesiologist (such as vasopressors), and biochemical endpoints of resuscitation, because, even when the operation is going well, the biochemical profile of the patient may not be optimal, or even acceptable, and this may directly affect the outcome of the surgery. This patient, a 41-year-old man, did very well and was discharged home having had his gastro-intestinal tract fully restored and functional.

In addition to the surgeon's training, education, leadership ability, physiologic and mental state, creativity (or simply making things up at times) might be the most critical element of all. Creativity in the service of excellence does not come easily, however. It takes dedication. It takes a lifetime of continuously studying the art and science of surgery.

The Surgeons' Physiology and State of Mind

As outlined earlier in this chapter, the surgical decision-making process (SDMP) depends on several factors, but most importantly, nothing will affect the outcome of a surgical procedure more than the decisions of the surgeon, and the state of mind and the physiology of the surgeon, followed by the patient's condition and physiologic state and the gravity of the disease. Patients or their families very often ask us: "Doctor, please get a good night's rest." or "Doc, have you had a good night's sleep?" We will discuss this topic in more detail in Chap. 3, but let us stress that the optimal physiology and the optimal state of mind of the surgeon often set the stage for the entire surgical symphony to function optimally or to become a chaotic state.

The lifestyle of us surgeons is intricately tied to the demanding nature of our profession. This role comes with a set of challenges that significantly influence the lifestyle choices and experiences of surgeons. Among the lifestyle elements, sleep is the most important one, affecting well-being and performance of surgeons. A study published in the Journal of the American College of Surgeons found that sleep deprivation negatively impacts surgical skill performance and decision-making. Adequate sleep is essential for maintaining cognitive function, concentration, and decision-making skills, all of which are critical in the high-stakes environment of surgery [23]. Here are some key points regarding the role of sleep in a surgeon's lifestyle:

1. **Cognitive Performance**: Sleep plays a vital role in cognitive functions such as memory consolidation, problem-solving, and attention. Surgeons need to be sharp and focused during procedures, and lack of sleep can impair these cognitive abilities. Another study in the Archives of Surgery emphasized the importance of ensuring surgeons get adequate sleep to maintain optimal cognitive and motor skills during surgeries [24]. Sleep loss can lead to impaired cognitive function, affecting memory, attention, and decision-making, which are critical aspects of surgical performance [25].
2. **Precision and Coordination**: Surgical procedures require precise movements and coordination. Fatigue and sleep deprivation can affect fine motor skills, leading to a potential increase in errors and complications during surgery.
3. **Reaction Time**: Quick and accurate decision-making is crucial in the operating room. Sleep deprivation can slow down reaction times and impair judgment, putting both the surgeon and the patient at risk.
4. **Emotional Well-being**: Lack of sleep can contribute to mood disturbances, irritability, and increased stress levels. Surgeons often work in high-pressure situations, and adequate sleep is essential for maintaining emotional resilience and overall mental health.
5. **Patient Safety**: Sleep-deprived surgeons are more prone to errors, which can compromise patient safety. Adherence to proper sleep hygiene is not only important for the well-being of the surgeon but also for ensuring the best outcomes for patients.
6. **Long Working Hours**: Surgeons often have demanding and unpredictable schedules, involving long working hours, night shifts, and on-call responsibilities. Balancing work and personal life while ensuring sufficient sleep can be challenging.

7. **Adaptability:** Surgeons need to be adaptable to varying work schedules and unexpected emergencies. Establishing healthy sleep patterns and finding effective strategies to manage fatigue becomes crucial for maintaining performance under different circumstances.

The role of sleep in a surgeon's lifestyle is pivotal for maintaining optimal cognitive function, precision, and overall well-being. Surgeons must prioritize adequate sleep to ensure they can perform at their best and provide safe and effective care to their patients.

There is a multifaceted relationship between a surgeon's professional responsibilities and their personal lifestyle, considering factors such as work hours, stress, and the pursuit of work-life balance.

Most surgeons often face demanding work schedules that extend beyond the conventional 9-to-5 timeframe. The nature of surgical emergencies and the unpredictability of cases mean that surgeons frequently work long hours, including evenings, nights, and weekends. This irregular work schedule can lead to challenges in maintaining a healthy work-life balance. The constant demand for availability and the pressure to respond promptly to emergencies contribute to a lifestyle that is often characterized by high levels of stress.

The stress associated with surgical practice is not only a result of long working hours but also stems from the inherent responsibility that comes with making critical decisions during surgeries. The life-and-death nature of surgical procedures, coupled with the intense focus required, can lead to significant mental and emotional strain. Surgeons must cope with the stress of making split-second decisions, managing unexpected complications, and dealing with the emotional toll of patient outcomes.

Research indicates that the lifestyle of surgeons can be physically demanding as well. Prolonged hours in the operating room, coupled with the need for precision and concentration, can contribute to musculoskeletal issues and physical fatigue. Maintaining peak physical and mental condition is crucial for surgeons, as any lapse in focus or physical capability can have severe consequences.

Despite the challenges, many surgeons find fulfillment in their work, deriving a sense of purpose from the positive impact they have on patients' lives. The satisfaction of successfully performing a complex surgery and contributing to a patient's recovery can offset some of the stresses associated with the profession. This intrinsic motivation often plays a significant role in shaping the lifestyle choices of surgeons.

Efforts to address the impact of a surgeon's lifestyle on their well-being have led to increased awareness of burnout within the profession. Burnout, characterized by emotional exhaustion, depersonalization, and a reduced sense of personal accomplishment, is a prevalent issue among surgeons. It is essential to acknowledge the importance of mental health and well-being in the medical profession and implement strategies to mitigate burnout.

In recent years, there has been a growing recognition of the need for work-life balance in surgical practice. Hospitals and healthcare institutions are implementing measures to support surgeons in maintaining a healthier lifestyle. These measures include implementing flexible scheduling, providing mental health resources, and encouraging a culture that prioritizes self-care.

In conclusion, the lifestyle of surgeons is a complex interplay between the demands of their profession and their personal well-being. The long hours, high stress levels, and physical demands of surgical practice shape the lifestyle choices of surgeons. While the profession brings unique challenges, it also offers a sense of purpose and fulfillment. Efforts to address burnout and promote work-life balance are essential to ensuring the long-term well-being of surgeons. As the healthcare landscape evolves, it is crucial to continue exploring ways to support surgeons in navigating the delicate balance between professional and personal life [26, 27, 28].

Overlooked Behaviors Impacting Surgical Decision-making Outcomes

When we discuss the outcomes of surgical patients in our quality improvement (Kaizen conference, formerly known as Morbidity and Mortality), we classify some of the complications as "potentially preventable" or what we say nowadays "room for improvement", however, whatever we call them, technically these are errors. I have identified several errors or omissions that I have called "Under radar behaviors," which are a de-facto part of surgical decision-making, and which do not get reported at all, or are barely mentioned during quality review of clinical outcomes.

1. Time from patient arriving in the emergency department to being seen by the surgeon.
2. Time from decision to operate to actually making an incision.
3. Time from when the patient is in the operating room till we actually make an incision (surgeon does not follow the patient to OR).
4. The use of useless CT scans, and/or other tests called "on the way to operating room."
5. "Dropping" of the patient in the ICU to the ICU team without proper communication, proper involvement, and complete ownership of patient, while working together with the team at the bedside.
6. Use proper vocabulary when we review quality issues and avoid entirely such worlds like: "perhaps," "probably," "maybe" when we should teach our trainees and tell our colleagues what happen exactly. Be ready always to have evidence ready, and say how would you have done it.
7. Audit the test ordered and decision made based on useless tests ordered daily. These test that most of the time go unnoticed adds greatly to the hospital cost.
8. Audit communication with anesthesia (patients is placed on vasopressors, and the surgeons does not know that).

The majority of these are under the radar of omissions or frank errors, but silenced or simply ignored, and do not get mentioned anywhere. Occasionally, there are some serious errors that become the subject of intense study both by surgeons and non-surgeons alike. These "errors" have been classified by a number of organizations. Yet, not everything that goes wrong occurs due to an error; such instances have been called "adverse events", "a near miss", and "a mistake". Other classifications of the errors include technical (i.e., one should have done a different move, or used a different approach), error in judgment (i.e., one did not realize how sick the patient was, or totally missed the diagnosis), or pure negligence (we need not dwell on this one, but suffice it to say it occurs far less than attorneys would have the world believe).

Recently, I observed a senior surgeon getting lost somewhat in the abdominal wall. He was "too concentrated on one point" and was clearly missing a bigger picture of the reconstruction. Getting "lost" is not that difficult, however. This is why surgical decision is constantly changing and is very dynamic. Yesterday, I observed a surgeon maturing, clearly an ischemic colostomy, but he was thinking that it will be alright. It will not. It did not. The other day, frank necrotic ileostomy was being watched for an entire week. "He was placed on vasopressor, and mucosa died" was explained to me. Not so. The stoma had technical issues impeding blood supply. There are a number of factors that may cause disruption of the surgical procedures that comprise the "symphony" of standard perioperative care. The researchers from Mayo Clinic prospectively analyzed flow disruptions by a trained observer in thirty-one cardiac surgeries, and described teamwork/communication failures, equipment and technology problems, extraneous interruptions, training-related distractions, and issues in resource accessibility. Surgical errors increased significantly with increases in flow disruptions; teamwork/communication failures were the strongest predictor of surgical errors [29]. In order to ensure a perfectly conducted surgical symphony, the goal of every surgeon should be pursuing a high-quality safety program. The type of errors that disrupt surgical symphony has been reported [30]. In this study, 78.3% of complications that occurred in 332 patients (3.4%) were attributed to errors in surgical technique (63.5%), errors in judgment (29.6%), inattention to detail (29.3%), and incomplete understanding (22.7%). In 34.4% of cases, patients had a prolongation of hospitalization, 25.1% had temporary disability, 8.4% permanent disability, and 16.0% died. In 20%, the error was a "mistake" (the wrong thing), and in 58% a "slip" (the right thing done incorrectly). System errors (2%) and communication errors (2%) were infrequently identified [30]. The authors of this excellent study concluded that after surgical technique, most surgical errors were caused by human factors: judgment, inattention to detail, and incomplete understanding, and not to organizational/system errors or breaks in communication.

The Never Event

In order to continue to improve the quality of our services the medical/surgical community have coined a new terminology: the never event, and we have gone to great lengths (rightly so, perhaps) to establish "never event" notion. Surgical never events are defined as errors such as wrong-procedure, wrong-site, retained foreign body, and wrong-patient events. Such errors are evaluated continually, and have received great public interest. While the consensus among surgeons, administrators, patients and their attorneys is that these events are completely avoidable, they occur quite often. According to the data from the National Practitioner Bank (NPDB) of the United States reviewed by Mehtsun et al. [31], between 1990 and 2010, over $1.3 billion was spent on malpractice lawsuits associated with surgical never events. A total of 9,744 malpractice cases related to never events occurred, with an estimated of 4,082 surgical never events occurring each year in the United States alone. The most common type of event was retained foreign body (n = 4,857; 49.8%), followed by wrong-procedure (n = 2,447; 25.1%); wrong-site (n = 2,413; 24.8%); and wrong-patient surgery (n = 27, 0.3%). Approximately 7% of these cases ended in death, 32% had permanent injuries, and 59% had temporary injuries. Perhaps most disturbing about this report is the fact that of physicians named in a surgical never event claim, 62% were named previously in a malpractice claim, and 12.4% were later named in at least one future surgical never event claim [31]. This is a truly a disturbing trend. Even worse, we do not know the extent of this major problem worldwide, particularly in the developing world. Factors related to the individual physician seem to be the most important items to consider in never events. The physician's age (40–49), <20 years from graduation, additional malpractice reports, state licensure disciplinary reports and clinical privileges reports were all statistically significant ($p = 0.001$) for physicians involved with surgical never events in this study.

The Institute of Medicine provided even more startling statistics that exemplify the gravity of the situation. On an annual basis in the United States, more people die from medical errors than from motor vehicle accidents, breast cancer, or AIDS [4]. According to a report published by IOM, between 44,000 and 98,000 people may die in hospitals each year due to errors. The report was written to evaluate, quantify, and provide suggestions for what can be done to increase safety and quality in the health care system. The IOM suggested the development of checklists and protocols to combat common errors [32]. While the WHO [33] has provided a checklist to the surgical team for save surgery, but this does not reduce the overwhelming complexity of modern surgery, the mechanistic and cognitive processes that surgeons grapple with that are less understood. These data have been questioned and errors are the cause of death.

Even more significantly, factors, such as stress and physiological responses to stress that affect these processes and contribute to error rates, need to be more fully understood. Read again the above sentence: a senior surgeon was "lost" in the abdominal wall dissection. Was the senior surgeon stressed out, was he feeling well, was he all of a sudden overwhelmed?

Whatever the state of his mind, and physiology, let me repeat this: as surgeons, we must be in command, not only within the operating theater, but throughout the journey across the entire continuum of care. And as surgeons, we should pay special attention to every detail of the surgical symphony, recognizing the limitations of the human mind, and preventing disruptions that may occur. Only then, will the surgical symphony sound perfect.

As a junior attending surgeon, I was assisting two senior residents perform tracheostomy in a morbidly obese patient with severe Acute Respiratory Distress Syndrome (ARDS). I had just joined the hospital after finishing residency and I did not know the residents or their abilities yet. The patients' neck was very large, and we used deep retractors to expose the trachea. When I asked the anesthesiologist to pull back the endotracheal tube, she pulled it out entirely. The tracheostomy tube that we had at hand was short for his very thick neck, would not reach the trachea. I asked for the tube exchanger, but the nursing anesthetist student (and here I thought we had an anesthesiologist on the other side of the curtain—total miscommunication within the team) did not know where they were. The patient's oxygen saturation started to drop, and with it his heart rate. At this very desperate moment, I asked for a nasogastric tube, and intubated the trachea by placing it over the endotracheal tube, surely preventing a catastrophic event. Later I recalled that I had heard a surgeon talking about this procedure on an audio tape, but it was many years prior to the event. It's amazing that I was able to access this stored information somewhere in my brain precisely when I needed it most; I still believe that it was the stress of the situation that prompted the retrieval of that specific memory.

The Effect of Alcohol on Surgical Decision-Making

As outlined in this chapter, there are many more factors affecting surgical decisions. In addition to those factors, alcohol abuse has a major effect. A number of studies have addressed surgeons' and other physicians' impairment due to alcohol [34, 35, 36]. A 2010 cross-sectional study conducted on 7197 members of the American College of Surgeons on alcohol use disorders reported that 15.4% had a score consistent with alcohol abuse or dependence. This prevalence certainly underestimates the true magnitude of the issue, as only 28.7% of those surgeons originally sampled responded to the survey. This is not surprising considering both the social stigma and legitimate risk to one's professional career. The survey also described that emotional exhaustion (odds ratio, 1.25; $P = 0.01$) and feelings of depression (odds ratio, 1.48; $P < 0.001$) were more strongly associated with alcohol dependence [35]. Alcohol consumption above 0.1 levels contributes to the activation of the HPA axis and stimulates the production of glucocorticoids. One study documented that surgeons who had used alcohol within a 24-hour time period had a higher average time taken to respond and resolve problems and higher error rates [37]. Additionally, Dorafshar et al. reported that surgical performance was impaired in the short-term after moderate alcohol consumption, but this effect was not observed during performance the day after drinking moderately [38]. Other studies have shown that a combination of alcohol and sleep deprivation was seen to have the greatest number of errors. The results of the study suggested that the effect of sleep deprivation and prior alcohol consumption on performance varies with the time of day ($P = 0.02$), and there are discernable residual effects of alcohol consumption the following day, despite undetectable levels of alcohol measured on the breath the next morning [39].

Conclusion

In conclusion, the intraoperative decision-making process is complex, drawing on a surgeon's education, clinical experience, leadership ability, mental state, physiology, and creativity. Despite advancements, most intraoperative decisions are made on-the-fly, defying easy theorization, quantification, or categorization. While the future of surgical decisions will continue to evolve, the exponential superiority and ingenuity combined with the intuition of the human mind over current supercomputers suggests that the unique decision-making abilities of surgeons will still continue to play an important role. As technology advances, there is potential for machines to become the first assistants to replicate the intricate complexities of surgical decision-making [40, 41]. This ongoing interplay between human decision-making and technological progress warrants continuous exploration and study.

In summary, this introductory chapter acknowledges the challenges in standardizing surgical decision-making and highlights the need for ongoing research and collaboration to better understand and improve the intricate processes that define the art and science of surgery. The artificial intelligence (AI) and super computers will undoubtedly add more interesting discussions as to the role of AI in surgical decision-making. As of now, there is no doubt that surgical decision-making includes science, art, lifestyle, and intuition. Yet, for the time being, when it comes to surgical decision-making, still there are more questions than answers [42].

References

1. Surgical decision making: beyond the evidence based surgery | SpringerLink. https://link.springer.com/book/10.1007/978-3-319-29824-5. Accessed 23 Jan 2024.
2. 737_RTS_Summary.pdf. https://www.faa.gov/sites/faa.gov/files/2022-08/737_RTS_Summary.pdf. Accessed 23 Jan 2024.
3. Korenkov M, Troidl H, Sauerland S. Individualized surgery in the time of evidence-based medicine. Ann Surg. 2014;259(5):e76–7.
4. Lustosa SAS, Matos D, Atallah AN, Castro AA. Stapled versus handsewn methods for colorectal anastomosis surgery (Cochrane Review). Cochrane Libr. 2001;(3)
5. Wu Z, Vakalopoulos KA, Kroese LF, et al. Reducing anastomotic leakage by reinforcement of colorectal anastomosis with cyanoacrylate glue. Eur Surg Res. 2013;50(3-4):255–61.
6. Beitler AL, Urschel JD. Comparison of stapled and hand-sewn esophagogastric anastomoses. Am J Surg. 1998;175(4):337–40.
7. Shogan BD, Carlisle EM, Alverdy JC, Umanskiy K. Do we really know why colorectal anastomoses leak? J Gastrointest Surg. 2013;17(9):1698–707. https://doi.org/10.1007/s11605-013-2227-0.
8. How do surgeons make intraoperative decisions?—PMC. https://www.ncbi.nlm.nih.gov/pmc/articles/PMC2464983/. Accessed 24 Jan 2024.
9. Pauley K, Flin R, Yule S, Youngson G. Surgeons' intraoperative decision making and risk management. Am J Surg. 2011;202(4):375–81. https://doi.org/10.1016/j.amjsurg.2010.11.009.
10. Klein GA, editor. Decision making in action: models and methods. Ablex Pub; 1993.
11. The surgeon's mental load during decision making at various stages of operations | European Journal of Applied Physiology. https://link.springer.com/article/10.1007/BF00429080. Accessed 24 Jan 2024.
12. Critical factors influencing intra-operative surgical decision-making | IEEE Conference Publication | IEEE Xplore. https://ieeexplore.ieee.org/abstract/document/4811427. Accessed 24 Jan 2024.
13. Jalote-Parmar A, Badke-Schaub P. Workflow integration matrix: a framework to support the development of surgical information systems. Des Stud. 2008;29(4):338–68. https://doi.org/10.1016/j.destud.2008.03.002.
14. Surgery for complex abdominal wall defects: update of a nine-step treatment strategy—Abstract—Europe PMC. https://europepmc.org/article/med/35313000. Accessed 24 Jan 2024.
15. Latifi R, Rhee P, Gruessner R, editors. Technological advances in surgery, trauma, and critical care. Springer; 2015.
16. Dilek O, Uraneus S, Latifi R. Prophylcatic Surgery. Springer Nature, Switzerland: Springer; 2021.
17. Surgical decision making in geriatrics: a comprehensive multidisciplinary approach | SpringerLink. https://link.springer.com/book/10.1007/978-3-030-47963-3. Accessed 25 Jan 2024.
18. Arora S, Sevdalis N, Nestel D, Woloshynowych M, Darzi A, Kneebone R. The impact of stress on surgical performance: a systematic review of the literature. Surgery. 2010;147(3):318–330.e6. https://doi.org/10.1016/j.surg.2009.10.007.
19. Mentis HM, Chellali A, Manser K, Cao CGL, Schwaitzberg SD. A systematic review of the effect of distraction on surgeon performance: directions for operating room policy and surgical train-

ing. Surg Endosc. 2016;30(5):1713–24. https://doi.org/10.1007/s00464-015-4443-z.
20. Effect of distractions on operative performance and ability to multitask—A case for deliberate practice—Ahmed—2015—The Laryngoscope—Wiley Online Library. https://onlinelibrary.wiley.com/doi/abs/10.1002/lary.24856. Accessed 24 Jan 2024.
21. Flin R, Youngson G, Yule S. How do surgeons make intraoperative decisions? Qual Saf Health Care. 2007;16(3):235–9. https://doi.org/10.1136/qshc.2006.020743.
22. Klein G. A recognition-primed decision making (RPD) model of rapid decision making. In: Decision Making in Action. Ablex; 1993.
23. The impact of sleep deprivation in military surgical teams: a systematic review | BMJ Military Health. https://militaryhealth.bmj.com/content/early/2016/09/13/jramc-2016-000640?versioned=true. Accessed 24 Jan 2024.
24. Dolan R, Huh J, Tiwari N, Sproat T, Camilleri-Brennan J. A prospective analysis of sleep deprivation and disturbance in surgical patients. Ann Med Surg. 2016;6:1–5. https://doi.org/10.1016/j.amsu.2015.12.046.
25. The effects of two nights of sleep deprivation with or without energy restriction on immune indices at rest and in response to cold exposure | European Journal of Applied Physiology. https://link.springer.com/article/10.1007/s00421-010-1378-x. Accessed 24 Jan 2024.
26. Burnout and career satisfaction among American surgeons: annals of surgery. https://journals.lww.com/annalsofsurgery/abstract/2009/09000/burnout_and_career_satisfaction_among_american.15.aspx. Accessed 24 Jan 2024.
27. Stress and burnout among surgeons: understanding and managing the syndrome and avoiding the adverse consequences | Surgery | JAMA Surgery | JAMA Network. https://jamanetwork.com/journals/jamasurgery/article-abstract/404847. Accessed 24 Jan 2024.
28. Surgeon burnout: a systematic review—PMC. Accessed January 24, 2024. https://www.ncbi.nlm.nih.gov/pmc/articles/PMC4884544/
29. Wiegmann DA, ElBardissi AW, Dearani JA, Daly RC, Sundt TM. Disruptions in surgical flow and their relationship to surgical errors: an exploratory investigation. Surgery. 2007;142(5):658–65. https://doi.org/10.1016/j.surg.2007.07.034.
30. Fabri PJ, Zayas-Castro JL. Human error, not communication and systems, underlies surgical complications. Surgery. 2008;144(4):557–65. https://doi.org/10.1016/j.surg.2008.06.011.
31. Mehtsun WT, Ibrahim AM, Diener-West M, Pronovost PJ, Makary MA. Surgical never events in the United States. Surgery. 2013;153(4):465–72. https://doi.org/10.1016/j.surg.2012.10.005.
32. To err is human: building a safer health system | CiNii Research. https://cir.nii.ac.jp/crid/1571417125129273216. Accessed 24 Jan 2024.
33. Tool and Resources. https://www.who.int/teams/integrated-health-services/patient-safety/research/safe-surgery/tool-and-resources. Accessed 24 Jan 2024.
34. Prevalence of alcohol use disorders among American surgeons | Surgery | JAMA Surgery | JAMA Network. https://jamanetwork.com/journals/jamasurgery/article-abstract/1107783. Accessed 24 Jan 2024.
35. Female surgeons' alcohol use: a study of a national sample of norwegian doctors | Alcohol and Alcoholism | Oxford Academic. https://academic.oup.com/alcalc/article/40/5/436/188773. Accessed 24 Jan 2024.
36. Schermer CR, Gentilello LM, Hoyt DB, et al. National survey of trauma surgeons' use of alcohol screening and brief intervention. J Trauma Acute Care Surg. 2003;55(5):849. https://doi.org/10.1097/01.TA.0000091110.83692.38.
37. Gallagher AG, Boyle E, Toner P, et al. Persistent next-day effects of excessive alcohol consumption on laparoscopic surgical performance. Arch Surg. 2011;146(4):419–26. https://doi.org/10.1001/archsurg.2011.67.
38. Dorafshar AH, O'Boyle DJ, McCloy RF. Effects of a moderate dose of alcohol on simulated laparoscopic surgical performance. Surg Endosc. 2002;16(12):1753–8. https://doi.org/10.1007/s00464-001-9052-3.
39. Kocher HM, Warwick J, Al-Ghnaniem R, Patel AG. Surgical dexterity after a 'night out on the town.'. ANZ J Surg. 2006;76(3):110–2. https://doi.org/10.1111/j.1445-2197.2006.03664.x.
40. Machine Learning and Artificial Intelligence for Surgical Decision Making | Surgical Infections. https://www.liebertpub.com/doi/abs/10.1089/sur.2021.007. Accessed 24 Jan 2024.
41. Loftus TJ, Tighe PJ, Filiberto AC, et al. Artificial intelligence and surgical decision-making. JAMA Surg. 2020;155(2):148–58. https://doi.org/10.1001/jamasurg.2019.4917.
42. Latifi R. Surgical decision-making process: more questions than answers – 2013. https://journals.sagepub.com/doi/full/10.1177/1457496913499836. Accessed 24 Jan 2024.

Part II

The Complexity of Surgical Decision: Setting the Stage

4 The Anatomy of the Surgeon's Decision-Making

Rifat Latifi and Abbas Smiley

As I was completing one case, I was told that the next patient was ready in the adjacent room. We were just finishing up, so I left the resident with the first patient and walked to the next room and saw the next patient was being intubated. I looked at the paperwork which stated "abdominal hernia." I examined the patient, who was now asleep. She had no abdominal wall hernia. My handwritten clinic note read "Bilateral inguinal hernia." The informed consent, however, stated "abdominal hernia". Because the patient was asleep, I could not examine her properly. I decided to contact her husband, a taxi driver, but he did not return the repeated phone calls that I made. She was a woman in her mid-thirties, who had a bilateral inguinal hernia based on my note. However, my notes did not match the resident's note, or the consent, which had been reviewed and approved by pre-operative nurses, pre-op anesthesia, and finally the anesthesiologist of record. There was a discrepancy, and examining the patient under anesthesia for inguinal hernia provided would not provide definitive answers. (This was back before the mandatory "surgical pause" or "time-out"). In that moment, I made the decision to cancel the operation and wake up the patient. This was an error on our collective side. It was a Friday, and on Monday we operated on the patient and repaired the bilateral hernia, laparoscopically. The team and I learned a very valuable lesson. I did not oversee the resident's note, and did not ensure that everyone knows exactly what I planned to do. There were many stages when this error could have been caught, but it was continuously missed. The human wall to prevent an error, coupled with the multiple reliable processes did not work. Neither the patient, nor her family was upset, and they were very glad that we did not do the surgery on Friday.

Introduction

While we the surgeons claim to be and act as leaders in the operating room, this surgical symphony [1, 2] is created by so many people, organized in so many layers, that one would think that we can build a true wall that mistakes cannot pass through. Yet, they still happen, and there is so much that goes on between the perfection expected from us, and what often, unfortunately, occurs. In 2009, Atul Gawande published his best-selling book, "The Checklist Manifesto." This book documented the decrease in error-rates of surgeons with the use of checklists prior to sur-

R. Latifi (✉)
Department of Surgery, The University of Arizona, Tucson, AZ, USA

Tucson Medical Center, Department of Surgery, Tucson, AZ, USA
e-mail: Latifi@surgery.arizona.edu

A. Smiley
Department of Surgery, University of Arizona, Tucson, AZ, USA

R. Latifi (ed.), *Surgical Decision-Making*, https://doi.org/10.1007/978-3-031-67391-7_4

gery [3]. While the use of checklists provides surgeons with one tool that battles the overwhelming complexity of modern surgery, the mechanistic and cognitive processes that surgeons grapple with are less understood, and frankly greatly underestimated. The layers that have been placed as a way of reducing the fatal errors such as performing the wrong surgery on the wrong patients still may become permeable and let an error get through. This process is complex and requires that we surgeons and the entire team performs well and understands the following:

1. **Preoperative Evaluation**: Assess the patient's medical history, including any existing health conditions, allergies, previous surgeries, and current medications; perform a physical examination to evaluate the patient's overall health status: and order and review relevant diagnostic tests (e.g., blood work, imaging studies) to ensure the patient is suitable for surgery.
2. **Anesthesia Consultation**: Consult with an anesthesiologist to determine the most appropriate anesthesia method for the patient (e.g., general anesthesia, local anesthesia, regional anesthesia); and discuss any potential risks or complications related to anesthesia, considering the patient's medical history and current health status.
3. **Preoperative Instructions for the Patient**: Provide clear instructions regarding fasting requirements (e.g., no food or drink prior to surgery) to minimize the risk of complications during anesthesia; inform the patient about any specific medication adjustments or restrictions before the surgery; explain the need to remove certain items (e.g., jewelry, contact lenses, dentures) prior to the operation.
4. **Surgical Consent and Discussion**: Obtain informed consent from the patient, ensuring they fully understand the risks, benefits, and alternatives of the proposed surgery; discuss the surgical procedure, expected outcomes, and potential complications or side effects the patient and the family should be aware of.
5. **Preoperative Preparation:** Schedule any necessary preoperative tests (e.g., EKG, X-rays) and consultations; ensure the surgical team is aware of any relevant information regarding the patient's medical condition, allergies, and medications; and coordinate with the operating room staff to arrange necessary equipment, supplies, and instruments for the procedure.
6. **Preoperative Medications and Precautions:** Administer prescribed preoperative medications (e.g., antibiotics, anticoagulants) as appropriate; ensure the patient follows any additional precautions required before surgery, such as skin preparation or bowel preparation.
7. **Time-Out Procedure:** Conduct a time-out or surgical safety checklist before the operation, involving the entire surgical team to ensure correct patient identification, procedure verification, site marking (if applicable), and confirmation of necessary equipment and implants.

It's important to note that this checklist can vary depending on the type of surgery, the specific facility, and the individual patient's needs.

Master surgeons, often make decisions or question others without any seemingly apparent evidence to do so. Such was the case with the patient who had the bilateral inguinal hernia, illustrated in my case presentation. How did I decide to cancel the case? I could write a note in the chart stating the facts and any reasonable person would have seen this as an error that did not harm the patient. Instead, I saw this as a major system issue, and thus decided to cancel the case. I had seen many patients and had been very busy, but I had enough recollection to realize that this was the same patient I had seen quite some time before seeing her again. The most important error was that I had not seen the patient before surgery, and operating room staff was trying to help me finish the entire operative program on time. There was no site marked for operation. There has been no double or triple checking. Faced with this, I decided that proceeding with surgery, was not alright. But what made me do that? Intuition? Common sense? Good medicine?

Let me discuss intuition and surgical decision-making. I asked AI on January 1, 2024 what is surgical intuition? Here is the answer: Surgical intuition refers to the ability of a surgeon to make quick and accurate judgments based on their extensive training and experience. It is often described as a combination of expertise, pattern recognition, and subconscious decision-making that allows surgeons to navigate complex surgical situations effectively.

Surgical intuition is developed over years of practice, observation, and exposure to various surgical scenarios. As surgeons encounter similar situations repeatedly, they develop a deep understanding of the anatomy, physiology, and pathology involved. This familiarity allows them to recognize patterns, anticipate potential complications, and make decisions intuitively, often without explicit reasoning.

One aspect of surgical intuition is the ability to rapidly assess a patient's condition and make critical decisions during surgery. Surgeons can evaluate the visual and tactile cues they perceive, integrating a vast amount of information in real-time. This skill enables them to adapt their surgical technique, modify their approach, or address unexpected challenges.

The development of surgical intuition requires a combination of technical proficiency, knowledge base, and the ability to remain calm and focused under pressure. It allows surgeons to make split-second decisions when necessary, optimizing patient outcomes and minimizing risks.

Interestingly, AI adds: "However, it is important to note that surgical intuition is not infallible. Surgeons must always rely on evidence-based practices, clinical guidelines, and collaboration with colleagues to ensure the best possible outcomes. Additionally, advancements in technology and surgical techniques have supplemented surgical intuition with data-driven decision-making and objective assessment tools, further enhancing patient care."

While explaining the subject of surgical decision-making, Abernathy and Hamm [2] in the 1990s defended the role of intuition in the surgical decision-making process. They define intuition as the act of knowing without the use of rational process, or "immediate cognition." It is a part of thinking that cannot be explained by others, which I agree entirely with. Surgeons who appear to use intuition typically have many years of experience. While experience is an important component to gaining this skill, these authors state that it is not always necessary.

Yet, the word intuition is not readily received among the scientific community, although from time to time it has appeared on scientific journals. Yet, they and others argue for the use of clear, analytic decision-making [2, 4] in order to reduce error rates. Specifically, some surgeons argue for the use of decision tree diagrams. Decision-tree diagrams can also help surgeons for reference purposes with later cases; however, while tools such as decision tree diagrams or checklists may help surgeons organize their work, they do not capture the complexity of intuitive decision-making. They are rudimentary tools, which of course are useful, but are simply the tools that keep the work in order.

Physical Factors, Personality Factors, and Situational Factors

A limited number of studies have assessed the surgical decision-making process by asking surgeons to recall decisions made during complex surgery, watch videos of other surgeons during surgery, or instructing surgeons to view themselves to determine why they made specific decisions [5, 6] (see Table 4.1). For example, Mitchell examined the decision-making process by trainee surgeons compared to the decision-making process by consultants. The authors specifically compared their abilities to assess risk during two different time points while watching short videos of other surgeons. While she found no statistically significant differences in risk ratings, she did gather important data on what surgeons believe to contribute to decision-making [5] while in the operating room, specifically regarding how surgeon critique and evaluate surgeries. The real question is can we statistically define the surgeon's decisions? Can we have a p-value when

Table 4.1 Studies that have assessed surgical decision-making

Author and Year	Title	Methods	Results
Chatterjee et al [29]	Assessing the surgical decision-making abilities of novice and proficient urologists	Surgical Decision Making Assessment Tool on 25 medical students, urology residents, and staff viewed 8 videos of minimally complex to complex urological procedures	Surgical Decision making tool is useful assessment to see strengths and weaknesses of surgeons. Rating scale distinguished training level across domains
Dekker and Hugh [8]	Laparoscopic Bile Duct Injury: Understanding the Psychology and Heuristics of the Error	Reviewed literature for errors between 1997 and 2007; found 49 errors, 42 of 49 were misidentification of bile duct, not recognized during operation	Psychological characteristics related to misidentification: underestimation of risk, cue ambiguity, and "believing what you see"; training should include how to be alert for cues of wrong duct, learning how to stop yourself once you've made a decision
Massarweh et al. [7]	Risk tolerance and bile duct injury: surgeon characteristics, risk-taking preference, and common bile duct injuries	Risk Taking Assessment Survey; Demographics, Questionnaire on Injuries	Found that those who had highest level of risk taking preferences also had highest risk for CBDI injuries
Mitchell et al. [5]	Intraoperative Surgical Decision-Making: A Video Study	27 surgeons (trainee vs. consultant) interviewed while watching 3 videos	No difference for risk taking preferences between trainees and consultants
Moulton et al. [6]	Slowing down when you should: Initiators and transitions from the routine to the effortful	28 surgeons interviewed; using grounded theory design, explored emergent themes	Found specific characteristics associated with surgical errors: physical, personality, situational
Yule et al. [29]	Development of a rating system for surgeons' non-technical skills	Cognitive task analyses (critical incident surveys) were given to 27 surgeons NOTSS	Five categories of non-technical skills were discovered: situation awareness, decision-making, task management, leadership and communication, and teamwork; later reliability tested and found that with minimal training, surgeons can rate each other's non-technical skills

in a single case the surgeon decides to perform this versus the other procedure in the "heat of the moment?" In other words, can we quantify and measure intuition? I do not believe so.

Moulton and colleagues conducted a study that interviewed twenty-eight surgeons using a semi-structured interview design to test decision-making during operating procedures [6]. They analyzed these interviews using a grounded theory design and produced a conceptual framework that they describe as the *"slowing down phenomenon."* The slowing down phenomenon consists of evaluating a situation and switching from automatic mindset to effortful mindset. Every experienced surgeon has had the *"slow down moment"* and can recall it, and moreover can recognize when there is a need for such moments during a complex surgery. I call it the ability to *"slow down your heart rate"*. In other words, when a situation has the tendency to fall out of our control, such as in major traumas or unexpected injuries, there is a moment when you truly have to "*slow down your heart rate*" and put that final suture that you know will save the patient's life. In my practice, I lower my voice, and "slow down or hold the breath to heart rate." I become extremely focused on the task at hand.

Through the iterative process used to create the surgical decision-making framework, Moulton and colleagues discovered certain personality characteristics that may influence the surgical decision-making process and the ability to *"slow-down"* during surgery. These characteristics include adaptability, willingness to learn, and confidence. No known studies that research these characteristics have been conducted.

There are several factors that affect the ability to "*slow down*." These factors include physiological, personality, and situational factors. Physiological factors include fatigue, illness, and endurance. Personality factors include ego, adaptability, willingness to learn, and confidence. Situational factors include time pressure, availability of resources, and social pressures [6].

Personality Characteristics

Does the personality of the surgeon matter, or rather how does the personality of the surgeon affect the outcome of the surgery? One of the most commonly studied injuries caused by surgeons has been common bile duct injury caused during laparoscopic cholecystectomy. Massarweh et al. conducted a simple survey of members of the American College of Surgeons and asked them to review which factors contributed to bile duct injuries during routine laparoscopic cholecystectomy (LC) [7]. The survey included an assessment of demographics, injuries reported during surgical procedure, and a short risk-taking questionnaire. Out of the 1,412 respondents, 12.9% reported having contributed to more than one injury. These surgeons, on average, were slightly older than the general sample and had been in practice longer. Additionally, surgeons who did not report a common bile duct injury were more likely to have trained at a LC course. Surgeons who scored very high on the risk-taking assessment had a relative risk for CBDI that was 17% greater than the surgeons who were trained in LC. The authors concluded that the impact of extremes of risk-taking preference on surgical decision-making can be an important part of decreasing risk for injury during surgery. These authors felt that risk-taking propensity should be one characteristic that is evaluated among surgeons.

Dekker and Hugh [8] reviewed literature on bile duct misidentification between 1997 and 2007. They found that of the 49 surgical errors that were reported during this time period, 42 errors were related to misidentifying the bile duct. Dekker and Hugh attribute these errors to certain psychological phenomena that include inability to read cues, inability to slow oneself during surgical procedures, and a belief that the risk is low during operation. Dekker and Hugh also emphasize the need to train surgeons to apply *"stopping rules"* when necessary during an operation and to train surgeons to accept the need for plan modification, which reminds us that Moulton's personality characteristics may be an important consideration. This phenomenon has been described as cognitive fixation and plan continuation by these authors. For example, if a surgeon makes a decision to go in one direction, but it is not the correct decision, it is more difficult to modify the plan of action once the decision is made. In essence, the surgeon becomes biased in the direction of his/her first decision. I call this, as most experienced surgeons do, the first mistake leading to the next mistake. In other words, it is important that we as surgeons evaluate the cognitive fixation plan and re-evaluate by "*slowing down our own heart rate*" and adapt intraoperatively to new conditions and situations. Early in my surgical career, during the difficult cholecystectomy with Mirrizi syndrome, I asked the resident, what she and I thought was a cystic duct. Unfortunately, it was the common bile duct adhered to the cystic duct, which I recognized immediately, as we say two open lumens, converted into open; spoke with the family, and did an anastomosis of the common bile duct to a limb of jejunum (choledochojejunostomy) with the assistance of one my partners. In retrospect we convinced our own bias that this is the only structure going into the gallbladder.

Decision-Making and Situational Awareness

An important concept that may effectively describe the surgeon's decision-making ability and how he/she makes decisions in the operating room is that of situational awareness, which has not been studied adequately among surgeons. Military strategists have applied this concept to operating aircraft, ships, and in emergency military situations much more than surgeons [9–12]. Situational Awareness can briefly be described as "*the perception of elements within a volume of time and space, the comprehension of their meaning, and the projection of their status in the near future* [9]." Numerous studies looking at the effects of situational awareness in virtual and real environments among military personnel have been conducted [10–13]. Few studies have been conducted that look at how situational awareness can be applied in the medical field, however. Considering studies that have investigated situational awareness in the medical field, communication among surgical team members, or the usefulness of the concept of situational awareness have gained the most attention among anesthesiologists and emergency practitioners within the realm of surgical non-technical skills [13–15]. There are additional concepts that have been studied related to the decision-making process.

Flin et al. made the case for applying decision-making analysis concepts (i.e., naturalistic decision-making) in a two-step process that included: assessing and diagnosing the situation, then using one of four strategies to make a decision [16]. These strategies included *intuitive recognition, rule based, analytical, and creative decision-making.* According to Yule and colleagues, these strategies are selected based on a continuum of urgency. When the need to make a decision is urgent, intuitive recognition decision-making is used, whereas when the need to make a decision is not urgent, creative decision-making is used [16]. However, in real practice, the intuitive vs. creative decision-making process is difficult to separate. For example, while the patient is dying in the operating room from hypotension, the surgeon reaches for the aorta and presses with two fingers until the blood pressure comes up again. The most common response for hypotension training in surgery is to open the chest and clamp the aorta in these situations. Would a response made by the surgeon that differs from standard training procedures in this situation be considered intuitive or creative? Specifically, creative decision-making requires more time and less urgency. It appears that there is a blend of intuitive recognition decision-making and creative decision-making during surgery.

Herein lies a key component to the construct of surgical intuition. Because an expert surgeon has many levels of knowledge, he or she is able to step away from analytical decision-making, otherwise known as "*taking steps through a decision,'* and take shortcuts or cut corners. Abernathy and Hamm state that memories are formed in "chunks." Experts are able to use representations of situations whereas non-experts remember processes in steps. While everyone has only the capacity to remember in five to seven "chunks," experts do not need to remember the steps of these chunks, thus allowing them to make creative and flexible decisions when under pressure. Specifically, if a surgeon is presented with a familiar pattern, they have more flexibility to think around the steps needed to perform a task because they do not have to "remember" all of the steps. This allows them to make decisions that seem intuitive or creative [2].

Studies looking at the mechanics underlying these dynamic decision-making processes have not been conducted due to the difficulty of obtaining the "real time" data from surgeons while in the operating room. It would be unethical to possibly jeopardize a patient's safety and the surgical procedure for the sake of understanding how surgeons make decisions. However, some enlightening studies have been conducted that examine visual tracking of cancerous masses on mammograms as well as abnormalities on electrocardiograms (ECG) [17, 18]. For example, Kundel et al., found that radiologists detect cancers on medical images well before eye movement to the abnormal region occurs [18]. These authors propose that an expertise in medical image analysis results in a "look-detect-scan" fashion rather than a "scan-look-detect," indicating that expertise brings in an almost "gut level" form of analysis [17]. Additionally, Wood et al. found that experts in reading ECGs had a different visual scanning behavior than ten-year medical students [18]. These studies are useful in that they provide a foundation for investigating the mechanistic underpinnings of surgical decision-making. Of course, the major difference between detecting abnormalities in an image and in surgical decision-making is the timing; hence, the concept of situational awareness is relevant. Surgical decision-making occurs within an almost unmeasurable, difficult to quantify period of time. There is no time to change one's opinion while in the operating room.

Complex surgical procedures carry significant risks and complications, whether performed alone or in combination. Despite the most conscientious preoperative preparations, surprising events may still occur. If the operation takes an unplanned turn, the surgeon has to make difficult decisions. It is essential to be continuously aware of the patient's physiological status—including fluid status, urine output, use of blood and blood products, bleeding, current medications (such as vasopressors), and biochemical endpoints of resuscitation. Even when the operation is going well, the biochemical profile of the patient may not be optimal, or even satisfactory, and this may directly affect the outcome of the surgery. In addition, the surgeon must recognize his or her own physiological status; if tired, for example, cutting corners and making major errors are much more likely [1].

Yule et al. interviewed twenty-seven surgeons using a cognitive task survey [19]. Results revealed that many errors made by surgeons were not technical errors, but in fact, behavioral errors. For example, many errors were due to communication problems among team members. Yule et al. documented five areas of non-technical skills that impacted the effectiveness of a surgeon's performance in the operating room. These non-technical skills included situation awareness, decision-making, communication, teamwork, and task management [19].

Numerous studies involving patients with brain damage have shown that considerable unconscious processing of visual stimuli, such as emotional, facial, semantics, and visual illusions occurs [20–24]. Additionally, studies on patients without brain damage have shown unconscious processing of stimuli presented to masked healthy subjects [25–27]. Yule's study [19] that interviewed twenty-seven surgeons asked them to document why they made decisions during the surgical procedure, but only after the fact. These surgeons were, in effect, retrospectively describing what they had done with a rubric that was based upon what they had been taught; however, psychologists propose that many actions are in response to stimuli that the individual is not aware. The feed forward sweep (FFS) is a term used to describe how visual stimuli are incorporated into the brain through the retina and into cortical regions. Every time the information reaches a successive stage, higher-level areas send information back to lower-level areas for a process known as recurrent processing (RP). van Gaal and Lamme [20, 24] have proposed that the RP is required for consciousness and FFS remains unconscious. These authors suggest that this is the proposed route for allowing seemingly unconscious monitoring of environmental stimuli occurs. Abernathy and Hamm are making a similar argument for intuition [2]. Intuition is essentially the awareness of subtle cues; this awareness may not be effectively verbalized as it is sensory in nature.

One specific area that has been shown to be activated during complex decision-making is that of the anterior cingulate cortex, ACC [27].This area is activated during error detection and competitive complex tasks. The ACC has also been demonstrated to be involved in consciousness, such as emotional awareness [28].

The formation of memories and how knowledge is stored and accessed is crucial to understanding seemingly gut-level processes. Latent knowledge is knowledge that we've acquired through learning and experience, but we are not always consciously aware of this knowledge [2]. The ability to access it depends on several factors. This type of knowledge, in conjunction with attention to situational cues, is crucial to intuitive decision-making. How do we access it? Reliability of the memory of this knowledge is dependent upon the frequency of the use of particular knowledge and how recently this particular knowledge was acquired. Surgeons rely on knowledge gained over long periods of time and from varied experiences. Long-term memory is knowledge that is stored for long periods of time. It can be considered almost a concrete aspect of thought processes or even identity. For example, "What street did you grow up on?" is a question that most people can answer very quickly without much thought. This is a memory that has been built over a long period of time and used repetitively. Short-term memory has a smaller capacity and holds ideas for a short period of time, unless they are used for long periods, then they become part of the long-term memory pool. Short-term memory is responsible for what we are thinking of at a given moment and what we are paying attention to. Long-term memory is accessed through short-term memory because short-term is what an individual is currently thinking of and is connected to the activities that the individual is engaging in. Short-term memory acts almost as a gatekeeper to long-term memory [2].

Conclusion

The anatomy of such decisions is of great importance to all surgeons, including those who work with surgeons, and patients. The construct of situational awareness can be applied to these "gut feeling" evaluations. How situational awareness and decision-making are affected by factors such as sleep deprivation and alcohol consumption are also important in understanding the decision-making process. Additionally, the mechanics behind this complex decision-making process should be tested. Other elements of surgical decision-making process should be kept in mind as well [29, 30].

References

1. Latifi R. Surgical decision-making process: more questions than answers. Scand J Surg. 2013;102(3):139–40. https://doi.org/10.1177/1457496913499836.
2. Abernathy C, Hamm R. Surgical intuition. What it is and how to get it. Philadelphia: Hanley & Belfus; 1995.
3. Gawande A. The checklist manifesto: how to get things right. New York: Metropolitan Books, Henry Holt and Company, LLC; 2009.
4. Weinstein MC, Fineberg HV, Elstein AS, et al. Clinical decision analysis. Philadelphia: WB Sanders; 1980.
5. Mitchell L, Flin R, Youngson G, Malik M, Ahmed I. Intraoperative surgical decision-making: a video study. International conference on naturalistic decision making. Marseille; 2013.
6. Moulton C, Regehr G, Lingard L, Merritt C, Macrae H. 'Slowing down when you should': Initiators and influences of the transition from the routine to the effortful. J Gastrointest Surg. 2010;14:1019–26.
7. Massarweh N, Devlin A, Gaston Symons R, Broeckel EJ, Flum D. Risk tolerance and bile duct injury: surgeon characteristics, risk taking preference, and common bile duct injuries. Am J Surg. 2009;209:17–24.
8. Dekker S, Hugh TB. Laparoscopic bile duct injury: understanding the psychology and heuristics of the error. ANZ J Surg. 2008:1109–14.
9. Endsley MR. Towards a theory of situation awareness in dynamic environments. Hum Factors. 1995;37:32–64.
10. Endsley MR. A survey of situation awareness requirements in air-to-air combat fighters. Int J Aviat Psychol. 1993;3:157–68.
11. Endsley MR. Measurement of situation awareness in dynamic systems. Hum Factors. 1995;37:65–84.
12. Endsley MR. The application of human factors to the development of expert systems for advanced cockpits. In: Proceedings of the 7th international symposium on aviation psychology. Columbus: Ohio State University; 1987. p. 167–71.
13. Gaba DM, Howard SK, Small SD. Situation awareness in anesthesiology. Hum Fact J Hum Fact Ergonom Soc. 1995;37:20–33.
14. Durso FT, Sethumadhavan A. Situation awareness: understanding dynamic environments. Hum Fact J Hum Fact Ergonom Soc. 2008;50:442–50. https://doi.org/10.1518/001872008X288448.
15. Shah H, Hamid ABD, Waterson P, Hignett S. Situation awareness to support decision-making among emergency care practitioners. In: Proceedings of NDM9, the 9th international conference on naturalistic decision-making. London; 2009.
16. Flin R, Youngson G, Yule S. How do surgeons make intraoperative decisions? Qual Saf Health Care. 2007;16:235–9. https://doi.org/10.1136/qshc.2006.020743.
17. Wood G, Batt J, Appelboam A, Harris A, Wilson MR. Exploring the impact of expertise, clinical history, and visual search on electrocardiogram interpretation. Med Decis Mak. 2014;34:75–85. https://doi.org/10.1177/0272989X13492016.
18. Kundel HL, Nodine CF, Krupinski EA, Mello-Thoms C. Using gaze-tracking data and mixture distribution analysis to support a holistic model for the detection of cancers on mammograms. Acad Radiol 2008 Jul;15(7):881-886. doi: https://doi.org/10.1016/j.acra.2008.01.023.
19. Yule S, Flin R, Paterson-Brown S, Maran N, Rowley D. Development of a rating system for surgeons' non-technical skills. Med Educ. 2006;40:1098–104. https://doi.org/10.1111/j.1365-2929.2006.02610.x.

20. van Gaal S, Lamme VAF. Unconscious high-level information processing: implication for neurobiological theories of consciousness. Neuroscientist. 2012;18:287–303.
21. Cowey A. The blindsight saga. Exp Brain Res. 2010;200:3–24.
22. Tamietto M, Castelli L, Vighetti S, Perozzo P, Geminiani G, Weiskrantz L, et al. Unseen facial and bodily expressions trigger fast emotional reactions. Proc Natl Acad Sci USA. 2009;106:17661–6.
23. Tamietto M, de Gelder B. Neural bases of the nonconscious perception of emotional signals. Nat Rev Neurosci. 2010;11:697–709.
24. Lamme VAF, Roelfsema PR. The distinct modes of vision offered by feedforward and recurrent processing. Trends Neurosci. 2000;23:571–9.
25. Breitmeyer BG, Ogmen H, editors. Visual masking: time slices through conscious and unconscious vision. Oxford, UK: Oxford University Press; 2006.
26. Klotz W, Neumann O. Motor activation without conscious discrimination in metacontrast masking. J Exp Psychol Hum Percept Perform. 1999;25:976–92.
27. Bush G, Luu P, Posner MI. Cognitive and emotional influences in anterior cingulate cortex. Trends Cogn Sci. 2000;4(6):215–22.
28. Lane RD, Reiman EM, Axelrod B, Yun LS, Holmes A, Schwartz GE. Neural correlates of levels of emotional awareness. Evidence of an interaction between emotion and attention in the anterior cingulate cortex. J Cogn Neurosci. 1998;10(4):525–35.
29. Yule S, Flin R, Paterson-Brown S, Maran N, Rowley D, Youngson G. Surgeons' non-technical skills in the operating room: Reliability testing of the NOTSS behaviour rating system. World J Surg. 2008;32:548–56.
30. Chatterjee S, Ng J, Kwan K, Matsumoto E. Assessing the surgical decision making abilities of novice and proficient urologists. J Urol. 2009;181:2251–6.

The Role of the Surgeon's Physiology and the State of Mind in the Surgical Decision-Making Process: An Update

5

Rifat Latifi and Abbas Smiley

Introduction

No small surgery exists, or is ever performed. Even the minutest surgical procedure can potentially end in catastrophic consequences. In this instance, we are not considering such tragedies as performing the wrong surgery on the wrong site, or even on the wrong patient; also, we will not discuss a sponge or other foreign body left in the abdomen or chest or any other cavity. Even with these situations eliminated, it is highly doubtful that any of us would consider a surgical procedure performed on ourselves or a loved one to be "small or minor", and therefore, we should appreciate that all of our cases are very personal for the patients and their families.

What the crew of this ship, named "The Operating Theater", does, or does not do, will have profound consequences. A team of surgeons, nurses, an anesthesiologist, scrub technicians, a radiologist, and scheduling personnel, are all led by the surgeon to execute a surgical procedure affecting the patient's life, and the lives of their family, friends, and their community. Everyone expects that this orchestra will execute the set of tasks perfectly, just like a symphony would. After all, this is a hospital with highly-trained professionals. In reality, how the surgery goes will depend on several factors, as we will see in many of the subsequent chapters of this book, but nothing will affect the outcome of a surgical procedure more than the decisions of the surgeon, followed only by the patient's condition and physiological state. In this chapter, we will examine the state of mind of the surgeon as a major factor. On many occasions during my elective surgical cases, patients or their families have said: "Doc, please get a good night's rest." or "Doc, have you had a good night's sleep?" These will be some of the factors that will be examined in more detail.

The authors have no financial or proprietary interest in the subject matter or materials discussed in the manuscript.

R. Latifi (✉)
Department of Surgery, The University of Arizona, Tucson, AZ, USA

Tucson Medical Center, Department of Surgery, Tucson, AZ, USA
e-mail: Latifi@surgery.arizona.edu

A. Smiley
Department of Surgery, University of Arizona, Tucson, AZ, USA

Primum Non Nocere

As mentioned in the commencement of this chapter, there are no such things as "minor or small surgeries." Each patient, "surgical case," or procedure needs to be treated with the utmost care as, while it is expected to go "smooth", it can and may be complicated. The well-known saying amongst surgeons is "only surgeons who do not operate enough" do not have complications! If

R. Latifi (ed.), *Surgical Decision-Making*, https://doi.org/10.1007/978-3-031-67391-7_5

things can go wrong, they probably will go wrong, but that does not diminish our commitment to do the best that we can for our patients and their families. And if for whatever reason, one cannot do the best, one should not do it all. Our primary role as surgeons is to not hurt the patient, hence the Latin maxim: "Primum non nocere" ("First, do no harm"), and help people live longer and lead better quality lives, free of pain, whenever possible. One only needs to consider the impact of the potential complications to appreciate that no surgery should be dismissed as minor or merely routine [1–4].

The Never Event

In order to continue to improve the quality of our services we in the medical/surgical community have coined a new terminology: the never event; and we have gone to great lengths (rightly so, perhaps) to establish the "never event" notion. Surgical never events are defined as errors such as wrong-procedure, wrong-site, foreign body, and wrong-patient events. Such errors are evaluated continually, and have received great public interest. While the consensus among surgeons, administrators, patients and their attorneys is that these events are completely avoidable, they occur quite often. According to the data from the National Practitioner Bank (NPDB) of the United States reviewed by Mehtsun et al., between 1990 and 2010, over $1.3 billion was spent on malpractice lawsuits associated with surgical never events. A total of 9744 malpractice cases related to never events occurred, with an estimated 4082 surgical never events occurring each year in the United States alone. The most common type of event was retained foreign body (n = 4857; 49.8%), followed by wrong-procedure (n = 2447; 25.1%); wrong-site (n = 2413; 24.8%); and wrong-patient surgery (n = 27, 0.3%). Approximately 7% of these cases ended in death, 32% had permanent injuries, and 59% had temporary injuries. Perhaps most disturbing about this report is the fact that of physicians named in a surgical never event claim, 62% were named previously in a malpractice claim, and 12.4% were later named in at least one future surgical never event claim [3]. This is a truly disturbing trend. Even worse, we do not know the extent of this major problem worldwide, particularly in the developing world. Factors related to the individual physician seem to be the most important items to consider in never events. The physician's age (40–49), years since graduation (<20), additional malpractice reports, state licensure disciplinary reports and clinical privileges reports were all statistically significant ($p = 0.001$) for physicians involved with surgical never events in this study.

The Institute of Medicine provided even more startling statistics that exemplify the gravity of the situation. On an annual basis in the United States, more people die from medical errors than from motor vehicle accidents, breast cancer, or AIDS [4]. According to a report published by IOM, between 44,000 and 98,000 people may die in hospitals each year due to errors. The report was written to evaluate, quantify, and provide suggestions for what can be done to increase safety and quality in the health care system. The IOM suggested the development of checklists and protocols to combat common errors [4]. Personally, based on my experience, I aways thought that this number was grossly an underestimation. Makary and Daniel have estimated medical error have become the third cause of death in the US [1].

As suggested by Atul Gawande, checklists provide a powerful tool for combating the occurrence of never events and other forms of surgical errors [5]. While the use of checklists provides surgeons with one tool that battles the overwhelming complexity of modern surgery, the mechanistic and cognitive processes that surgeons grapple with are less understood. Even more significantly, the factors, such as stress and physiological responses to stress that affect these processes and contribute to error rates need to be more fully understood.

As surgeons, we are in command, not only within the operating theater, but throughout the journey across the entire continuum of patient's care. And as surgeons, we should pay special attention to every detail of the surgical symphony, recognizing the limitations of the human mind, and preventing disruptions that may occur. Only then will the surgical symphony sound perfect.

Stress: The Positives and the Negatives

The term stress is often associated with negative outcomes [6]. This chapter reviews the physiological effects of stress, including sleep deprivation, on cognitive function and how these factors can affect the abilities of a surgeon [6]. Driskell and Salas (2006) define stress as a process by which certain environmental demands (i.e., performance in front of others, or taking an exam) evoke an appraisal process in which perceived demand exceeds resources and results in undesirable physiological, psychological, or behavioral outcomes [7]. However, certain amounts of stress can increase performance responses [8]. While stress can increase effectiveness for certain tasks, specific forms and amounts of stress have been shown to impair decision-making as well [7].

Walter Cannon was one of the first scientists to begin analyzing how the adrenal gland was responsive to emotional stimuli. He observed the similar physiological reactions between emotional stress and sympathetic nervous system (SNS) arousal [8–12]. Cannon coined the phrase "fight or flight", which has now been used extensively. The SNS aids in the control of most of the body's internal organs, particularly during preparation for the fight or flight response. The SNS is thought to counteract the parasympathetic system, which generally works to promote maintenance of the body at rest. He also proposed the emergency function theory of adrenal-medulla function that offered a purposeful explanation of the stress response in that the release of adrenaline made an animal more efficient in their struggle with fear, rage, or pain [8]. Cannon was one of the first to explain that stress and the physiological stress response could be positive inducers of peak performance in individuals. However, this peak performance can be adversely affected by other stressors, such as lack of sleep, negative emotions, diet, and alcohol intake.

Surgeons experience a specific form of stress that includes time pressure, task pressure, and coordination among team members to complete a task. While in the operating theater, surgeons are under immense, time-dependent pressure known as acute stress [7]. How does stress affect a surgeon and their decisions? For surgeons, stress in the right amount is useful, and prepares them for the pressures associated with surgery. As proposed by Cannon and observed by many others, the stress response coordinated through the hypothalamic-pituitary-adrenal (HPA) axis actively prepares the individual for specific activities. Glucocorticoids and catecholamines are the primary hormones that are released when the stress response system is stimulated [6]. Glucocorticoids have the function of increasing the availability of energy substrates and allowing for optimal adaptations to the changing demands of the environment. Specifically, it has been found that low levels of circulating glucocorticoids and catecholamines enhance memory function and high levels of these hormones disrupt memory function [13]. Furthermore, according to Mendl, an inverted U-shaped relationship exists between an individual's state of stress or arousal and its ability to perform a cognitive task effectively, the so-called Yerkes–Dodson law, is commonly encountered [13]. Empirical research on attention and memory processes reveals more specific findings. Stressors appear to cause shifts, lapses and narrowing of attention, and can also influence decision speed. There is conflicting evidence as to whether hormones involved in the hypothalamic–pituitary–adrenal stress response play a part in these processes. These hormones, and those involved in the sympathetic-adrenomedullary stress response, do appear to play an important role in memory formation. Low or moderate concentrations of circulating glucocorticoids and catecholamines can enhance memory formation, while excessively high or prolonged elevations of these hormones can lead to memory disruption [13].

Each individual surgeon will vary on what they identify as a potential stressor, but those commonly reported include laparoscopic (versus robotic) surgery, procedural complexity, distractions, and lack of time [14]. While distractions in particular may lead to an increase in surgical errors, due to tasks that require more concentration, they tend to be more stressful; it has been shown that the deliberate practice and minimization of intermittent auditory distractions can help a surgeon better multitask during a procedure [15, 16]. Since there is no single tool to assess stress directly, an individual may choose to either measure their subjective perceptions of stress, and/or objectively assess their physiological state during moments of stress [14]. The Imperial Stress Assessment Tool (ISAT) is a non-intrusive approach to assessing stress during surgery that measures both objective (i.e., salivary cortisol and continuous heart rate) and subjective (self-reported levels) components of stress. Validation studies have determined that the subjective indicators of stress were associated with high cortisol levels 70% of the time, and continuous rapid heart rate 84% of the time [17].

Another important element of surgical decision-making involves learning and memory. How much can one recall from past training or when one reads an article or book and later has to apply it to their clinical practice? Data are particularly lacking when it comes to the field of surgery. However, what is known already is that learning and memory retention can be enhanced under certain forms of stress. For example, Joels et al. proposed that stress facilitates learning and memory processes when stress is experienced in the context and around the time of the event that needs to be remembered and when the hormones and neurotransmitters, released in response to stress, exert their actions on the same circuits as those activated by the situation [18]. Specifically, physical and psychological challenges, such as those presented during surgery, will enhance the information-gathering type of behavior that is useful in assessment of the stressor [18]. For residents and surgeons, extensive medical training prepares them to form a cognitive representation for comparison that stimulates arousal, alertness, and focused attention. Brain structures involved when confronting a stressor are the hippocampus (involved in retention and memory), the amygdala (emotional stimuli processing), and the prefrontal cortex (part of the executive function control). All of these regions are connected to the HPA, which is responsible for the secretion of corticosteroids and other "stress hormones." These hormones activate glucocorticoid receptors when stress occurs to help face an immediate threat as well as preparing an individual for challenging situations in the future. Psychological stressors, such as performing complex surgery, will activate regions such as the amygdala which promotes the memory of salient, but not neutral information. For example, when faced with a surgical procedure, a surgeon may recall key complex procedures more accurately than procedures that are not as pressing or salient. Can one extract a memory that has been stored somewhere in the brain, under stress?

As a junior attending surgeon, I was assisting two senior residents perform a tracheostomy in a morbidly obese patient with severe Acute Respiratory Distress Syndrome (ARDS). I had just joined the hospital, and I did not know the residents or their abilities yet. The neck was very large, and we used deep retractors to expose the trachea. When we asked the anesthesiologist to pull back the endotracheal tube, she pulled it out entirely. The tracheostomy tube that we had at hand would not reach the trachea. I asked for the tube exchanger, but the nursing anesthetist student (and here I thought we had an anesthesiologist on the other side of the curtain), did not know where they were. The patient's oxygen saturation was dropping, and with it his heart rate. At this very desperate moment, I asked for a nasogastric tube, and intubated the trachea by placing it over the endotracheal tube, surely preventing a catastrophic event. Later I recalled that I had heard a surgeon talking about this procedure on an audio tape, but it was many years prior to the event. It's amazing that I was able to access this stored information somewhere in my brain precisely when I needed it most; I still believe that it was the stress of the situation that prompted the retrieval of that specific memory.

Inhibitors of Performance in Stressful Situations

Numerous studies have shown that factors, such as sleep deprivation and alcohol consumption, can affect glucocorticoid production, memory recall, and mood [6, 13, 19]. Many studies also documented how these factors affect performance through memory disruption. Sleep, alcohol consumption, and other forms of stress will affect memory recall and peak performance functioning.

Sleep

Sleep deprivation causes slower response times, reduced learning acquisition in cognitive tasks, and loss of situational awareness [20]. Additionally, individuals with chronic sleep disturbances have significantly worse memory consolidation overnight as compared to control subjects [21, 22].

Scoville and Milner discovered that certain forms of long-term memory rely on the hippocampus [23]. Explicit memory, such as memory of facts, events, people, and places, which are all important aspects of surgical procedures, involves human conscious awareness and requires the hippocampus. Sleep deprivation disrupts hippocampal function and plasticity. In particular, long-term memory consolidation is impaired by sleep deprivation, which suggests that a specific critical period exists following learning during which sleep is necessary [24].

The effects of sleep deprivation on medical staff functioning have been studied over the years [21, 25–28]. Deary and Tait found that those who were on-call or working rotating shifts had less short-term memory recall and higher rates of mood disruption [26]. Harrison and Horne reported that one of the major consequences of sleep deprivation is impaired memory [29]. Specifically, sleep deprivation affects the acquisition of memory [21, 25, 30]. Goldman, McDonough, and Rosemond documented that junior doctors were less focused when suffering from sleep deprivation [27]. Additional studies with clinical staff have shown that sleep deprivation affects innovative thinking and verbal fluency [28].

While the conditions that surgeons are operating under should be considered to be of primary importance, the excessive demands placed on them by long work schedules have only recently begun to gain attention by the medical association. For example, it has been documented that sleep deprivation associated with long working hours will affect performance in areas such as recall, decision-making strategies, spatial abilities, and metacognitive abilities (i.e., appraisal of one's own performance under pressure), and this sleep deprivation will affect individuals differently [31]. Thus, there is no single formula for predicting performance in response to sleep deprivation.

In 2009, the Institute of Medicine (IOM) published a report entitled, "Resident duty hours: Enhancing Sleep, Supervision, and Safety." The report called for revising the requirements for hospital resident working hours, time off between shifts, and more stringent training procedures because it documented a decline in performance among residents due to sleep deprivation [4]. Additional evidence for effects of sleep-disturbance on cognitive processing is provided by studies that assessed mechanistic underpinnings during cognitive activity. By using functional magnetic resonance imaging (fMRI) methods, Drummond and colleagues found that the anterior cingulate cortex (ACC) was active for cognitive tasks in non-sleep deprived subjects; whereas it was not active in sleep-deprived subjects, indicating a mechanistic explanation of how sleep patterns may disrupt the ability of surgeons [32]. Blum and colleagues issued a paper that established effective ways to implement the IOM's suggestions [33].

Alcohol Consumption and Surgeons

A number of studies have addressed surgeons' and other physicians' impairment due to alcohol [34–36]. A 2010 cross-sectional study conducted on 7197 members of the American College of

Surgeons on alcohol use disorders reported that 15.4% had a score consistent with alcohol abuse or dependence. This prevalence certainly underestimates the true magnitude of the issue, as only 28.7% of those surgeons originally sampled responded to the survey. This is not surprising considering both the social stigma and legitimate risk to one's professional career. The survey also described that emotional exhaustion (odds ratio, 1.25; P = 0.01) and feelings of depression (odds ratio, 1.48; P < 0.001) were more strongly associated with alcohol dependence [34].

Alcohol consumption above 0.1 levels contributes to the activation of the HPA axis and stimulates the production of glucocorticoids [19]. While alcohol consumption appears to reduce anxiety, the activation of the HPA axis over time contributes to the habituation of the body to stress hormones. In humans and other animals, the magnitude and duration of the glucocorticoid response depends on the amount of alcohol consumed [19, 37]. In response to alcohol, the levels of cortisol, which is the main glucocorticoid hormone in humans, can be substantial and even surpass the levels typically seen in response to various stressful circumstances [38].

One study documented that surgeons who had used alcohol within a 24 hour time period had higher average time taken to respond and resolve problems and higher error rates [39]. Additionally, Dorafshar et al. reported that surgical performance was impaired in the short-term after moderate alcohol consumption, but this effect was not observed during performance the day after drinking moderately [40].

A small study of five male surgeons between the ages of 31–40 compared the effects of alcohol and/or partial sleep deprivation on surgical dexterity as measured on a laparoscopic surgical simulator (by the time taken to complete tasks, number of errors, diathermy time, and injury time). There were three experimental states that were described: a control state where no alcohol was consumed and subjects received a full night of undisturbed sleep; a sleep-deprived group that consumed no alcohol, and finally, sleep deprivation combined with ad libitum alcohol consumption. Those who underwent sleep deprivation averaged 3.75 hours of sleep (range 3–5 hours), while 10.33 units (range 6–15) of alcohol (equivalent to 100 ml of pure ethanol) were consumed on average by those during this respective treatment. Repeated measures were taken at three time points for each subject, and breath alcohol analyses for all participants were 0% by the next morning, but it is unclear if there were adequate washout periods or randomization of the treatment order. Based on these results from five individuals who demonstrated large interpersonal variations, alcohol consumption seemed to have the greatest adverse effect on surgical performance, particularly with diathermy and injury time. A combination of alcohol and sleep deprivation was seen to have the greatest number of errors. The results of the study suggested that the effect of sleep deprivation and prior alcohol consumption on performance varies with the time of the day (P = 0.02), and there are discernable residual effects of alcohol consumption the following day, despite undetectable levels of alcohol measured on the breath the next morning [41].

Conclusion

There is ample evidence for how the physiology and state of mind of surgeons, such as sleep deprivation and alcohol consumption, can affect the surgeon and interfere with his/her performance during stressful events such as complex surgery. Surgeons should be more aware of these factors and make life style changes accordingly.

References

1. Makary MA, Daniel M. Medical error-the third leading cause of death in the US. BMJ. 2016;353:i2139. https://doi.org/10.1136/bmj.i2139.
2. Wiegmann DA, et al. Disruptions in surgical flow and their relationship to surgical errors: an exploratory investigation. Surgery. 2007;142(5):658–65.
3. Mehtsun WT, et al. Surgical never events in the United States. Surgery. 2013;153(4):465–72.
4. Kohn LT, Corrigan JM, Donaldson MS. To err is human:: building a safer health system, vol. 6. National Academies Press; 2000.
5. Gawande A, Lloyd JB. The checklist manifesto: how to get things right, vol. 200. Metropolitan Books New York; 2010.

6. Lupien SJ, et al. The effects of stress and stress hormones on human cognition: implications for the field of brain and cognition. Brain Cogn. 2007;65(3):209–37.
7. Driskell JE, Salas E, Johnston JH. Decision making and performance under stress. In: Britt TW, Adler A, Castro CA, series editors, Britt TW, Castro CA, Adler A, editors. Military life: the psychology of serving in peace and combat; 2006. 1: pp. 128–154.
8. Cannon WB. The emergency function of the adrenal medulla in pain and the major emotions. Am J Physiol Legacy Content. 1914;33(2):356–72.
9. Cannon WB. The influence of emotional states on the functions of the alimentary canal. Am J Med Sci. 1909;137(4):480–6.
10. Cannon WB, Shohl AT, Wright W. Emotional glycosuria. Am J Physiol Legacy Content. 1911;29(2):280–7.
11. Cannon WB. Studies on the conditions of activity in endocrine glands: the isolated heart as an indicator of adrenal secretion induced by pain, Asphyxia and Excitement V. 1919: publisher not identified.
12. Cannon WB. Studies on the conditions of activity in endocrine glands: the influence of motion and emotion on medulliadrenal secretion. XX. 1927: publisher not identified.
13. Mendl M. Performing under pressure: stress and cognitive function. Appl Anim Behav Sci. 1999;65(3):221–44.
14. Arora S, et al. The impact of stress on surgical performance: a systematic review of the literature. Surgery. 2010;147(3):318–30. e6
15. Ahmed A, et al. Effect of distractions on operative performance and ability to multitask—a case for deliberate practice. Laryngoscope. 2015;125(4):837–41.
16. Mentis H, et al. A systematic review of the effect of distraction on surgeon performance: directions for operating room policy and surgical training. Surg Endosc. 2015:1–12.
17. Arora S, et al. The Imperial stress assessment tool (ISAT): a feasible, reliable and valid approach to measuring stress in the operating room. World J Surg. 2010;34(8):1756–63.
18. Joels M, et al. Learning under stress: how does it work? Trends Cogn Sci. 2006;10(4):152–8.
19. Spencer R, McEwen B. Adaptation of the hypothalamic-pituitary-adrenal axis to chronic ethanol stress. Neuroendocrinology. 1990;52(5):481–9.
20. Durmer JS, Dinges DF. Neurocognitive consequences of sleep deprivation. Semin Neurol. 2005;
21. Abel T, Lattal KM. Molecular mechanisms of memory acquisition, consolidation and retrieval. Curr Opin Neurobiol. 2001;11(2):180–7.
22. Backhaus J, et al. Impaired declarative memory consolidation during sleep in patients with primary insomnia: influence of sleep architecture and nocturnal cortisol release. Biol Psychiatry. 2006;60(12):1324–30.
23. Scoville WB, Milner B. Loss of recent memory after bilateral hippocampal lesions. J Neurol Neurosurg Psychiatry. 1957;20(1):11.
24. Prince T-M, et al. Sleep deprivation during a specific 3-hour time window post-training impairs hippocampal synaptic plasticity and memory. Neurobiol Learn Mem. 2014;109:122–30.
25. Abel T, et al. Sleep, plasticity and memory from molecules to whole-brain networks. Curr Biol. 2013;23(17):R774–88.
26. Deary IJ, Tait R. Effects of sleep disruption on cognitive performance and mood in medical house officers. Br Med J (Clin Res Ed). 1987;295(6612):1513–6.
27. Goldman LI, McDonough MT, Rosemond GP. Stresses affecting surgical performance and learning: I. correlation of heart rate, electrocardiogram, and operation simultaneously recorded on videotapes. J Surg Res. 1972;12(2):83–6.
28. Nelson CS, et al. Residents' performance before and after night call as evaluated by an indicator of creative thought. J Am Osteopath Assoc. 1995;95(10):600–3.
29. Harrison Y, Horne JA. The impact of sleep deprivation on decision making: a review. J Exp Psychol Appl. 2000;6(3):236–49.
30. Saletin JM, van der Helm E, Walker MP. Structural brain correlates of human sleep oscillations. NeuroImage. 2013;83:658–68.
31. Rocklage M, et al. White matter differences predict cognitive vulnerability to sleep deprivation. Sleep. 2009;32(8):1100–3.
32. Drummond S, Gillin JC, Brown GG. Increased cerebral response during a divided attention task following sleep deprivation. J Sleep Res. 2001;10(2):85–92.
33. Blum AB, et al. Implementing the 2009 Institute of Medicine recommendations on resident physician work hours, supervision, and safety. Nat Sci Sleep. 2011;3:47.
34. Oreskovich MR, et al. Prevalence of alcohol use disorders among American surgeons. Arch Surg. 2012;147(2):168–74.
35. Rosta J, Aasland OG. Female surgeons' alcohol use: a study of a national sample of norwegian doctors.[Erratum appears in Alcohol Alcohol. 2005 Nov-Dec;40(6):590]. Alcohol Alcohol. 2005;40(5):436–40.
36. Schermer CR, et al. National survey of trauma surgeons' use of alcohol screening and brief intervention. J Trauma-Injury Inf Crit Care. 2003;55(5):849–56.
37. Groote Veldman R, Meinders AE. On the mechanism of alcohol-induced pseudo-Cushing's syndrome. Endocr Rev. 1996;17(3):262–8.
38. Mendelson JH. Biochemical mechanisms of alcohol addiction. In: The biology of alcoholism. Springer; 1971. p. 513–44.
39. Gallagher AG, et al. Persistent next-day effects of excessive alcohol consumption on laparoscopic surgical performance. Arch Surg. 2011;146(4):419–26.
40. Dorafshar AH, O'Boyle D, McCloy R. Effects of a moderate dose of alcohol on simulated laparoscopic surgical performance. Surg Endosc Other Interv Tech. 2002;16(12):1753–8.
41. Kocher H, et al. Surgical dexterity after a 'night out on the town'. ANZ J Surg. 2006;76(3):110–2.

Surgeons and Pilots: What Do We Have in Common?

6

Rifat Latifi

Introduction

Flying a plane (or riding in a plane for that matter) can be dangerous business, but still much safer than a number of things we do regularly. In fact, it is one the safest thing that we do. There were 37.4 million flights in 2014, the highest number ever, and this equates to more than 100,000 flights per day. Given the low number of fatal crashes that year (1), you would statistically have to fly 5,342,857 times for every accident. The average for 2010–2014 is lower, but still better than any previous five-year period; one fatal crash per 2,925,000 flights. That means a 0.000034% risk. You have never been less likely to fly on a plane that will crash and experience fatalities [1]. Still the list of fatalities is extensive and often high-profile [2]. Recent fatalities include the AF Andrade Empreendimentos e Participações Cessna 560XLS+ Citation Excel in Guarujá, Brazil, where five passengers and a pilot were killed after crashing into a residential area on 13 August 2014. On 10 August 2014, Sepahan Airlines HESA IrAn 140, flight 217, near Nardaran, Azerbaijan, five crew members and 18 passengers were killed when the aircraft crashed shortly after takeoff. On 24 July 2014, Air Algerie MD83, EC-LTV, flight AH5017, near Gossi, Mali, crashed after the pilot contacted the control tower to request a different route due to weather conditions, killing six crew members and 119 passengers. Last few crashes have been mentioned in the introduction chapters.

Pilots and surgeons undergo intensive training. However, the question is do long and intensive trainings determine who will commit errors and who will handle emergency situations effectively, in surgery or aviation. Numerous factors play a part in how these situations are handled in both fields. Some basic factors are similar and include communication, technical skill, mental state, and external distracting factors.

Once, in an interview, John O'Connell, a pilot with more than 18,000 hours of pilot in command time, provided a brief vision of what a pilot may have to encounter, and what that pilot perceives he has to do in emergency situations. O'Connell claims that there is a plan A, then a B, then a C and D. More than one backup plan is necessary, and it is good to have these plans mentally available during a time of crisis. Similarly, in complex surgeries there must be a plan A, a plan B, and at least a plan C, but in a flight, the public does not see these plans. On the other hand, we surgeons discuss these plans with a patient and family all the time. The most important thing is to know the basics of flying, down to a point where you don't even think about them, and to perform a surgery plan A and not think about plan B and C, unless it

R. Latifi (✉)
Department of Surgery, The University of Arizona, Tucson, AZ, USA

Tucson Medical Center, Department of Surgery, Tucson, AZ, USA
e-mail: Latifi@surgery.arizona.edu

R. Latifi (ed.), *Surgical Decision-Making*, https://doi.org/10.1007/978-3-031-67391-7_6

is really needed. But if you need them, you have to play them down clearly. That way, in a time of crisis, you address the crisis, and not the basic activity of flying, or performing surgery in the operating room. O'Connell states that the use of checklists during specific situations is helpful. For example, if the engine loses power, there is a standard checklist that pilots go through in order to systematically identify the problems that may be causing the engine failure [3]. However, if the patient has a cardiac arrest on the operating table, while we surgeons do not have a written checklist for that scenario hanging on the wall of the operating room, it is expected that we all know what to do. That is, every surgeon should know what to do, or call for help.

The safety of airlines is clearly multifactorial, but both pilots and surgeons, as captain of the "ship" play a major role and both are in charge of the situation.

Performing surgery could be a dangerous and complex process. The training that goes into becoming a surgeon is even more intensive than becoming a pilot. Surgeons typically have between eleven to sixteen years of training, including residency. The training is very complex and it is not an easy process. Such training is necessary in order for the doctor to become a surgeon, an expert who is ready to deal with the unexpected. Much like the scenario of a pilot who does not have to think about the basics when an emergency occurs, a surgeon cannot waste time on thinking through basics of operating when things get out of hand. It should be effortless.

It takes many years of training before one can independently take on a complex surgical case. The training is so difficult that a recent anonymous survey of 371 categorical general surgery residents and evaluation of 10-year attrition rates for thirteen residency programs in the USA revealed that 58.0% seriously considered leaving training [4]. The most frequent reasons for wanting to leave were sleep deprivation on a specific rotation (50.0%), an undesirable future lifestyle (47.0%), and excessive work hours on a specific rotation (41.4%). Factors most often cited that kept residents from leaving were support from family or significant others (65.0%), support from other residents (63.5%), and perception of being better rested (58.9%). Interestingly, on univariate analysis, older age, female sex, postgraduate year, training in a university program, the lack a faculty mentor, particularly in female residents, lack of female faculty mentors, and lack of Alpha Omega Alpha status were associated with serious thoughts of leaving surgical residency. On multivariate analysis, only female sex was significantly associated with serious thoughts of leaving residency (odds ratio, 1.2; $P = 0.003$), while married male, and especially married male with children were more satisfied in their residency program and did not think of leaving.

The authors [4] conclude that: "*The training of surgical residents is a long and arduous process that necessitates an immense investment of time for the trainee and the faculty. As such, resident attrition is a tremendous loss for all involved parties. In this multi-institutional survey of surgical residents, a majority seriously considered leaving their training, and most had such thoughts more than once. Given that prior investigations indicate that surgical residents who think of quitting are more likely to subsequently do so, the survey results herein are sobering. With the increasing number of women entering surgical training, the fact that female sex predicted thoughts of quitting in the present study is similarly concerning. Surgical training programs should take heed of these findings and work in a cooperative fashion to address factors that increase residents' desire to leave surgical residency.*"

It is unclear what the true attrition rate is among aircraft pilots, as the recent addition of navigators of unmanned aircrafts has complicated things a bit. However, recent articles suggest that attrition of trainees from the aviation program is a continuing concern for the U.S. Navy, and each late-stage navy aviator training failure costs the taxpayer over $1000,000, and ultimately results in decreased operational readiness of the fleet [5]. Over the past 20 years, the attrition rate of incoming aviation students has been between 15–25%. As with surgical trainees, attrition among pilot trainees occurs for a variety of reasons including medical problems. However, most attritions result from academic or flight performance failures or requests to be dropped from the program. Naval aviation is a highly stressful occupation requiring the ability to respond quickly and appropriately in dangerous situations. While there is no measure of the impact of psychological stress on attrition from the program, it makes a clear contribution to academic/flight performance failures and drop out request. Biological screening of potential aviators based on performance under psychological stress could reduce all of the major contributing factors of attrition, thus saving the Navy millions of dollars.

There is a difference between how surgical residents and pilots are selected. Potential aviators are currently selected using the Aviation Selection Test Battery (ASTB). The ASTB is a written test designed to evaluate math and verbal skills, mechanical comprehension, aviation and nautical information and spatial apperception. The ASTB has a strong predictive validity through primary flight training. While the ASTB evaluates many skills necessary to aviation, and is correlated with performance, it does not account for the natural genetic variation in physiological stress response. Once selected by the ASTB, all naval pilot trainees undergo water survival training in the Modular Egress Training Simulator (METS) device, a highly demanding and stressful test. In contrast, potential surgical residents are interviewed, and have to demonstrate that they have done well in their past education, show dedication, but there is no physical test. Actually, once I observed a chief resident struggling while removing a gallbladder. I asked him to see an optometrist, as I thought his glasses were old and maybe he needed a new prescription. To my huge surprise, he admitted that he had a depth perception problem that could not be fixed. Since then I have wondered why we do not give a real comprehensive screening test for our future surgeons.

Human performance under psychological stress has been studied extensively, and it has been primarily done psychometrically or using reductionist biological methods such as blood cortisol measurements [6]. Moreover, a study published in 1999 that looked at the neuroendocrine responses among students suggested that neuroendocrine reactions as a response to the psychological workload of military flying could be used for identifying stress tolerance in military pilots [7].

Both pilots and surgeons work under highly stressful jobs, so identifying specific biomarkers to predict who will make it through training, and identify those who will not, would be quite useful. Such work would also provide potential biomarkers for screening humans for capability of superior performance under stress. If this testing is proved in the future to predict who will be able to adapt better to high intensity situations, we believe that such protocols should be extended to future surgeons as well.

While there are a number of similarities among pilots and surgeons, still there are some other significant differences between surgeons and pilots with respect to public involvement. Every pilot error is recorded, scrutinized, analyzed and made public; rarely are the errors of surgeons made public. There is no recording of the procedures, and, thus, it is impossible or very difficult to replay the surgery and make it public. Furthermore, because of privacy issues, only a few major mistakes by surgeons ever make it to the news.

Pilots and Surgeons: The Dangerous Jobs

Both pilots and surgeons have dangerous jobs; these types of careers take the lives of other people in their hands while engaging in tasks that are played out in dynamic, ever-changing contexts. Paying attention to all available cues is of the utmost importance. After all, people's lives depend on it! Like pilots, surgeons work in dynamic environments, while taking responsibility for the lives of individuals and managing to complete difficult tasks such as a pancreaticoduodenectomy, liver or lung resection, or takedown of complex multiple fistulas or managing a patient major abdominal trauma after a high-speed head-on collision in patient in severe shock spiraling down, without knowing in advance what you will find in the abdomen. While these and the countless other surgical procedures may seem very difficult for non-surgeons or novice and inexperienced trainees, and surgeons, the well-trained surgeon can complete these procedures safely, but when a crisis arrives, things change dramatically. Maybe as we surgeons have a bit "more time" to address our crises, as our operating room is not flying at 1000 km/hour. Still, the environments of surgeons and pilots are considered dynamic, meaning there is continual change occurring within the environment. Often, however, we do not have much time, as in patients with cardiac stab or even blunt trauma in cardiac tamponade.

When broken down by steps, work within dynamic environments can be fitted into three major categories. First, the pilot or surgeon must continually monitor and assess the situation. While this is the first step in the process, it is also continual. The pilot or surgeon has to assess the situation with each development in order to process how to respond and which step to take next. He or she must then take appropriate reactions based on assessment. Once appropriate action is taken, evaluation of results must be made. The cycle then repeats itself [8, 9]. These jobs are intensely stressful, not only because people's lives are dependent upon decisions that are made, but there is no "down-time" while performing these jobs. A surgeon can't go take a break during a long and intense surgery. A pilot can't stop flying a plane if he doesn't feel well. Additionally, a key aspect to functioning successfully in complex dynamic environments is the ability not only to observe and seek information, but to understand what that information means in the larger context of a task goal [10]. Moreover, an ability to then anticipate events in that environment leads to better prediction and understanding of future events. The cognitive components of these processes are of interest to researchers and will briefly be discussed in this chapter. While these cognitive components are of interest, a major goal of this chapter is to establish what may be occurring when a surgeon or pilot seemingly makes a "gut-level" decision. There is a whole host of other factors that the operator is not aware of, such as the integration of the information they have learned through training and experience. This phenomenon can be called situational awareness, sense-making, or unconscious processing of environmental cues. Regardless of the term used, the concept has been reviewed in a number of ways, particularly in the literature on the abilities of pilots [10–13].

Situational Awareness and Common Sense-Making

Situational Awareness is a concept that has been studied extensively for pilots and can be applied to surgeons in the operating room. Military strategists have applied this concept to operating aircraft, ships, and in emergency military situations. As described in chapter two of this book, situational awareness can briefly be described as "*the perception of elements within a volume of time and space, the comprehension of their meaning, and the projection of their status in the near future* [9]." Numerous studies looking at the effects of situational awareness in virtual and real environments among military personnel have been conducted [9]. Few studies have been conducted that look at how situational awareness can be applied in the medical field.

Of the few studies that investigate situational awareness (SA) in the medical field, either communication among surgical team members or the usefulness of the concept of situational awareness has gained most attention; these aspects are also termed non-technical skills. Postgraduate training in the medical field is extensive, but especially in surgical disciplines. With this postgraduate training, several technical skills are acquired from how to approach and examine the patient and identifying problems that need an intervention, to highly technical procedures for various operations. However, non-technical skills are somewhat individually-based, and not every surgeon is trained for the same, although the basics are fairly similar. These skills are just as valuable as technical ones, and are a common subject of investigation for surgical never-events. As described earlier in the book, surgical never events are events that include operating on the wrong patient, performing the incorrect surgery, operating on the wrong limb, etc. These errors are substantially high and are easily remedied if the proper precautions are taken [14]. Specifically, the use of non-technical skills, such as communication and organization, is required in order to prevent surgical never events.

The concept of situational awareness has been investigated in order to prevent these forms of errors. For example, Gaba et al. discusses potential application of the concept among anesthesiologists [14]. Flin et al. make a case for applying decision-making analysis concepts (i.e., naturalistic decision-making) in a two-step process that includes: assessing and diagnosing the situation, then using one of four strategies to make a decision [15]. These strategies are selected based on a continuum of urgency, and include intuitive recognition, rule-based, analytical, and creative decision-making. When the need to make a decision is urgent, intuitive recognition decision-making is used, whereas when the need to make a decision is not urgent, creative decision-making is used [15]. For example, creative decision-making requires more time and less urgency. It appears that there is a blend of intuitive recognition decision-making and creative decision-making during surgery.

According to Mica Endsley, a pioneer in the field of SA, there are different levels of SA [11, 12]. At the lowest level of SA, a person needs to perceive relevant information (Level 1 SA). Integrating various pieces of information, while keeping the overall objective of the task in mind, allows the individual to form an understanding of the meaning of that information within context, forming Level 2 SA. Based on this understanding, future events can then be predicted (Level 3), allowing for timely and effective decision-making. Several processing mechanisms have been hypothesized to be related to SA, including attention and working memory limitations, attention distribution, current goals, mental models, schemata, and automaticity [10–12]. In addition to characteristics of individuals, the design of a system, for example, how patient information flows to the surgeon prior to surgery, and the team environment can affect SA.

Situation Awareness, Perception, Comprehension, Projection

The three main factors that drive or underlie SA are perception, comprehension, and projection [16–19]. These can easily be mapped onto the levels described by Endsley. These concepts allow for awareness to be parceled out into tractable portions for further understanding. One of the cognitive processes associated with SA is that of working memory (WM). Personally, from very busy surgical practice, I took a leave of absence from surgery for 18 months, while serving as the Minister of Health for the Republic of Kosova and taking a few months off after that. When I returned to operating, I performed as the first case, a major complex abdominal wall reconstruction, and was fascinated how I my working memory took place immediately, and I had no problems asking for the instruments that I had not even thought about for 18 months. I guess there is a reason why we say "It's like riding a bike" to mean that that once you learn how to do something, you never forget it. Working memory can be defined as the system that actively holds multiple pieces of transitory information in the mind, where they can be manipulated. Working memory includes subsystems that store and manipulate visual images or verbal information, as well as a central executive that coordinates the subsystems. It includes visual representation of the possible moves, and awareness of the flow of information into and out of memory, all stored for a limited amount of time. Working memory tasks require monitoring, which is a component of SA, as part of completing goal-directed actions in dynamic environments. The cognitive processes needed to achieve this include the executive and attention control of short-term memory, which permit interim integration, processing, disposal, and retrieval of information. These processes are sensitive to age: working memory is associated with cognitive development, and research shows that its capacity tends to decline with old age. In addition, neurological studies demonstrate a link between working memory and learning and attention, as well as being an underlying component of SA [17].

Conclusion

Both pilots and surgeons have to make serious decisions that are time dependent and may have serious consequences. While the pilot is supported by the most sophisticated technologies of the flying machine, which now a days have full control on their own, the surgeon has to make decisions that are highly dependent on his or her experience, knowledge, and often this decision is gut based. Overall, these decisions are made in highly dynamic and changing environments. Awareness of the individual state of the surgeon and pilot is crucial, together with awareness of the operating environment, such as communication dynamics among the teams. Not being aware of certain subtleties in communication may be detrimental to both surgical and piloting outcomes. Additionally, extensive training will allow for a surgeon and a pilot to be prepared for unexpected events. Checklists, while possibly viewed as something to be used by novices only, have been shown to be helpful with pilots and surgeons [20, 21, 22]. Finally, there is much to learn regarding how and why individuals make decisions, particularly decisions that appear to be gut-level or unconscious. The research in this field is valuable and informative for professions that make decisions in dynamic environments that will affect the lives of other individuals.

Still major errors or so called "human errors" are attributed to major catastrophes in aviation, both commercial and private, while in surgery we attribute "technical errors", "error in judgment" to surgeons, and it is not uncommon, to mix with "the patients' disease" as a major attribution to bad outcome. Imagine, if the pilots fly really old airplanes, with no updated software or hardware, like surgeons operating in a geriatric population which has, in addition to being old, several comorbidities. And we surgeons do this day in and day out.

References

1. Garfors G. Is it safe to fly? Globetrotting Galore. 2015. Retrieved October 20, 2015, from http://www.garfors.com/2015/03/is-it-safe-to-fly-dangerous.html
2. ABC News. In wake of emergency landings, pilot simulates situations. 2014. Retrieved October 20, 2015, from http://www.abc-7.com/story/26293414/in-wake-of-emergency-landings-pilot-simulates-situations#.VibA6H6rSUl
3. Federal Aviation Administration (FAA). Federal Aviation Administration (FAA). 2015. Retrieved October 20, 2015, from http://www.faa.gov/
4. Gifford E, Galante J, Kaji AH, et al. Factors associated with general surgery residents' desire to leave residency programs: a multi-institutional study. JAMA Surg. 2014;149(9):948–53. https://doi.org/10.1001/jamasurg.2014.935.
5. Cooksey AM, Momen N, Stocker R, Burgess SC. Identifying blood biomarkers and physiological processes that distinguish humans with superior performance under psychological stress. PLoS One. 2009;4(12):e8371. https://doi.org/10.1371/journal.pone.0008371.
6. Schedlowski M, Wiechert D, Wagner TO, Tewes U. Acute psychological stress increases plasma levels of cortisol, prolactin and TSH. Life Sci. 1992;50:1201–12051.
7. Leino TK, Leppäluoto J, Ruokonen A, Kuronen P. Neuroendocrine responses to psychological workload of instrument flying in student pilots. Aviat Space Environ Med. 1999;70(6):565–70.
8. Endsley MR. Towards a theory of situation awareness in dynamic environments. Hum Factors. 1995;37:32–64.
9. Endsley MR. A survey of situation awareness requirements in air-to-air combat fighters. Int J Aviat Psychol. 1993;3:157–68.
10. Endsley MR. Measurement of situation awareness in dynamic systems. Hum Factors. 1995;37:65–84.
11. Endsley MR. The application of human factors to the development of expert systems for advanced cockpits. In: Proceedings of the 7th international symposium on aviation psychology. Columbus: Ohio State University; 1987. p. 167–71.
12. Durso FT, Sethumadhavan A. Situation awareness: understanding dynamic environments. Hum Fact J Hum Fact Ergonom Soc. 2008;50:442–50. https://doi.org/10.1518/001872008X288448.

13. Mehtsun WT, et al. Surgical never events in the United States. Surgery. 2013;153(4):465–72.
14. Gaba DM, Howard SK, Small SD. Situation awareness in anesthesiology. Hum Fact J Hum Fact Ergonom Soc. 1995;37:20–33.
15. Flin R, Youngson G, Yule S. How do surgeons make intraoperative decisions? Qual Saf Health Care. 2007;16:235–9. https://doi.org/10.1136/qshc.2006.020743.
16. Gutzwiller RS, Clegg BA. The role of working memory in levels of situation awareness. J Cogn Eng Decis Making. 2013;7(2):141–54.
17. Durso FT, Sethumadhavan A. Situation awareness: understanding dynamic environments. Hum Fact J Hum Fact Ergonom Soc. 2008;50:44.
18. Bedny G, Meister D. Theory of activity and situation awareness. Int J Cogn Ergon. 1999;3:63–72.
19. Smith D. Introduction to aeronautical decision making. Retrieved 08 October 2009 from the World Wide Web: ADM; 2002.
20. Aircare. An aviators guide to good decision making. Welligton: Aircareå; 2006.
21. Gawande A. The checklist manifesto: how to get things right. New York: Metropolitan Books, Henry Holt and Company, LLC; 2009.
22. Anwer M, Manzoor S, Muneer N, Qureshi S. Compliance and effectiveness of WHO surgical safety check list: A JPMC Audit. Pak J Med Sci. 2016;32(4):831–5. https://doi.org/10.12669/pjms.324.9884. PMID: 27648023; PMCID: PMC5017086.

7 Planning and Preparing for the Operation: The Role of Artificial Intelligence in Modern Surgery

J. Esteban Foianini and Genna Beattie

Introduction

As surgeons, we have to make surgical decisions based on multiple variables. Often, these decisions are not based on evidence. Irrespective of how one makes the decisions, it will affect the course of the surgical intervention and may impact the patient's eventual outcome.

As we plan for an operation, surgeons have historically used hypothetical reasoning based on current literature, surgical training, mentors, and previous experience. This reasoning is called clinical "gestalt" and is the method by which many clinical decisions are still made.

In the era of evidenced-based surgery and data-driven results, there has been an attempt to generate predictive models to plan surgical procedures and predict outcomes in our patients. However, complex and cumbersome decision trees or unreliable algorithms have hindered the application of these tools in everyday surgical practice. Survival data is typically studied using linear models [1, 2]. Unfortunately, we know that surgical complications are non-linear [3].

J. E. Foianini (✉)
Surgeon and Medical Director, Clinica Foianini, Santa Cruz, Bolivia
e-mail: efoianini@clinicafoianini.com

G. Beattie
Clinical Fellow (PGY-9), Trauma & Acute Care Surgery, University of California San Francisco, San Francisco, CA, USA
e-mail: genna.beattie@ucsf.edu

Artificial Intelligence (AI) and machine learning have begun to revolutionize all aspects of our lives, and most recently, there has been increased interest in its role in medicine. One of the advantages of AI is its non-linear properties, which allow it to perceive relationships that are not readily apparent. AI is particularly suited to analyzing large datasets, computing complex interactions, identifying hidden patterns, and generating actionable predictions in clinical settings [4]. At present, AI's role in interpreting imaging studies has been one of its first incursions into the medical field. However, AI is poised to alter how we diagnose and treat patients, and it will become prevalent in our daily and professional lives shortly.

With the ready availability of electronic medical records (EMR) and storage of immense amounts of health data, it seems logical that AI should integrate with these systems to obtain the data and inform the provider of potential risks and outcomes. Ideally, the EMR would notify the provider of possible adverse outcomes, calculate risks when the patient's EMR is accessed, and send alerts for critical events to ensure a prompt and adequate response by the healthcare provider.

Surgeons have been taught to rely on current evidence, past clinical experiences, mentor teachings, and institutional protocols. These experiences are critical to surgical decision-making but also introduce a degree of surgical bias. AI will not remove all of these potential biases, but it can

R. Latifi (ed.), *Surgical Decision-Making*, https://doi.org/10.1007/978-3-031-67391-7_7

collect a large amount of data and variables and find patterns that can assist us in predicting outcomes and defining treatment.

Since AI is an emerging technology, its application within surgery is still limited. As of this writing, it is clear that AI can potentially allow for risk stratification in surgical treatments or procedures and their associated complications. It may also serve to predict treatment outcomes, morbidity, and survival. AI is altering how we look at and process data, which will directly impact how we conduct medical research in the future.

Furthermore, models are being developed that will allow us to predict subgroups of patients at a higher risk for complications. Then, we can tailor treatment to mitigate the possibility of specific complications. In this chapter, we will review several applications of AI in surgical and clinical practice. As it stands currently, knowing fully that the role of AI will expand dramatically in every aspect of modern surgery.

Definitions

Artificial Intelligence refers to computer systems capable of performing complex tasks that historically only humans could do, such as reasoning, making decisions, or solving problems [5]. It emulates human cognition and can learn from training examples to predict future events [6].

Three common terms are associated with AI: machine learning, neural networks, and deep learning. Machine learning (ML) is a branch of AI and computer science where machines can recognize patterns and learn from their experiences without being explicitly programmed [7–9].

ML is the most widely applied arm of AI in medicine. ML is particularly useful in settings where signals and data are produced faster than the human brain can interpret and in identifying subtle patterns in large datasets [10]. It can identify patterns imperceptible to humans performing manual analysis as it allows for more indirect and complex non-linear relationships [11].

Neural networks are a sub-field of machine learning, and deep learning (DL) is a sub-field of neural networks [12]. Neural networks process signals in layers of single computational units. Deep learning networks are neural networks composed of many layers and can learn more complex patterns [11].

XGBoost, which stands for Extreme Gradient Boosting, is a scalable, distributed gradient-boosted tree machine learning library. It is the leading machine-learning library for regression, classification, and ranking problems [13].

The Area Under the Curve (AUC) measures the accuracy of a quantitative diagnostic test [14]. It has critical applications in various fields, such as statistics, machine learning, and analyzing real-life data [15]. The higher the AUC, the better the model's performance at distinguishing between the positive and negative classes.

Augmented Reality During Surgery

AI can provide augmented reality (AR) during surgery. The technology superimposes images onto structures, allowing it to highlight critical anatomical structures and point out potential pitfalls. In this sense, it assists the surgeon but is not poised to replace the surgeon during the procedure. A typical example of AR is during laparoscopic cholecystectomy, as it can identify areas of potential harm or injury to vital structures. A recent publication described a DL model that provided real-time intraoperative guidance. This model identified safe and dangerous zones of dissection during laparoscopic cholecystectomy [16]. These systems intend to provide real-time guidance and minimize the risk of adverse events. The incorporation of AR during laparoscopic cholecystectomy could potentially lead to a reduction in the risk of bile duct injury during these procedures in the future.

Another example of AR is during oncological surgery for a liver tumor. The AR allows the surgeon to visualize the tumor and determine its relationship to major intra-parenchymal vascular structures in real time [17]. In the future, AR should become widespread in modern operating theaters and will probably be applied to most minimally invasive procedures.

Overall Surgical Complications

AI will significantly impact how we analyze and predict surgical complications. Surgical complications occur in as many as 34% of procedures. Importantly, underestimating complication risks can lead to the under-triage of high-risk patients, impacting their clinical outcomes [18, 19].

Several models have been developed to determine the risk of postoperative complications. Accurate predictions of complications are essential for precise clinical decision-making, shared decisions between the patient and the surgeon, allocation of resources, quality benchmarking, and planned postoperative disposition (general ward versus intensive care unit). Most current models suffer from suboptimal performance, limitations of manual data entry, and a lack of clinical workflow integration [19].

Surgical Risk Models

The American College of Surgeons Surgical Risk Calculator (ACS-SRC)

One of the most utilized risk calculators is the American College of Surgeons Surgical Risk Calculator (ACS-SRC), which uses data from the American College of Surgeons National Surgical Quality Improvement Program (ACS-NSQIP). The ACS-SRC risk calculator can be assessed at https://riskcalculator.facs.org/RiskCalculator/. ACS-SRC is an excellent tool widely used to inform treatment and support clinical decisions [20]. One of its limitations is that it is an online platform requiring manual data entry, which is not integrated into the clinical workflow. The report can be emailed to the clinician or printed as a PDF (Fig. 7.1).

Images are obtained from the ACS-SCR calculator, which is a web-based platform. The latest version of the ACS-SCR provides the following quote: "The Risk Calculator's risk-estimating methodology has now transitioned from regression to machine learning. This change in methodology will improve the calculator's already excellent accuracy, though differences in estimated risk should not be large." [21]

The Predictive OpTimal Trees in Emergency Surgery Risk Calculator (POTTER)

The Predictive OpTimal Trees in Emergency Surgery Risk Calculator (POTTER) was introduced in 2018. The ACS-SRC is tailored to elective surgical patients, while the POTTER calculator is geared towards emergency surgery. This ML risk calculator for emergency surgery is available for iOS and Android smartphones at no expense. The developers intend to integrate the calculator into the EMR in the future.

The calculator predicts 30-day postoperative mortality, morbidity, and each one of the 18 individual postoperative complications of the ACS-NSQIP, such as renal failure, respiratory failure, myocardial infarction, or deep vein thrombosis. With regard to 30-day postoperative morbidity, the c-statistic of the POTTER algorithms was the highest at 0.8414, outperforming the American Society of Anesthesiology (ASA) (0.7842), Emergency Surgery Score (ESS) (0.7768), and the ACS-SRC (0.8063). The POTTER calculator predicted the occurrence of individual 30-day postoperative complications with a moderate to extremely high accuracy (c-statistic range from 0.7358 to 0.9338). It performed best in predicting postoperative septic shock (c-statistic 0.9338), postoperative ventilator dependence for longer than 48 hours (0.9254), and postoperative renal failure (0.9126) [3]. In a follow-up article, the lead authors compared the POTTER calculator with surgeon gestalt. The POTTER calculator outperformed surgeon gestalt in predicting postoperative mortality and outcomes in Emergency General Surgery cases. Surgeon-predicted estimates were mostly higher and significantly more dispersed than POTTER estimates (Fig. 7.2) [22].

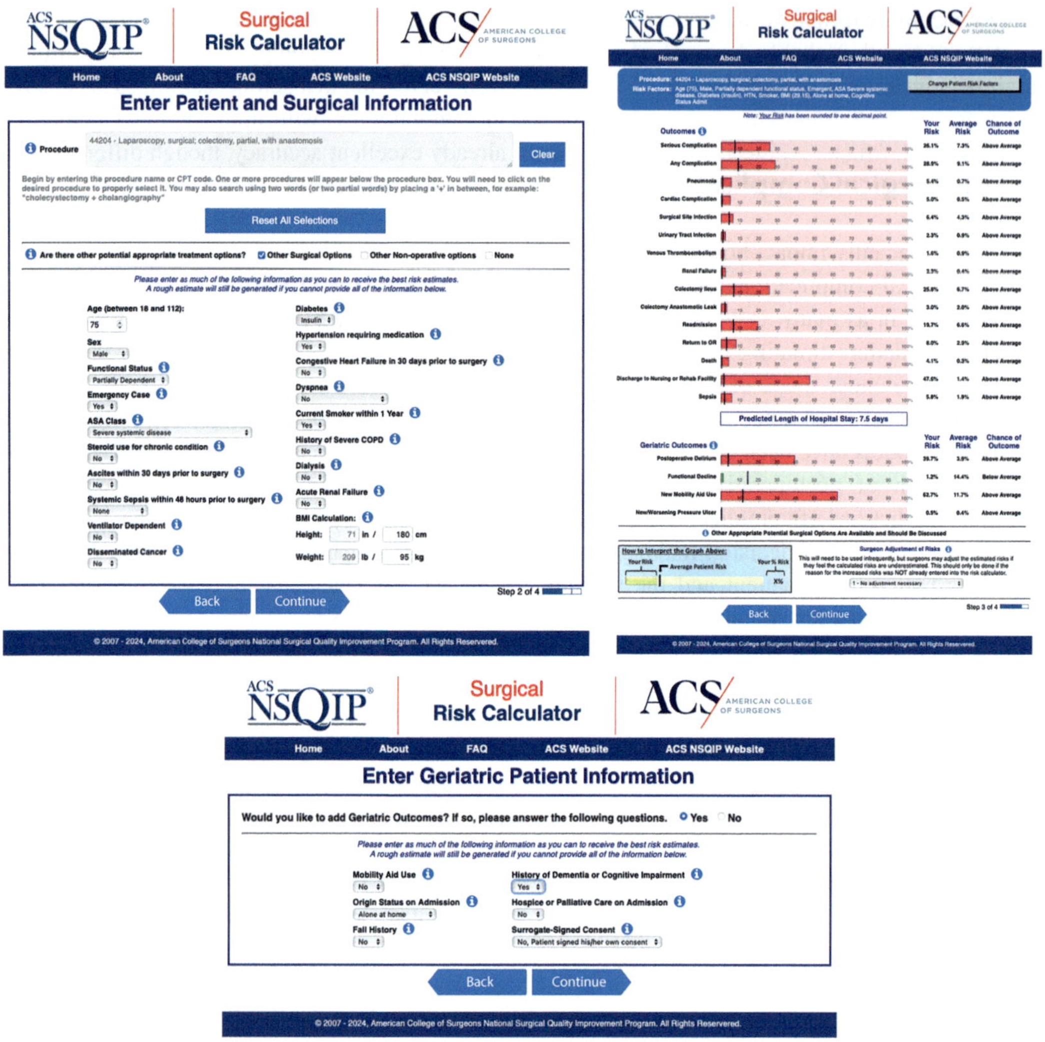
ACS NSQIP
Surgical Risk Calculator
ACS AMERICAN COLLEGE OF SURGEONS
Home About FAQ ACS Website ACS NSQIP Website
Enter Patient and Surgical Information
Procedure
44204 - Laparoscopy, surgical; colectomy, partial, with anastomosis
Clear
Reset All Selections
Are there other potential appropriate treatment options?
Other Surgical Options
Other Non-operative options
None
Age (between 18 and 112):
75
Sex
Male
Functional Status
Partially Dependent
Emergency Case
Yes
ASA Class
Severe systemic disease
Steroid use for chronic condition
No
Ascites within 30 days prior to surgery
No
Systemic Sepsis within 48 hours prior to surgery
None
Ventilator Dependent
No
Disseminated Cancer
No
Diabetes
Insulin
Hypertension requiring medication
Yes
Congestive Heart Failure in 30 days prior to surgery
No
Dyspnea
No
Current Smoker within 1 Year
Yes
History of Severe COPD
No
Dialysis
No
Acute Renal Failure
No
BMI Calculation:
Height: 71 in / 180 cm
Weight: 209 lb / 95 kg
Back
Continue
Step 2 of 4
© 2007 - 2024, American College of Surgeons National Surgical Quality Improvement Program. All Rights Reserved.
Outcomes
Your Risk
Average Risk
Chance of Outcome
Serious Complication
Any Complication
Pneumonia
Cardiac Complication
Surgical Site Infection
Urinary Tract Infection
Venous Thromboembolism
Renal Failure
Colectomy Ileus
Colectomy Anastomotic Leak
Readmission
Return to OR
Death
Discharge to Nursing or Rehab Facility
Sepsis
Predicted Length of Hospital Stay: 7.5 days
Geriatric Outcomes
Postoperative Delirium
Functional Decline
New Mobility Aid Use
New/Worsening Pressure Ulcer
Other Appropriate Potential Surgical Options Are Available and Should Be Discussed
How to Interpret the Graph Above:
Surgeon Adjustment of Risks
Back
Continue
Step 3 of 4
Enter Geriatric Patient Information
Would you like to add Geriatric Outcomes? If so, please answer the following questions.
Yes
No
Please enter as much of the following information as you can to receive the best risk estimates.
A rough estimate will still be generated if you cannot provide all of the information below.
Mobility Aid Use
No
Origin Status on Admission
Alone at home
Fall History
No
History of Dementia or Cognitive Impairment
Yes
Hospice or Palliative Care on Admission
No
Surrogate-Signed Consent
No, Patient signed his/her own consent
Back
Continue
© 2007 - 2024, American College of Surgeons National Surgical Quality Improvement Program. All Rights Reserved.

Fig. 7.1 ACS-SRC calculator. Example of data entry and risk prediction

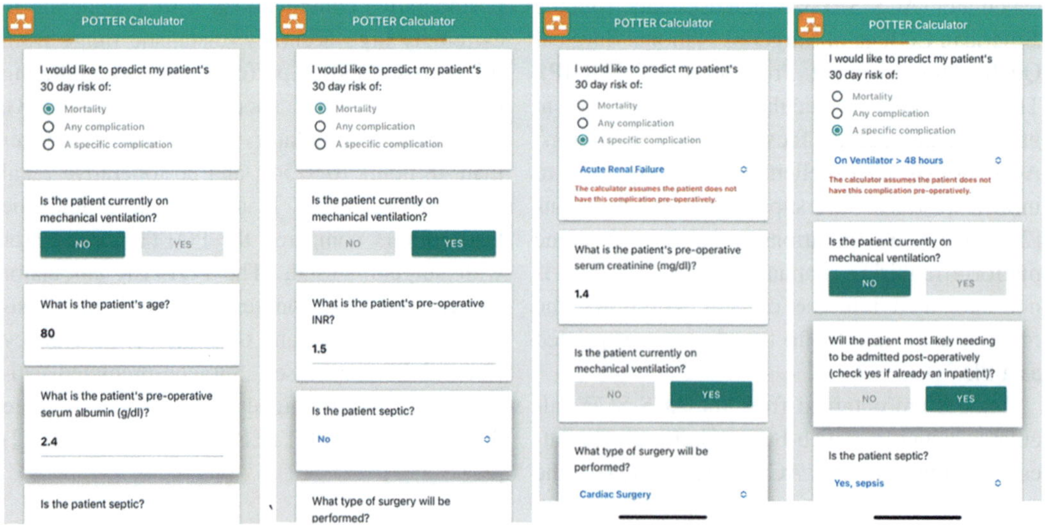

Fig. 7.2 POTTER calculator. Example of data entry and risk prediction

Images are obtained from simulated patients using the IOS app. Note that the POTTER calculator prompts change based on the information that is added. The Potter calculator differs from the ACS-SRC, which requires the user to input all the info linearly to provide the estimated outcome.

The POTTER calculator can provide the percentage risk for three variables: mortality, any complication, or a specific complication.

The MySurgeryRisk Platform

A group from the University of Florida developed the MySurgeryRisk platform, which utilizes automated EMR data to make predictions of postoperative complications and mortality directly uploaded to the surgeon's smartphone [18]. The eight postoperative complications that are included were prolonged (>48 hours) ICU stay, prolonged mechanical ventilation, and neurological complications, including delirium, cardiovascular complications, acute kidney injury, venous thromboembolism, sepsis, and wound complications. When the investigators compared the AUC of the MySurgeryRisk algorithm versus the initial physician risk assessment, the AUC ranged between 0.73 and 0.85 versus 0.47 and 0.69 [23]. A significant advantage of this model is that it predicts major complications using existing clinical data in the EMR.

Specific Complications Measured by AI

AI has been used to predict specific complications related to surgery. These include specific models to predict the onset of sepsis and technical complications associated with a given operation.

Sepsis

Sepsis is one of the leading causes of death in critically ill patients. Predicting which patients are at risk, to institute prompt treatment, is essential for improved outcomes. AI models can be applied to multiple stages of sepsis and can help with early prediction, mortality, and optimal management. An algorithm based on EMR was able to detect sepsis six hours before its onset with an AUC of 0.782 [24]. Another group was able to develop a similar model using 40 clinical variables, including eight vital signs, 26 laboratory values, and six demographics, to realize a 6-hour ahead early-onset prediction of sepsis [25].

Pancreatic Fistula

Clinically relevant postoperative pancreatic fistula (CR-POPF) is a significant complication after pancreaticoduodenectomy. Many models have been developed to help predict this complication, but most risk calculators use intraoperative and postoperative variables. Two commonly used models to predict CR-POPF use pancreatic gland texture and drain fluid amylase [26, 27]. The need to obtain intra-operative and postoperative findings hinders their utility in the preoperative setting. A group of surgeons at the University of California San Francisco developed the first risk calculator using ML algorithms and only preoperatively known variables. Using XGBoost, they were able to obtain an AUC = 0.72. The authors identified the five main preoperative variables for CR-POPF (non-adenocarcinoma histology, lack of neoadjuvant chemotherapy, pancreatic duct size less than 3 mm, higher Body Mass Index, and higher preoperative serum creatinine) [28].

Hepatic Surgery

Liver resection is commonly employed for both benign and malignant liver disease. Post-hepatectomy liver failure (PHLF) is one of the most dreaded complications after a major liver resection. Multiple models have been developed to attempt to predict PHLF. These include indocyanine green clearance, model for end-stage liver disease (MELD) system, Child-Pugh grade, "0–50 Criteria," and Future liver remnant

(FLR) volume. Each model has shortcomings, and there is no universally accepted model for clinical application. A group of investigators at Zhejiang University School of Medicine developed a deep learning model for predicting post-hepatectomy liver failure. The authors used preoperative contrast-enhanced computed tomography and were able to create a DL model on the prediction of PHLF with an accuracy value of 84.15%, an AUC value of 79.27%, sensitivity of 72.53%, and a specificity of 90.23%. The authors concluded that the DL could be useful for predicting PHLF based on preoperative CT images. The model could help to improve the selection of patients and offer alternative treatments to patients at high risk of PHLF [29]. Another group of investigators from Guangxi Medical University Cancer Hospital developed an artificial neural network model (ANN) to predict severe PHLF after major hepatectomy in patients with hepatocellular carcinoma. This study used five selected risk factors (platelet count, prothrombin time, total bilirubin, aspartate aminotransferase, and standardized FLR) as the input neurons. These risk factors are easily obtained before hepatectomy and can be derived from the EMR. The ANN model had significantly better predictive capabilities than commonly used scoring systems. The AUC for ANN was 0.880 vs. Child-Pugh of 0.568 and MELD of 0.608 [30].

Transplant

AI has multiple uses in Transplant Surgery. These include applications in donor-recipient matching, waitlist prioritization, and prediction of outcomes. In the pre-transplant setting, ML could provide 3-, 6-, and 12-month waitlist mortality, determine organ quality by evaluating obtained images, assist the pathologists in evaluating donor pathology, and identify the best donor-recipient matches by discovering hidden non-linear relationships. Using the data received from the donor and recipients, ML models can predict short and long-term survival post-transplant with higher accuracy than conventional methods [31]. ML models can also help predict graft failures and aid organ allocation [32]. Several studies have looked at the use of DL to predict hepatocellular cancer recurrence after transplantation [33–35]. Identifying these patients could help clinicians select the most appropriate candidates for liver transplantation.

Frailty

Frailty is characterized by a cumulative decline of physiological resilience across several body systems [36]. Frailty has become an essential concept in Emergency General Surgery and Trauma care as it increases perioperative and postoperative morbidity and mortality in these patients. Evaluating the frailty risk in aging patients before surgery is critical since these patients are at risk of significant functional, physical, and cognitive decline following an episode of illness or injury [37]. Age is still used as a suboptimal surrogate for frailty. Many frailty assessment tools require functional status history-taking through patient or surrogate interviews, which can be time-consuming and impractical for rapid prognostication [38]. It is suggested that approximately 37% of major trauma patients aged 65 years or older are frail [36]. Unfortunately, the commonly used tools to determine frailty (gait speed, handgrip strength, or extensive checklists) are cumbersome and ill-suited to real-time clinical assessments [39].

The Hospital Frailty Risk Score (HFRS) and Operation Frailty Risk Score (OFRS) are commonly applied frailty measurements. A recent article compared HFRS and OFRS against a predictive model utilizing XGBoost as a machine learning technique. The XGBOOST algorithm model showed the highest prediction performance, while OFRS and HFRS showed relatively low prediction. The authors concluded that the predictive performance of the machine learning method's modeling is superior to the statistical modeling of the existing traditional method [39].

The recently developed TROUT index, a point-of-care, machine-learning-based tool, was created to have a geriatric trauma frailty index that captures only baseline conditions and is readily implementable and accurate. The TROUT index looks to replace age as a more precise marker of frailty. Instead of using age, one should consider underlying physical reserve and stamina. The authors highlighted that their tool should be used with injury patterns, clinical management, and institution-specific workflows. Institutions could use the TROUT index to assist in predicting the need for ICU beds, nursing facility disposition, inpatient mortality, and need for prolonged hospitalization (>5 days). The TROUT index is a mobile application (iOS and Android) allowing bedside use (Table 7.1, Fig. 7.3) [38].

TROUT index scores range from 0 to 100, stratified as low [0–19.9], medium [20.0–37.1], and high [37.2–100] frailty risk [38].

Images taken from simulated patients with the iOS app. The app provides information in a timely fashion with limited input. It gives information on the need for mechanical ventilation, hospitalization >5 days, inpatient mortality, and the possibility of disposition to a nursing facility.

Table 7.1 Baseline conditions and mechanism of injury constituting the Trout index

	Elements	Points
General	"do not resuscitate" status	8.7
	Dependent on supplemental O2/dialysis/wheelchair	4.1
Neurological	Vascular dementia	4.5
Cardiovascular	Multiple valve diseases	5.2
	Aortic valve disease	1.9
	Atrial fibrillation/flutter	18.7
	Atrioventricular/left bundle-branch block	3.1
	Heart failure	2.4
	Ischemic heart disease or the presence of cardiovascular implants/grafts	11.7
	Hypertensive heart/kidney disease	5.5
Renal	Chronic kidney disease	2.3
Endocrine	Type 2 diabetes mellitus	13.2
Hematological	Chronic anemia	2.3
Musculoskeletal	Leg ulcer (non-pressure)	2.8
Mechanism of Injury	Ground-level fall	13.8

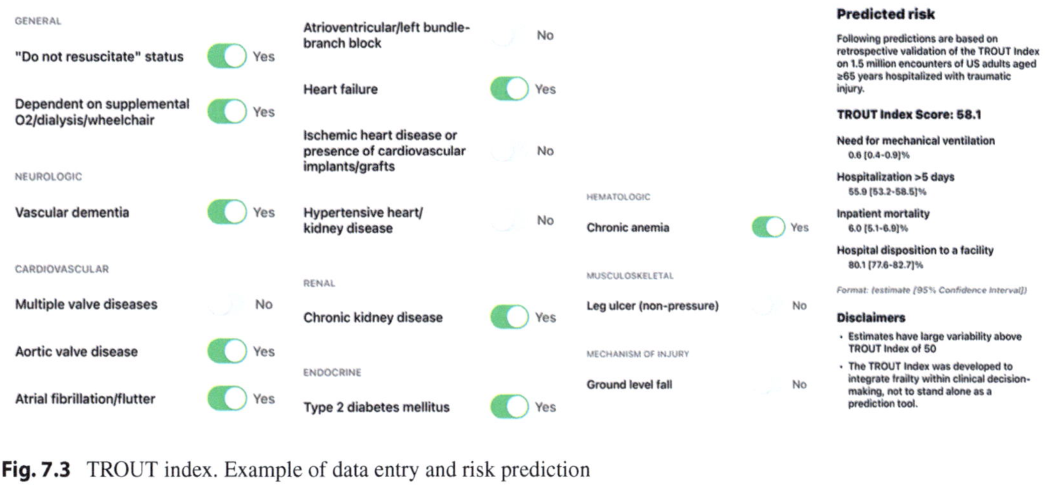

Fig. 7.3 TROUT index. Example of data entry and risk prediction

Disposition

The correct postoperative discharge of patients to the general surgical ward or intensive care unit is paramount. Inappropriate disposition can lead to over and under-triage with perilous risks or inadequate resource allocations for our patients. A group of investigators from Adelaide, Australia, developed a machine learning algorithm (Adelaide Score) to predict discharge within 12 and 24 hours after general surgical procedures. The investigators felt that reliance on human interpretation of data would likely create variability in postoperative discharge planning. They developed a machine learning algorithm with extensive data inputs, including recorded vital signs, pain scores, recent bowel movements, and laboratory parameters in the previous 48 hours. The random forest model was the best-performing model for the prediction of discharge within 12 hours, with an AUC of 0.84, while the logistic regression model classification had an AUC of 0.72 [40].

Anesthesia

Robots that utilize AI are poised to be incorporated into operating theaters. They are intended to free the anesthesiologist from repetitive tasks. These robots are divided into pharmacological, mechanical, and cognitive robots. The pharmacological robots would assist with fluid management and medication delivery. In comparison, mechanical robots are intended for intubation or the application of regional anesthesia. Cognitive robots detect abnormal laboratory findings, ensure drug compliance, conduct checklists, monitor alarms, and accurately identify appropriate prophylactic antibiotics [41]. AI may create a safer surgical environment as it has the potential to predict outcomes from anesthesia and may assist the anesthesiologist in controlling mechanical ventilation and weaning of anesthetized patients.

Pain Management

There is ongoing research in utilizing AI to predict the correct opioid dose, assist in better management of postoperative pain, and predict which patients would benefit from evaluation by a specialty pain service. Utilizing historical data in EMR, machine learning classifiers could predict which surgical cases would require a preoperative request for acute pain service consultation in 92% of the cases [42]. In a recent study, the researchers were able to create a model that predicted postoperative opioid requirements with an accuracy of around 70% [4].

Cancer Treatment

AI may significantly assist clinicians in diagnosing and treating specific malignancies. It may determine if surgery or neoadjuvant therapy should be applied first based on tumor biology and multiple data points.

Gastric Cancer

A group of investigators developed an artificial neural network (ANN) model to predict long-term survival in gastric cancer patients. The model was superior to clinical TNM ($p < 0.05$) and equivalent to pathological TNM ($p = 0.130$) in predicting long-term survival in this group of patients [43]. The preoperative data provides an advantage over the TNM system, which relies on postoperative findings for better accuracy. In this study, the authors developed the predictive ANN model based on preoperative inflammatory markers obtained from peripheral blood (neutrophil-lymphocyte ratio, platelet-lymphocyte ratio, and albumin-globulin ratio). The accuracy of the ANN model in predicting the 3-year survival rate was 92% [43].

Detecting Preinvasive Occult Pancreatic Ductal Adenocarcinoma

The authors developed an automated 3-dimensional (3D) Convolutional Neural Network (CNN) to detect visually occult pancreatic cancers not detected on routine CT scans. Their model was able to detect occult pancreatic ductal adenocarcinoma (PDA) on pre-diagnostic CT with an AUC of 0.91 [95% CI, 0.86–0.94]; sensitivity, 0.75 [95% CI, 0.67–0.84]; and specificity, 0.90 [95% CI, 0.85–0.95]) at a median 475 days (range, 93-1082 days) before clinical diagnosis. The authors used incidental portal-venous phase CT obtained for unrelated conditions between 3 to 36 months before the clinical diagnosis of PDA. All of these CTs had been previously interpreted to be negative for PDA. These studies were then utilized to train and validate the model. The ability to detect PDA early has the potential to assist with screening and should have a favorable impact on patient outcomes [44].

Colorectal Cancer

Realizing that the majority of patients with T1 colorectal cancer (CRC) undergo lymph node resection despite a low prevalence (10%), a group of investigators from Japan opted to develop an ANN to detect patients with T1 CRC at risk for lymph node metastasis. The ANN model (AUC=0.83) outperformed both the American (0.73) and Japanese (AUC = 0.57) guidelines in prediction of lymph node metastasis in patients with T1 CRC [45]. This model can alter our approach to these tumors and limit the degree of dissection in selected cases, potentially limiting the operative time and associated morbidity.

Conclusions

Artificial Intelligence and machine learning have begun to revolutionize all aspects of our lives. AI will also globally impact and transform surgical care and how we evaluate and treat patients with surgical conditions. As these technologies get implemented, we need to be cognizant that these "tools" are here to assist surgeons and physicians in improving the level of care by identifying patients at risk of complications, better selecting patients to undergo organ transplantation and cancer treatment, improving patient disposition and pain management, and assisting surgeons in decreasing intraoperative complications via augmented reality. The question remains: Will AI simplify or complicate further surgical decision-making by surgeons and patients? We sincerely hope and believe that AI will contribute to better patient care and outcomes in the foreseeable future.

References

1. Cox DR. Regression models and life-tables. J R Stat Soc Series B Stat Methodol. 1972;34(2):187–220. https://doi.org/10.1111/j.2517-6161.1972.tb00899.x.
2. Armitage P, Berry G, Matthews JNS. Statistical methods in medical research. Oxford: John Wiley & Sons; 2008.
3. Bertsimas D, Dunn J, Velmahos GC, Kaafarani HMA. Surgical risk is not linear: derivation and validation of a novel, user-friendly, and machine-learning-based predictive OpTimal trees in emergency surgery risk (POTTER) calculator. Ann Surg. 2018;268(4):574–83. https://doi.org/10.1097/sla.0000000000002956.
4. Nair AA, Velagapudi MA, Lang JA, Behara L, Venigandla R, Velagapudi N, et al. Machine learning approach to predict postoperative opioid requirements in ambulatory surgery patients. PLoS ONE. 2020;15(7):e0236833. https://doi.org/10.1371/journal.pone.0236833.
5. https://www.coursera.org/articles/what-is-artificial-intelligence#
6. Bose I, Mahapatra R. Business data mining-a machine learning perspective. Inf Manage. 2001;39:211–25.
7. Carlos RC, Kahn CE, Halabi S. Data science: big data, machine learning, and artificial intelligence. J Am Coll Radiol. 2018;15(3 Pt B):497–8. https://doi.org/10.1016/j.jacr.2018.01.029.
8. Syeda-Mahmood T. Role of big data and machine learning in diagnostic decision support in radiology. J Am Coll Radiol. 2018;15(3 Pt B):569–76. https://doi.org/10.1016/j.jacr.2018.01.028.
9. Jiang F, Jiang Y, Zhi H, Dong Y, Li H, Ma S, Wang Y, Dong Q, Shen H, Wang Y. Artificial intelligence

in healthcare: past, present and future. Stroke Vasc Neurol. 2017;2(4):230–43. https://doi.org/10.1136/svn-2017-000101.
10. Meyer A, Zverinski D, Pfahringer B, Kempfert J, Kuehne T, Sündermann SH, Stamm C, Hofmann T, Falk V, Eickhoff C. Machine learning for real-time prediction of complications in critical care: a retrospective study. Lancet Respir Med. 2018;6(12):905–14. https://doi.org/10.1016/S2213-2600(18)30300-X.
11. Hashimoto DA, Rosman G, Rus D, Meireles OR. Artificial intelligence in surgery: promises and perils. Ann Surg. 2018;268(1):70–6. https://doi.org/10.1097/SLA.0000000000002693.
12. https://www.ibm.com/topics/machine-learning
13. https://www.nvidia.com/en-us/glossary/xgboost/
14. https://analyse-it.com/docs/user-guide/diagnostic-performance/auc
15. https://testbook.com/maths/area-under-the-curve
16. Madani A, Namazi B, Altieri MS, Hashimoto DA, Rivera AM, Pucher PH, Navarrete-Welton A, Sankaranarayanan G, Brunt LM, Okrainec A, Alseidi A. Artificial intelligence for intraoperative guidance: using semantic segmentation to identify surgical anatomy during laparoscopic cholecystectomy. Ann Surg. 2022;276(2):363–9. https://doi.org/10.1097/SLA.0000000000004594.
17. Phutane P, Buc E, Poirot K, et al. Preliminary trial of augmented reality performed on a laparoscopic left hepatectomy. Surg Endosc. 2018;32:514–5.
18. Ren Y, Loftus TJ, Datta S, Ruppert MM, Guan Z, Miao S, Shickel B, Feng Z, Giordano C, Upchurch GR Jr, Rashidi P, Ozrazgat-Baslanti T, Bihorac A. Performance of a machine learning algorithm using electronic health record data to predict postoperative complications and report on a mobile platform. JAMA Netw Open. 2022;5(5):e2211973. https://doi.org/10.1001/jamanetworkopen.2022.11973.
19. Shickel B, Loftus TJ, Ruppert M, Upchurch GR Jr, Ozrazgat-Baslanti T, Rashidi P, Bihorac A. Dynamic predictions of postoperative complications from explainable, uncertainty-aware, and multi-task deep neural networks. Sci Rep. 2023;13(1):1224. https://doi.org/10.1038/s41598-023-27418-5.
20. Bilimoria KY, Liu Y, Paruch JL, et al. Development and evaluation of the universal ACS NSQIP surgical risk calculator: a decision aid and informed consent tool for patients and surgeons. J Am Coll Surg. 2013;217:833–842.e3.
21. https://riskcalculator.facs.org/RiskCalculator/index.jsp
22. El Moheb M, Gebran A, Maurer LR, Naar L, El Hechi M, Breen K, Dorken-Gallastegi A, Sinyard R, Bertsimas D, Velmahos G, Kaafarani HMA. Artificial intelligence versus surgeon gestalt in predicting risk of emergency general surgery. J Trauma Acute Care Surg. 2023;95(4):565–72. https://doi.org/10.1097/TA.0000000000004030. Epub 2023 Jun 14
23. Brennan M, Puri S, Ozrazgat-Baslanti T, et al. Comparing clinical judgment with the MySurgeryRisk algorithm for preoperative risk assessment: a pilot usability study. Surgery. 2019;165(5):1035–45. https://doi.org/10.1016/j.surg.2019.01.002.
24. Lee BT, Kwon OY, Park H, Cho KJ, Kwon JM, Lee Y. Graph convolutional networks-based noisy data imputation in electronic health record. Crit Care Med. 2020;48:e1106–11. https://doi.org/10.1097/CCM.0000000000004583.
25. He Z, Du L, Zhang P, Zhao R, Chen X, Fang Z. Early sepsis prediction using ensemble learning with deep features and artificial features extracted from clinical electronic health records. Crit Care Med. 2020;48(12):e1337–42. https://doi.org/10.1097/CCM.0000000000004644.
26. Al Abbas AI, Borrebach JD, Pitt HA, et al. Development of a novel pancreatoduodenectomy-specific risk calculator: an analysis of 10,000 patients. J Gastrointest Surg J Soc Surg Aliment Tract. 2021;25(6):1503–11. https://doi.org/10.1007/s11605-020-04725-0.
27. Nassour I, AlMasri S, Hodges JC, Hughes SJ, Zureikat A, Paniccia A. Novel calculator to estimate the risk of clinically relevant postoperative pancreatic fistula following distal pancreatectomy. J Gastrointest Surg J Soc Surg Aliment Tract. 2022;26(7):1436–44. https://doi.org/10.1007/s11605-022-05275-3.
28. Ashraf Ganjouei A, Romero-Hernandez F, Wang JJ, Casey M, Frye W, Hoffman D, Hirose K, Nakakura E, Corvera C, Maker AV, Kirkwood KS, Alseidi A, Adam MA. A machine learning approach to predict postoperative pancreatic fistula after pancreaticoduodenectomy using only preoperatively known data. Ann Surg Oncol. 2023;30(12):7738–47. https://doi.org/10.1245/s10434-023-14041-x. Epub 2023 Aug 7
29. Xu X, Xing Z, Xu Z, Tong Y, Wang S, Liu X, Ren Y, Liang X, Yu Y, Ying H. A deep learning model for prediction of post hepatectomy liver failure after hemihepatectomy using preoperative contrast-enhanced computed tomography: a retrospective study. Front Med (Lausanne). 2023;10:1154314. https://doi.org/10.3389/fmed.2023.1154314.
30. Surel AA, Tez M. Re: Artificial neural network model for preoperative prediction of severe liver failure after hemihepatectomy in patients with hepatocellular carcinoma. Surgery. 2021;169(4):1000. https://doi.org/10.1016/j.surg.2020.08.038. Epub 2020 Oct 12
31. Bhat M, Rabindranath M, Chara BS, Simonetto DA. Artificial intelligence, machine learning, and deep learning in liver transplantation. J Hepatol. 2023;78(6):1216–33. https://doi.org/10.1016/j.jhep.2023.01.006.
32. Wingfield LR, Ceresa C, Thorogood S, Fleuriot J, Knight S. Using artificial intelligence for predicting survival of individual grafts in liver transplantation: a systematic review. Liver Transplant. 2020;26(7):922–34. https://doi.org/10.1002/lt.25772.
33. Liu Z, Liu Y, Zhang W, Hong Y, Meng J, Wang J, et al. Deep learning for prediction of hepatocellular carcinoma recurrence after resection or liver trans-

plantation: a discovery and validation study. Hepatol Int. 2022;16(3):577–89. https://doi.org/10.1007/s12072-022-10321-y.
34. Nam JY, Lee JH, Bae J, Chang Y, Cho Y, Sinn DH, Kim BH, Kim SH, Yi NJ, Lee KW, Kim JM, Park JW, Kim YJ, Yoon JH, Joh JW, Suh KS. Novel model to predict HCC recurrence after liver transplantation obtained using deep learning: a multicenter study. Cancers (Basel). 2020;12(10):2791. https://doi.org/10.3390/cancers12102791.
35. He T, Fong JN, Moore LW, Ezeana CF, Victor D, Divatia M, Vasquez M, Ghobrial RM, Wong STC. An imageomics and multi-network based deep learning model for risk assessment of liver transplantation for hepatocellular cancer. Comput Med Imaging Graph. 2021;89:101894. https://doi.org/10.1016/j.compmedimag.2021.101894. Epub 2021 Mar 11
36. Jarman H, Crouch R, Baxter M, et al. Frailty in major trauma study (FRAIL- T): a study protocol to determine the feasibility of nurse- led frailty assessment in elderly trauma and the impact on outcome in patients with major trauma. BMJ Open. 2020;10:e038082. https://doi.org/10.1136/bmjopen-2020-038082.
37. Clegg A, Young J, Iliffe S, Rikkert MO, Rockwood K. Frailty in elderly people. Lancet. 2013;381(9868):752–62. https://doi.org/10.1016/S0140-6736(12)62167-9. Epub 2013 Feb 8. Erratum in: Lancet. 2013 Oct 19;382(9901):1328
38. Choi J, Anderson T, Tennakoon L, Spain DA, Forrester JD. Explainable machine learning to bring database to the bedside: development and validation of the TROUT (Trauma fRailty OUTcomes) index, a point-of-care tool to prognosticate outcomes after traumatic injury based on frailty. Ann Surg. 2023;278(1):135–9. https://doi.org/10.1097/SLA.0000000000005649. Epub 2022 Aug 3
39. Lee SW, Lee EH, Choi IC. An ensemble machine learning approach to predict postoperative mortality in older patients undergoing emergency surgery. BMC Geriatr. 2023;23(1):262. https://doi.org/10.1186/s12877-023-03969-0.
40. Kovoor JG, Bacchi S, Gupta AK, Stretton B, Malycha J, Reddi BA, Liew D, O'Callaghan PG, Beltrame JF, Zannettino AC, Jones KL, Horowitz M, Dobbins C, Hewett PJ, Trochsler MI, Maddern GJ. The Adelaide score: an artificial intelligence measure of readiness for discharge after general surgery. ANZ J Surg. 2023;93(9):2119–24. https://doi.org/10.1111/ans.18546. Epub 2023 Jun 1
41. Singh M, Nath G. Artificial intelligence and anesthesia: a narrative review. Saudi J Anaesth. 2022;16(1):86–93. https://doi.org/10.4103/sja.sja_669_21. Epub 2022 Jan 4
42. Tighe PJ, Lucas SD, Edwards DA, Boezaart AP, Aytug H, Bihorac A. Use of machine-learning classifiers to predict requests for preoperative acute pain service consultation. Pain Med. 2012;13(10):1347–57. https://doi.org/10.1111/j.1526-4637.2012.01477.x. Epub 2012 Sep 7
43. Que SJ, Chen QY, Qing-Zhong LZY, Wang JB, Lin JX, Lu J, Cao LL, Lin M, Tu RH, Huang ZN, Lin JL, Zheng HL, Li P, Zheng CH, Huang CM, Xie JW. Application of preoperative artificial neural network based on blood biomarkers and clinicopathological parameters for predicting long-term survival of patients with gastric cancer. World J Gastroenterol. 2019;25(43):6451–64.
44. Korfiatis P, Suman G, Patnam NG, Trivedi KH, Karbhari A, Mukherjee S, Cook C, Klug JR, Patra A, Khasawneh H, Rajamohan N, Fletcher JG, Truty MJ, Majumder S, Bolan CW, Sandrasegaran K, Chari ST, Goenka AH. Automated artificial intelligence model trained on a large data set can detect pancreas cancer on diagnostic computed tomography scans as well as visually occult preinvasive cancer on prediagnostic computed tomography scans. Gastroenterology. 2023;165(6):1533–1546.e4. https://doi.org/10.1053/j.gastro.2023.08.034. Epub 2023 Aug 30
45. Kudo SE, Ichimasa K, Villard B, Mori Y, Misawa M, Saito S, Hotta K, Saito Y, Matsuda T, Yamada K, Mitani T, Ohtsuka K, Chino A, Ide D, Imai K, Kishida Y, Nakamura K, Saiki Y, Tanaka M, Hoteya S, Yamashita S, Kinugasa Y, Fukuda M, Kudo T, Miyachi H, Ishida F, Itoh H, Oda M, Mori K. Artificial intelligence system to determine risk of T1 colorectal cancer metastasis to lymph node. Gastroenterology. 2021;160(4):1075–1084.e2. https://doi.org/10.1053/j.gastro.2020.09.027. Epub 2020 Sep 24

Decision-Making in Critical Care Rescue for Re-operative Surgery

8

Diane N. Haddad and Gary A. Bass

Principles of Critical Care Rescue in the Re-operative Patient

Re-operative surgery can be the intended progression of staged operations, such as a damage-control open cavity approach to hemostasis and source control. Re-intervention may also be unplanned, however, due to ischemic insult, hollow viscous perforation, or anastomotic disruption consequent upon unanticipated pathophysiology or technical failure [1] (Fig. 8.1). Patients requiring urgent or emergent re-operative surgery may experience hemodynamic instability, respiratory failure, acute blood loss anemia, end-organ dysfunction or other physiologic perturbation. Resuscitation, enhanced monitoring and repair or support of organ dysfunction mandate critical care rescue before, during and after re-operative surgery [2] (Fig. 8.2).

D. N. Haddad
Division of Traumatology, Surgical Critical Care and Emergency Surgery, Department of Surgery, Perelman School of Medicine, University of Pennsylvania, Philadelphia, PA, USA
e-mail: Diane.haddad@pennmedicine.upenn.edu

G. A. Bass (✉)
Division of Traumatology, Surgical Critical Care and Emergency Surgery, Department of Surgery, Perelman School of Medicine, University of Pennsylvania, Philadelphia, PA, USA

European Society for Trauma and Emergency Surgery, Vienna, Austria
e-mail: Gary.Bass@Pennmedicine.upenn.edu

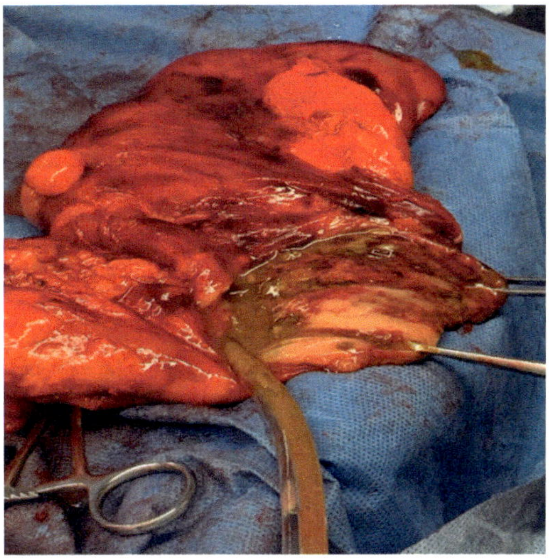

Fig. 8.1 Photograph courtesy of Dr Latifi

Principles of resuscitation include maintenance of adequate oxygen delivery, restoration of circulating volume and support of vascular tone and forward flow with vasoactive agents [3]. In patients undergoing re-operation for surgical complications, specific vigilance should be given to intravascular volume expansion and augmented vascular tone in mitigation of hemodynamic collapse upon induction of general anesthesia. Patients with peritonitis requiring emergency re-operative surgery often present with physiologic derangements, such as electrolyte abnormalities or renal failure in the setting of hypovolemia due to septic shock with large fluid shifts. Markers of resuscitation include but are

R. Latifi (ed.), *Surgical Decision-Making*, https://doi.org/10.1007/978-3-031-67391-7_8

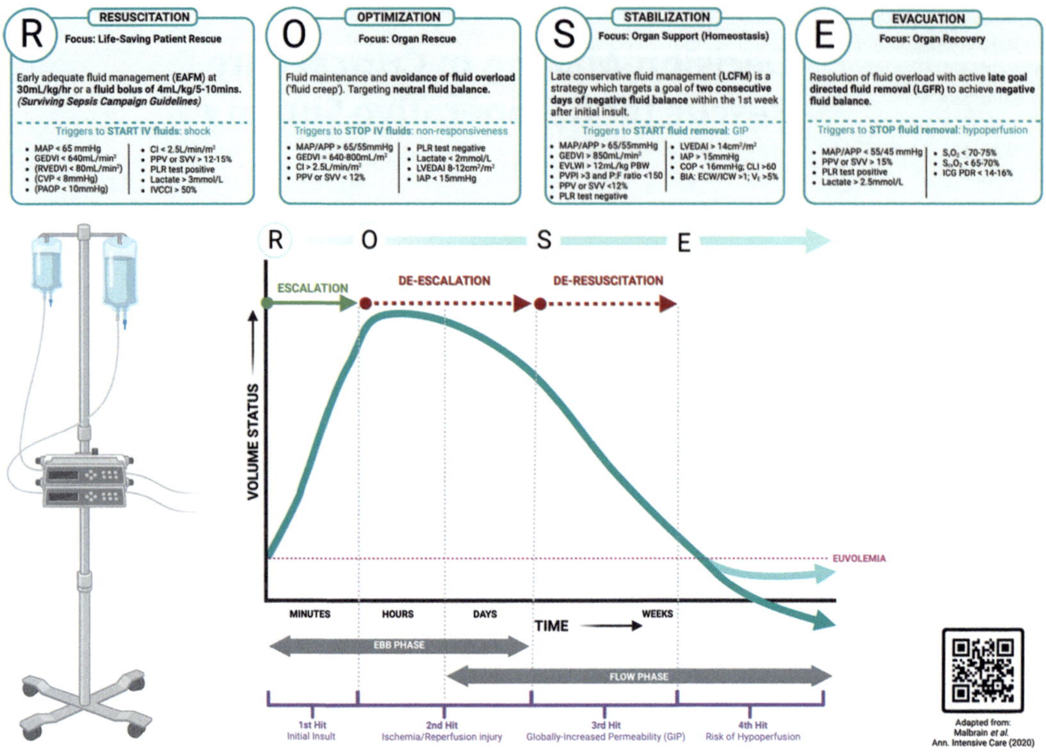

Fig. 8.2 ROSE model (Malbrain et al. Ann Intensive Care 2020) describing the phases of targeted volume expansion and contraction therapy to support critically-ill patients undergoing re-operation. (Figure is authors' original)

not limited to: serum hemoglobin, pH, lactic acid, base deficit, and mixed venous oxygen saturation [4]. Upon recognition of the need for emergency re-operative surgery, initiation of broad-spectrum antibiotics is recommended by guidelines from the Surviving Sepsis Campaign [5]. However, pre-operative resuscitation should not delay prompt progression to the operating room, endoscopy or interventional radiology suite in pursuit of expedient source control in septic patients and hemorrhagic control in bleeding patients [6].

Phases of Resuscitation

Resuscitation should follow four broad phases: resuscitation, optimization, stabilization and evacuation (ROSE) [3]. Ideally, re-operation should occur in the resuscitation phase, where the goal is maintenance of perfusion pressure during lifesaving interventions such as source or hemorrhage control. During the optimization phase, emphasis shifts to promoting adequate oxygen delivery by maintaining and optimizing adequate blood pressure and cardiac output. Stabilization refers to the phase after hemodynamic stability has been achieved, where the goal shifts to prevention of ongoing organ dysfunction. Finally, through active de-resuscitation in the evacuation phase, vasoactive agents are weaned and a negative fluid balance is achieved in pursuit of restored homeostasis. Data-driven strategic timing of fluid administration and removal, as encapsulated in the ROSE model, has been associated with improved outcomes in critically-ill surgical patients [7] (Fig. 8.3).

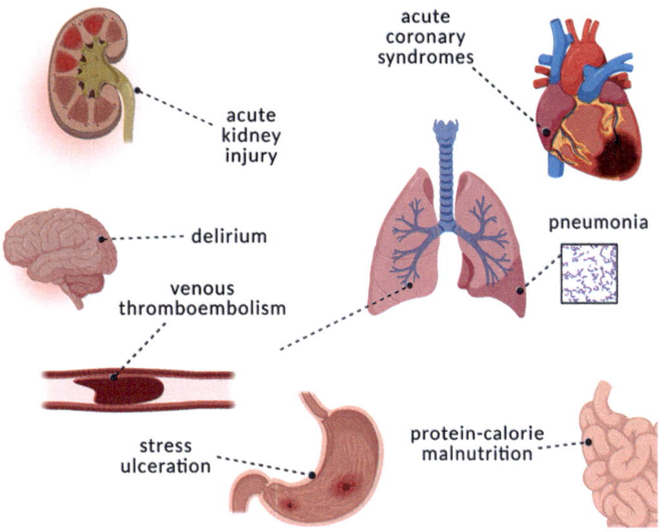

Fig. 8.3 Nonsurgical complications in the operated or re-operated patient, which will require perioperative critical care support. (Original figure by the authors)

Technological Adjuncts

Perioperative Monitoring

Enhanced monitoring of critically ill patients before, during, and after interventional rescue from complications provides actionable data to guide effective resuscitation. Technological advancements providing cues such as trended cardiac output (CO), stroke volume variation (SVV) and systemic vascular resistance (SVR) can help guide resuscitation endpoints. The pulmonary artery catheter (PAC), historically the gold standard for CO monitoring in the ICU, has fallen out of favor in the past decades [8], due to a combination of factors including the risk of procedural complications related to the insertion of invasive monitors (arrhythmia, infection, pulmonary artery injury), and the more recent observation that universal PAC monitoring was not associated with improved survival outcomes in the critically ill [8–10]. More recently, non-invasive cardiac output monitoring devices that can be attached to peripherally-inserted arterial lines, such as the FloTrac or LiDCO systems, have gained in popularity [11], although the accuracy of these devices is currently limited in unstable patients with severe aortic valve pathology or severe arrhythmias [12]. Ongoing randomized validation studies, such as the "Non-Invasive Cardiac Output Monitor (NICOM) for Goal-directed Fluid Resuscitation for Inpatients With Hypotension and/or Septic Shock" randomized control trial (RCT) out of the University of Minnesota (NCT05630716) are attempting to answer the association between the use of non-invasive cardiac output monitors and the reproducible and clinically-useful outcome measures, such as hospital mortality, hospital and ICU lengths of stay, duration of vasopressor use, change from baseline serum creatinine and net and cumulative fluid balance at 72 hours or ICU discharge. Previous RCT data showed no causal association between early continuous cardiac output and stroke volume monitoring and improved hemodynamic rescue of hemodynamically bioinappropriate patients admitted to the ICU [13]. However, goal directed hemodynamic therapy, particularly in the operating room utilizing similar non-invasive devices have been associated with decreased postoperative complications, particularly in abdominal surgery and very high-risk patients [14]. Identifying the optimal use case and population for these devices has the potential to improve the care of critically ill re-operative patients.

Point of Care Ultrasound

Point of Care Ultrasound (POCUS) is a useful non-invasive adjunct increasingly available to ICU providers to determine dynamic changes in inferior vena caval caliber as a surrogate for response to intravascular volume expansion. Rapid evaluation of life-threatening pathology such as pneumothorax, cardiac tamponade and right ventricular strain from a massive pulmonary embolism are accessible at bedside with the use of heart and lung ultrasonography. While this skill requires dedicated training, it is readily deployable across all levels of learners and is now recognized as an essential component of critical care training [15].

Functional Coagulation Assay Driven Resuscitation

Fluid imbalance, acute blood loss anemia, and sepsis are all associated with an acquired coagulopathy in patients with post-operative complications. Thromboelastographic (TEG) and rotational thromboelastometric (ROTEM) analysis of clot kinetics, clot strength, and fibrinolysis provide real-time guidance for perioperative blood component-based balanced resuscitation with whole blood, packed red cells, fresh frozen plasma, platelets, clotting factor concentrates, tranexamic acid (TXA), and cryoprecipitate [16, 17].

Acute Kidney Injury

Acute kidney injury (AKI) is a frequent occurrence when complications following surgical intervention induce sustained hypotension, with approximately 50% of postoperative patients developing AKI while in the ICU [18, 19] (Fig. 8.4). Sepsis-related acute kidney injury or disease are associated with short- and long-term morbidity and mortality [20]. Irrespective of speculation regarding causality or "which came first", renal malperfusion is the likely sequel of systemic shock, but can itself further exacerbate systemic dysregulation. Initiation of renal replacement therapy in the ICU is indicated if noninvasive management fails. Indications for dialysis include volume overload, impacting other organ systems, metabolic acidosis, electrolyte abnormalities (including hyperkalemia and

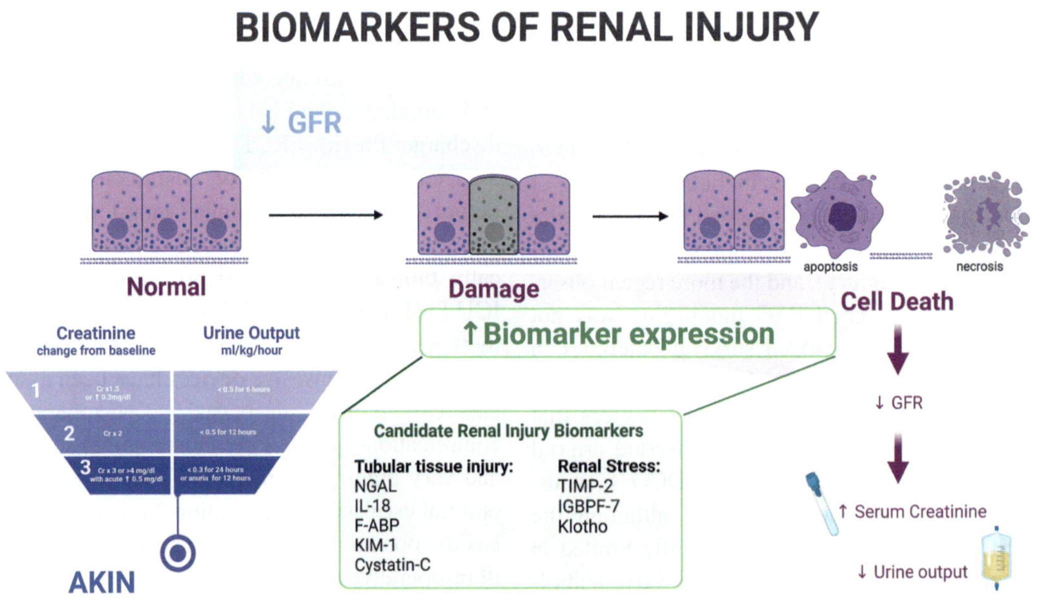

Fig. 8.4 Acute kidney injury progression in the perioperative period. (Original figure by the authors [Ref: Bass GA, et al. Cameron's Current Surgical Therapy14th Edition; 2022; pp.: 1554–1563])

hyperphosphatemia), uremia contributing to worsening encephalopathy and pericarditis, and drug and toxin removal. The use of Continuous Renal Replacement Therapy (CRRT) may be preferred over intermittent Hemodialysis (iHD) as it allows for slower removal of fluids with less hemodynamic lability [21, 22]. However, existing evidence suggests no difference in survival between CRRT and iHD despite propensity and other adjustment for disease severity [25–27].

The types of CRRT vary by the method of solute removal. Appropriate renal replacement prescription requires specialized knowledge, as well as a trained nurse capable of supervising and maintaining therapy delivery. Continuous Venovenous Hemofiltration (CVVH) removes a large volume of water across a semipermeable membrane, using hydrostatic pressure to facilitate removal of solutes in a process called ultrafiltration or convection. Continuous Venovenous Hemodialysis (CVVHD) removes smaller waste molecules by diffusion using a transmembrane concentration gradient created by dialysate fluid. Continuous Venovenous Hemodiafiltration (CVVHDF) combines both ultrafiltration and diffusion methods of filtration. When CRRT is utilized just for volume removal via ultrafiltration, it is referred to as slow continuous ultrafiltration (SCUF). Choice of CRRT modality takes into account patient indication, however depends on provider preferences and local resource availability [23].

Initiation of CRRT requires central vascular access, ideally via the right internal jugular or femoral vein. Subclavian venous access should be avoided due to risk of developing central stenosis in patients who may go on to need long-term dialysis. The choice of systemic anticoagulation (heparinization) versus regional anticoagulation (citrate) should take into account the patient's condition, planned procedures, and risk factors for bleeding. However, citrate is contraindicated in patients with liver failure, due to inability to hepatically convert citrate to bicarbonate for excretion. Frequent, intermittent saline flushes can be employed if other methods of anticoagulation are contraindicated [24].

Despite complexity in distinguishing the etiology of AKI along the causal pathway, supporting renal failure in critical illness is essential in managing acidosis, electrolyte abnormalities and volume overload in patients requiring re-operative surgery.

Extracorporeal Membrane Oxygenation

Extracorporeal membrane oxygenation (ECMO), when used appropriately, may provide cardiopulmonary rescue in critically-ill surgical patients. Extracorporeal life support can also be used as an adjunct to cardiopulmonary resuscitation (CPR) in the case of refractory cardiac arrest, commonly referred to as extracorporeal CPR or ECPR [31]. Cannulation has been reported by prehospital personnel, as well as inpatient intensivists, surgeons and cardiologists, but must be coordinated with a team of critical care intensivists and perfusionists. Time to ECMO initiation has been identified as the strongest predictor of mortality for patients receiving ECPR [32]. Insertion of cannulas is currently recommended within 10–20 min after failed resuscitation efforts to avoid risk of anoxic brain injury. Venovenous (VV) ECMO is used in cases of severe respiratory failure with preserved cardiac function. VV ECMO is indicated in severe hypoxia refractory to conventional management—when the partial pressure of oxygen (PaO_2) is less than 80 mmHg on 100% fraction of inspired oxygen (FiO_2) with or without hypercarbia (pH <7.20). VV ECMO has demonstrated benefit in conditions of reversible respiratory failure, including acute respiratory distress syndrome (ARDS), trauma, bacterial or viral pneumonia, including COVID-19 and aspiration pneumonia. This involves percutaneous insertion of either two cannulas or one dual-lumen cannula into the central veins for transfer of deoxygenated blood through an oxygenator and then back to the right side of the heart (Fig. 8.5). Contraindications are determined by institution specific protocols and include conditions such as advanced age, active malignancy,

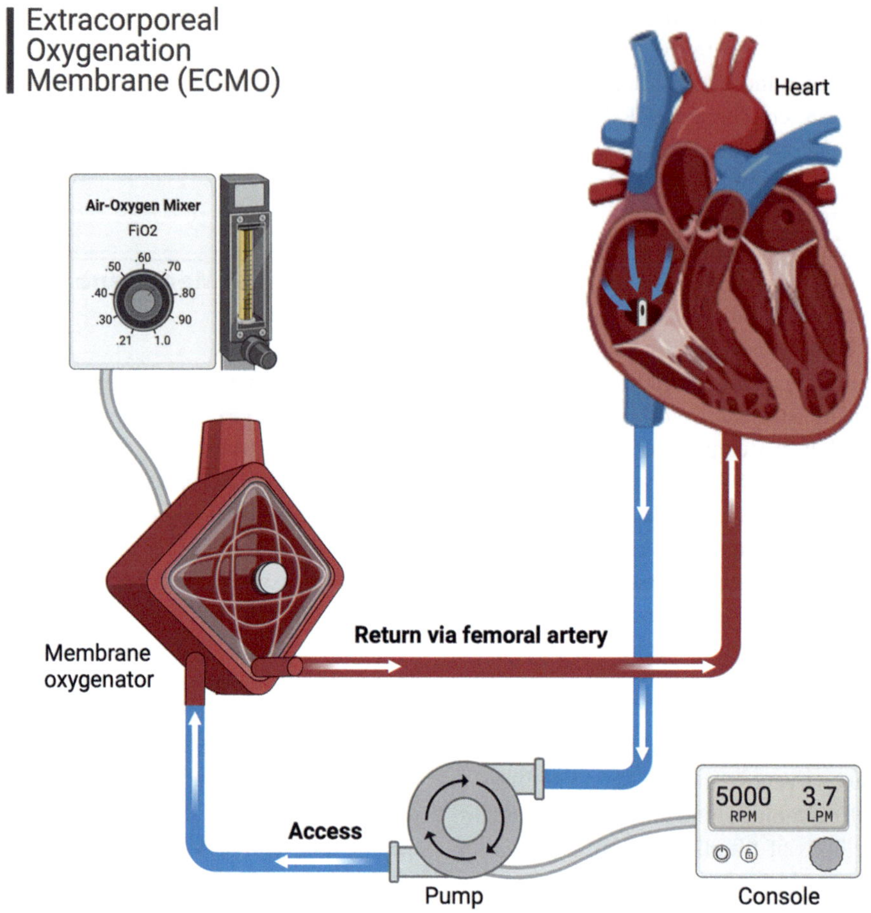

Fig. 8.5 Schematic representation of extracorporeal membrane oxygenation (ECMO) for heart and/or lung support

liver failure, non-recoverable brain injury, prolonged ventilator dependence, and severe obesity. Use of VV ECMO for refractory hypoxia has demonstrated mixed results regarding improving mortality, however randomized control trials have been complicated by high crossover rates and intention-to-treat analysis. [28, 29]

Venoarterial (VA) ECMO, also referred to as extracorporeal life support, is indicated in cardiogenic shock with refractory hypotension and depressed cardiac output, despite maximum inotropic and intra-aortic balloon pump support. Causes of cardiogenic shock where VA ECMO is indicated include acute coronary syndrome, refractory cardiac arrythmia, sepsis-induced cardiomyopathy, myocarditis, pulmonary embolism, drug toxicity, cardiac trauma, anaphylaxis and heart failure. Arterial and venous access cannulas are inserted percutaneously or centrally with drainage of deoxygenated blood and return of oxygenated blood to the systemic circulation. Recent randomized trials have not demonstrated improved outcomes in patients with cardiogenic shock secondary to myocardial infarction [30].

Bedside Laparotomy

As the spectrum of bedside therapeutic interventions are limited by illumination, equipment availability, and staff familiarity, re-operation is usually preferable to transporting the patient to the operating room (OR), where intervention rather than exploration will be more readily feasible. Infrequently, severe hemodynamic or respiratory instability precludes transportation of the decompensating surgical patient to the OR [6]. In this circumstance, rescue efforts may require bedside surgical intervention in the ICU. Common indications for bedside exploratory laparotomies include but are not limited to re-exploration in the setting of severe, refractory shock, where there is concern for uncontrolled hemorrhage, irreversible bowel ischemia, or abdominal compartment syndrome [33].

While studies have demonstrated the safety of operative intervention in the ICU, the operating surgeon must be aware of several essential logistic elements to ensure availability of all necessary equipment. [33] Safe and effective emergent re-operation, albeit in the OR or at the patient bedside in the ICU, requires close coordination with not only the ICU team administrating the intravenous general anesthetic, but also the ICU nursing staff, as well as the operating room scrub and circulating staff. Preparation should include provision for continuous ICU monitoring with frequent recording of the vitals, appropriate sedation, and analgesia to facilitate paralysis, availability of personnel familiar with operating room equipment and logistics, including adequate lighting and electrocautery. We recommend that each institution establishes its own protocol to facilitate safe bedside laparotomies when indicated in critically ill patients. Recognizing that these rare high-stake interventions are rescue therapy with high associated mortality, abbreviated operation is vital, and temporary abdominal closure with a negative pressure wound system is preferred [34].

Management of the Open Abdomen

During re-operative surgery, disrupted intestinal continuity, ischemia, or visceral edema in the presence of adverse physiology (hypothermia, acidosis and coagulopathy) should prompt consideration of a damage control surgery approach incorporating laparostomy(open abdomen) with negative pressure wound therapy and recovery to the ICU with a plan for interval serial surgical re-explorations to manage bacterial bioburden and progress toward conditions favorable for abdominal closure [6]. This approach serves to minimize the risk of intraabdominal hypertension or abdominal compartment syndrome and allow for easy access to the peritoneal cavity [35, 36]. Advances in resuscitation efforts away from massive crystalloid resuscitation have helped avoid these potentially fatal complications. However, the overutilization of the damage control open abdomen approach is not without risk [37, 38]. Rates of primary fascial closure and postoperative complications increase with prolonged duration of open abdomen [39].

Multiple strategies have been explored to facilitate abdominal closure. Decreasing the number of subsequent laparotomies as well as time to first re-laparotomy have both been associated with improved rates of primary fascial closure [40]. The use of intravenously administered hypertonic saline has been demonstrated to increase primary fascial closure in single center observational studies, however recent randomized control trials have questioned the generalizability this finding [41, 42] (Fig. 8.6). Additionally, hypertonic saline carries a risk of renal dysfunction due to the high chlorine load and patients should be monitored closely for worsening renal function and hypernatremia. Direct peritoneal resuscitation has been demonstrated in certain centers to facilitate abdominal closure through the reduction in local inflammatory mediators and minimize visceral edema [43]. Direct peritoneal resuscitation (DPR) provides targeted volume resuscitation into the splanchnic microcirculation using direct intraperitoneal delivery of a hyperosmolar glucose-based solution. The goal is to reverse vasoconstriction and prevent hypoperfusion at the splanchnic cellular level and simultaneously reduce endothelial dysfunction and organ necrosis mitigated by the local inflammatory cytokines [43]. A percutaneous catheter, placed with its tip at the root of the mesentery or the pelvis, instills the hyperosmolar solution into the peritoneal cavity, and continuous suction applied using commercial or non-commercial negative pressure wound vacuum options continuously drain the effluent. Infusion rates are described at 400 mL/h or 1.5 ml/kg/h until definitive closure is obtained [44].

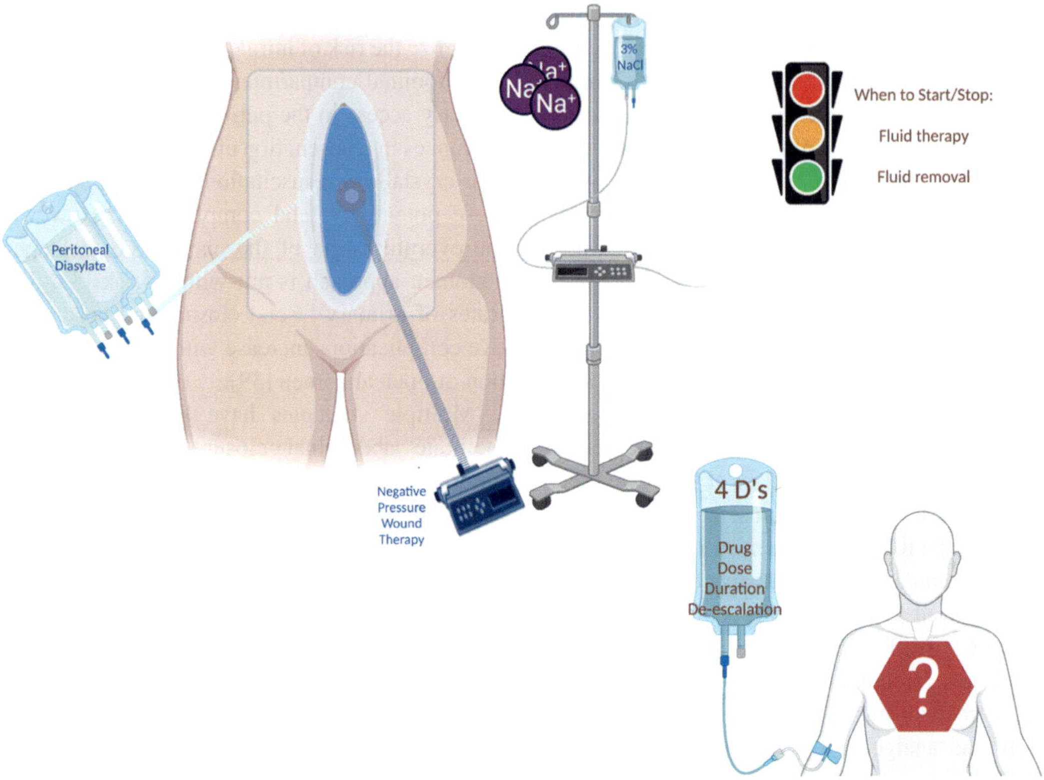

Fig. 8.6 Fluid management in the open abdomen. The most-studied adjuncts to current care are direct peritoneal resuscitation and parenteral hypertonic saline. Thoughtful optimal care revolves around determining optimal timing for resuscitation and de-resuscitation. (Original figure by the authors)

Maintaining a cautious fluid balance is necessary to avoid abdominal compartment syndrome, as is warming of the fluid to avoid hypothermia, which would worsen coagulopathy.

In both animal and human models, use of DPR not only improves splanchnic blood flow and vascular organ perfusion, but also decreases local tissue hypoxia and injury. Decreased levels of inflammatory markers, including proinflammatory cytokines, have also been observed [43, 45]. Benefits of DPR include improved timing and successful rates of primary fascial closure, as well as decreased ICU related duration of stay [46]. The best outcomes for DPR occur when it is coupled with targeted conventional resuscitation, optimizing local and systemic tissue perfusion. Lack of familiarity with DPR protocols, rather than lack of evidence appears to be the major barrier to widespread use. Future, multicenter, randomized studies will help to test the efficacy across broader populations.

Nutritional Considerations

Nutrition is an essential component of recovery for critically ill patients undergoing re-operation. Ischemia, inflammation and tissue edema facilitate gut bacterial translocation, antimicrobial therapy compromises commensal bacterial defense, while prolonged fasting depletes luminal brush border enzymes required for digestion (Fig. 8.7). Guidelines for critical illness recommend early enteral nutrition initiated within 48 h of admission and advancing to goal during the early phase of critical illness [47]. Early use of enteral nutrition has been demonstrated to be superior to either parental nutrition or late enteral

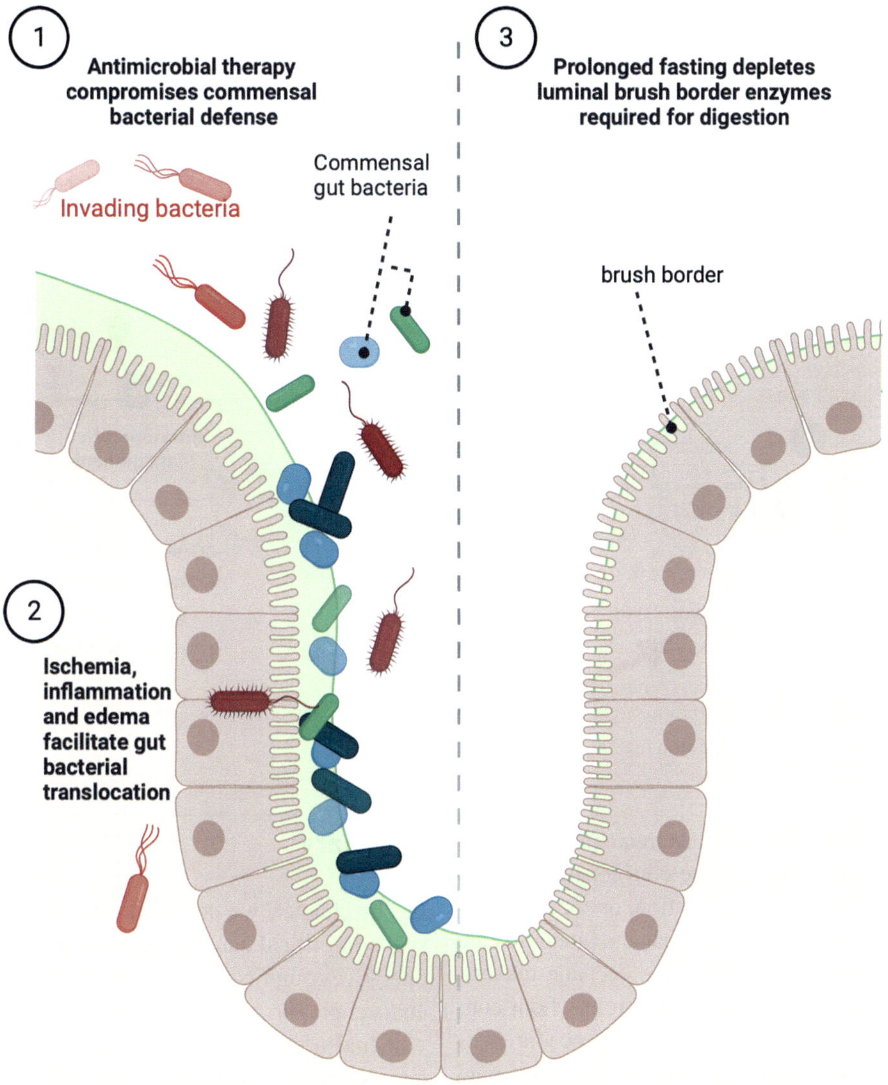

Fig. 8.7 Consequences of critical illness on gut function

nutrition. Early enteral nutrition has not only been demonstrated to be safe, but also associated with improved outcomes in critically-ill patients with temporary abdominal closure where there is intestinal continuity [48]. Supplementation of amino acids, omega-3 fatty acids and Vitamin C and D may further help counteract the inflammatory catabolism associated with critical illness [6]. Any nutrition strategy must account for the additional catabolic state associated with the open abdomen. Parenteral nutrition remains inferior to enteral nutrition, and should only be considered if enteral nutritional is not feasible in malnourished patients with expected 7 days without adequate nutrition [49–51].

Patient Centered Care Goals

Critical illness provides a challenging time for both patients and their families on whom physicians often rely to make life-or-death decisions

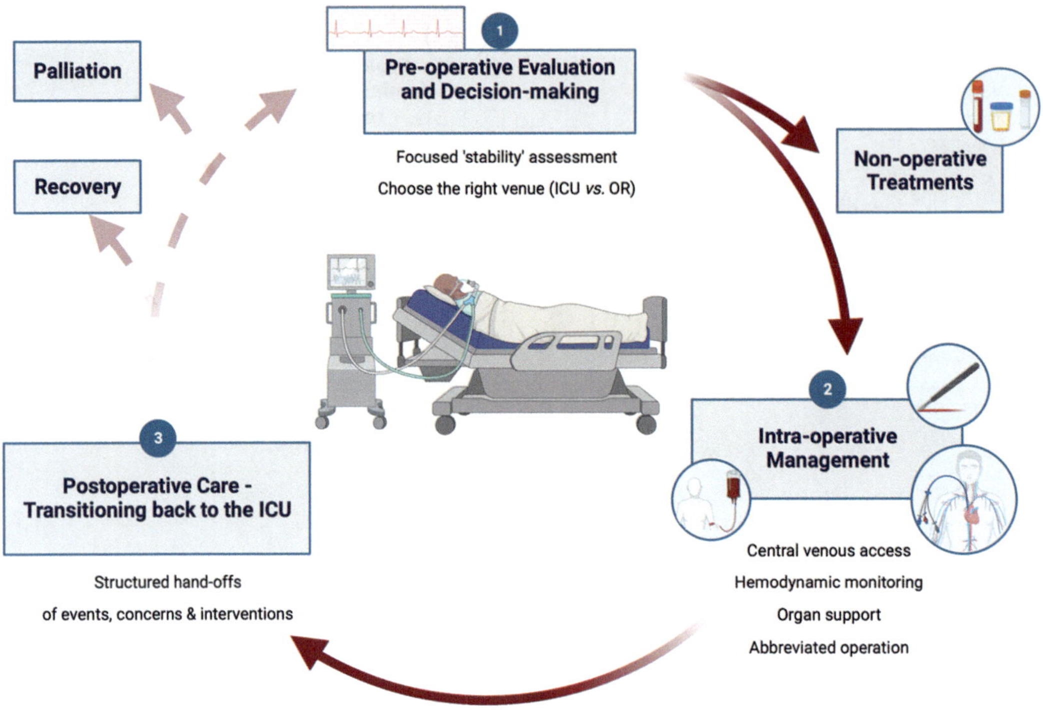

Fig. 8.8 Patient-centered decision making

(Fig. 8.8). Often patients are frequently unable to participate in complex care conversations due to mechanical ventilation, sedation, or encephalopathy. Discussions by the surgical and intensive care teams should include surrogate decision-makers, such as close family members, from whom consent for invasive, life-altering procedures is obtained. Mobilizing all the available hospital resources to support patients and families during this time is imperative. Support from social workers, chaplains, and palliative care consultation can all enhance the families' experience regardless of the outcome. Engaging the services of the Palliative Care Medicine consultation team early and often helps to establish support for the individual and the family for the impending life changes, as well as facilitate discussions regarding patient preferences and goals of care [52]. Maintaining patient dignity while supporting multisystem organ failure in patients requiring re-operative surgery is a team endeavor leveraging expertise across multiple specialties.

Summary

In this chapter, we delve into the intricate landscape of critical care for patients in whom post-operative complications require repeat radiologic, endoscopic or surgical intervention. Surgeons will find a comprehensive analysis of the challenges inherent in managing critically ill patients before, during, and after re-operation, with a focus on decision-making, optimization strategies, technological advances, ethical considerations, and a glimpse into future innovations. This review aims to equip surgeons with a nuanced understanding to enhance the care and outcomes of these complex patients.

References

1. De Waele J, Lipman J, Sakr Y, et al. Abdominal infections in the intensive care unit: characteristics, treatment and determinants of outcome. BMC Infect Dis. 2014;14:420.

2. Vincent JL, Rello J, Marshall J, et al. International study of the prevalence and outcomes of infection in intensive care units. JAMA. 2009;302(21):2323–9.
3. Vincent JL, De Backer D. Circulatory shock. N Engl J Med. 2013;369(18):1726–34.
4. Fouche Y, Sikorski R, Dutton RP. Changing paradigms in surgical resuscitation. Crit Care Med. 2010;38(9 Suppl):S411–20.
5. Rhodes A, Evans LE, Alhazzani W, et al. Surviving sepsis campaign: international guidelines for management of sepsis and septic shock: 2016. Intensive Care Med. 2017;43(3):304–77.
6. Bass GA, Dzierba AL, Taylor B, Lane-Fall M, Kaplan LJ. Tertiary peritonitis: considerations for complex team-based care. Eur J Trauma Emerg Surg. 2022;48(2):811–25.
7. Dhondup T, Tien JC, Marquez A, Kennedy CC, Gajic O, Kashani KB. Association of negative fluid balance during the de-escalation phase of sepsis management with mortality: a cohort study. J Crit Care. 2020;55:16–21.
8. Gershengorn HB, Wunsch H. Understanding changes in established practice: pulmonary artery catheter use in critically ill patients. Crit Care Med. 2013;41(12):2667–76.
9. Barnett CF, Vaduganathan M, Lan G, Butler J, Gheorghiade M. Critical reappraisal of pulmonary artery catheterization and invasive hemodynamic assessment in acute heart failure. Expert Rev Cardiovasc Ther. 2013;11(4):417–24.
10. Binanay C, Califf RM, Hasselblad V, et al. Evaluation study of congestive heart failure and pulmonary artery catheterization effectiveness: the ESCAPE trial. JAMA. 2005;294(13):1625–33.
11. Sangkum L, Liu GL, Yu L, Yan H, Kaye AD, Liu H. Minimally invasive or noninvasive cardiac output measurement: an update. J Anesth. 2016;30(3):461–80.
12. Mayer J, Boldt J, Poland R, Peterson A, Manecke GR Jr. Continuous arterial pressure waveform-based cardiac output using the FloTrac/Vigileo: a review and meta-analysis. J Cardiothorac Vasc Anesth. 2009;23(3):401–6.
13. Takala J, Ruokonen E, Tenhunen JJ, Parviainen I, Jakob SM. Early non-invasive cardiac output monitoring in hemodynamically unstable intensive care patients: a multi-center randomized controlled trial. Crit Care (London, England). 2011;15(3):R148.
14. Jessen MK, Vallentin MF, Holmberg MJ, et al. Goal-directed haemodynamic therapy during general anaesthesia for noncardiac surgery: a systematic review and meta-analysis. Br J Anaesth. 2022;128(3):416–33.
15. Expert Round Table on Ultrasound in ICU. International expert statement on training standards for critical care ultrasonography. Intensive Care Med. 2011;37(7):1077–83.
16. Brill JB, Brenner M, Duchesne J, et al. The role of TEG and ROTEM in damage control resuscitation. Shock. 2021;56(1s):52–61.
17. Bogert JN, Harvin JA, Cotton BA. Damage control resuscitation. J Intensive Care Med. 2016;31(3):177–86.
18. Hoste EA, Bagshaw SM, Bellomo R, et al. Epidemiology of acute kidney injury in critically ill patients: the multinational AKI-EPI study. Intensive Care Med. 2015;41(8):1411–23.
19. Ronco C, Bellomo R, Kellum JA. Acute kidney injury. Lancet. 2019;394(10212):1949–64.
20. Peerapornratana S, Manrique-Caballero CL, Gómez H, Kellum JA. Acute kidney injury from sepsis: current concepts, epidemiology, pathophysiology, prevention and treatment. Kidney Int. 2019;96(5):1083–99.
21. Legrand M, Darmon M, Joannidis M, Payen D. Management of renal replacement therapy in ICU patients: an international survey. Intensive Care Med. 2013;39(1):101–8.
22. Bagshaw SM, Darmon M, Ostermann M, et al. Current state of the art for renal replacement therapy in critically ill patients with acute kidney injury. Intensive Care Med. 2017;43(6):841–54.
23. Saunders H, Rehan A, Sanghavi DK. Continuous renal replacement therapy. In: StatPearls. StatPearls Publishing, Treasure Island (FL); 2023. PMID: 32310488.
24. Peng B, Lu J, Guo H, Liu J, Li A. Regional citrate anticoagulation for replacement therapy in patients with liver failure: a systematic review and meta-analysis. Front Nutr. 2023;10:1031796.
25. Schefold JC, von Haehling S, Pschowski R, et al. The effect of continuous versus intermittent renal replacement therapy on the outcome of critically ill patients with acute renal failure (CONVINT): a prospective randomized controlled trial. Crit Care (London, England). 2014;18(1):R11.
26. Gaudry S, Grolleau F, Barbar S, et al. Continuous renal replacement therapy versus intermittent hemodialysis as first modality for renal replacement therapy in severe acute kidney injury: a secondary analysis of AKIKI and IDEAL-ICU studies. Crit Care (London, England). 2022;26(1):93.
27. Rabindranath K, Adams J, Macleod AM, Muirhead N. Intermittent versus continuous renal replacement therapy for acute renal failure in adults. Cochrane Database Syst Rev. 2007(3):Cd003773.
28. Combes A, Hajage D, Capellier G, et al. Extracorporeal membrane oxygenation for severe acute respiratory distress syndrome. N Engl J Med. 2018;378(21):1965–75.
29. Peek GJ, Mugford M, Tiruvoipati R, et al. Efficacy and economic assessment of conventional ventilatory support versus extracorporeal membrane oxygenation for severe adult respiratory failure (CESAR): a multicentre randomised controlled trial. Lancet. 2009;374(9698):1351–63.
30. Thiele H, Zeymer U, Akin I, et al. Extracorporeal life support in infarct-related cardiogenic shock. N Engl J Med. 2023;389(14):1286–97.
31. Richardson AS, Schmidt M, Bailey M, Pellegrino VA, Rycus PT, Pilcher DV. ECMO Cardio-Pulmonary

Resuscitation (ECPR), trends in survival from an international multicentre cohort study over 12-years. Resuscitation. 2017;112:34–40.
32. Zakhary B, Nanjayya VB, Sheldrake J, Collins K, Ihle JF, Pellegrino V. Predictors of mortality after extracorporeal cardiopulmonary resuscitation. Crit Care Resusc. 2018;20(3):223–30.
33. Piper GL, Maerz LL, Schuster KM, et al. When the ICU is the operating room. J Trauma Acute Care Surg. 2013;74(3):871–5.
34. Schreiber J, Nierhaus A, Vettorazzi E, et al. Rescue bedside laparotomy in the intensive care unit in patients too unstable for transport to the operating room. Crit Care (London, England). 2014;18(3):R123.
35. Coccolini F, Roberts D, Ansaloni L, et al. The open abdomen in trauma and non-trauma patients: WSES guidelines. World J Emerg Surg. 2018;13(1):7.
36. Person B, Dorfman T, Bahouth H, Osman A, Assalia A, Kluger Y. Abbreviated emergency laparotomy in the non-trauma setting. World J EmergSurg. 2009;4(1):41.
37. Montalvo JA, Acosta JA, Rodríguez P, Alejandro K, Sárraga A. Surgical complications and causes of death in trauma patients that require temporary abdominal closure. Am Surg. 2005;71(3):219–24.
38. Cheatham ML, Safcsak K, Llerena LE, Morrow CE Jr, Block EF. Long-term physical, mental, and functional consequences of abdominal decompression. J Trauma. 2004;56(2):237–41; discussion 241–232.
39. Hatch QM, Osterhout LM, Podbielski J, et al. Impact of closure at the first take back: complication burden and potential overutilization of damage control laparotomy. J Trauma. 2011;71(6):1503–11.
40. Kwon E, Krause C, Luo-Owen X, et al. Time is domain: factors affecting primary fascial closure after trauma and non-trauma damage control laparotomy (data from the EAST SLEEP-TIME multicenter registry). Eur J Trauma Emerg Surg. 2022;48(3):2107–16.
41. Harvin JA, Mims MM, Duchesne JC, et al. Chasing 100%: the use of hypertonic saline to improve early, primary fascial closure after damage control laparotomy. J T Acute Care Surg. 2013;74(2):426–30; discussion 431–422.
42. García AF, Manzano-Nunez R, Carrillo DC, et al. Hypertonic saline infusion does not improve the chance of primary fascial closure after damage control laparotomy: a randomized controlled trial. World J Emerg S. 2023;18(1):4.
43. Ribeiro-Junior MAF, Costa CTK, de Souza AS, et al. The role of direct peritoneal resuscitation in the treatment of hemorrhagic shock after trauma and in emergency acute care surgery: a systematic review. Eur J Trauma Emerg Surg. 2022;48(2):791–7.
44. Smith JW, Garrison RN, Matheson PJ, Franklin GA, Harbrecht BG, Richardson JD. Direct peritoneal resuscitation accelerates primary abdominal wall closure after damage control surgery. J Am Coll Surg. 2010;210(5):658–64, 664–657.
45. Smith JW, Matheson PJ, Franklin GA, Harbrecht BG, Richardson JD, Garrison RN. Randomized controlled trial evaluating the efficacy of peritoneal resuscitation in the management of trauma patients undergoing damage control surgery. J Am Coll Surg. 2017;224(4):396–404.
46. Smith JW, Neal Garrison R, Matheson PJ, et al. Adjunctive treatment of abdominal catastrophes and sepsis with direct peritoneal resuscitation: indications for use in acute care surgery. J Trauma Acute Care Surg. 2014;77(3):393–8; discussion 398–399.
47. Reintam Blaser A, Starkopf J, Alhazzani W, et al. Early enteral nutrition in critically ill patients: ESICM clinical practice guidelines. Intensive Care Med. 2017;43(3):380–98.
48. Collier B, Guillamondegui O, Cotton B, et al. Feeding the open abdomen. JPEN J Parenter Enteral Nutr. 2007;31(5):410–5.
49. Jeejeebhoy KN. Total parenteral nutrition: potion or poison? Am J Clin Nutr. 2001;74(2):160–3.
50. Bohl CJ, Parks A. A mnemonic for pharmacists to ensure optimal monitoring and safety of total parenteral nutrition: I AM FULL. Ann Pharmacother. 2017;51(7):603–13.
51. McClave SA, Martindale RG, Vanek VW, et al. Guidelines for the provision and assessment of nutrition support therapy in the adult critically ill patient: Society of Critical Care Medicine (SCCM) and American Society for Parenteral and Enteral Nutrition (A.S.P.E.N.). JPEN J Parenter Enteral Nutr. 2009;33(3):277–316.
52. Ito K, George N, Wilson J, Bowman J, Aaronson E, Ouchi K. Primary palliative care recommendations for critical care clinicians. J Intensive Care. 2022;10(1):20.

Part III

Surgical Decision Making in Difficult Scenarios of Acute Care Surgery

Surgical Decision-Making in Postinjury Multiple Organ Failure

9

Ryan S. Ting, Kate L. King, and Zsolt J. Balogh

Postinjury Multiple Organ Failure (MOF)

Postinjury multiple organ failure (MOF) was first described in the late 1970s. During this period, advances in trauma and critical care meant that traumatologists were able to keep patients with previously unsurvivable injuries and isolated organ failures alive long enough for a new late peak in postinjury mortality to develop—the deadly syndrome of MOF [1, 2]. MOF is the sequential failure of vital organs, which includes those that were not damaged in the initial injury. This lethal series of vital organ decompensation demands intensive resource utilization and generally poor outcomes regardless.

The epidemiology of MOF has continued to evolve along with the at-risk population, which is now a decade older than historical controls [3, 4]. However, depending on the study cited, the mortality of MOF in contemporary cohorts has remained similar or decreased, despite a presumably more comorbid study population, which is a credit to the advances in modern trauma care [3, 5]. Nonetheless, MOF patients still have a three- to fourfold higher mortality rate than risk-matched patients who do not develop MOF [6, 7]. It is disappointing, therefore, that the incidence of this high-acuity, high mortality syndrome has remained unchanged in the last 50 years [8].

The greatest impediment to our study of the epidemiology of MOF is that there is no consensus on how we objectively define the syndrome. In fact, a recent systematic review found that there were 40 different definitions for MOF, many of which have not been validated in trauma cohorts. In addition, even when using the same scoring system, different studies utilized different cut-off values to define MOF [8]. The MOF definition of a Denver score >3 after at least 48 h postinjury is well validated in trauma cohorts and is a specific method of defining MOF that the authors recommend to standardize reporting, to facilitate the study of its epidemiology and benchmark our progress in the prevention and management of MOF [9].

Decision-Making to Identify Patients at Risk of MOF

MOF is a rare syndrome among the general population, affecting less than one in every 100,000 people [5]. Its incidence, however, rises rapidly the more severely injured the study population (denominator) becomes, and ranges between

R. S. Ting
St George & Sutherland Clinical School, University of New South Wales, Sydney, NSW, Australia
e-mail: R.Ting@unsw.edu.au

K. L. King · Z. J. Balogh (✉)
Department of Traumatology, Division of Surgery, John Hunter Hospital & University of Newcastle, Newcastle, NSW, Australia
e-mail: Kate.King@health.nsw.gov.au; Zsolt.Balogh@health.nsw.gov.au

R. Latifi (ed.), *Surgical Decision-Making*, https://doi.org/10.1007/978-3-031-67391-7_9

13% and 59% based on previous investigations in polytrauma cohorts [8].

The Denver group were the first to describe the early predictors of MOF, and their findings formed the basis of much of our current understanding on the population at risk. They found that in trauma patients admitted to the ICU who survived for longer than 24 h, that the independent predictors of MOF were: age older than 55 years, an Injury Severity Score (ISS) of 25 or more, receiving more than 6 units of packed red blood cells within 12 h, a base deficit greater than 8 mEq/L within the first 12 h, and a lactate level over 2.5 mmol/L between 12 and 24 h [10].

However, a subsequent investigation two decades later by the Newcastle group, who used similar inclusion criteria, found that the epidemiology and predictors of MOF had fundamentally changed. They found that MOF patients were a decade older and presumably more comorbid. Injury and shock parameters no longer predicted MOF in their study. However, theirs was a uniformly severely injured cohort, with mean ISS of 32 and 30 in the MOF and non-MOF groups respectively. Interestingly, they found that hematological parameters, in particular relative thrombocytopenia (less than 150×10^9/L) on emergency department presentation, greater maximum serum creatinine (greater than 150×10^9/L) on day 1, and minimum bilirubin (greater than 10×10^9/L), had become the new predictors of MOF [11]. Acute traumatic coagulopathy is an early endogenous phenomenon that is catalyzed by massive tissue death and shock and is associated with increased mortality in trauma patients [12]. Although acute traumatic coagulopathy is often defined as INR >1.2, a multicenter prospective observational study found that coagulopathy only predicted MOF when INR >1.5 [13].

Trauma cohorts are typically male-predominated, and this trend is sustained in the MOF study population [6, 14–17]. Furthermore, obesity has been identified as an independent risk factor for MOF [18, 19]. Obesity is a complex chronic systemic disease, often associated with other comorbidities that predispose its host to pro-inflammatory states like MOF. In the midst of the modern obesity epidemic, the prototypical trauma patient, and by extension the majority of MOF patients, are likely to be the obese male [20].

While traumatologists are well aware that the risk of MOF in polytrauma cohorts is high, the heterogeneity of MOF definitions and study populations in the published literature makes it challenging to estimate just how likely a patient is to develop the syndrome. Nonetheless, the incidence of MOF per the Denver score >3 definition in trauma patients admitted to the ICU ranges from 13% to 25% [4, 6, 10, 11]. Furthermore, as population demographics evolve and as trauma systems continue to advance from the prehospital level to advances in critical care, so too does the epidemiology of postinjury MOF. The clinical significance and dynamic nature of MOF demand funding for continuous focused research into its predictors in contemporary cohorts [21].

In practical terms today, the high-risk MOF trauma patients are males, especially ones with severe tissue injury, obesity, and coagulopathy, requiring shock resuscitation, and being older than the average age of the local polytrauma population. Early subclinical renal impairment and thrombocytopenia also remained statistically validated predictors from different sites.

Decision-Making Around Interventions

Interventional Radiology

Interventional radiological procedures such as angioembolization are critical treatment options for the exsanguinating trauma patient. Endovascular interventions have become the first line management in surgically challenging scenarios like the hemodynamically unstable pelvic fracture patient [22]. As such, the American College of Surgeons Committee on Trauma guidelines recommend that interventional radiology should be ready to perform emergency procedures within 30 minutes in all designated Level I and Level II trauma centers [23]. Furthermore, advances in technology and the proven effectiveness of interventional radiology in management of shock in trauma patients have led to the development of hybrid trauma operating rooms like the Resuscitation Angiography Percutaneous Treatments and Operative Resuscitations (RAPTOR) suite, which further expedites the provision of definitive care [24].

Surgery

Surgical interventions have long been proposed as risk factors for MOF, and are frequently discussed in review articles and expert opinions as "second hits" that precipitate the syndrome. However, there is no quality data on their frequency or possible temporal relationship with MOF [25–27]. In the current era of hemostatic resuscitation that commences early from the prehospital phase, and without cyclic supranormal crystalloid resuscitation, we do not have evidence that definitive musculoskeletal stabilization makes patients sick if physiologically maintained [17, 28, 29]. In fact, the opposite is true. A study of 162 MOF patients who underwent surgery during their ICU admission by the Newcastle group found that preoperatively optimized laboratory physiological parameters were not compromised by surgery—contrary to historical assumptions. Furthermore, they concluded that the effect of optimizing surgical timing in MOF patients would be modest, potentially decreasing the ICU length of stay by 7 days with no difference in mortality [29].

Ultimately, it is critical to underscore that nothing can replace sound, consultant-led surgical decision-making [30]. Catchy terms like "damage control" and "early total care" have pervaded the literature, and the pendulum has swung between these two extremes through the decades. Lately terms like "early appropriate care" and "safe definitive surgery" have emerged, perhaps to acquiesce that the correct decision is rarely the absolute adherence to one therapeutic mode over another, but rather frequently lies in the expanse between.

Each surgical decision needs to be tailored to the individual patient using the resources available at that specific point in time, making every scenario unique. Early definitive surgical intervention is desirable and often produces superior patient outcomes and reduced healthcare resource utilization than delayed surgery [31, 32]. Acute fracture fixation in polytraumatized patients helps with positioning, mobilization, and decreasing morbidity and can help to reduce the time spent on the ventilator and in the ICU. However, this must be balanced against the insult of surgical interventions, which may further push patients off the precipice into MOF. Ultimately, the underlying principle is to perform definitive surgery as early as it is safe to do so.

Not all patients, however, are fit to undergo early definitive surgery. Patients with hemodynamic instability, severe pulmonary injuries, or head injuries and those with compromised general health, such as the elderly, are poor candidates for acute fixation. It is in these unstable or in extremis patients where damage control surgery would be the appropriate lifesaving option [33]. In borderline or stable patients, the priority should be on early resuscitation to optimize polytrauma patient physiology. While life-, limb-, or vital organ-saving operations are clear indications to proceed with surgery, the decision to operate on other injuries should be guided by whether or not physiological homeostasis can be achieved preoperatively and maintained or improved intraoperatively. Notably, temperature, coagulation, metabolic acidosis, ventilation parameters, tissue perfusion, and inotrope requirements are perhaps the most vital indicators of patient physiology and can easily be monitored on the operating table. In the polytraumatized patient, planning surgery in such a way that allows continuous reassessment between procedures on different body regions is critical. Compromise of any of these key parameters is an indication to bail out to an abbreviated, staged procedure.

Decision-Making Around Surgical Critical Care

Contemporary studies on the epidemiology of postinjury MOF show that the at-risk cohort is now a decade older than they were 20 years ago [5, 7, 11]. This change is reflective of an aging population in the developed world. Yet, the decreasing mortality of MOF, despite an older and presumably more comorbid study population, is a reflection of the advances in surgical critical care but also an important reminder that our sickest polytrauma patients may be coming in sicker than ever before.

Pulmonary

Pulmonary failure has historically been observed to be the catalyst behind a patient's deterioration into MOF [14, 34]. Pulmonary dysfunction itself is often caused by acute respiratory distress syndrome (ARDS). There are several theories behind the pathophysiology of ARDS in trauma patients [35]. However, the most relevant, potentially modifiable, cause from surgical decision-making perspective involves the use of crystalloids during trauma resuscitation, intraoperatively and in ICU. Crystalloid boluses have historically been used to achieve hemodynamic stability, assess "fluid responsiveness" and/or generate a Starling curve, and its deleterious effects are especially pronounced after protracted operations with significant and frequently underestimated blood loss, which contribute to dilution anemia and ARDS [17]. Crystalloids are therefore not inert but proinflammatory substances with specific indications and potentially deadly side effects [36].

As most MOF patients suffer from pulmonary failure, it is unsurprising that the majority of MOF patients require mechanical ventilation in the ICU. Since 1998, the incidence of ARDS in trauma cohorts has gradually decreased, partially due to lung protective ventilation, but also as crystalloid use has decreased - such that more recent studies have shown that cardiac failures are now more common than pulmonary failures in polytrauma patients [5, 17, 37].

Veno-venous extracorporeal membrane oxygenation (ECMO) has been shown to improve survival rates in trauma patients with severe refractory hypoxic respiratory failure [38–40]. It achieves this by relieving the lungs by performing gas exchange extracorporeally, which facilitates lung-protective ventilation and pulmonary recovery [41]. Therefore, in patients with severe pulmonary failure refractive to lung-protective ventilation, simultaneous veno-venous ECMO should be considered. The exception to this is for patients with massive post-traumatic pulmonary emboli, who should instead receive veno-arterial ECMO [42].

Cardiac

Achieving and maintaining cardiocirculatory homeostasis in postinjury MOF patients is complicated by often severe hemorrhage, systemic inflammation, metabolic acidosis, coagulopathy, hypothermia, and overall physiological derangements that compromise the body's ability to maintain adequate cardiac output and tissue perfusion. There are many possible causes of cardiac injury in trauma patients. Cardiac events may have preceded and may potentially lead to the traumatic event, or direct cardiac injuries might occur as a result of thoracic trauma [43, 44]. Indirect cardiac injuries associated with systemic inflammation, takotsubo cardiomyopathy, and preexisting chronic heart disease are all possible causes of cardiac dysfunction in trauma patients, and the presence of cardiovascular risk factors is independently associated with increased postinjury mortality [45, 46].

A laboratory study in rodent models showed that severe hemorrhage and injury compromised cardiac output and stroke volume, which remained depressed despite resuscitation. Furthermore, myocardial injury, widespread ultrastructural disorganization of sarcomeres and mitochondria, immunohistochemical evidence of catabolism and an oxidative stress response, and elevated troponin-I and heart fatty acid-binding protein levels were found in injured animal models versus controls and mirrored the pattern of postinjury cardiac dysfunction seen in trauma patients [47, 48].

Interestingly, a recent multicenter prospective study of MOF patients found that cardiac failures were the first and most common organs to fail, in contrast to historical precedents [5]. Again, these severely injured patients may show a transient response in mean arterial pressure to crystalloid infusions, but vigorous boluses eventually extravasate from the circulation and flood the interstitial tissues, increasing polycompartment pressures and further compromising tissue perfusion [17, 49].

In these patients, invasive cardiac output monitoring is often required. We can achieve this using continuous cardiac output pulmonary artery catheters and trans-pulmonary thermodilution, which also allow us to administer vasoactive and inotropic drugs in tandem [50].

These are invasive interventions with side effects, and once our strict physiological targets are reached and the patient begins to improve, our resuscitation should be adjusted accordingly.

In patients with postinjury cardiac insufficiency, veno-arterial ECMO can be utilized if prior attempts at resuscitation with inotropes and volume reconstitution fail [51]. Veno-arterial ECMO is not the first-line treatment for postinjury cardiac dysfunction due to the severity of its associated complications, which include ipsilateral lower limb ischemia secondary to femoral artery damage from large bore cannulas, iatrogenic pseudoaneurysm and potential vessel perforation, and/or incorrect placement [52]. However, it is still a potentially lifesaving intervention that merits consideration in trauma patients with refractory cardiac dysfunction [51]. In addition, utilization of ECMO requires a carefully designed anticoagulation strategy to balance the risk of intra-circuit thrombotic complications and bleeding in an already coagulopathic trauma patient, although this has been mitigated to some degree recent years by heparin-coated circuits [53].

In recent years, however, a lower proportion of patients get invasive cardiac monitoring compared to previous eras. Furthermore, a limitation of all the major MOF scoring systems is their use of inotropes as a surrogate for cardiac failure, which may contribute to the high cardiac failure numbers. Thus, it may be time to update the cardiac scoring systems to reflect changes in critical care practices to support the circulatory system.

Renal

The incidence of acute renal failure in trauma cohorts varies greatly. This is because it suffers from the same heterogeneity in definitions as MOF does [54]. Renal failure typically presents after day 4, later in the course of a MOF patient's ICU journey than cardiac or respiratory failures, and is associated with increased mortality in comparison [5]. Early renal failure carries a poor prognosis, with the Denver group showing that early acute renal failure (creatinine >159 × 10^9/L by day 2) was a stronger predictor for MOF and mortality than dysfunction in either of the three other vital organs that we monitor for the diagnosis of MOF [55].

There are multiple causes of renal failure in the polytraumatized patient, and its integral role in maintaining homeostasis, interorgan cross-talk, and its major endocrine functions, particularly with respect to blood pressure regulation, makes it unsurprising that mortality is so high when the kidneys are compromised. Shock is most commonly the culprit in prerenal renal failure in trauma patients [56]. While the treatment for this is volume resuscitation, the effect of overzealous fluid reconstitution can lead to major complications; to stay relevant, ARDS and abdominal compartment syndrome are particularly important in the MOF patient. While positive end-expiratory pressure ventilation is critical in ARDS by preventing alveolar collapse, excessive pressures can increase intrathoracic pressures, reduce cardiac output, and decrease renal perfusion [57]. Abdominal compartment syndrome, which can be secondary to supranormal trauma resuscitation or from intra-abdominal hemorrhage, also compromises renal blood supply, and 42% of these patients end up with renal failure [28].

Radiocontrast agents are frequently implicated as the cause of iatrogenic renal insufficiency. A recent investigation showed that repeat contrast studies in trauma patients at risk of MOF was not associated with the development of acute kidney injury, disproving the historical dogma [58]. While we must remain vigilant in our management of our patients, the data suggests that contrast-induced acute kidney injury is unlikely to be caused by essential secondary imaging in trauma patients.

The management of renal failure begins with avoiding it early by providing balanced, target-based resuscitation and involves continuous reassessment of our therapeutic modes. Renal replacement therapy, however, is the mainstay of treatment when prevention has failed and the underlying cause cannot be otherwise reversed [59]. Renal replacement therapy may also be considered in fluid-overloaded patients to reduce edema and improve respiratory function and for the management of electrolytes, even in the absence of renal failure [60]. Diuretic use should be used with extreme caution, as its use in ICU patients with renal failure has been associated with increased mortality and non-recovery of renal function [61].

Hepatic

Acute liver failure the postinjury setting is typically the consequence of direct liver injury, or secondary to shock, both of which are deadly, especially in trauma patients with preexisting hepatic cirrhosis [62]. Indirect liver injury may occur as a consequence secondary to the systemic inflammatory stress response to trauma. Postinjury liver failure in the acute phase is typically the consequence of ischemia reperfusion injury, a syndrome precipitated by shock liver and caused by the release of proinflammatory cytokines and reactive oxygen species after reperfusion [63, 64].

Management of postinjury liver failure in the ICU is a challenging clinical entity because it is often complicated by cardiac, respiratory, and/or renal dysfunction [65]. Hepatic failures in MOF patients occur after day 5—the latest onset relative to the other vital organs [5]. Acute hepatic failures without preexisting liver disease that occur in MOF patients before this time are rare and are likely to be the result of incomplete resuscitation.

Due to its numerous functions, the liver is a likely culprit for interorgan cross-talk in MOF, and hepatic failure can exacerbate the function of other already dysfunctional organs. For example, relative adrenal insufficiency and an inadequate cortisol response can dampen the vascular pressor response, compromising cardiocirculatory function, which itself has downstream effects on renal perfusion [65–67].

Management of hepatic failure includes compensating for its role in hematological detoxification. Hepatic encephalopathy is the consequence of toxic accumulation of ammonia and is pathognomonic for hepatic failure [68, 69]. Therefore, hemodialysis or hemofiltration may be utilized to remove toxins from the circulation. Therapeutic plasmapheresis effectively reduces the circulating levels of proinflammatory cytokines and large albumin-bound and water-soluble toxins and has been shown to reduce vasopressor requirements and increase transplant survival in patients with acute hepatic failure [70, 71].

Current guidelines recommend enteral feeds, but do not advocate for specific feed formulations [72–74]. However, because hepatic gluconeogenesis is compromised in patients with liver failure, continuous intravenous glucose for nutritional support and insulin for stable glycemic control has become a nearly universal practice [72]. Water-soluble vitamins, particularly vitamins B-complex and C, and trace element supplementation is also recommended for patients throughout their admission [75].

Decision-Making in Survivors of MOF

While MOF is a high-acuity, high-mortality, resource-intensive syndrome, it often evolves into a chronic disease among the patients whom we manage to save. In these patients, it is critical that a multidisciplinary approach targeted at holistic, individualized patient-centered care is employed to ensure that the appropriate medical, nutritional, psychological, and physical rehabilitation and/or supports are accounted for during discharge planning [76].

Survivors of MOF often suffer from permanent disability and are 3.9 times as likely to require personal assistance in activities of daily living than risk-matched patients who did not get MOF [77]. This places significant social and financial strains on our patients and their families. A chronic critical illness (CCI) is defined as spending ≥14 days in ICU with persistent organ dysfunction [78]. It was found that at 12 months post-ICU discharge, 40% of CCI patients were dead and that survivors with CCI had significantly inferior physical function and health-related quality of life than those who did not develop CCI [79].

Persistent inflammation, immunosuppression, and catabolism syndrome (PICS) was described by the Gainesville group in 2012 as a subgroup of CCI that included patients who had suffered inflammatory insults, and is a more modern problem faced by the survivors of MOF [78]. Our understanding of the pathomechanism that drives PICS is still developing. However, the data shows that that elderly, sarcopenic patients are at increased risk for PICS and that this persistent catabolic disease contributes to the poor physical and overall prognostic outcomes in these patients [80]. Therefore, these patients may benefit from consultation with a dietitian to design an anabolic nutritional meal plan, which should include a high protein intake, leucine supplementation, and anti-inflammatory supplements like fish oil-derived specialized pro-resolving mediators [81, 82].

References

1. Baue AE. Multiple, progressive, or sequential systems failure. A syndrome of the 1970s. Arch Surg. 1975;110(7):779–81.
2. Eiseman B, Beart R, Norton L. Multiple organ failure. Surg Gynecol Obstet. 1977;144(3):323–6.
3. Frohlich M, Lefering R, Probst C, Paffrath T, Schneider MM, Maegele M, et al. Epidemiology and risk factors of multiple-organ failure after multiple trauma: an analysis of 31,154 patients from the TraumaRegister DGU. J Trauma Acute Care Surg. 2014;76(4):921–7; discussion 7.
4. Ciesla DJ, Moore EE, Johnson JL, Burch JM, Cothren CC, Sauaia A. A 12-year prospective study of postinjury multiple organ failure: has anything changed? Arch Surg. 2005;140(5):432–40.
5. Ting RS, Weaver NA, King KL, Way TL, Sarrami P, Daniel L, et al. Epidemiology of postinjury multiple organ failure: a prospective multicenter observational study. Eur J Trauma Emerg Surg. 2024. [In Press].
6. Sauaia A, Moore EE, Johnson JL, Chin TL, Banerjee A, Sperry JL, et al. Temporal trends of postinjury multiple-organ failure: still resource intensive, morbid, and lethal. J Trauma Acute Care Surg. 2014;76(3):582–92, discussion 92–3.
7. Dewar DC, Mackay P, Balogh Z. Epidemiology of post-injury multiple organ failure in an Australian trauma system. ANZ J Surg. 2009;79(6):431–6.
8. Ting RS, Lewis DP, Yang KX, Nguyen TA, Sarrami P, Daniel L, et al. Incidence of multiple organ failure in adult polytrauma patients: a systematic review and meta-analysis. J Trauma Acute Care Surg. 2023;94(5):725.
9. Dewar DC, White A, Attia J, Tarrant SM, King KL, Balogh ZJ. Comparison of postinjury multiple-organ failure scoring systems: Denver versus Sequential Organ Failure Assessment. J Trauma Acute Care Surg. 2014;77(4):624–9.
10. Sauaia A, Moore FA, Moore EE, Haenel JB, Read RA, Lezotte DC. Early predictors of postinjury multiple organ failure. Arch Surg. 1994;129(1):39–45.
11. Dewar DC, Tarrant SM, King KL, Balogh ZJ. Changes in the epidemiology and prediction of multiple-organ failure after injury. J Trauma Acute Care Surg. 2013;74(3):774–9.
12. Davenport R. Pathogenesis of acute traumatic coagulopathy. Transfusion. 2013;53(Suppl 1):23s–7s.
13. Peltan ID, Vande Vusse LK, Maier RV, Watkins TR. An international normalized ratio-based definition of acute traumatic coagulopathy is associated with mortality, venous thromboembolism, and multiple organ failure after injury. Crit Care Med. 2015;43(7):1429–38.
14. Faist E, Baue AE, Dittmer H, Heberer G. Multiple organ failure in polytrauma patients. J Trauma. 1983;23(9):775–87.
15. Moore FA, Sauaia A, Moore EE, Haenel JB, Burch JM, Lezotte DC. Postinjury multiple organ failure: a bimodal phenomenon. J Trauma. 1996;40(4):501–10; discussion 10–2.
16. Hardy BM, King KL, Enninghorst N, Balogh ZJ. Trends in polytrauma incidence among major trauma admissions. Eur J Trauma Emerg Surg. 2022;50:623.
17. King KL, Dewar DC, Briggs GD, Jones M, Balogh ZJ. Postinjury multiple organ failure in polytrauma: more frequent and potentially less deadly with less crystalloid. Eur J Trauma Emerg Surg. 2023;50:131.

18. Andruszkow H, Veh J, Mommsen P, Zeckey C, Hildebrand F, Frink M. Impact of the body mass on complications and outcome in multiple trauma patients: what does the weight weigh? Mediat Inflamm. 2013;2013:345702.
19. Ciesla DJ, Moore EE, Johnson JL, Burch JM, Cothren CC, Sauaia A. Obesity increases risk of organ failure after severe trauma. J Am Coll Surg. 2006;203(4):539–45.
20. Hruby A, Hu FB. The epidemiology of obesity: a big picture. Pharmacoeconomics. 2015;33(7):673–89.
21. Tyagi D, Ting RS, Balogh ZJ. Postinjury multiple organ failure: Proposal of the rare syndrome approach. Injury. 2024;55(7):111599.
22. Devaney GL, Balogh ZJ. We asked the experts: traumatic shock from pelvic trauma: eliminating pelvic hemorrhage-related mortality. World J Surg. 2024;48(1):11–3.
23. Rotondo M, Cribari C, Smith R, American College of Surgeons, Committee on Trauma. Resources for optimal care of the injured patient. Chicago: American College of Surgeons; 2014. p. 6.
24. Kirkpatrick AW, Vis C, Dubé M, Biesbroek S, Ball CG, Laberge J, et al. The evolution of a purpose designed hybrid trauma operating room from the trauma service perspective: the RAPTOR (Resuscitation with Angiography Percutaneous Treatments and Operative Resuscitations). Injury. 2014;45(9):1413–21.
25. Giannoudis PV, Tzioupis C, Pape HC. Fat embolism: the reaming controversy. Injury. 2006;37(Suppl 4):S50–8.
26. Lasanianos NG, Kanakaris NK, Dimitriou R, Pape HC, Giannoudis PV. Second hit phenomenon: existing evidence of clinical implications. Injury. 2011;42(7):617–29.
27. Dewar D, Moore FA, Moore EE, Balogh Z. Postinjury multiple organ failure. Injury. 2009;40(9):912–8.
28. Balogh Z, McKinley BA, Cocanour CS, Kozar RA, Valdivia A, Sailors RM, et al. Supranormal trauma resuscitation causes more cases of abdominal compartment syndrome. Arch Surg. 2003;138(6):637–42; discussion 42.
29. Ting RS, King KL, Lewis DP, Weaver NA, Balogh ZJ. Modifiability of surgical timing in postinjury multiple organ failure patients. World J Surg. 2024;48(2):350–60.
30. King KL, Balogh ZJ. Catchy code names in trauma care cannot replace surgical decision-making. ANZ J Surg. 2023;93(4):802–3.
31. Pape H-C, Giannoudis P, Krettek C. The timing of fracture treatment in polytrauma patients: relevance of damage control orthopedic surgery**This manuscript is dedicated to Harald Tscherne, who has influenced the discussion and the standards of fracture treatment substantially. Am J Surg. 2002;183(6):622–9.
32. Bone LB, Johnson KD, Weigelt J, Scheinberg R. Early versus delayed stabilization of femoral fractures. A prospective randomized study. J Bone Joint Surg Am. 1989;71(3):336–40.
33. Pape HC, Giannoudis PV, Krettek C, Trentz O. Timing of fixation of major fractures in blunt polytrauma: role of conventional indicators in clinical decision making. J Orthop Trauma. 2005;19(8):551–62.
34. Regel G, Grotz M, Weltner T, Sturm JA, Tscherne H. Pattern of organ failure following severe trauma. World J Surg. 1996;20(4):422–9.
35. Tsukamoto T, Chanthaphavong RS, Pape HC. Current theories on the pathophysiology of multiple organ failure after trauma. Injury. 2010;41(1):21–6.
36. Joshi S, Balogh ZJ. Haemoglobin drift or crystalloid flood? ANZ J Surg. 2023;93(7–8):1740–1.
37. Acute Respiratory Distress Syndrome Network, Brower RG, Matthay MA, Morris A, Schoenfeld D, Thompson BT, Wheeler A. Ventilation with lower tidal volumes as compared with traditional tidal volumes for acute lung injury and the acute respiratory distress syndrome. N Engl J Med. 2000;342(18):1301–8.
38. Swol J, Brodie D, Napolitano L, Park PK, Thiagarajan R, Barbaro RP, et al. Indications and outcomes of extracorporeal life support in trauma patients. J Trauma Acute Care Surg. 2018;84(6):831–7.
39. Swol J, Cannon JW, Barbaro RP, Fanning JJ, Zonies D. Extracorporeal membrane oxygenation in Trauma. ASAIO J. 2022;68(4):e62.
40. Zhang Y, Zhang L, Huang X, Ma N, Wang P, Li L, et al. ECMO in adult patients with severe trauma: a systematic review and meta-analysis. Eur J Med Res. 2023;28(1):412.
41. Trivedi JR, Alotaibi A, Sweeney JC, Fox MP, van Berkel V, Adkins K, et al. Use of extracorporeal membrane oxygenation in blunt traumatic injury patients with acute respiratory distress syndrome. ASAIO J. 2022;68(4):e60.
42. Amos T, Bannon-Murphy H, Yeung M, Gooi J, Marasco S, Udy A, et al. ECMO (extra corporeal membrane oxygenation) in major trauma: a 10 year single centre experience. Injury. 2021;52(9):2515–21.
43. Kavi KS, Gall NP. Trauma and syncope: looking beyond the injury. Trauma Surg Acute Care Open. 2023;8(1):e001036.
44. Tran H-V, Charles M, Garrett RC, Kempe PW, Howard CA, Khorgami Z. Ten-year trends in traumatic cardiac injury and outcomes: a trauma registry analysis. Ann Thorac Surg. 2020;110(3):844–8.
45. Uribarri A, Núñez-Gil IJ, Conty DA, Vedia O, Almendro-Delia M, Cambra AD, et al. Short- and long-term prognosis of patients with takotsubo syndrome based on different triggers: importance of the physical nature. J Am Heart Assoc. 2019;8(24):e013701.
46. Ferraris VA, Ferraris SP, Saha SP. The relationship between mortality and preexisting cardiac disease in 5,971 trauma patients. J Trauma Acute Care Surg. 2010;69(3):645.
47. Wall J, Naganathar S, Praditsuktavorn B, Bugg OF, McArthur S, Thiemermann C, et al. Modeling cardiac dysfunction following traumatic hemorrhage injury: impact on myocardial integrity. Front Immunol. 2019;10:2774.

48. Simpson R, Praditsuktavorn B, Wall J, Morales V, Thiemermann C, Tremoleda JL, et al. Myocardial alterations following traumatic hemorrhagic injury. J Trauma Acute Care Surg. 2023;95(4):481–9.
49. Balogh ZJ, Martin A, Van Wessem KP, King KL, Mackay P, Havill K. Mission to eliminate postinjury abdominal compartment syndrome. Arch Surg. 2011;146(8):938–43.
50. Mehta Y, Arora D. Newer methods of cardiac output monitoring. World J Cardiol. 2014;6(9):1022–9.
51. Zonies D, Codner P, Park P, Martin ND, Lissauer M, Evans S, et al. AAST critical care committee clinical consensus: ECMO, nutrition. Trauma Surg Acute Care Open. 2019;4(1):e000304.
52. Burrell A, Kim J, Alliegro P, Romero L, Serpa Neto A, Mariajoseph F, et al. Extracorporeal membrane oxygenation for critically ill adults. Cochrane Database Syst Rev. 2023;9:CD010381.
53. Chlebowski MM, Baltagi S, Carlson M, Levy JH, Spinella PC. Clinical controversies in anticoagulation monitoring and antithrombin supplementation for ECMO. Crit Care. 2020;24(1):19.
54. Kellum JA, Levin N, Bouman C, Lameire N. Developing a consensus classification system for acute renal failure. Curr Opin Crit Care. 2002;8(6):509–14.
55. Wohlauer MV, Sauaia A, Moore EE, Burlew CC, Banerjee A, Johnson J. Acute kidney injury and posttrauma multiple organ failure: the canary in the coal mine. J Trauma Acute Care Surg. 2012;72(2):373–8; discussion 9–80.
56. Eachempati SR, Wang JC, Hydo LJ, Shou J, Barie PS. Acute renal failure in critically ill surgical patients: persistent lethality despite new modes of renal replacement therapy. J Trauma. 2007;63(5):987–93.
57. Kuiper JW, Groeneveld AB, Slutsky AS, Plötz FB. Mechanical ventilation and acute renal failure. Crit Care Med. 2005;33(6):1408–15.
58. Giles T, Weaver N, Varghese A, Way TL, Abel C, Choi P, et al. Acute kidney injury development in polytrauma and the safety of early repeated contrast studies: a retrospective cohort study. J Trauma Acute Care Surg. 2022;93(6):872–81.
59. Tandukar S, Palevsky PM. Continuous renal replacement therapy: who, when, why, and how. Chest. 2019;155(3):626–38.
60. Cordemans C, De Laet I, Van Regenmortel N, Schoonheydt K, Dits H, Huber W, et al. Fluid management in critically ill patients: the role of extravascular lung water, abdominal hypertension, capillary leak, and fluid balance. Ann Intensive Care. 2012;2(Suppl 1 Diagnosis and management of intra-abdominal hyperten):S1.
61. Mehta RL, Pascual MT, Soroko S, Chertow GM, PICARD Study Group. Diuretics, mortality, and nonrecovery of renal function in acute renal failure. JAMA. 2002;288(20):2547–53.
62. Dangleben DA, Jazaeri O, Wasser T, Cipolle M, Pasquale M. Impact of cirrhosis on outcomes in trauma. J Am Coll Surg. 2006;203(6):908–13.
63. Tacke F, Luedde T, Trautwein C. Inflammatory pathways in liver homeostasis and liver injury. Clin Rev Allergy Immunol. 2009;36(1):4–12.
64. Helling TS. The liver and hemorrhagic shock. J Am Coll Surg. 2005;201(5):774–83.
65. Bernal W, Auzinger G, Sizer E, Wendon J. Intensive care management of acute liver failure. Semin Liver Dis. 2008;28(2):188–200.
66. Harry R, Auzinger G, Wendon J. The clinical importance of adrenal insufficiency in acute hepatic dysfunction. Hepatology. 2002;36(2):395–402.
67. Marik PE. Mechanisms and clinical consequences of critical illness associated adrenal insufficiency. Curr Opin Crit Care. 2007;13(4):363–9.
68. Tofteng F, Hauerberg J, Hansen BA, Pedersen CB, Jørgensen L, Larsen FS. Persistent arterial hyperammonemia increases the concentration of glutamine and alanine in the brain and correlates with intracranial pressure in patients with fulminant hepatic failure. J Cereb Blood Flow Metab. 2006;26(1):21–7.
69. Bernal W, Hall C, Karvellas CJ, Auzinger G, Sizer E, Wendon J. Arterial ammonia and clinical risk factors for encephalopathy and intracranial hypertension in acute liver failure. Hepatology. 2007;46(6):1844–52.
70. Larsen FS, Schmidt LE, Bernsmeier C, Rasmussen A, Isoniemi H, Patel VC, et al. High-volume plasma exchange in patients with acute liver failure: an open randomised controlled trial. J Hepatol. 2016;64(1):69–78.
71. Nagaki M, Hughes RD, Keane HM, Lau JY, Williams R. In vitro plasma perfusion through adsorbents and plasma ultrafiltration to remove endotoxin and cytokines. Circ Shock. 1992;38(3):182–8.
72. Schütz T, Bechstein WO, Neuhaus P, Lochs H, Plauth M. Clinical practice of nutrition in acute liver failure--a European survey. Clin Nutr. 2004;23(5):975–82.
73. Charlton M. Branched-chain amino acid enriched supplements as therapy for liver disease. J Nutr. 2006;136(1 Suppl):295s–8s.
74. Plauth M, Cabré E, Riggio O, Assis-Camilo M, Pirlich M, Kondrup J, et al. ESPEN guidelines on enteral nutrition: liver disease. Clin Nutr. 2006;25(2):285–94.
75. Marin A, Hardy G. Practical implications of nutritional support during continuous renal replacement therapy. Curr Opin Clin Nutr Metab Care. 2001;4(3):219–25.
76. Mira JC, Brakenridge SC, Moldawer LL, Moore FA. Persistent inflammation, immunosuppression and catabolism syndrome. Crit Care Clin. 2017;33(2):245–58.
77. Ulvik A, Kvåle R, Wentzel-Larsen T, Flaatten H. Multiple organ failure after trauma affects even long-term survival and functional status. Crit Care. 2007;11(5):R95.
78. Gentile LF, Cuenca AG, Efron PA, Ang D, Bihorac A, McKinley BA, et al. Persistent inflammation and immunosuppression: a common syndrome and new horizon for surgical intensive care. J Trauma Acute Care Surg. 2012;72(6):1491.

79. Gardner AK, Ghita GL, Wang Z, Ozrazgat-Baslanti T, Raymond SL, Mankowski RT, et al. The development of chronic critical illness determines physical function, quality of life, and long-term survival among early survivors of sepsis in surgical ICUs. Crit Care Med. 2019;47(4):566–73.
80. Efron PA, Brakenridge SC, Mohr AM, Barrios EL, Polcz VE, Anton S, et al. The persistent inflammation, immunosuppression, and catabolism syndrome 10 years later. J Trauma Acute Care Surg. 2023;95(5):790.
81. Baum JI, Kim IY, Wolfe RR. Protein consumption and the elderly: what is the optimal level of intake? Nutrients. 2016;8(6):359.
82. Rosenthal MD, Patel J, Staton K, Martindale RG, Moore FA, Upchurch GR Jr. Can specialized pro-resolving mediators deliver benefit originally expected from fish oil? Curr Gastroenterol Rep. 2018;20(9):40.

The Unplanned Return to the Operating Room in Acute Setting

10

Rifat Latifi

Introduction

Most surgical procedures done either electively or even emergently go well, and postoperatively, patients recover nicely. However, despite our best efforts and highest levels of preparation for elective surgery, or even in emergent cases, complications can and do occur, with one or more complications occurring in 16.4% of the patients in various grades [1]. These complications can be simple and easily remedied (grade I), but they can also be serious (grade II and III) and/or fatal (grade IV). On occassions, patients need to be returned to the operating room at once or acutely (bleeding, burst abdomen), or in less urgent basis ,in a semi-planned fashion, but still need reoperation and increases the length of hospital stay (HLOS. In fact, the grading of complications (grades I–V) significantly correlates with the duration of the hospital stay [1]. In this study, the median length of hospitalization in patients without complication was 7 days (range 1–28), while HLOS in patients with complications increases to 14 days (range 1–44 days) when patients developed grade I complications only, 17 days (range 1–68 days) in those with grade II, 20 days (range 5–59 days) in presence of grade IIIa, 23 days (range 4–137 days) in grade IIIb, 26 days (2–74 days) in grade IVa, and, finally, 53 days (14–175 days) in grade IVb complications. The length of hospitalization of patients with grade V was 18 days (1–81 days). Not surprisingly, a strong correlation was found between the complexity of surgery (and assumed higher complication rates) and outcome of surgery, in particular emergency surgery.

The burden and the profile of emergency general surgery (EGS) patients or procedures, likely to have complications, have been studied and reported [2] and have received major attention [3]. In a large study [2] of 421,476 patient encounters associated with operative emergency general surgery (EGS), representing 2.1 million patients over the 4-year study period, the mortality rate was 1.23%, the complication rate was 15.0%, and mean cost per admission was $13 241. The largest contribution to EGS mortality and morbidity burden was attributed to seven operative EGS procedures that collectively accounted for 80.0% of procedures, 80.3% of deaths, 78.9% of complications, and 80.2% of inpatient costs nationwide. These seven procedures included partial colectomy, small-bowel resection, cholecystectomy, operative management of peptic ulcer disease, lysis of peritoneal adhesions, appendectomy, and laparotomy [2].

An unplanned surgery becomes necessary due to various complications arising after the initial or subsequent surgery. These complications can

R. Latifi (✉)
Department of Surgery, The University of Arizona, Tucson, AZ, USA

Tucson Medical Center, Department of Surgery, Tucson, AZ, USA
e-mail: Latifi@surgery.arizona.edu

R. Latifi (ed.), *Surgical Decision-Making*, https://doi.org/10.1007/978-3-031-67391-7_10

include infections, bleeding, organ dysfunction, wound complications, or other unexpected events. However, not all complications have the same impact [4].

The authors of this study of 79,183 patients from ACS-NSQIP database who underwent an EGS procedure found that the most common complications in these patients were bleeding (6.2%), incisional surgical site infection (SSI) (3.4%), pneumonia (2.7%), and organ/space SSI (2.6%). Bleeding was the complication with the greatest overall impact on mortality and end-organ dysfunction. The only other complication with the major impact on mortality was pneumonia. On the other hand, complications such as urinary tract infection, venous thromboembolism, myocardial infarction, and incisional SSI had negligible impacts on these outcomes [4].

Similarly, on the bariatric surgery population, bleeding and leak were the complications with the largest overall effect on end-organ dysfunction, reoperation, and intensive care unit admission after bariatric surgery [5]. Overall serious complications (grades II–VI), for the most part, require unplanned surgical or other intervention – such as minimally invasive intervention by interventional radiology done using ultrasound or CT-guided [6, 7].

Postoperative Complications Requiring Reoperation

The decision to proceed with an unplanned surgery if complication occurs is based on several factors, including the patient's physiologic status, the severity of the complications, what is required to eliminate the complication, and the potential risks and benefits of surgical intervention.

The first thing that the surgeon should do when postoperative complications occur is to determine if returning to the operating room is necessary. Most surgeons, unless it is a true emergency, such as massive bleeding, will work up the patient and decide what to do next. This assessment of the patient should be done by the same operating surgeon whenever possible. This may not be always possible, due to conversion of surgeons into shift doctors and practice changes. If the previous operating surgeon is not available for whatever reason, the "du jour" should contact the operating surgeon. The surgeon assesses the patient's condition and symptoms in detail, conducting physical examinations and deciding on the plan of action. Most often, patients do not need excessive studies and imaging but needs a surgeon's "eye scan."

If, on the other hand, diagnostic investigations are required to determine the underlying cause of the complications, these studies should be done promptly. Source control (bleeding, infection, dehiscence, compartment syndrome) should be also the modus operandi. On occasion, you may need blood work, microbiological cultures, or consultations with other specialists to aid in the accurate diagnosis, and all these tests need to be reviewed by the surgeon.

Often, we need to consult with a multidisciplinary team, but in the end it is the surgeon's decision in collaboration with the patient and family. These conversations should be straightforward, with no ambiguity. Collaboration allows for a comprehensive assessment and a well-informed decision and help with shared surgical decision-making.

Irrespective how slow or how fast you make a decision, you must analyze risk benefits of the procedure by thoroughly considering the potential risks and benefits associated with returning to the operating room, considering factors such as the immediate threat to the patient's condition, the likelihood of successful intervention, the potential for complications during the second surgery, and the overall impact on the patient's long-term outcome.

For all this, you have to be honest and straightforward and speak in the language that the patient and the family understand by explaining the complications, treatment options, associated risks, and potential benefits. Informed consent ensures that the patient is aware of the situation, understands the proposed course of action, and can actively participate in the decision-making process.

Finally if the decision is made to proceed with an (unplanned) surgery, you should have detailed plans A, B, and even C based on the specific approach and how will you deal with the complications. This plan may involve revisiting the surgical site, controlling bleeding, repairing or removing damaged tissue, negotiating the risks associated with anesthesia, and addressing any other issues identified. Intraoperatively, during all cases, but particularly unplanned surgery, you must decide on a resuscitation model and lead this process, based on what you find during in the reoperation, such as asking for blood and blood product or abbreviating the procedure altogether.

Adequate postoperative management plays a vital role in the patient's recovery and outcome; thus the postoperative management including the monitoring, pain management, further resuscitation, nutrition support, length and choice of antibiotics, wound care, and rehabilitation process must be directed by the operating surgeon.

It is important to highlight that the decision to return to the operating room for postoperative complications is made on a case-by-case basis. For younger surgeons and even seasoned surgeons, my advice is to consult other surgeons who may have different views and different clinical judgments and better experience and have collaborative discussions with the team to ensure the best possible care for the patient. The primary consideration is always the patient's safety and well-being. When surgeons are faced with the decision to unplanned return back to the operating room for complications, there are several important considerations they need to keep in mind, but the most important fact is to stay as objective as possible. Although it is difficult to control your emotions and "think straight," not doing so, can lead to more complications. Here is where the value of the second opinion comes in very handy. If not, you risk making the same "error" as before, as illustrated in the following case:

A 43-year-old patient being treated actively for lymphoma had a perforation of mid-small bowel. He undergoes segmental SB resection and damage control laparotomy (DCL). Subsequently he has anastomosis and has undergone reoperation two more times, due to leak of the anastomosis. Finally he becomes critically ill and is taken to the operation room, but they did not see a leak. Temporary abdominal closure (TAC) is performed, and the patient is transferred to another hospital, where he is taken to the operating room for exploration. This surgeon too did not see the stigmata off the leak, looking at the omentum covering the small bowel and the anastomosis, despite the murky fluid around the liver, and decided to re-pack him and bring back in a day or two, as he was still on multiple pressors. The next trip was to the operating room, after the omentum was lifted from the small bowel and large amount of succus became evident. The surgeon, decided to redo the anastomosis for the third time. Fortunately, a senior surgeon walks in the OR and advised for the third time anastomosis in a very sick patient, takes down this anastomosis, and performs an ileostomy and TAC. The direct peritoneal resuscitation (DPR) was initiated and after few more trips to OR, closed his skin only, and the patient recovered very nicely.

The moral of the story in this difficult case is this: if you return to OR yourself on your patient, or you re-explore the patient who has had one or multiple operations and most did not go well, you must start from the beginning. You must explore every cm of the gastrointestinal (GI) tract and every corner of intra-abdominal cavity. The initial surgeon(s) lost objectivity and did not "eye-scan" the anastomosis. The same happen with two other surgeons. The last surgeon, too, fell on the same trap due to lack of experience.

In summary, when the unplanned return to the operating room becomes necessary, such as in the case of early hemorrhage or abdominal catastrophe (our case discussed), there are a number of issues that surgeons need to address.

Discussing the plan with a patient and his/her family as well as other members of the surgical and anesthesia team is paramount. If the situation is clearly emergent, this conversation may not happen preoperatively but needs to occur after the procedure. Other times, the clues are subtle, and the decision to return early to the operating room needs to be taken seriously and in a timely fashion, rather than procrastinating the inevitable. This decision, however, is a combination of experience, intuition, sometimes art, and evidence but always (when possible) should be done by the operating surgeon of the index operation.

Unplanned trips to the operating room are not very common (< 3.5%) [8–10], but all surgeons will encounter these at some point in their careers, and knowing when and how best to perform these operations can make the difference in the survival and outcomes of our patients.

In recent years, a textbook outcome concept [11–13] has become another tool for the measurement of quality in esophagectomy [11], pancreaticoduodenectomy [12], colon cancer [13], and many other conditions. The textbook outcome was recently divided into early and late outcomes [14]. The early textbook outcome was defined as "Discharged from hospital without serious postoperative complications (Clavien–Dindo ≥ grade III; including intra-abdominal sepsis, organ failure, unplanned reoperation or death)." For trauma patients, on the other hand, it was defined as "Discharged from hospital without unexpected transfusion after haemostasis, and no serious postoperative complications (adapted Clavien–Dindo for trauma ≥ grade III; including intra-abdominal sepsis, organ failure, unplanned re-operation on or death)." The longer-term textbook outcome for both non-trauma and trauma was "Achieved the early Textbook Outcome, and restoration of baseline quality of life at 1 year" [14].

Reasons for Reoperative Surgery in the Early Postoperative Period

As mentioned earlier, the need to return to the operating room in the early postoperative period can be for a variety of reasons, and it also depends on the surgical discipline. I will discuss these indications in the acute phase unplanned and planned return to the operating room – that is, immediately or soon after patient is discharged home and later (up to 90 days or later but related to the index operation). While most complications are counted within 30 days of the index operation, we have suggested that we should look past 90 days [15]. In this study of patients undergoing complex abdominal wall reconstruction with biologic mesh, we found that readmitted patients had higher surgical site infections ($p < 0.01$) and wound necrosis ($p = 0.01$). Higher CCI, past or concomitant pelvic surgery, and the presence of enterocutaneous fistula were independent predictors of earlier days to readmission [15].

Examples of type of complications have been described by Claivien's group and are widely cited. The most common causes for acute unplanned surgery [16, 17] have been reported and have been used as a quality indicator for hospitals. In a prospective cohort study for five causes of unplanned reoperations, the authors found that the reasons for unplanned return to operation room were (1) bleeding, (2) infection, (3) wound-related, (4) anastomosis-related, and (5) others, with an overall return rate for an unplanned operations that was 3.5% [17]. The most common procedure requiring unplanned reoperations in this study included colon resection (18% of total reoperations), renal transplant (9%), gastric bypass (6%), and pancreatic resection (6%), which are associated with higher mortality rates: pancreatic resection (33% vs 3.7%; $P = .04$), esophagogastrectomy (100% vs 4.2%; $P = .002$), and laparoscopic Nissen fundoplication (50% vs 0%; $P = .01$). Overall, 91 reoperations (85%) were for complications occurring at the original surgical site, including those related to anastomosis (n = 16), surgical wound (n = 21), infection (n = 16), bleeding (n = 12), and others (n = 26). Patients requiring unplanned reoperation have significantly higher mortality (11.63% vs 5.23%) [16].The unplanned return to operating room rates varies from clinical disciplines [2, 4, 18, 19].

In general, in major abdominal surgeries, one major, albeit, not so frequent, reason of return to the operation room is abdominal dehiscence or burst abdomen. A burst abdomen is a severe surgical complication characterized by the complete or partial separation of the layers of the abdominal incision. This condition usually occurs due to errors in technique of the closure (rare), or when the incision fails to heal properly, resulting in a separation at the surgical site, but the most common reasons are intraperitoneal infection, bleeding, and anastomotic leak.

Poor wound healing and excessive strain on the incision such as sudden forceful movements (coughing perioperatively due to COPD or other reasons) can contribute to an abdominal dehiscence and error in suture technique and need prompt surgical intervention. Early recognition, timely surgical intervention, and diligent postoperative care are crucial for managing this condition and ensuring favorable patient outcomes.

The big question, in these situations, is how does one manage burst abdomen? Keep the patient with an open abdomen management, reclose primarily, or reclose using retention suture or something else? In my practice, how I deal with this difficult problem depends on the reason and etiology of burst abdomen. If there is a major septic cause, I will initiate DPR and return back in few days (3–4 days) for relook and examination (eye scan). If sepsis has been cleared, I will perform complex abdominal wall reconstruction with posterior component separation including cases with burst abdomen [20, 21].

Planned Return to the Operation Room

The planned return to the operating room, such as in cases of continuous surgical management, that is, damage control laparotomy (DCL) or damage control surgery (DCS) in other body compartments (head, chest, extremity), burns, multiple plastic surgery reconstruction, or staged Complex Abominal Wall Reconstruction (CAWR), debridement for necrotizing soft tissue infections, and other planned returns to OR such as vascular or transplant surgery, is common when there is physiologic instability in the patient manifested grossly as the lethal triad of coagulopathy, hypothermia, and acidosis. Damage control surgery (DCS) is used as a temporizing measure to control hemorrhage, prevent ongoing contamination from perforated intestines, and prevent further issues from profound systemic inflammatory response. While the "norm" when to return back is the normalization of end-point resuscitations, one cannot and should wait too long to bring back the patient for another exploration or definitive surgery [22, 23], unless you have initiated DPR [24, 25].

The major tenant of a DCL is that the underlying problems that are leading to the lethal triad need to be corrected. Coagulopathy, acidosis, and hypothermia need to be resolved, if not already corrected before a definitive operation is performed. In the instance of a DCL, temporizing measures are applied to the abdomen, and the patient is taken to the ICU for rewarming, ongoing fluid and blood product resuscitation, and shock management [26].

In the face of major trauma with major edema from resuscitation or with contamination or non-traumatic catastrophe, I start these patients on direct peritoneal resuscitation (DPR) [24, 25], which has shown significant improvement of APACHE-IV score and Acute Physiology Score (APS) in patients with peritonitis/septic abdomen, as well as advances in definitive closure of the abdomen. In our prospectively collected data on 37 patients between August 2020 and October 2021 who underwent DCL with open abdomen after the index operation and DPR, 86% required DCL and DPR due to septic abdomen/bowel ischemia. The median (interquartile range [IQR]) age was 62 years (53–70), 62% were male, and median (IQR) body mass index was 30.0 kg/m2 (25.5–38.4). On DPR initiation, the median (IQR) APACHE-IV score was 48 (33–64), and the median (IQR) Acute Physiology Score (APS) was 31 (18–54). After initiation, the median (IQR) APACHE-IV score and the median (IQR) APS were 39 (21–62) and 19 (11–56), respectively, and both showed significant improvement in survivors ($p < 0.05$). The median (IQR) DPR duration was 4 days (2–8), and primary abdominal closure was achieved in 30 patients (81%). Twenty-four patients (67%) were discharged home/transferred to a rehab center/nursing home. This adjunct technique has become a standard adjunct of DCL for intra-abdominal catastrophe.

Overall, in DCL, depending on the severity of the injury or infection, most of these issues start improving within 12–48 hours of the initial operation. The best time for considering the second operation tends to be in the first 24- to 48-hour window. Prior to the 24-hour window, patients may still be too unstable for an operation, and subjecting them to prolonged surgeries or anesthesia is not advisable. At the same time, waiting longer than 48 hours may increase further morbidity and mortality as it can lead to organ failures, prolonged need for ventilatory support, nutritional deficits, and open abdomens which are a source of fluid loses, and it puts patients at higher risk for serosal injuries, enterocutaneous (EC) fistulas and anastomotic leaks. Loss of domain is also a concern with an open abdomen, and delaying closure of the abdominal wall past 48 hours may lead to large hernias and need for future surgeries for abdominal wall reconstruction, unless you perform CAWR [21].

One exception to the 24- to 48-hour window is when source control has not been established, such as with profound contamination or necrotizing soft tissue infections or in the case of ongoing hemorrhage. Often in these cases, patients continue to do poorly or worsen in the first 12 hours after the initial operation, and they may need a second procedure sooner to establish better source control or complete disruption of infectious cascade. In these cases, the risk of a second surgery is less than the risk of death from ongoing septic shock, and a second operation should be performed before 12 hours.

Infection Complications: Source Control

Unfortunately, despite having perioperative optimization, infectious complications such as wound infection and other intra-abdominal catastrophes do occur [27]. One major cause of intra-abdominal catastrophes is anastomotic leaks that range anywhere from 3% to 15% of all bowel anastomoses [28–32] and have high morbidity and mortality if not addressed immediately. Most anastomotic failures occur around days 3–7 after initial resection and anastomosis and have been described as early leaks (<5 days) [32], but some of these anastomotic leaks occur at a later time [33]. In this study of 1223 patients, the leaks occurred in 33 patients (2.7%), diagnosed in the majority of cases within a mean of 12.7 days postoperatively, but 4 patients (12.1%) were diagnosed past postoperative day > 30. A total of 14 of 33 (42%) patients had their leak diagnosed only after readmission. Fifteen patients required fecal diversion, whereas 18 were managed non-operatively. There have been other cases reported though, of late anastomotic failures occurring weeks after the primary operation [33].

The intestinal leaks have been classified [34]. Grade A anastomotic leakage results in no change in patients' management, whereas grade B leakage requires active therapeutic intervention but is manageable without re-laparotomy. Grade C anastomotic leakage requires re-laparotomy. Management of this dreaded complication can range anywhere from observation to percutaneous drainage to the need for unplanned surgery. While some surgeons hesitate to go back in grades A and B and attempt to use "conservative management," I believe that the best approach is to return to OR, revise the anastomosis altogether if needed, and lavage the abdomen, because there is a real possibility that these leaks actually will develop in full disruption or cause major peritonitis, and prolong hospital stay. If you decide to return to the operating room, definitely do not "just place another suture or two." If, on the other hand, you do not have an experience with complex reoperative surgery, or you do not have the required resources available to you in your institution, transfer a patient to another surgeon and or institution.

Missed Enterotomies

Another rare complications, requiring unplanned return to the operating room, are missed enterotomies or incomplete or improperly fixed enterotomy, either from open or a laparoscopic lysis of adhesions (most commonly). These injuries declare themselves within 24–48 hours from surgery, and intra-abdominal abscesses typically present about 5–7 days from surgery. Some may end up inspetic shock. There should be a surgical approach just like the one I described above for anastomosis leak, although some do have expectant management with antibiotics, serial abdominal exams, and drain placement by interventional radiologists [35, 36]. Any patient who becomes septic or goes into septic shock after intra-abdominal surgery for example for small bowel or large bowel surgery, the major intestinal leak is number 1, number 2 and number 3 potential reason, thus immediate complete exploration is mandatory. It is not myocardial infarction; you do not need a CT scan, but you need an "eye scan."

If you decide that your patient is a candidate for observant management (this author rarely recommends), you need to be vigilant to continually reassess for any clinical worsening or instability, and you the senior surgeon (not your intern or medical student) need to examine the patient.

If at any point your patient displays any worsening of clinical exam, the patient needs to be operated upon immediately, because anastomotic leaks, intra-abdominal infections, or missed enterotomies can be life-threatening and definitely will seriously prolong hospital stay, particularly in elderly patients. In summary of this section, if the patient in the postoperative period has any hemodynamic instability, severe acidosis, or shock, re-exploration should be performed as soon as possible. Immediate source control is necessary, with or without temporary diverting ostomy as needed.

Postoperative Hemorrhage: Need to Stop the Bleeding

Bleeding can and does occur in the perioperative period. Typically, bleeding will present or recur within the first few hours to days from surgery. The mainstay of treatment depends on a number of factors – hemodynamic stability of the patient, resources available in your institution (blood bank, for example), the location, and the cause of the bleeding.

Postoperative hemorrhage can be from a number of sources, and identifying the source can often help determine which management will be appropriate. In the instance of arterial bleeding, these patients are often acutely unstable, showing evidence of hemorrhagic shock, and transiently respond to blood transfusions. In these cases, the patient needs to be brought back for an immediate reoperation or embolization by a trained team [37]. If you do decide to proceed with embolization, you need to be constantly monitoring your patient and providing aggressive resuscitation with blood and blood products. If at any point your patient is no longer responding to blood transfusions or medical management in the preparation of doing an embolization procedure, then the patient should be taken immediately for the operating room. Occasionally, postoperative hemorrhage can be due to venous bleeding or oozing from raw operative surfaces. Typically, patients with this type of bleeding will be more responsive to resuscitation with blood and coagulation factors and overall tend to be more hemodynamically stable, although not always. This type of bleeding is not amenable to direct surgical or interventional radiology interventions; therefore the options for management are observation vs. re-exploration. In severe bleeding from the retroperitoneum raw surface, packing with one of several hemostatic agents, resuscitation with balanced transfusions, utilizing clotting factors, allowing for mild permissive hypotension, and correction of coagulopathies. If the patient responds to resuscitation, I would consider observation and correction of coagulation factors. A repeat operation often may not identify the source of bleeding, and patient needs to be packed and his or her coagulopathy reversed. There may be a role of nonselective angio-embolization for the management of venous bleeding, especially in the setting of pelvic injury or surgery with ongoing hemorrhage. Access to the region can be difficult, and identification of the source of bleeding can often be near impossible with an open procedure. This technique has gained a lot of attention in the literature in recent years and involves nonselective embolization of the feeding artery with a temporary substance.

The site where the operative bleeding is occurring from can also be a guide to management. In the case that the bleeding is coming from the pelvis, a strong consideration should be for intervention radiological (IR) intervention to address this. As previously discussed, access and visibility within the pelvis can often be difficult, even in the situation of an open laparotomy. Preperitoneal packing may be required as well.

If the bleeding occurs from the intestines or a staple line from a bowel resection, reoperation is required. The use of embolization for the management of bleeding after an anastomosis should not be done. Embolization, either selective or nonselective, can compromise blood flow to the area of the healing anastomosis. If this occurs, an anastomotic leak or breakdown can occur and would lead to life-threatening complications. Also, expanding hematomas in and around the intestines could lead to compression of the lumen and bowel obstructions. In this instance, re-exploration is recommended.

Early Bowel Obstruction: When Waiting Is No Longer an Option

The most common long-term unplanned reason for reoperation after abdominal surgery is adhesive small bowel disease. Just the opening of the peritoneal cavity leads to adhesions forming in 95% of patients. Of this, approximately 4% of all patients who undergo abdominal surgery will go on to have a clinically significant bowel obstruction. These obstructions often occur months to years after an operation. Occasionally, these obstructions occur within the first few days to weeks after initial surgery. It has been reported that 30% of all bowel obstructions occur within the first 30 days of surgery, but the way to manage is debated [38].

Adhesion formation occurs from a local response of the peritoneum and serosa to ischemia, desiccation, and trauma that can originate from the primary disease process or surgery itself (contact with instruments, gloves, sponges, suture, or other irritants). When this occurs, the normally fluid bowel can become twisted or kinked leading to a bowel obstruction. Adhesions and inflammation tend to be at their worst at 14 days to 1-month post-op and then slowly improve over months.

Post-op ileus is unfortunately a frequently encountered condition after intra-abdominal surgery. The symptoms of ileus (distention, lack of flatus, belching, abdominal pain, nausea, and vomiting) mimic the bowel obstruction. It is recommended that to start, nasogastric (NG) tube decompression and bowel rest should be utilized. A GI imaging, starting first with abdominal X-ray and then a CT scan with oral contrast versus small bowel follow-through, looking for potential sources of obstruction, should be performed if symptoms persist. If a diagnosis of ileus is decided, watchful waiting is recommended. Typically, this will resolve within 3–7 days. Surgeons should try to "restrain" themselves and manage the patient, family, and your own team.

In the setting of an early small bowel obstruction, the majority of these will also resolve within 7–14 days after initial surgery. A study by Chessin et al. showed that the need for reoperation on early small bowel obstruction was only 0.8% [39].

With that being said, though, if a bowel obstruction persists beyond 14 days post-op, the likelihood it will resolve without a reoperation is extremely low, <10% (39 Pickleman) [40], and reoperation should be strongly considered. With these statistics in mind, if imaging reveals that a patient has a bowel obstruction, especially within the first 10 days of surgery, it would be recommended to proceed with watchful waiting and conservative management including NG tube decompression, limitation of narcotics, parenteral nutrition, and serial abdominal exams, as the majority of these will resolve with this treatment. One point that is extremely important to remember, though, is if at any point, the patient shows evidence of bowel ischemia (increasing abdominal pain, elevated white blood cell (WBC), increasing lactate, evidence of sepsis), immediate operative intervention should be undertaken to prevent irreversible bowel death and or perforation.

One hot topic that continues to be debatable in the ligature and in the corridors of surgical wards is the question does water-soluble contrast medium (gastrografin) decrease the need for operative intervention nor the duration of hospital stay in uncomplicated acute adhesive small bowel obstruction? While some have suggested that it is a safe and effective treatment and correlated with a significant reduction in the need for surgery and in the length of hospital stay [41], others report results of the present study, and those of our systematic review suggest that gastrografin administration is of no benefit in patients with adhesive small bowel obstruction [42]. Despite the debate, it is a common practice to use water-soluble contrast in these patients [43].

Summary

The need for early unplanned surgery after intra-abdominal surgery is rare but can be due to multiple different etiologies, with bleeding, as the most common cause.

References

1. Dhindo D, Demartines N, Clavien PA. Classification of surgical complications: a new proposal with evaluation in a cohort of 6336 patients and results of a survey. Ann Surg. 2004;240(2):205–13. https://doi.org/10.1097/01.sla.0000133083.54934.ae. PMID: 15273542; PMCID: PMC1360123
2. Scott JW, Olufajo OA, Brat GA, Rose JA, Zogg CK, Haider AH, Salim A, Havens JM. Use of national burden to define operative emergency general surgery. JAMA Surg. 2016;151(6):e160480. https://doi.org/10.1001/jamasurg.2016.0480. Epub 2016 Jun 15. PMID: 27120712
3. Paul MG. The public health crisis in emergency general surgery: who will pay the price and bear the burden? JAMA Surg. 2016;151(6):e160640. https://doi.org/10.1001/jamasurg.2016.0640.
4. Scarborough JE, Schumacher J, Pappas TN, McCoy CC, Englum BR, Agarwal SK Jr, Greenberg CC. Which complications matter most? Prioritizing quality improvement in emergency general surgery. J Am Coll Surg. 2016;222(4):515–24. https://doi.org/10.1016/j.jamcollsurg.2015.12.038. Epub 2016 Jan 14. PMID: 26916129; PMCID: PMC5131647
5. Daigle CR, et al. Which postoperative complications matter most after bariatric surgery? Prioritizing quality improvement efforts to improve national outcomes. Surg Obes Relat Dis. 2018;14(5):652–7. https://doi.org/10.1016/j.soard.2018.01.008. Epub 2018 Jan 12
6. Zhao N, et al. CT-guided special approaches of drainage for intraabdominal and pelvic abscesses: One single center's experience and review of literature. Medicine (Baltimore). 2018;97(42):e12905. https://doi.org/10.1097/MD.0000000000012905. PMID: 30335020; PMCID: PMC6211865
7. Ballard DH, Gates MC, Hamidian Jahromi A, Harper DV, Do DV, D'Agostino HB. Transrectal and transvaginal catheter drainages and aspirations for management of pelvic fluid collections: technique, technical success rates, and outcomes in 150 patients. Abdom Radiol (NY). 2019;44(7):2582–93. https://doi.org/10.1007/s00261-019-01974-9. PMID: 30868244; PMCID: PMC6561799
8. Lepor H, Nieder AM, Ferrandino MN. Intraoperative and post-operative complications of radical retropubic prostatectomy in a consecutive series of 1,000 cases. J Urol. 2001;166(5):1729–33.
9. Nelson J. Reoperations within the first 30 days after pelvic surgery. In: Billingham RP, Kobashi K, Peters WA, editors. Reoperative pelvic surgery. New York: Springer; 2009.
10. Augustin T, Aminian A, Romero-Talamas H, Rogula T, Schauer PR, Brethauser SA. Reoperative surgery for management of early complications after gastric bypass. Obes Surg. 2015:1–5.
11. Buchholz V, et al. Textbook outcomes after oesophagectomy: a single-centre observational study. BMC Surg. 2023;23(1):368. https://doi.org/10.1186/s12893-023-02253-7. PMID: 38066440; PMCID: PMC10704701
12. Kulshrestha S, et al. Textbook oncologic outcome in pancreaticoduodenectomy: Do regionalization efforts make sense? J Surg Oncol. 2022;125(3):414–24. https://doi.org/10.1002/jso.26712. Epub 2021 Oct 7. PMID: 34617590; PMCID: PMC8799483
13. Yang CC, Tian YF, Liu WS, Chou CL, Cheng LC, Chu SS, Lee CC. The association between the composite quality measure "textbook outcome" and long term survival in operated colon cancer. Medicine (Baltimore). 2020;99(40):e22447. https://doi.org/10.1097/MD.0000000000022447. PMID: 33019430; PMCID: PMC7535643
14. Naumann DN, Bhangu A, Brooks A, Martin M, Cotton BA, Khan M, Midwinter MJ, Pearce L, Bowley DM, Holcomb JB, Griffiths EA, BEACON Collaborative. Novel textbook outcomes following emergency laparotomy: delphi exercise. BJS Open. 2024;8(1):zrad145. https://doi.org/10.1093/bjsopen/zrad145.
15. Gogna S, Latifi R, Choi J, Con J, Prabhakaran K, Smiley A, Anderson PL. Predictors of 30- and 90-day readmissions after complex abdominal wall reconstruction with biological mesh: a longitudinal study of 232 patients. World J Surg. 2020;44(11):3720–8. https://doi.org/10.1007/s00268-020-05714-9. Epub 2020 Jul 30
16. Kao F-C, et al. Risk factors for unplanned return to the operating room within 24 hours: a 9-year single-center observational study. Medicine. 2021;100(49):e28053. 10.1097/MD.0000000000028053
17. Birkmeyer JD, Hamby LS, Birkmeyer CM, Decker MV, Karon NM, Dow RW. Is unplanned return to the operating room a useful quality indicator in general surgery? Arch Surg. 2001;136(4):405–11. https://doi.org/10.1001/archsurg.136.4.405).
18. Gale SC, Shafi S, Dombrovskiy VY, Arumugam D, Crystal JS. The public health burden of emergency general surgery in the United States: a 10-year analysis of the Nationwide Inpatient Sample—2001 to 2010. J Trauma Acute Care Surg. 2014;77(2):202–8.
19. Ogola GO, Gale SC, Haider A, Shafi S. The financial burden of emergency general surgery: national estimates 2010 to 2060. J Trauma Acute Care Surg. 2015;79(3):444–8.

20. Kajmolli A, Azim A, McGuirk M, Prabhakaran K, Samson DJ, Rhee P, Latifi R. Early abdominal wall reconstruction with biologic mesh is feasible after catastrophic abdominal wall disruption from blunt trauma. Surg Technol Int. 2021;38:193–8. https://doi.org/10.52198/21.STI.38.HR1435. PMID: 33830494
21. Gogna S, Latifi R, Choi J, Con J, Prabhakaran K, Anderson PL, Policastro AJ, Klein J, Samson DJ, Smiley A, Rhee P. Early versus delayed complex abdominal wall reconstruction with biologic mesh following damage-control surgery. J Trauma Acute Care Surg. 2021;90(3):527–34. https://doi.org/10.1097/TA.0000000000003011.).
22. Sharrock AE, Barker T, Yuen HM, Rickard R, Tai N. Management and closure of the open abdomen after damage control laparotomy for trauma. A systematic review and meta-analysis. Injury. 2015;
23. Dubose JJ, Scalea TM, Holcomb JB, Shrestha B, Okoye O, Inaba K, Bee TK, Fabian TC, Whealan J, Ivatury RR. AAST open abdomen study group. J Trauma Acute Care Surg. 2013;74(1):113–20.
24. Okumura K, Latifi R, Smiley A, Lee JS, Shnaydman I, Zangbar B, Bronstein M, Con J, Prabhakaran K, Rhee P, Klein J, Shivaraj K, Klein MD, Miller DM. Direct Peritoneal Resuscitation (DPR) improves Acute Physiology and Chronic Health Evaluation (APACHE) IV and acute physiology score when used in damage control laparotomies: prospective cohort study on 37 patients. Surg Technol Int. 41:sti41/1620. https://doi.org/10.52198/22.STI.41.GS1620. Epub ahead of print
25. McGuirk M, Kajmolli A, Gachabayov M, Haider A, Bronstein M, Spatz D, Gwardshaladse C, Latifi R. Use of direct peritoneal resuscitation for intra-abdominal catastrophes: a technical note. Surg Technol Int. 2020;37:127–31.
26. Jenoff JS, Kim P. Management of the difficult abdomen and damage control surgery. In: Flint L, Meridith JW, Schwab CW, Trunkey DD, Rue LW, Taheri PA, editors. Trauma: contemporary principles and therapy. Philadelphia: Lippincott Williams & Wilkins; 2008.
27. Kassahun CW, Melekamu S, Alemu MT. Clinical anastomosis leakage and associated factors among patients who had intestinal anastomosis in northwest referral hospitals, Ethiopia. PLoS One. 2022;17(12):e0275536. https://doi.org/10.1371/journal.pone.0275536. PMID: 36584017; PMCID: PMC9803163
28. Brundage SI, Jurkovich GJ, Hoyt DB, Patel NY, Ross SE, Marburger R, Stoner M, Ivatury RR, Ku J, Rutherfort EJ, Maier RV. Stapled versus sutured gastrointestinal anastomoses in the trauma patient: a multicenter trial. J Trauma Acute Care Surg. 2001;51:1054–61.
29. Catena F, La Donna M, Gagliardi S, Avanzolini A, Taffurelli M. Stapled versus hand-sewn anastomosis in emergency intestinal surgery: results of a prospective randomized study. Surg Today. 2004;34:123–6.
30. Farrah JP, Lauer CW, Bray MS, McCartt JM, Chang MC, Meredith JW, Miller PR, Mowery NT. Stapled versus hand-sewn anastomosis in emergency general surgery: a restrospective review of outcomes in a unique patient population. J Trauma Acute Care Surg. 2013;74(5):1187–94.
31. Shekarriz H, Eigenwald J, Shekarriz B, Upadhyay J, Shekarriz J, Zoubie D, Wedel T, Wittenburg H. Anastomotic leak in colorectal surgery: are 75% preventable? Int J Colorectal Dis. 2015;30(11):1523–31.
32. Li YW, Lian P, Huang B, Zheng HT, Wang MH, Gu WL, Li XX, Xu Y, Cai SJ. Very early colorectal anastomotic leakage within 5 post-operative days: a more severe subtype needs relaparatomy. Sci Rep. 2017;7:39936. https://doi.org/10.1038/srep39936. PMID: 28084305; PMCID: PMC5233968
33. Hyman N, Manchester TL, Osler T, Burns B, Cataldo PA. Anastomotic leaks after intestinal anastomosis: it's later than you think. Ann Surg. 2007;245(2):254–8. https://doi.org/10.1097/01.sla.0000225083.27182.85. PMID: 17245179; PMCID: PMC1876987
34. Rahbari NN, Weitz J, Hohenberger W, Heald RJ, Moran B, Ulrich A, Holm T, Wong WD, Tiret E, Moriya Y, Laurberg S, den Dulk M, van de Velde C, Büchler MW. Definition and grading of anastomotic leakage following anterior resection of the rectum: a proposal by the International Study Group of Rectal Cancer. Surgery. 2010;147(3):339–51. https://doi.org/10.1016/j.surg.2009.10.012. Epub 2009 Dec 11. PMID: 20004450
35. Nicksa GA, Dring RV, Johnson KH, et al. Anastomotic leaks: what is the best diagnostic imaging study? Dis Colon Rectum. 2007;50(2):197–203.
36. Gray M, Marland JRK, Murray AF, Argyle DJ, Potter MA. Predictive and diagnostic biomarkers of anastomotic leakage: a precision medicine approach for colorectal cancer patients. J Personal Med. 2021;11(6):471. https://doi.org/10.3390/jpm11060471.
37. Young JL, Lachance JA, Rice LW, Foley EF. Reoperation and management of postoperative pelvic hemorrhage and coagulopathy. In: Billingham RP, Kobashi K, Peters WA, editors. Reoperative pelvic surgery. New York: Springer; 2009.
38. Duron JJ, Da Silva NJ, Tezenas du Montcel S, Berger A, Muscari F, Hennet H, Veyrieres M, Hay JM. Adhesive postoperative small bowel obstruction: incidence and risk factors of recurrence after surgical treatment. Ann Surg. 2006;244:750–7.
39. Chessin DB, Enker BD, Wong WD, Guillem JG. Complications after preoperative combined modality therapy and radical resection of locally advanced rectal cancer: a 14 year experience from a specialty service. J Am Coll Surg. 2005;200:876–82.
40. Pickleman J, Lee RM. The management of patients with suspected early postoperative small bowel obstruction. Ann Surg. 1989;210(2):216–9.
41. Ceresoli M, Coccolini F, Catena F, Montori G, Di Saverio S, Sartelli M, Ansaloni L. Water-soluble contrast agent in adhesive small bowel obstruction: a systematic review and meta-analysis of diagnostic and therapeutic value. Am J Surg. 2016;211(6):1114–25.

https://doi.org/10.1016/j.amjsurg.2015.06.012. Epub 2015 Aug 12
42. Scotté M, Mauvais F, Bubenheim M, Cossé C, Suaud L, Savoye-Collet C, Plenier I, Péquignot A, Yzet T, Regimbeau JM. Use of water-soluble contrast medium (gastrografin) does not decrease the need for operative intervention nor the duration of hospital stay in uncomplicated acute adhesive small bowel obstruction? A multicenter, randomized, clinical trial (Adhesive Small Bowel Obstruction Study) and systematic review. Surgery. 2017;161(5):1315–25. https://doi.org/10.1016/j.surg.2016.11.026. Epub 2017 Jan 10
43. Cohen RB, Olafson SN, Krupp J, Parsikia A, Kaplan MJ, Moran B, Leung PS. Timing of gastrografin administration in the management of adhesive small bowel obstruction (ASBO): does it matter? Surgery. 2021;170(2):596–602. https://doi.org/10.1016/j.surg.2021.03.008. Epub 2021 Apr 6

11 Surgical Decision-Making in Complex Clinical Scenarios in Abdominal Surgery: A Case-Based Discussion and Approach to the Eight Most Common Problems with Nine Patients

Trista Rosing and Rifat Latifi

Introduction

Acute care surgery has become a well-recognized model of surgical emergency care mostly delivered by trauma and general surgeons. In fact, it is nothing else but surgery in the emergency setting that has been done for centuries, but now it is performed, by general surgeons, or, in the case of the USA, by trauma and general surgeons more commonly. In emergency surgery, surgical decision-making is often fast-paced and high-stake, as we surgeons must quickly assess the patient's condition, determine the most appropriate course of action, and proceed with the surgical intervention to address the urgent medical issue. This process requires a combination of clinical expertise, critical thinking, and the ability to make quick, informed decisions under pressure to ensure the best possible outcome for the patient. Surgeons must weigh factors such as the patient's overall health, the severity of the condition, and the risks and benefits of different treatment options in order to provide timely and effective care in emergency situations.

There are a number of major and complex issues that we surgeons deal with, particularly we the "acute care surgeons" when you have little support in the middle of the night. In this chapter, we will review some of the most complex and difficult conditions of common clinical scenarios that we face and where surgical decision-making requires both intuition and experience and of course an open-minded approach.

Postoperative Enterocutaneous Fistulas

Patient # 1*

You get a phone call from your resident that the patient you performed an emergency abdominal exploration who presented with mechanical intestinal obstruction due to severe adhesive disease had small bowel gangrene requiring resection and handsewn anastomosis, 7 days earlier. Your resident continues; well he has murky fluid coming out of the lower portion of the incision, but "do not worry, he looks good, although his

T. Rosing
Abrazo Health Network General Surgery Residency, Phoenix, AZ, USA

R. Latifi (✉)
Department of Surgery, The University of Arizona, Tucson, AZ, USA

Tucson Medical Center, Department of Surgery, Tucson, AZ, USA
e-mail: Latifi@surgery.arizona.edu

R. Latifi (ed.), *Surgical Decision-Making*, https://doi.org/10.1007/978-3-031-67391-7_11

body temperature is slightly up, and the WBC count is 17,000 this morning." You know exactly what will happen next. Or at least you fear you know what will happen next: fascial dehiscence, due to a missed intestinal injury that you caused while dissecting those severe adhesions. What else it could be? Multiple fistulas, but why?

** Several patients used as examples have been created for illustrations, and some are real.*

How many times have you taught your residents and students that wound infection and dehiscence are almost always from the intra-abdominal infection, and not simply from the superficial wound infection? But those infections, followed by the dehiscence or burst abdomen almost always have happened in the patients of "your partners," right? Now it may be your turn. The next phone call confirms all your fears: multiple fluid collections filled with air, too many to be drained percutaneously. To make things even worse, you are at a conference or perhaps on vacation with your family. Your rule is to never do a "big case" before leaving town, but this happened to be an emergency when you were last on-call overnight.

Enterocutaneous fistulas (ECFs) are arguably one of the most complex issues a surgeon can treat, and given that more than three-quarters of fistulas are postoperative complications, surgeons also play a major role in their origin [1]. Fortuitously, the overall incidence of ECF is low [2], but their etiology varies, and unfortunately there is a lack of randomized clinical trials in the literature, and therefore management guidelines tend to be based upon expert opinion rather than evidence-based, Grade A recommendations. A 15-year study reviewing the application of the SOWATS treatment guideline (comprised of *s*epsis, *o*ptimization of nutritional state, *w*ound care, *a*natomy (of the fistula), *t*iming of surgery, and *s*urgical strategy) in 135 patients treated for ECFs demonstrated an overall closure rate of 87.4% (n = 118) [3]. Spontaneous closure occurred in 21 of patients, usually those with an intact abdominal wall and on total parenteral nutrition (TPN), while surgical closure was achieved in the remaining 97 individuals [3]. Our surgical group has expanded the SOWATS guideline to nine steps, and we call it "ISOWATS PL," where the additional components are I, identification and diagnosis of postoperative fistula; P, postoperative care; and L, long-term follow-up [4].

While the reported mortality rate resulting from treating ECFs has dropped from 44% in 1960 [5] to around less than 10% presently [6], patients with ECFs still present the most difficult and complex challenge to any patient and a general surgeon. Despite the developments in surgical techniques, wound care, nutritional support, and overall intensive and surgical care, patients with high-output fistulas (>500 ml/d) are still at risk of severe malnutrition, bloodstream catheter-related sepsis, intra-abdominal sepsis, and death [2, 7]. Dealing with ECF or entero-atmospheric fistula (EAF) is considerably complex and will test the skills of even the most experienced surgeon [8].

Identification and Diagnosis of Fistulas

The diagnosis, that is the early identification of the fistulas, needs to be established in a timely fashion and without much delay, while the presentation depends on the clinical situation [9]. The cause of postoperative wound infections and abdominal dehiscence is not straightforward, and one has to fear intra-abdominal catastrophe before "blaming" technical reasons for suture failure of the closure. The first cause of abdominal wound dehiscence, with or without fistula after the creation of a single or multiple anastomoses, with or without lysis of adhesions, should be sought in some other sort of abdominal catastrophe, such as severe infection (abscess), due to missed injury or anastomotic leak.

The choice of action to take, while resuscitation is ongoing, is to prepare for emergent return to the operating room (my practice, in the majority of such cases) or obtain a computerized tomography (CT) scan. What is really needed is, what I call it, an "eye-scan," which is an intraoperative evaluation and correction of whatever the cause is. We prefer that in fresh postoperative patients, wound exploration should be done in the operating room in order to completely assess the wound (as well as the subfascial collections and intestines lying under the sutures, which could easily erode into the lumen and cause new fistulas). However, most of these patients in practice receive a CT scan as well, although magnetic resonance imaging (MRI) is also being increasingly used [10]. The CT scan or MRI will identify any deep peritoneal or pelvic collections that could be drained, guided by CT, MRI, or ultrasound. In the first few postoperative days (and in my experience the first 10–14 days), one should not hesitate to take the patient back to the operating room for an exploration and direct assessment, if clinically warranted.

Over the years, the senior author (RL) has observed an interesting phenomenon in surgeons' behavior. As surgeons, we not only behave differently in novel situations, but we also vary our behavior in the same scenarios with different patients. The best examples are among acute care surgeons or trauma surgeons. When a trauma patient is not doing well postoperatively, we, the trauma surgeons, immediately think that we have missed an injury or there is something new happening and take the patient back to the operating room for an "eye-scan" exploration. And we do that exact thing, most of the time. Yet, when we perform an elective surgery, or even emergency general surgery, such as the patient with elective colostomy take-down described later on in this chapter, and they develop a severe complication like a wound infection, even with questionable fascial integrity, we hesitate and use any possible imaging technique to avoid returning to the operating room, often causing significant delays in dealing with the problem at hand. I cannot entirely explain such a change in a surgeon's behavior. Perhaps it is an ego thing.

The basic treatment strategy for patients with acute postoperative wound dehiscence, severe soft tissue infections, or simple wound infections, as well as of those with ECFs (and/or EAFs) includes source control, proper antibiotic therapy, electrolyte and fluid normalization, correction of coagulation factors and hemoglobin levels, achievement of hemodynamic stability, and provision of nutritional support while the patient undergoes diagnostic or therapeutic interventions, or simply being observed for any reason. In the last few decades, the achievement of sepsis and source control has undergone significant changes [8].

Provision and Optimization of Nutrition in Patient with Fistula

Initiating, maintaining, and optimizing the nutrition for patients with fistulas or other postoperative complications are not easy matters either. Let us consider our patient with the take-down colostomy again. Most of us have changed the practice when we do straightforward colon surgery. We no longer leave a nasogastric (NG) tube in for 7 days, starving the patient until the gastrointestinal function is returned postoperatively before initiating oral or enteral nutrition. Yet, when we lyse adhesions, but particularly when we perform small bowel resection, even if we do not leave an NG tube, we often will not advance the feeding for days.

The patient from our example was barely started on a clear liquid diet by day 5. On the 6th postoperative day, he was not feeling well, and now you receive the call on day 7. At this point, the patient has developed complications, and this process of starvation will be prolonged ever further. One has to remember that we should initiate and maintain nutritional therapy enterally or parenterally throughout the hospitalization. However, in a very busy practice, it is easily forgotten that a patient who underwent a major surgical operation needs aggressive nutritional support.

Management for Fistulas

One of the most important elements in the management of complex open wounds, with or without fistula and/or stomas, is continuous wound care and reduction of the overall infectious bioburden. Therefore, avoiding skin excoriations from the bile salts, intestinal fluids, or stool is essential. The vacuum-assisted closure (VAC) and proper stoma equipment have revolutionized wound care; how-

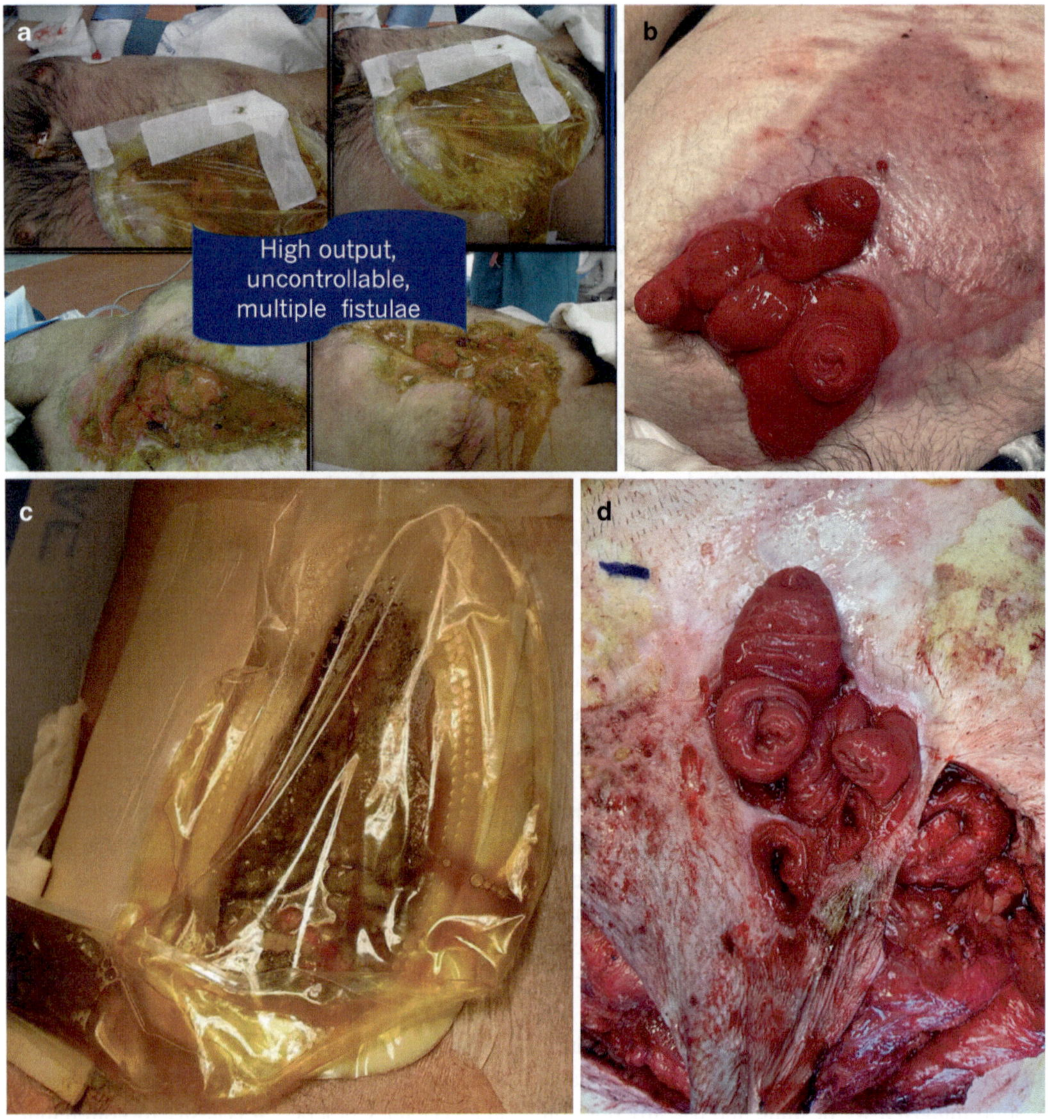

Fig. 11.1 (**a–c**) "Fistula City"—these types of fistulas need surgical resection, as they will not close otherwise. (Courtesy of Dr. Latifi)

ever, collecting all the fluids from patients with large open abdominal wall defects (which the senior author (RL) has termed "a fistula city") (Fig. 11.1) may prove extremely difficult. Controlling sepsis, providing adequate wound care and tissue coverage (native or biologic) of the abdominal wall, and maintaining nutritional support will result in patient improvement. They may of course eventually develop a major hernia that also needs to be fixed at a later time. One major aspect of this surgical decision-making process is the involvement of the patient and their families in every aspect of care. Remember, the patient is the main decision-maker in this triangle consisting of the disease process, the patient (and their families), and the surgeon. We need to make sure that all involved work together to both inform and empower the patient, while we the surgeons continue to advise the patient and family and implement the shared decisions.

The biggest question in the treatment of fistulas is the timing of surgery. Factors that favor surgical treatment of a fistula include high output and the presence of multiple fistulas [1]. To reestablish intestinal continuity, the bowel segment giving rise to the fistula is resected, and some have recommended long intestinal tube stenting of the entire small bowel afterward [11]. The surgery for ECFs should be timed after sepsis has been addressed and nutritional status improved, but there are cases when neither intra-abdominal infections nor malnutrition will not resolve until you resolve the source of the problem. In order to protect the surrounding skin from the caustic effects of intestinal contents, the output of the fistula needs to be controlled [12]. Patients who develop a fistula at the anastomosis (Fig. 11.2a,b) or elsewhere, following dense adhesions release, in the perioperative phase, should be operated on at once. That segment of the intestines should be resected completely and never close with just one or two stitches. For patients with an abdominal wound that cannot immediately be closed and are at high risk for complications, a vacuum-assisted closure (VAC) device can be utilized both pre- and postoperatively and maintained on a continuous mode with a negative pressure high enough to keep a good seal, between 50 and 75. The wound dressings should be changed daily, but use of wound VAC devices reduces the frequency of required dressing changes [7, 12]. For high-output ECFs, a 10-year review of vacuum-compaction devices demonstrated that the treatment was effective in controlling output among 89 out of 91 (97.8%) patients, with output being entirely suppressed within a week for 37 patients (40.7%), and spontaneous closure being achieved in 42 patients (46.2%) [2]. Knowing the anatomy of the fistula is also important to the surgeon, as visualization of the complete bowel tract and the length and quality of the remaining bowel are mandatory [3]. The incidence of spontaneous closure for a fistula is greater when there is a greater distance between the bowel and the skin and when etiologic factors of the fistula are corrected [7].

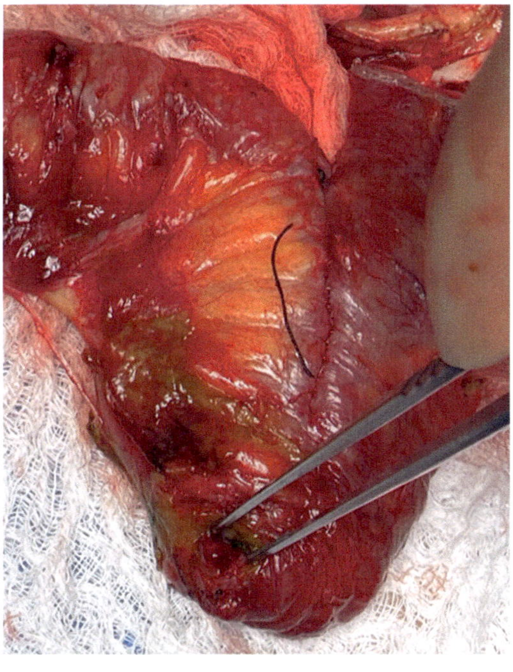

Fig. 11.2 (**a**) Post-operative leak, identified on CT scan, postoperative day # 6 and operated immediately with takedown complete stapler/hand-sewn anastomoses and creation of new hand-sewn anastomoses. (Courtesy of Dr. Latifi)

Summary

When one is dealing with difficult situations such as postoperative fistulas, the priorities are management of sepsis, nutritional optimization also being crucial (including rehydration and electrolyte correction), and wound care, while you prepare the patient for the definitive surgery. Sources of sepsis should be identified and treated quickly, using appropriate radiological investigation and culture of all potential sites of infection [7]. We will elaborate more on the chapter dedicated to complex abdominal wall reconstruction (CAWR).

Necrotizing Soft Tissue Infections

Patient #2

You performed a take-down colostomy on a 51-year-old female with a permanent tracheostomy and on steroids, which one of your partners did an end colostomy for perforated diverticulitis. (She no longer wants to deal with your partner after he told her to stop smoking! "How dare he tell me?" she says vividly upset.) You performed a very low hand-sewn, two-layer anastomosis, but there is a huge filled uterus lying right on top of the anastomosis. You consider inviting the gynecologist to take her uterus out but decided against the first instinct and did not call. The operation went well, but the feeling that you should have removed the uterus was bothering you. You were concerned that the large uterus will compress the blood supply of the anastomosis and it will fall apart. It will be a disaster. You manage the stoma site by packing it with gauze soaked in Betadine and normal saline, and put in four sutures, for a delayed closure on day 5 or 6.

She was doing well until postoperative day 4, when she develops a fever and a foul-smelling wound. The first thought that came to your mind was that anastomosis has fallen apart. You order an emergency rectal contrast study, pack the stoma site wound, and wait. When you review the study and there is no contrast leaking from the recto-sigmoid anastomosis, you are relieved. "It is just a wound infection that can be treated non-operatively," your partner tells you. You opened the wound, and the fascia was fine at the previous stoma site with the sutures still in place. But the smell! It was an awful smell.

While you are dining with family, your partner called back to tell you that the patient had coughed vigorously, as her tracheostomy was clogged with a mucus plug and she eviscerated most of her intestines. He took her to the operating room but was really surprised when he found a necrotizing soft tissue infection (NSTI) of her stoma site, requiring resection of a large portion of her left abdominal wall. "At least, she did not have a leak, and there was no injury to the bowel," he tells you, but you continued to ponder about the infection. "I had used the proper antibiotics, and packed the stoma site with betadine and saline" you keep thinking all night. And you used recommended bowel prep too. The patient underwent multiple debridements, open abdomen management, skin coverage of the defect, and wound VAC and had subsequently repair of large abdominal defect, for which she required complex abdominal reconstruction.

It was a colostomy take-down that ended up with major complications, despite all preparations. Moreover, one does not think of NSTI of this magnitude, when taking down colostomy as the first complication.

Postoperative Necrotizing Soft Tissue Infections (NSTIs)

Postoperative necrotizing soft tissue infections (NSTIs) are rare entities but can occur after any operation. An example of postoperative necrotizing fasciitis (NF) is depicted (Fig. 11.3) in a patient who underwent exploratory laparotomy and small bowel resection, which could lead to catastrophic outcomes if not dealt with immediately and of course in this case will lead to burst

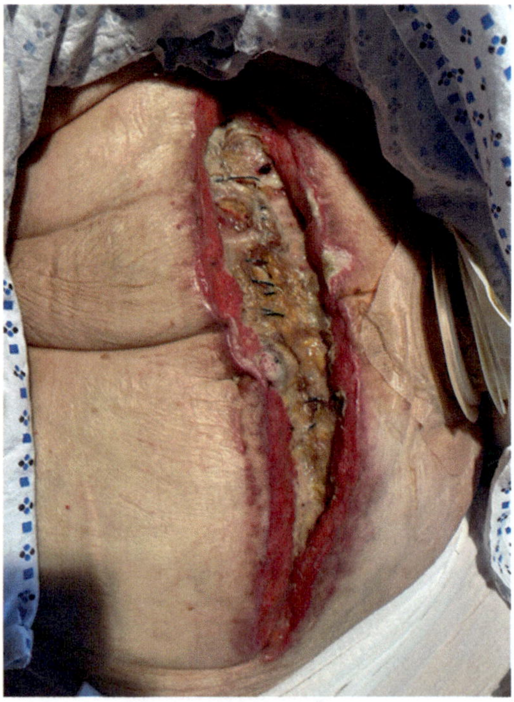

Fig. 11.3 Wound infection with partial necrosis of the abdominal wall, secondary to intra-abdominal cavity abscess, secondary to a small anastomotic leak. This type of complications should be managed immediately with aggressive debridement and staged early closure of the abdominal wall using posterior component separation and biologic mesh. (Courtesy of Dr. Latifi)

abdomen first, discussed later in this chapter. Necrotizing soft tissue infections (NSTIs) are rapidly progressing conditions with high mortality and include fasciitis, gas gangrene, Fournier gangrene, or anaerobic myositis, but postoperative NSTIs, while rare, have high mortality if not addressed immediately and without delay [13] and require multidisciplinary approach, including intensive care unit (ICU) [14]. Patients with NSTI classically present with fever, signs of systemic toxicity, and severe pain that is disproportionate to the clinical findings [14–16]. Common risk factors include diabetes mellitus, obesity, peripheral vascular disease, chronic renal failure, intravenous drug use (particularly black tar heroin), alcoholism, immunosuppression, and old age (>50 years) [15–17]. While the overall pathophysiology is common among all necrotizing infections, the rate at which clinical symptoms develop are dependent upon the particular pathogen [15].

The US Food and Drug Administration (FDA) excludes necrotizing soft tissue infections from therapeutic trials, and therefore current recommendations have been inferred from complicated skin and soft tissue infections (cSSTIs) [18]. Complicated SSTIs are generally classified by either their anatomical site, microbial etiology, or severity, with complicated cases being those requiring surgery [14]. The management applied to NSTI includes a combination of aggressive surgical debridement and antibiotic management [14, 19, 20]. However, prompt recognition of NSTIs is essential, and delay in treatment is associated with increased mortality, particularly if surgery is delayed [13, 16]. Antibiotic therapy should initially be broad, as the necrotizing infection may be the result of multiple organisms, and targeted at the most likely pathogen but then quickly adjusted after culture and sensitivity laboratory results become available [20, 21].

The Management

The aforementioned case example and data from our own clinical practice group demonstrate that surgical intervention within the first 6 hours after diagnosis of NSTI improves hospital outcomes in terms of shortening both the hospital length of stay (LOS) and intensive care unit (ICU) LOS [22]. In our study, the overall mortality was (11/87 or 12.5%), which is less than what has been reported in many previous studies [13, 23–25]. Although there was a clinically significant difference in the mortality between the groups based on the timing of surgical intervention (17.5% in late vs. 7.5% in early intervention group), this did not reach statistical significance.

NSTI, in particular necrotizing fasciitis, remains the deadliest of surgical infections if not treated aggressively with resuscitation and surgical debridement. Early diagnosis, early antibiotic treatment, and early surgical debridement remain the cornerstone of care for these patients. While "early" has not been clearly defined, we believe that surgery in these patients should be performed within the first few hours, but no longer than 6 hours from diagnosis [22]. In a study by McHenry et al., the mean time from admission to operation was 45 hours (range: 1.7–312 hours), while the average time from admission to operation was 90 hours for non-survivors *versus* 25 hours in the survivors group ($p = 0.0002$) [26]. In our study, we found that patients with NSTI underwent an operation as soon as possible, but certainly no later than 6 hours after their arrival or presentation to the emergency department. In fact, most of our Group I patients underwent an operation even earlier, within a mean time of 2.95 ± 1.1 hours.

In patients with NSTI, the most common reason for a delay in surgery is difficulty in making the correct diagnosis. Erythema, tenderness, and swelling are all common. The clinical presentation can be deceiving, particularly in immunocompromised patients, ranging from indolent wound infections to severe gangrene with septic shock, as defined with end-organ failure requiring vasopressors despite adequate fluid resuscitation [27]. Some clinicians often think that "patients are too sick to be immediately operated on," so they attempt to resuscitate them first, resulting in significantly delayed surgery, or the clinical presentation is deceiving, particularly in immunocompromised patients [28]. However, one must keep in mind that the source control of the infection is the number one priority in the management of any critically ill patients. These patients should be treated with the same urgency as a gunshot wound or any other major insult to the body.

Despite numerous scoring systems and models introduced to discriminate between NSTI and non-necrotizing soft tissue infections, making the diagnosis and predicting mortality and limb loss in NSTI are still difficult [29, 30] and the most important element remains early clinical recognition. Yet, there can be considerable diagnostic challenges when one is faced with "bad-looking" cellulitis and trying to distinguish it from NSTI. While we do not suggest that every patient with suspected NSTI undergo CT scan, in practice most patients will get a CT scan or even an MRI, before the surgeons ever meets these patients. On occasion, the patient may get a plain film radiograph to rule out gas in the tissue, but this is rare. As a rule, we use imaging techniques more often to assure ourselves and the patient that there is no immediate indication for an operation.

Laboratory test results in patients with NSTI have been well studied by a number of authors. The Laboratory Risk Indicator for Necrotizing Fasciitis (LRINEC) scoring system has been advocated to be helpful in distinguishing between NSTI and non-necrotizing soft tissue infections [31], as well as in differentiating between severe and not severe NSTI; however, in our study, we found that no single laboratory value independently predicted early diagnosis of NSTI. Furthermore, a study of a small group of patients strongly suggested that the LRINEC system is too insensitive for diagnosis of NSTIs [32]. Although hypoalbuminemia (< 2 g/dl) is a known factor for postoperative complications, in our study, the albumin level did not significantly differ between our two groups (2.1 ± 0.7 vs. 1.9 ± 0.5; P = 0.579). Our microbiologic findings were similar to those of other reported series and reflected a wide spectrum of bacteria. In a retrospective cohort study of 115 patients of NSTI with a mean age of 55 ± 18 years, 41% were females, 55% were diabetics, and 30% of patients underwent early surgery (< 6 h). While there were no significant differences between groups in baseline characteristics, the late group (≥ 6 h) had prolonged hospital stay (38 vs. 23 days, p < 0.008) in comparison to the early group (< 6 h). With every 1 h delay in time to surgery, there is a 0.268 day increase in length of stay, adjusted for these other variables: alcohol abuse, number of debridement's, peripheral vascular disease, previous infection, and clinical necrosis. Mortality was 16.5%. Multivariable analysis revealed that alcohol abuse, peripheral vascular disease, diabetes, obesity, hypothyroidism, and presence of chronic obstructive pulmonary disease (COPD) were associated with an increase in mortality [33].

We believe that rapid surgical treatment of our patients once the diagnosis was established was the main reason for our low mortality rate. The overall mortality rate has been reported to be very high (up to 72%) if the patient does not undergo surgical debridement as soon as possible. A median time to surgery of 8.4 hours had a relatively low mortality rate of 16.4% [23], while an interval > 14 hours from diagnosis to surgery in patients with septic shock was independently associated with in-hospital death [13]. The in-house presence of a trauma surgeon (acute care surgeon) ensures that these patients are seen almost immediately after the surgical resident is consulted by emergency medicine or internal medicine colleagues. This in turn ensures early intervention for patients with NSTI, although, for this study, we did not specifically assess the impact of our own practice style.

Hyperbaric oxygen therapy for NSTI, despite all its commercial activities, continues to be controversial [34] but certainly can be used once the debridement is performed and the patient can tolerate being in the hyperbaric chamber. While there were a number of lower extremity NSTIs at our institutions, NSTIs are managed by trauma or acute care surgeons.

While early surgical intervention is crucial in reducing morbidity and mortality in necrotizing fasciitis (NF) patients, there is still lack of a clear definition on what exactly defines "early."

Therefore, together with future studies, our work may contribute to the definition of early intervention [26, 35].

Summary

Early and aggressive emergency debridement of necrotic and poorly perfused tissue (and all tissues that can be easily lifted off the fascia with gentle pressure) removes the source of infection and toxins, improves the penetration of antibiotic therapy, and is a life-saving treatment [15–17]. Be sure to obtain gram stains and cultures from the wound. Early surgical treatment is essential and may minimize tissue loss and reduce the need for extremity amputation; however, there will still likely be a large area that needs covering [15, 16]. After initial debridement, monitor the wound every 24–48 hours, and if there is concern about the tissue viability, the patient should be returned to the operating room promptly for additional surgical debridement, necrosectomy, and fasciotomy in cases presenting with the compartment syndrome [16, 17]. Enteral nutritional feedings should be initiated as soon as possible to offset malnutrition, but parenteral nutrition support should be undertaken if more aggressive therapy is warranted after multiple debridements. If available, hyperbaric oxygen may be of benefit to a hemodynamically stable patient with certain infections, particularly *Clostridium* species; however, the evidence regarding the benefit for its use in non-clostridial infections is weak [15].

Postoperative Enterotomy Repair and Anastomotic Leaks

Patient # 3

A 73-year-old female with history of multiple previous intra-abdominal surgeries and major comorbidities undergoes laparoscopic exploration and partial laparoscopic lysis of adhesion and repair of one small recognized enterotomy. Postoperative day 5 she develops full-blown septic shock, and an emergent re-exploration reveals a leak at the enterotomy site. She undergoes damage control surgery (DCS) and primary repair of the leak. A few days later, she is taken back for re-exploration and drainage of the leak site, but you are unable to perform resection and anastomosis due to inflammation and cocoon abdomen. She left the hospital with a small manageable fistula a couple of months later but continued to have a persistent (Fig. 11.4a) drainage and multiple visits to various emergency departments, always triggering work-up including CT scans.

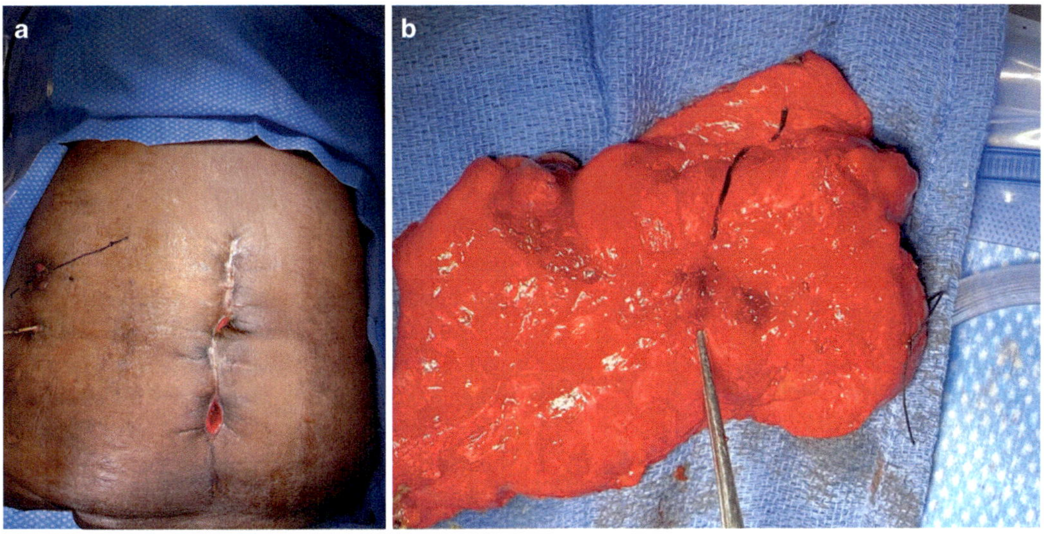

Fig. 11.4 (**a**) Persistent small fistula; (**b**) resected. (Courtesy of Dr. Latifi)

She was taken back to the operating room for final resection of the fistula and of the anastomosis (Fig. 11.4b).

Patient # 4

A 62-year-old underwent post-multiple abdominal explorations, damage control surgery, direct peritoneal resuscitation, and skin closure and underwent ileostomy take-down, small bowel stapler anastomosis, and complex abdominal wall reconstruction (CAWR) with biologic. Postoperative day # 5, while clinically was doing excellent, his drain output placed over the fascia changed to bilious. Emergency CT scan revealed a small anastomotic leak. On immediate re-exploratory laparotomy, a pinpoint 3 mm leak was identified, anastomosis was resected, and a handsewn new anastomosis was performed. CAWR was redone, and biologic was not removed (Figs. 11.2 and 11.5).

One of the most dreaded complications of general surgery is the anastomotic leak following small or large bowel resection. These postoperative anastomotic leaks are serious complications of colorectal surgery, and while their incidence is reported to be below 20%, their associated mortality can be as high as 39% [35, 36]. Advanced tumor stage, distal site (particularly with rectal tumors), and need for postoperative blood transfusion have been independently associated with increased rates of anastomotic disruption [35], and the rates of anastomotic dehiscence are similar between open versus laparoscopic techniques [36]. Those leaks that are diagnosed through imaging, without signs or symptoms, are usually considered subclinical, whereas clinical leaks present with signs of peritonitis and/or septicemia [37], which represent a major surgical challenge often resulting in sepsis, reoperation, and increased length of hospital stay [36–39].

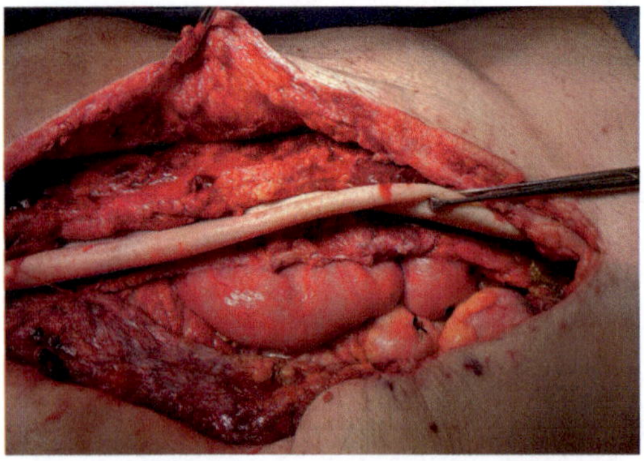

Fig. 11.5 Patient on Fig. 11.2, final re-reconstruction of abdominal wall, without the need to remove the biologic mesh. (Courtesy of Dr. Latifi)

The decision on how to approach this potentially catastrophic complication is not entirely straightforward. For patients with previous surgeries and intestinal resection and/or obese patients, an anastomotic leak may be lethal if not recognized immediately. Patients with intraperitoneal leaks with clinical generalized peritonitis or high-grade sepsis require immediate surgical intervention after receiving appropriate resuscitation [37]. If evidence of ischemia at the site of the anastomosis is recognized intraoperatively, the anastomosis should be redone immediately (Fig. 11.2) and require redo of the anastomosis. When identified postoperatively with significant peritoneal contamination, or if the anastomotic defect is large, the patient should undergo a resection of the anastomosis with the formation of an end stoma [37]. If the leak is at the sigmoid colon or rectum, a Hartmann's procedure may minimize the possibility of further abdominal catastrophe. Some surgeons may instead opt to perform a reanastomosis with a proximal section of bowel, but this should only be attempted in those patients who are not septic, well-nourished, and do not suffer from inflammatory bowel disease. In this situation, our preference is to divert the patient, either with an end stoma or with a loop diversion. Regardless of the technique, it is important to ensure that both bowel ends allow for a tension-free anastomosis. While others suggest the use of drains [37], this is not our practice.

If the intraperitoneal leakage is instead accompanied with localized peritonitis or abscess, a diagnostic imaging work-up using a triple-phase computerized tomography (CT) scan of the abdomen and pelvis should be performed and appears to be far more helpful than contrast enema in diagnosing a leak [38]. If a large abscess or multiple abscesses are noted, then the patient should be managed surgically as described before if the site of the abscess is inaccessible for draining. However, if the observed abscess is small (<3 cm), broad-spectrum intravenous antibiotics are recommended instead [37]. Distinguishing an anastomotic leak from a postoperative abscess can be difficult [38]. If the patient has an extra-peritoneal leak but is experiencing generalized sepsis, they should be managed in a similar way to those with intraperitoneal leaks.

The basic principles of patient management are similar to fistula management for the most part. At times, the surgeon may get "too close" to the patient and family over the long course of their care, and it may be beneficial to have a partner to look after the patient for a while. This is not an abandonment of the patient but simply one taking a "break" to gain some perspective and later approach the case more objectively to prevent a potentially catastrophic event.

Intestinal Ischemia

Patient # 5

A 76-year-old female with long-standing recurrent abdominal pain, with multiple trips to the emergency department, previous abdominoplasty, and hysterectomy, presents with worsening abdominal pain. A CT scan demonstrated a long, enlarged, and fecalized loop of small bowel in the pelvis and part of her bladder in the inguinal hernia, worsening kidney function, and severe acidosis. Exploratory laparotomy revealed a 50 cm gangrenous segment of small bowel secondary to a single band of adhesion in the pelvis (Fig. 11.6). She underwent damage control surgery and resuscitation for 36 hours and subsequently, primarily abdominal closure. She recovered nicely but was sent to a rehab center.

Every general surgeon has had a memorable case of intestinal ischemia, because the surgeon either missed the diagnosis altogether or simply intervened too late (Fig. 11.6). Intestinal ischemia, due to an obstruction secondary to adhesions, but particularly major acute mesenteric ischemia (AMI), is a complex problem commonly faced by general surgeons, with high complications and mortality around 60% [39]. Patients are typically elderly, with clinical histories consisting of atrial fibrillation, recent myocardial infarction, congestive heart failure (CHF), or other risks for superior mesenteric artery (SMA) embolism [40]. There are a number of underlying causes for AMI, but arterial thrombosis is the most common pathophysiology, accounting for about half of the cases [40]; other causes include arterial or venous thrombosis and nonobstructive causes (such as systemic coagulation disorders), leading to intestinal hypoxia, irreversible bowel damage, and potentially death [39].

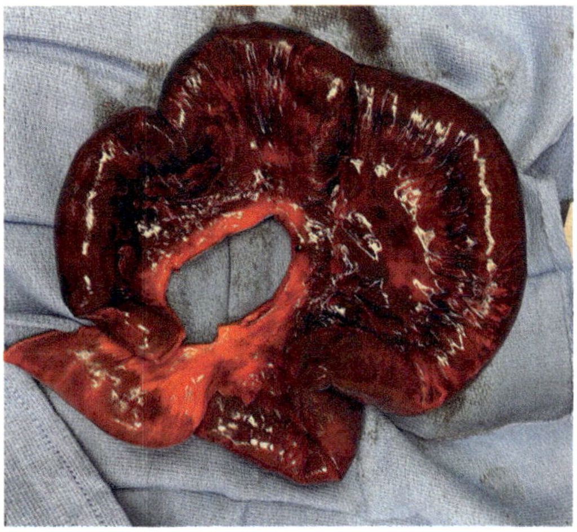

Fig. 11.6 Neglected bowel ischemia, not developed full blown gangrene, secondary to a pelvic adhesion. (Courtesy of Dr. Latifi)

The blood supply to the intestines is mainly provided by three large vascular systems stemming from the abdominal aorta: the celiac axis, the superior mesenteric artery (SMA), and the inferior mesenteric artery (IMA). Arterial emboli are more commonly localized in the SMA due to its wider angle of origin compared with the celiac artery and its parallel course to the abdominal aorta [39]. The SMA and celiac axis systems communicate via the gastroduodenal artery and pancreaticoduodenal arcades at the pancreatic head region, and since routine pancreaticoduodenectomy (PD) involves resection of these branches, ischemic complications may also arise in this patient group [41].

Timely diagnosis is critical to prevent ischemic complications and improve odds of survival; however, the diagnosis of patients with AMI can be difficult, as the abdominal pain is often accompanied by nonspecific symptoms such as fever, vomiting, diarrhea, and loss of bowel sounds. Therefore, the patient's history is important to consider, particularly if they are elderly and have cardiovascular or peripheral vascular disease [39]. Computerized tomography (CT) scan is both highly sensitive and specific for diagnosing AMI and can visualize both the occlusions and the consequences of the intestinal hypoxia; in situations where it is not available, mesenteric angiography or duplex ultrasonography can be utilized [39, 40].

Particularly difficult is the situation of a patient with multiple abdominal surgeries, requiring significant amounts of pain medication. When these patients develop ischemia, it is difficult to discern pain associated with ischemia from their "usual pain." Such an example is an obese patient with multiple previous abdominal operations and large ventral hernia (Fig. 11.7), who presented with the exacerbation of the abdominal pain.

Surgical exploration is warranted for all patients who have any suspected mesenteric ischemia and signs of peritonitis, regardless of its cause. These patients are high-risk for irreversible bowel infarction and abdominal sepsis, and bowel that is approaching irreparable necrosis can seem normal in appearance. In contrast, bowel that may appear "dusky" may be viable after revascularization. For these reasons, the priority of the surgeon should be to reestablish vascularization and then reassess the viability of before making decisions about intestinal resection.

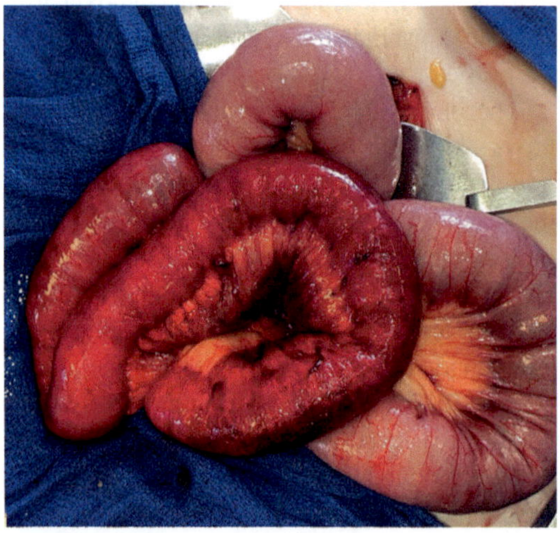

Fig. 11.7 Patient with obese obesity post with multiple previous abdominal operations and large ventral hernia. (Courtesy of Dr. Latifi)

When to Resect Intestines and When to Watch?

Patient # 6

"A 52-year-old female with stage 3 kidney disease is evaluated in the ED with abdominal pain and septic shock, requiring pressors. Exploratory laparotomy reveals multiple points of ischemia (Fig. 11.8a,b), verified by ICG. She has good pulses of the mesentery. The surgeon decided to continue with resuscitation and DCS. She was brought back 24 hours later, and her ischemia now has become worse, in a larger segment of SB, but no clear zone of resection. Now the surgeon decides to place her on DPR and bring her back 72 hours later. Her intestinal ischemia improved dramatically (Fig. 11.8c), resection was avoided, and her abdomen was closed".

This case illustrates two of the biggest and most difficult questions: (1) How much intestines should one resect? and (2) When to perform an anastomosis, in cases when ischemia is not clear-cut like in patient # 5? (Fig. 11.8a,b). Until recently, a good rule of thumb was to perform a temporary abdominal closure (TAC) and return to the operating room within 24–48 hours while you continue resuscitating the patient, following acid-base balance and lactate level. In recent years the use of indocyanine green (ICG) dye to evaluate perfusion has become popular [42, 43], both robotically, laparoscopically, and in open surgery. Use of ICG and direct peritoneal resuscitation (DPR) and DCS, when re-evaluation is required [44], has become a standard practice. Focal ischemia of small bowel can resolve using DPR (Fig. 11.8c) and resuscitation. Small bowel ischemia if neglected and delayed laparotomy may have catastrophic consequences (Fig. 11.8).

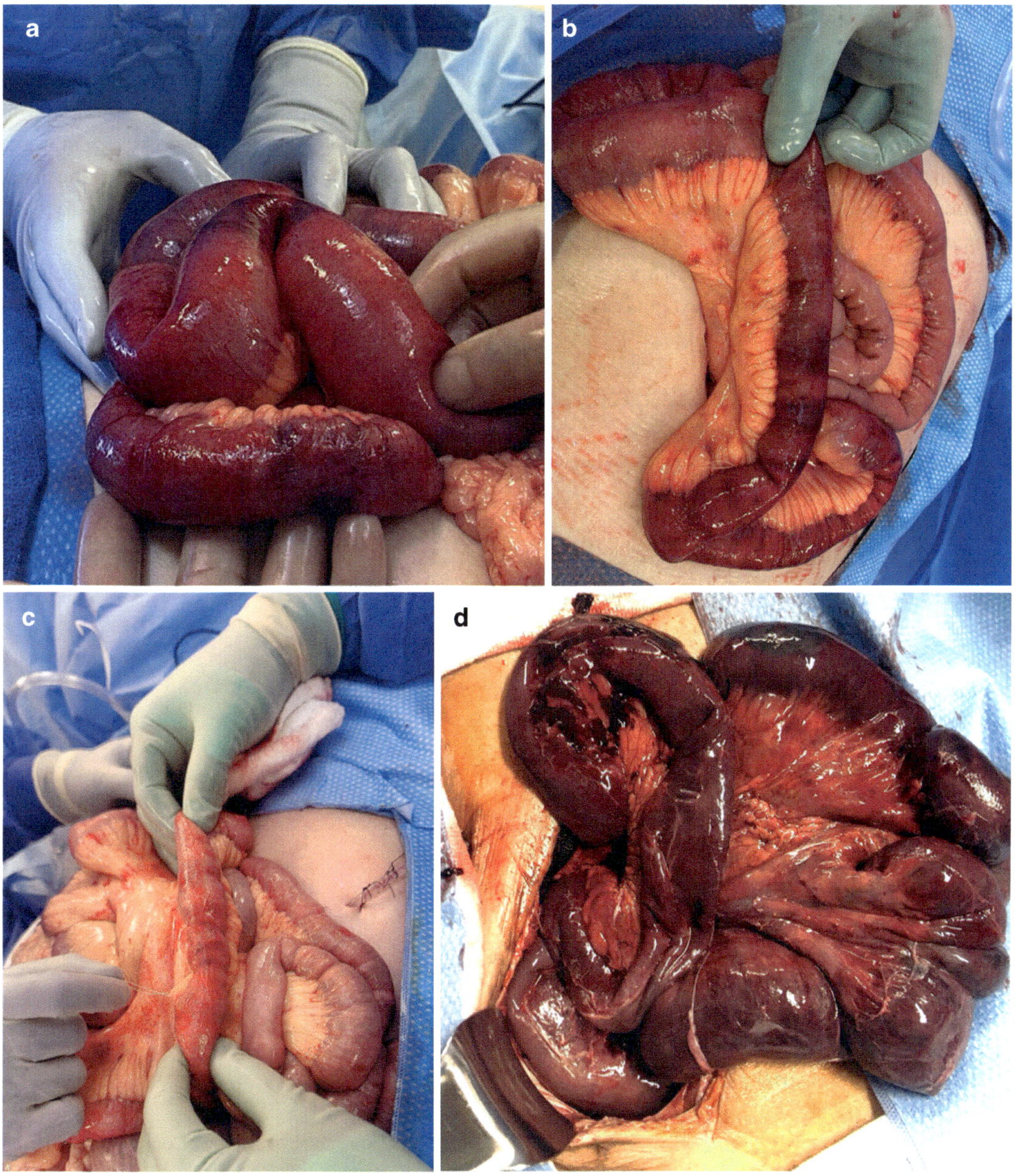

Fig. 11.8 (**a–c**) When unclear margins of full-blown ischemia, the patients should be observed and return back for second or even third look. In this patient, as it is our practice, we initiated direct peritoneal resuscitation, and patient did not require resection. (**d**) Catastrophic delay addressing small bowel ischemia. (Courtesy of Dr. Latifi)

Summary

Dealing with real difficult situations in general surgery is challenging and requires a thoughtful and meticulous approach, yet expeditious action. However, we cannot become paralyzed with the fear of failing or having complications or a potentially negative laparotomy. Fistulas, necrotizing soft tissue infections, and intestinal ischemia are all dramatic and can have significant mortality if not addressed appropriately. As general surgeons, we are expected to deal with situations that often are very difficult. However, when we face a complicated patient, either during re-operative surgery (when others have operated beforehand) or for whatever reason your patients' postoperative course gets truly complicated, then things get difficult on more than one level. The situation becomes personal. These personal complications sometimes make it difficult to return to the operating room, but one must do it, to start the fight again and remember that we must get back in the saddle.

The Difficult Cholecystectomy: Approaches and Bailout Strategies

Patient Example 7

Patient is a 54-year-old female with no significant past medical history who presents with right upper quadrant abdominal pain for the past 3 days. Patient has had similar episodes of abdominal pain over the past 2 years. This time the pain has progressively worsened, and she has associated nausea and emesis. Ultrasound is performed which demonstrates cholelithiasis, no pericholecystic fluid, and common bile duct measures 4mm. You take her to the operating room for a laparoscopic cholecystectomy and discover a tense gallbladder with significant edema covered with multiple dense adhesions. You attempt to carefully dissect out the critical view of safety but are unable to safely identify the cystic duct. You must decide between performing a subtotal cholecystectomy or converting to an open procedure in order to avoid the most feared complication, an iatrogenic common bile duct injury.

In the multifaceted landscape of abdominal surgery, navigating the intricacies of a stubborn gallbladder presents an arduous challenge. Regardless of the dexterity and proficiency intrinsic in surgical practice, there inevitably arises an occasion where continued dissection of the cystohepatic triangle becomes hazardous due to factors like dense adhesions, inflammation, and scarring. Distortion of the surgical dissection planes creates a phenomenon known as "frozen Calot's," limiting the possibility of safe identification of the biliary structures and rendering isolation of the critical view of safety unattainable [42]. Termed as encountering a "difficult gallbladder," this scenario inherently carries a significant threat for surgical mishaps secondary to several factors including necrosis, gangrene, empyema, Mirizzi syndrome, dense adhesions, intraoperative bleeding, distorted anatomy, and known perforation [43, 45]. Other occasions that required transition to an open procedure included discovering a cholecystoenteric fistula, concern for malignancy, common bile duct (CBD) exploration for stones, and iatrogenic enterotomy [45]. These factors have historically led to conversion to open (Fig. 11.9), subtotal cholecystectomy (Fig. 11.10).

It is critical to acknowledge that the incidence of confronting a "difficult gallbladder" is not a rarity, with rates reported up to 26% [45].

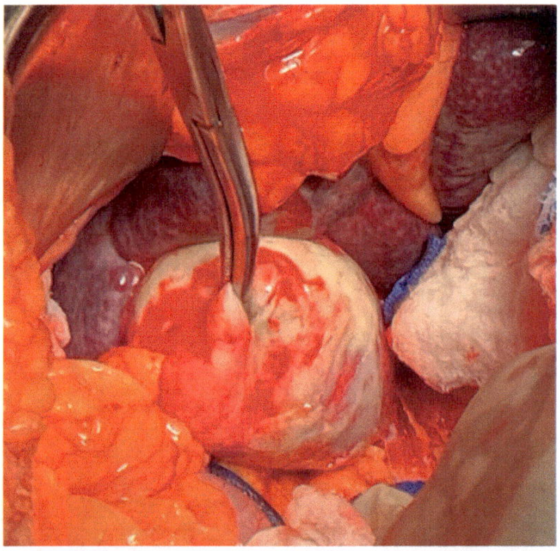

Fig. 11.9 Open cholecystectomy. (Courtesy of Dr. Latifi)

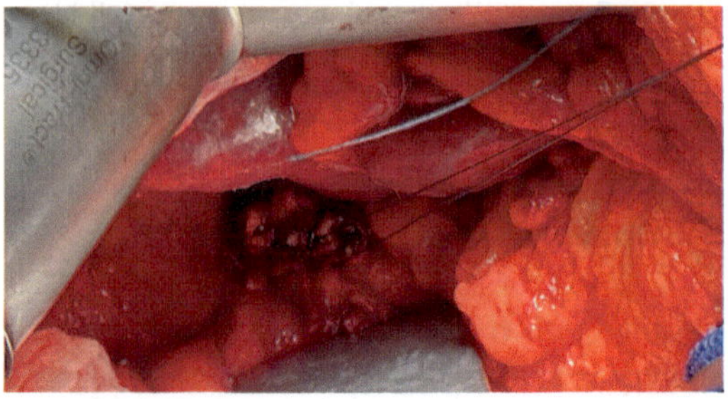

Fig. 11.10 Partial or near complete open cholecystectomy. (Courtesy of Dr. Latifi)

Moreover, procedure-related complications include subhepatic fluid collections requiring drainage (7.7%), postoperative hemorrhage requiring transfusion (4.8%), pneumonia (4.6%), sepsis requiring vasopressor support (6%), and wound infection (4.3%) [45].

Addressing a difficult gallbladder requires a strategic approach combined with technical expertise. Despite the challenges presented, contemporary surgical practice favors continued laparoscopic dissection over conversion to open surgery, especially in the modern era where open cholecystectomies in training programs are diminishing in frequency. Converting to an open cholecystectomy has become a rarity and now presents new unfamiliar technical challenges for ascending surgeons than the more familiar laparoscopic dissection. Despite the opposition of a bad gallbladder, difficult cholecystectomies have a laparoscopic completion rate of 96%, with rates of conversion to open procedures nearing 4–10.5% [46].

Persisting laparoscopically in the face of a challenging gallbladder can dispose one to catastrophic injuries including vascular injury to the hepatic arteries, or injury to the extrahepatic biliary tree [43]. Therefore, knowing when to abort a completion laparoscopic cholecystectomy is crucial to every surgeon, and the strategic utilization of bailout techniques becomes essential when faced with this hazardous situation. According to several studies, employing a laparoscopic subtotal cholecystectomy technique is not only a suitable alternative to completed laparoscopic cholecystectomy but in current practice has become the preferred a bail-out technique to replace conversion to open.

Preoperatively diagnosing challenging gallbladders and their pathologies can support operative planning by employing the 2018 Tokyo Guidelines which delineate specific criteria for the diagnosis of acute cholecystitis [47]. These guidelines include a combination of the following quantifications: (A) local signs of inflammation, either Murphy's sign or Right Upper Quadrant (RUQ) tenderness or mass; (B) systemic signs of inflammation including fever, elevated CRP, and leukocytosis; and (C) imaging findings suggestive of acute cholecystitis [47]. High suspicion for acute cholecystitis arises if criteria is present in categories A and B, while definitive diagnosis mandates that all three categories' criteria have been involved [47]. Additionally, the guidelines introduce a severity scale, categorizing the disease into mild, moderate, and severe based on systemic effects and end-organ damage that coincide with 30-day mortality rates of Grade I (1.1%), Grade II (0.8%), and Grade III (5.4%) [47].

Additionally, the 2018 Tokyo Guidelines also propose management bundles for treatment of acute cholecystitis [48]. Per these guidelines, patients should undergo assessment every 6–12 hours utilizing the previously discussed diagnostic criteria until the diagnosis is firmly established [48]. Abdominal ultrasound serves as the standard imaging modality for diagnosis, with CT and MRI reserved for cases that remain inconclusive [48]. The severity scale aids in quantifying disease severity and guiding further treatments. Grade I recommendations are to perform a laparoscopic cholecystectomy within 7 days of diagnosis but preferably within 72 hours [48]. For Grade II patients, urgent laparoscopic cholecystectomy is recommended for suitable surgical candidates, while early drainage followed by delayed laparoscopic cholecystectomy is advised for those deemed unsuitable [48]. In Grade III disease, patients that are good surgical candidates should be taken for emergent laparoscopic cholecystectomy, while immediate drainage is recommended for those unable to tolerate surgery [48]. Additionally, cultures from blood, bile, or both should be acquired for Grade II and higher cases [48]. In cases where urgent drainage, laparoscopic cholecystectomy, or ICU facilities are unavailable, patients should be promptly transferred to capable facilities [48]. Adherence to these guidelines can aid surgeons in diagnosing, treating, and surgical planning for complex gallbladder cases.

The integration of indocyanine green (ICG) as an adjunctive tool in cholecystectomy procedures has recently gained traction, particularly for enhancing visualization and identification of the extrahepatic biliary ducts during dissection of the hepatocystic triangle [49]. As laparoscopic surgery has become the standard of care, there has been a concordant increase in common bile duct (CBD) injuries, primarily accredited to inadequate visualization of the extrahepatic ducts. ICG has emerged as a validated supplemental tool to enhance bile duct visualization and has demonstrated noteworthy reductions in CBD injury rates during laparoscopic procedures as well as decreasing the necessity for conversion to open procedures [50]. The utilization of ICG results in a 4-fold decrease in bile duct injuries and a 17-fold decrease in the requirement for conversion to open procedures [50]. Deliberation regarding the optimal dosing and timing of ICG administration has led to more standardized guidelines. A comparative study assessed the administration of ICG between 20 and 30 minutes prior to anesthesia induction, 2–6 hours prior, or over 6 hours prior. The group receiving ICG 2–6 hours prior to surgery achieved successful visualization of the CBD in 97.1% of cases, compared to 85.4% in the group receiving ICG at the time of anesthesia. This contrasted with the group-administered ICG greater than 6 hours prior to surgery with visualization of the CBD achieved only 65.5% of the time [49]. This evidence concludes that ICG administration in the preoperative area up to 30 minutes prior to the operation adequately facilitates successful visualization of the extrahepatic ducts during a difficult dissection. Additionally, a comparison of dosing strategies between weight-based (0.05 mg/kg) and a standardized dose of 1cc of 25 mg diluted in 10 mL saline (2.5 mg/mL) identified the standardized dose as superior, achieving CBD visualization in 87.3% of cases [49]. This suggests that utilizing a standardized dose of 2.5 mg/mL is sufficient to achieve adequate visualization of the extrahepatic ducts particularly in the presence of inflammation, anatomical distortions, and aberrant anatomy. When grappling with a difficult gallbladder, adjuncts like ICG should be utilized to accurately identify anatomical variations and ensure a safer dissection process.

The introduction of robotic surgery has represented a significant technological advancement to the minimally invasive cholecystectomy. However, the role of robotic technology in emergency surgery, particularly in cases of acute cholecystitis, is still being deliberated. The World Society of Emergency Surgery does not consider emergency surgery a specific contraindication for utilizing a robotics approach, with the caveat that the operating room is fully staffed with robotically trained personnel and that the surgeon has sufficient robotic experience [51]. The technological capabilities of robotic platforms, including 3D stereoscopic vision, instrument stabilization, and wrist technology, enhances dissection of inflamed or aberrant anatomy, potentially averting iatrogenic injury, or the need for conversion to an open procedure [51]. One study examining single-port robotic cholecystectomy in both emergent and elective cases reported a low CBD injury rate (0.7%), an overall complication rate of 8.7%, and an increased operative time (95 +/– 4.4 minutes) for robotic cholecystectomies in the emergent setting compared to elective cases [52].

We believe that robotic technology has been ultimately the most important advancement that is ideal for "bad" gallbladders. Ultimately, the decision to opt for robotic cholecystectomy in urgent cases of acute cholecystitis hinges on the surgeon's expertise and the availability of support personnel, pending further research to establish comparative outcomes. A significant number of acute care surgery services continue to adopt robotic cholecystectomy, as the training of nursing and technical staff is expanding.

Open Cholecystectomy

Although the current standard of care favors laparoscopic approaches, open cholecystectomy remains relevant in select scenarios as an indication of strong surgical judgment to mitigate iatrogenic injuries. Risk factors for conversion to an open procedure have been reported including gallbladder wall width >4 mm, pericholecystic fluid, male sex, age >60 years old, acute cholecystitis, neurologic disorders, and diabetes [53,

54], but ultimately the determining factor is the individual surgeon who makes the surgical decision to convert. The three main reasons identified for surgeons deciding to convert to an open procedure include unusual anatomy, inflammatory adhesions, and prolonged dissection [55].

The senior author prefers early conversion to open cholecystectomy if the operations do not flow as expected and one does not make progress. The decision to convert to open, while decided early, should not be made until after four ports have been placed and the gallbladder has been identified with the fundus grasped and elevated [55]. At this point should dissection prove to be too difficult or risky, early conversion to an open approach prevents longer operating times and decreases the risk of iatrogenic injury. While contemporary trends may veer toward minimally invasive techniques, open cholecystectomy continues to remain a valuable adjunct in the armamentarium of surgeons navigating the difficult gallbladder. However, just the fact that you have converted to open may not make the procedure any easier.

Summary

The successful management of difficult gallbladder cases hinges on a balanced integration of technical proficiency and strategic decision-making. At times, the gallbladder may look difficult, but if it continues to make progress, then the operation can be safely completed (Fig. 11.11). Subtotal cholecystectomy, whether employing a fenestrated or reconstituted approach, is an acceptable and safe alternative. Advances in technology, especially robotic surgery, have revolutionized acute care surgery, particularly common procedures such as cholecystectomy and colon surgery [51]. Adjuncts such as ICG are now indicated to aid the surgeon in visualization of complex anatomy. Finally, utilization of the open approach remains a gold-standard technique in the toolbox of any surgeon approach to safely managing the difficult gallbladder.

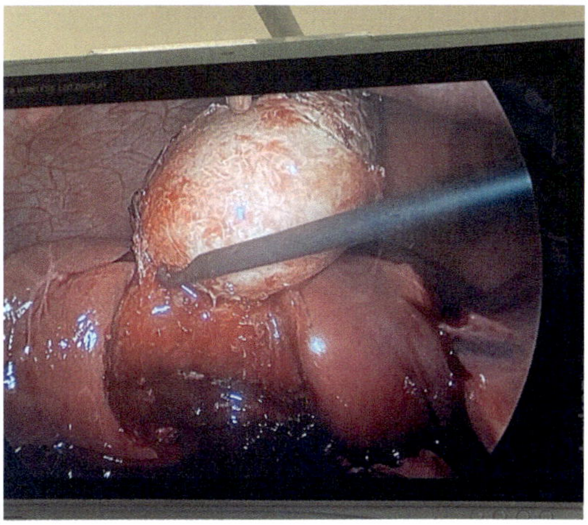

Fig. 11.11 Difficult, but doable laparoscopic cholecystectomy. (Courtesy of Dr. Latifi)

The Burst Abdomen

Patient 7

Patient is an 84-year-old female with past medical history of hypertension and diabetes who is status post-screening colonoscopy 1 day ago presenting now with abdominal pain. She has diffused pain across the abdomen and leukocytosis of 13.2, associated with free air on CT. She underwent an exploratory laparotomy and discovered a perforation in the sigmoid colon. You perform a segmental sigmoid resection with primary anastomosis. The procedure is uncomplicated. On postoperative day # 3, her GI functions return of and tolerating a soft diet. Her leukocytosis has resolved to 9.8. She is cleared for discharge and pending placement. On POD #5 has a rising leukocytosis of 12.3, but she is afebrile. Her midline wound has new "soupy pink" discharge. You remove a couple of staples and wash out the incision leaving wet to dry packing. The next day you get a call from the nurse that the patients' incision has opened. On examination her midline incision has completely dehisced, exposing matted bowel (Fig. 11.12). You take her urgently back to the operating room. She made your surgical decision very easy. The diagnosis: A burst abdomen.

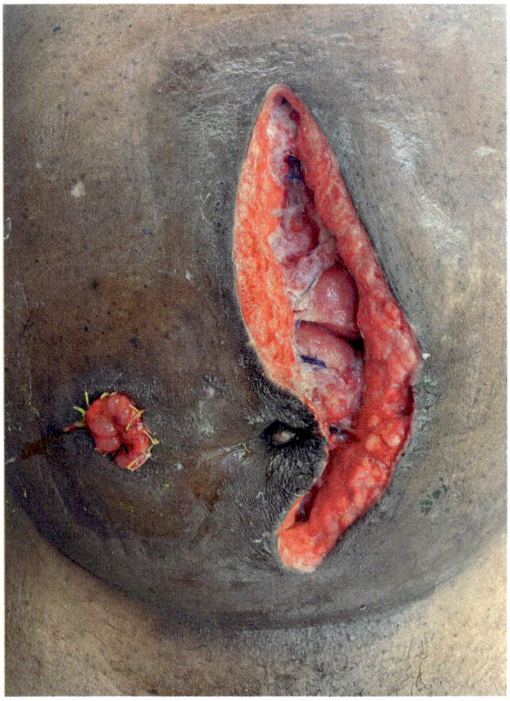

Fig. 11.12 Wide dehiscence of the abdominal wound. (Courtesy of Dr. Latifi)

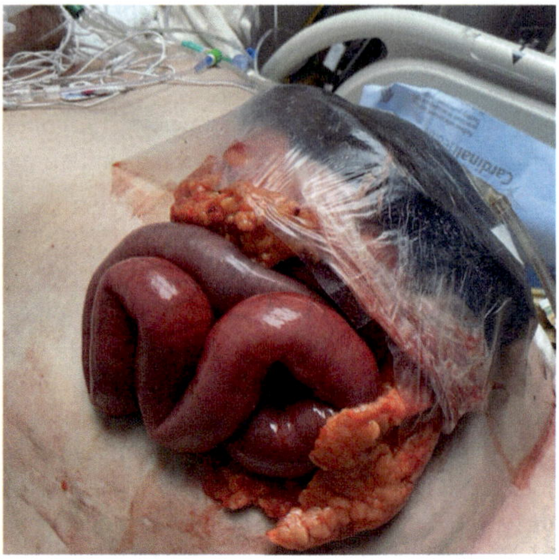

Fig. 11.13 Evisceration of the abdominal content in a patient with temporary abdominal closure, due to lack of proper sedation. (Courtesy of Firas Madbak, MD)

Consequences of Burst Abdomen

The burst abdomen is defined by the breakdown of reapproximated wound edges of a closed surgical incision and represents a grave complication with significant morbidity and mortality [56]. The acute burst of the abdomen when intestines are found in the dressing, while very dramatic for the patient and nursing staff, is not common, although it may often occur in patients with temporary closure with wound VAC on a ventilator and not properly sedated (Fig. 11.13, Courtesy of Firas Madbak, MD). More commonly it is as a result of infection, followed by dehiscence and eventually a burst abdomen (Figs. 11.3 and 11.12). Surgical wound dehiscence can be classified as either superficial or deep and can involve an infectious etiology or not [56]. The incidence of abdominal wound dehiscence is around 1% within the 30-day postoperative period but has very high mortality rates of up to 40% [56]. Wound dehiscence typically manifests between the 5th and 12th postoperative days, with the initial presentation often including drainage of serosanguinous "salmon-colored" fluid from the wound [57].

While there are multiple factors contributing abdominal wound dehiscence, decreased tissue strength and infection are the most common [53]. However, infection is the most common factor predisposing patients to abdominal wound dehiscence [53, 57]. Increased rates of wound infection are often associated with an emergency operation [57]. Specific risk factors include age over 50, male gender, peritonitis, and emergency laparotomy [53]. Additionally, postoperative increases in intra-abdominal pressures with coughing, vomiting, and distention from ileus, along with comorbidities such as hypoproteinemia, sepsis, ascites, and steroid use, further predispose individuals to this complication [57].

Can Burst Abdomen Be Prevented?

Preventive measures in the initial laparotomy play a crucial role in averting the occurrence of burst abdomen. Employing mesh during emergent laparotomies can preempt future fascial dehiscence, particularly in cases where there are concerns regarding weak fascia or infection risks are high [54]. Additionally, employing long-lasting monofilament sutures in a running technique during primary fascial closure has been shown to reduce incisional hernia rates compared to interrupted suture techniques [58].

The Management

In managing the burst abdomen, emergent reclosure in the operating room remains the cornerstone. The eviscerated abdominal contents should be washed with warm saline and returned to the abdominal cavity.

The choice of closure technique and the timing of closure is a crucial surgical decision. The current evidence favors fascial closure reinforced with mesh [59], which results in lower incisional hernia rates (12.5%) compared to primary suture closure (30.7%) [54, 59]. The mesh reinforcement has similar outcomes in terms of surgical site infection, recurrence, and mortality rates [59].

We prefer use of biologic mesh reinforcement, placed in the retro rectus space and complex abdominal wall reconstruction [8]. In the case of a burst abdomen, utilizing size 0 polydioxanone (PDS) suture material in a running fashion with each bite encompassing the entire abdominal wall excluding the skin and subcutaneous tissue has been shown to effectively prevent recurrent dehiscence [60]. Each bite should be 3 cm from the fascial edge and should travel no more than 5 mm creating a wound-suture ratio of 1:10 [60].

Summary

The management of burst abdomen represents a rare but a great challenge in acute care surgery. Burst abdomen, characterized by the breakdown of surgical incisions, poses significant challenges, with mortality rates reaching 40% and an incidence of 1% within 30 days postoperatively (Fig. 11.14). The closure technique of burst abdomen should include mesh reinforcement, placed in the retro rectus space, but the timing is based on the edema and present of contamination level. If there is significant edema present, we prefer use of DPR (Fig. 11.15) and temporary closure for 48–72 hours [45], followed by CAWR (Figs. 11.16 and 11.17).

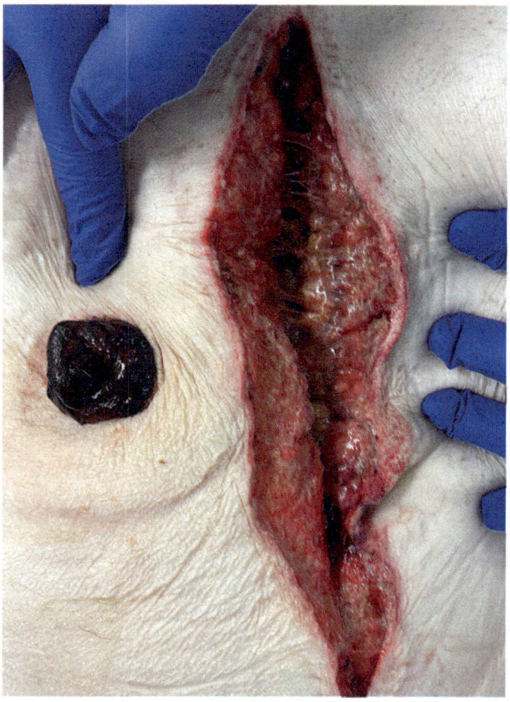

Fig. 11.14 Ischemia of the ileostomy and severe wound infection due to intra-abdominal process. (Courtesy of Dr. Latifi)

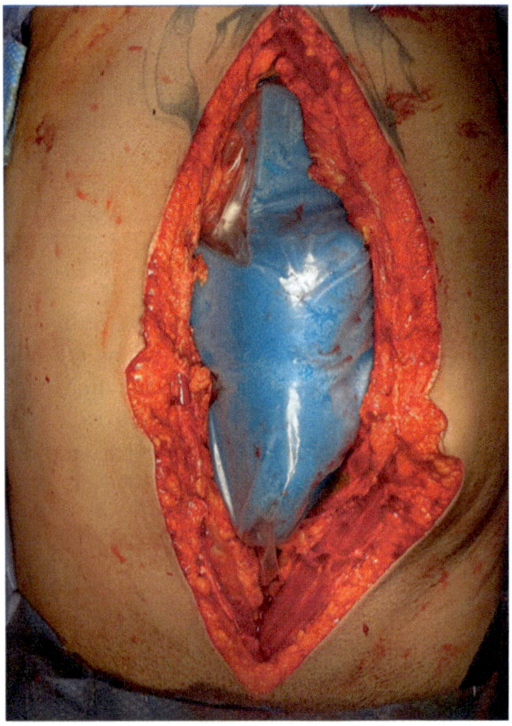

Fig. 11.15 Illustration of a patient undergoing DCL and DPR (Fig. 11.15). Temporary abdominal closure with DPR. Blake drain (not seen are placed for DPR, one on each side of superior abdomen, with final CAWR with biologic mesh) (Figs. 11.16 and 11.17). (Courtesy of Dr. Latifi)

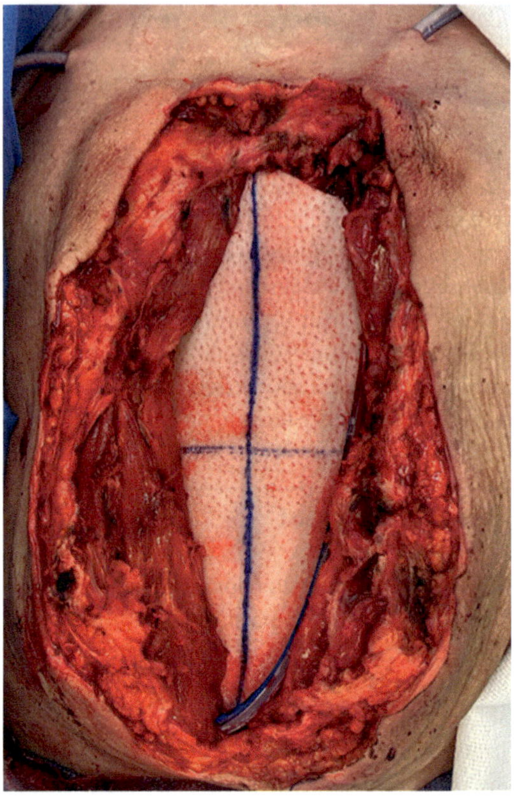

Fig. 11.16 Illustration of a patient undergoing DCL and DPR (Fig. 11.15), with final CAWR with biologic mesh (Figs. 11.16 and 11.17). Tailored biologic mesh size for CAWR. (Courtesy of Dr. Latifi)

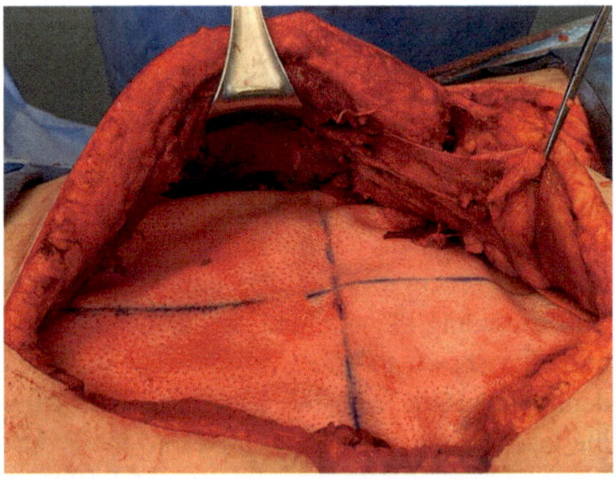

Fig. 11.17 Illustration of a patient undergoing DCL and DPR (Fig. 11.15), with final CAWR with biologic mesh (Figs. 11.16 and 11.17). Ensuring that biologic mesh is placed appropriately for proper coverage. (Courtesy of Dr. Latifi)

The Difficult Hernia Repair

Patient Example 8

Patient is a 47-year-old male with past medical history of obesity, hypertension, and GERD who presents to the emergency department with abdominal pain. Patient states that he has had an abdominal hernia ever since he underwent an exploratory laparotomy 1 year ago for GSW to the abdomen. He underwent two explorations and incomplete lysis of adhesions, and on the last exploration several years ago, the surgeon found a hostile abdomen and decided to bell out and declared that "abdomen was not operable." He has had multiple visits to the emergency department since then and refused to be operated on, the last one being two weeks prior to this visit. On CT scan patient has a large ventral hernia containing most of his small bowel. You evaluate the patient and note that the hernia is tender to palpation with erythematous skin changes. This time he agrees to let you take the patient urgently to the operating room. Diagnosis: Neglected ventral hernia.

Identification and Diagnosis

"Ventral hernia is a surgical disease, should be treated surgically, and one should die from it" – the senior author wrote in recent years on one editorial [61], but the timing and optimal repair technique intervention continue to be debated. In the context of strangulated hernias, reduction should be abstained from to prevent the introduction of compromised or necrotic bowel segments into the peritoneal cavity, potentially leading to diffuse peritonitis [62], and the patient should be operated on at once. The discomfort caused by neglecting it is obvious as illustrated in a 77-year-old male patient (Fig. 11.18) that was "shopping" for a surgeon for years but was refused, because he was "not symptomatic enough," and "he would die on the table." He did very well with a new abdominal wall. Another group of patients with hernia that are often neglected by surgeons are those with ascites due to cirrhosis (Fig. 11.19).

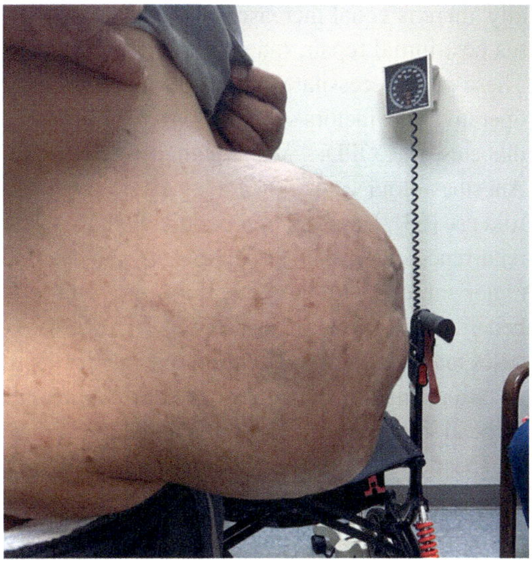

Fig. 11.18 Large neglected abdominal wall hernia on a patient that was seen by many surgeons, but was not operated because he did not have obstructive symptoms! (Courtesy of Dr. Latifi)

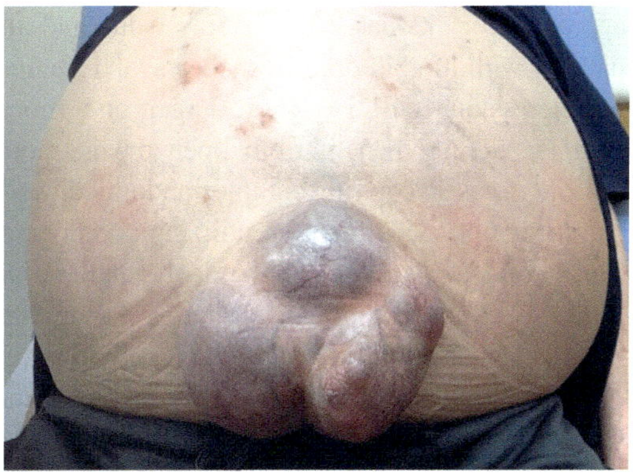

Fig. 11.19 Large neglected umbilical hernia in a patient with severe liver cirrhosis awaiting liver transplant. This patient underwent complex abdominal wall reconstruction with much improved quality of life, and about 6 months later, he received a liver transplant. (Courtesy of Dr. Latifi)

Management of the Disease

Preoperative considerations, including comorbidities and hernia complexity, are pivotal in determining the management of difficult hernias. With the prevalence of ventral hernias increasing annually, there is equal increase in recurrent rates status post-initial repair, ranging from 15% to 40%. These rates necessitate careful evaluation of preoperative risk factors such as BMI >30, smoking, diabetes, COPD, American Society of Anesthesiologist (ASA) Grades III–IV, and steroid use [63]. Having a preoperatively high risk of recurrence indicates that patients are subjected to major surgery with the potential of no long-term benefit. While ventral hernia repair for elective cases may benefit from preoperative medical optimization, emergency scenarios require immediate surgical intervention despite the associated risks.

The decision between open and laparoscopic approaches for ventral hernia repair has been rigorously debated. While an open approach is the mainstay for emergent repair of strangulated bowel, contemporary trends favor more minimally invasive approaches, supported by studies demonstrating reduced hospital stays, decreased chronic pain, and fewer analgesic requirements [64]. Current evidence suggest considering a laparoscopic approach for hernias <10 cm in width and in patients with morbid obesity, diabetes, and immunosuppression [64]. However, larger and more complex hernias benefit from open repair, most notably in cases requiring complex abdominal wall reconstruction. This involves utilizing component separation techniques which divide the myofascial layers to alleviate midline tension and facilitate midline closure [65]. While there is a broad array of mesh to choose from, ranging from permanent synthetic to absorbable synthetic and biologic, mesh selection is influenced by factors such as hospital inventory, surgeon preference, and the contamination level. In summary, while minimally invasive techniques have a modern role in ventral hernia repair, more complex and larger diameter hernias may necessitate an open approach utilizing component separation and complex abdominal wall reconstruction with mesh reinforcement.

Management of Intraoperative Surprises in Acute Care Surgery

Patient # 9

A 58-year-old male with obesity, hypertension, congestive heart failure (CHF) from an unknown etiology, and a pacemaker presented with deteriorating overall condition secondary to groin and scrotal pain related to a long-standing left inguinal hernia. Following years of the hernia being present, sudden onset swelling and pain in the left groin, and inability to reduce the hernia, he presented with hemodynamic instability and severe leukocytosis, and overall "real-sick look." CT scan imaging done prior to surgery team consultation uncovered an incarcerated left scrotal hernia containing the sigmoid colon. Upon evaluation by the surgical team, the patient not only had a strangulated inguinal hernia, but he also had a NSTI of the scrotum (Fig. 11.20).

In light of the patient's deteriorating hemodynamic status and unstable cardiac condition, an emergent exploratory laparotomy was undertaken to reduce the sigmoid colon. The reduction of the sigmoid colon and return to the abdomen was performed with many difficulties (Fig.

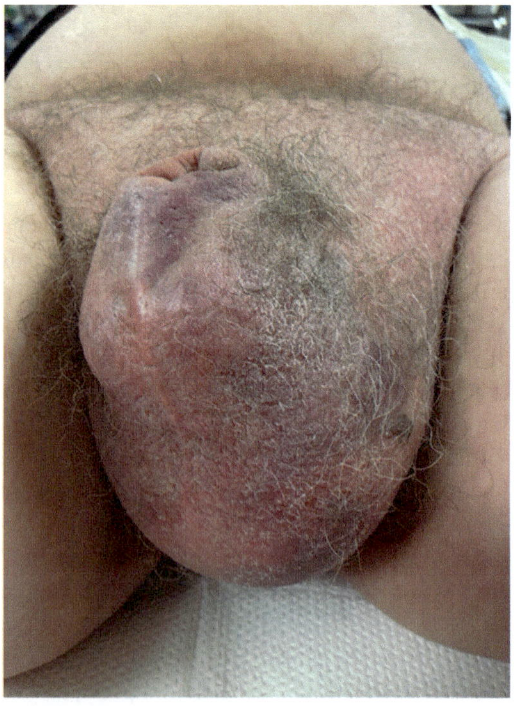

Fig. 11.20 Scrotum of the patient with NSTI secondary to incarcerated, non-reducible left colon into the scrotum, and neglected for at least 7 days. (Courtesy of Dr. Latifi)

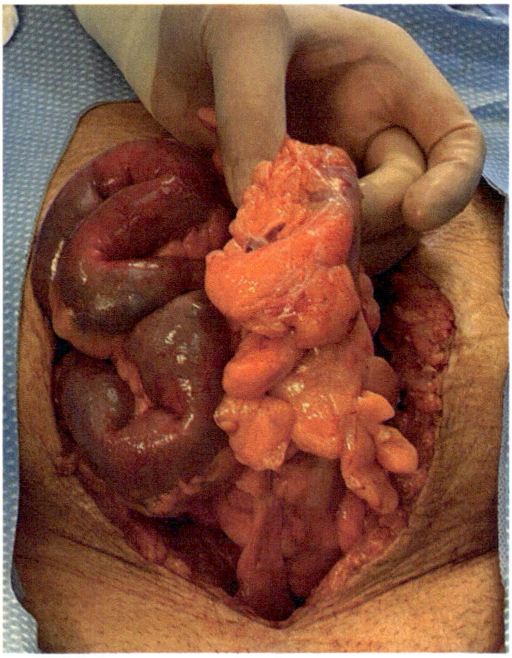

Fig. 11.21 Incarcerated left colon in the left scrotum, pulled out of the scrotum from the abdomen. (Courtesy of Dr. Latifi)

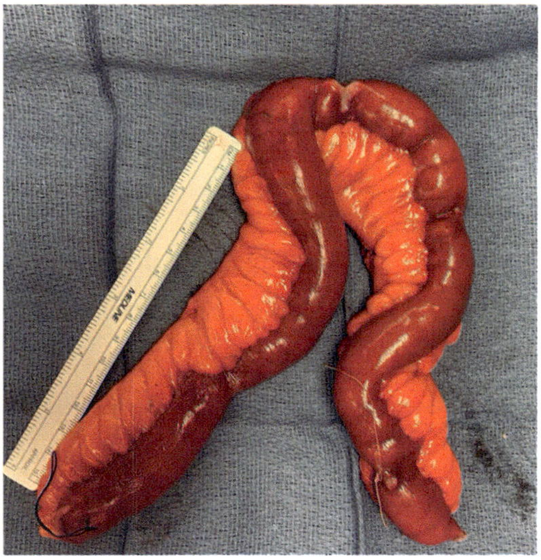

Fig. 11.22 A segment of small bowel with three lesions of endocrine tumor. (Courtesy of Dr. Latifi)

11.21). Intraoperatively, he developed significant hypotension and desaturation requiring ambo bagging and high doses of vasopressors, necessitating a swift transition to a damage control laparotomy and wide incision and debridement of the scrotum with placement of wound VAC both in the abdomen and scrotum, followed by surgical intensive care unit (ICU) admission for resuscitation.

Second-Look Procedures

The challenging nature of the case became further pronounced during second-look procedures, where intraoperative exploration revealed unforeseen white plaques on a 45 cm segment of small bowel, prompting a resection with primary anastomosis (Fig. 11.22). The identification of cirrhotic changes in the liver and an edematous, partially necrotic and calcified gallbladder (Fig. 11.23) prompted a partial cholecystectomy. A matted hepatocytic triangle during cholecystectomy posed additional unforeseen challenges leading to a reconstituted subtotal cholecystectomy. Additionally, an appendectomy was performed due to the presence of large fecaliths in the appendix which further underscored the theme of unexpected findings that highlight the complexity of this case. Multiple trips to the operating room were required including near completion of the cholecystectomy on the third exploration (Fig. 11.10) followed by meticulous wound management and wound VAC placement.

Pathology reports unveiled a well-differentiated neuroendocrine tumor in the small bowel segment, creating a new dimension in the patient's diagnostic journey. Elevated biomarkers such as plasma chromogranin A and serum serotonin levels pointed toward neuroendocrine tumor activity, introducing a new realm of complexity into the management plan. Additionally, pathological examination of the gallbladder and appendix uncovered chronic cholecystitis, cholelithiasis, and acute inflammation of the appendix, contributing further to the intricate nature of the case. Eventually we were able to save both of his testicles (Fig. 11.23) and close the scrotum and the abdominal wall. He was discharged from the hospital in very good condition (Fig. 11.24).

Management of unexpected findings in the operating room both electively but particularly in emergency surgery or acute care surgery often requires a change in operative planning and adaptation to a

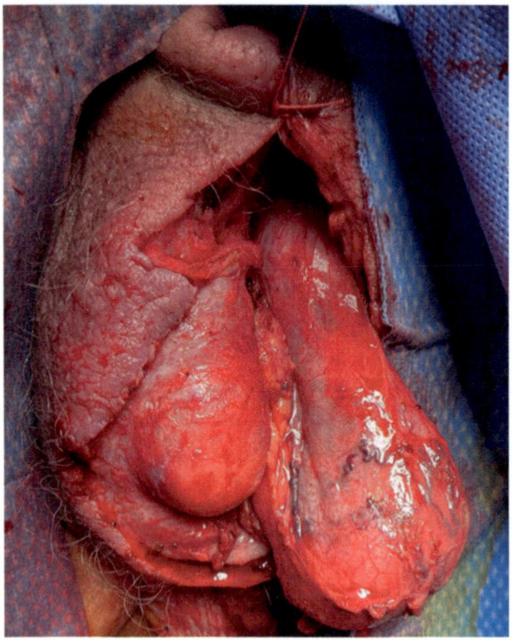

Fig. 11.23 Viable testicle following multiple debridement of scrotum for NSTI. (Courtesy of Dr. Latifi)

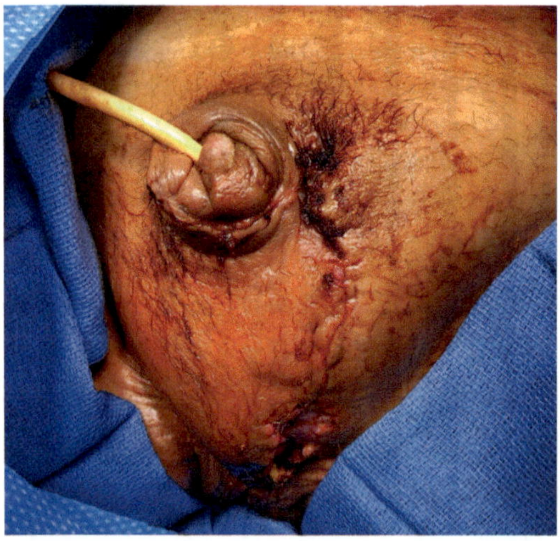

Fig. 11.24 Scrotum closed. Full recovery. Closed scrotum from Fig. 11.23. Patient had no complications and made a full recovery. (Courtesy of Dr. Latifi)

new environment and pathology. Despite meticulous preoperative planning and thorough imaging studies, unforeseen intraoperative surprises can present formidable challenges that demand immediate attention and innovative solutions. Surgeons must maintain a high level of vigilance and readiness to navigate through unanticipated discoveries, ranging from anatomical variations and hidden pathologies to unforeseen complications arising from the patient's unique physiological response to surgery. These surprises test the surgeon's expertise, decision-making skills, and the ability to think swiftly and strategically under pressure.

The ability to adeptly handle intraoperative surprises is a hallmark of surgical mastery, signifying a surgeon's capacity to pivot and adjust surgical strategies in real time to safeguard patient well-being. Whether encountering unexpected anatomical variations, unforeseen pathology, or unanticipated bleeding, surgeons must demonstrate adaptability, resilience, and quick thinking to ensure optimal outcomes for their patients. The art of surgical decision-making lies not only in meticulous planning and technical proficiency but also in the surgeon's capacity to remain calm, focused, and proactive in the face of unexpected challenges that may arise during the course of a surgical procedure. Embracing these surprises as opportunities for growth and learning, surgeons navigate through uncharted territory with skill and finesse, showcasing the dynamic and ever-evolving nature of the surgical art.

The above case that authors dealt with recently illustrates best such unexpected surprises. The case of the patient with a complex medical history and unfolding obstacles represented major challenges requiring new adaptation, such as small bowel resection, partial open cholecystectomy, initiation of DPR, and revision of the abdominal wound.

In other words, the presented case emphasizes the importance of adaptability and agility in surgical decision-making when faced with unknown and unexpected intraoperative findings. The ability to swiftly adjust the management plan in response to surprises encountered during the surgical procedure is crucial in ensuring the best possible outcome for the patient. The multidisciplinary collaboration and meticulous approach to addressing each unforeseen challenge underscore the complexity inherent in managing acute hernia complications in patients with significant comorbidities. This case serves as a poignant example of the intricate and dynamic nature of surgical decision-making in the face of unexpected clinical scenarios, highlighting the critical importance of remaining flexible, proactive, and thorough in the pursuit of optimal patient care.

When confronted with the challenging scenario of a large bowel being incarcerated in the scrotum, we firmly believe that an emergent exploratory laparotomy is the most prudent approach to ensure optimal patient outcomes. In our case we had to perform both laparotomy and groin incision to facilitate and make possible return of intact sigmoid colon. By opting for a laparotomy, surgeons can safely and effectively reduce the colon intact, with meticulous attention to detail to confirm the absence of ischemic changes and to alleviate any potential vascular compromise. This approach allows for a comprehensive assessment of the incarcerated bowel segment, facilitating timely intervention and minimizing the risk of complications associated with bowel compromise.

The laparotomy provides a controlled and well-visualized environment for surgeons to meticulously address the unique challenges posed by a large bowel herniating into the scrotum. By carefully maneuvering and reducing the colon back into the abdominal cavity, surgeons can assess the viability of the bowel, identify any signs of ischemia or necrosis, and intervene promptly to restore optimal blood supply and prevent further damage. The laparotomy approach not only ensures the safe reduction of the herniated bowel but also enables thorough exploration of the entire abdominal cavity to address any underlying pathology or associated complications, promoting a comprehensive and definitive resolution of the complex surgical dilemma.

References

1. Martinez JL, et al. Systematic management of postoperative enterocutaneous fistulas: factors related to outcomes. World J Surg. 2008;32(3):436–43.
2. Wainstein DE, et al. Treatment of high-output enterocutaneous fistulas with a vacuum-compaction device. A ten-year experience. World J Surg. 2008;32(3):430–5.
3. Visschers RG, et al. Treatment strategies in 135 consecutive patients with enterocutaneous fistulas. World J Surg. 2008;32(3):445–53.
4. Latifi R, Peralta R, Al Thani H. Surgery of complex abdominal wall defects. New York: Springer Science & Business Media; 2013.
5. Edmunds LH Jr, Williams G, Welch CE. External fistulas arising from the gastro-intestinal tract. Ann Surg. 1960;152(3):445.
6. Owen RM, et al. Definitive surgical treatment of enterocutaneous fistula: Outcomes of a 23-year experience. JAMA Surg. 2013;148(2):118–26.
7. Dionigi G, et al. Treatment of high output enterocutaneous fistulae associated with large abdominal wall defects: single center experience. Int J Surg. 2008;6(1):51–6.
8. Latifi R. Practical approaches to definitive reconstruction of complex abdominal wall defects. World J Surg. 2015; In Press
9. Girard E, et al. Anastomotic leakage after gastrointestinal surgery: diagnosis and management. J Visc Surg. 2014;151(6):441–50.
10. Lee JK, Stein SL. Radiographic and endoscopic diagnosis and treatment of enterocutaneous fistulas. Clin Colon Rectal Surg. 2010;23(3):149.
11. Singh B, et al. Surgery for high-output small bowel enterocutaneous fistula: a 30-year experience. Int Surg. 2008;94(3):262–8.
12. Schecter WP. Management of enterocutaneous fistulas. Surg Clin North Am. 2011;91(3):481–91.
13. Boyer A, et al. Influence of surgical treatment timing on mortality from necrotizing soft tissue infections requiring intensive care management. Intensive Care Med. 2009;35(5):847–53.
14. Dryden MS. Complicated skin and soft tissue infection. J Antimicrob Chemother. 2010;65(suppl 3):iii35–44.
15. Morgan M. Diagnosis and management of necrotising fasciitis: a multiparametric approach. J Hosp Infect. 2010;75(4):249–57.
16. Edlich RF, et al. Modern concepts of the diagnosis and treatment of necrotizing fasciitis. J Emerg Med. 2010;39(2):261–5.
17. Roje Z, et al. Necrotizing fasciitis: literature review of contemporary strategies for diagnosing and management with three case reports: torso, abdominal wall, upper and lower limbs. World J Emerg Surg. 2011;6(1):46.
18. May AK, et al. Treatment of complicated skin and soft tissue infections. Surg Infections. 2009;10(5):467–99.
19. Solomkin JS, et al. Diagnosis and management of complicated intra-abdominal infection in adults and children: guidelines by the Surgical Infection Society and the Infectious Diseases Society of America. Clin Infectious Dis. 2010;50(2):133–64.
20. Stevens DL, et al. Practice guidelines for the diagnosis and management of skin and soft tissue infections: 2014 update by the Infectious Diseases Society of America. Clin Infect Dis. 2014;59(2):e10–52.

21. Cainzos M. Review of the guidelines for complicated skin and soft tissue infections and intra-abdominal infections—are they applicable today? Clin Microbiol Infect. 2008;14(s6):9–18.
22. Hadeed GJ. et al. Early surgical intervention in patients presenting with necrotizing soft tissue infections: a single academic center experience. In Print, 2015.
23. Frazee BW, et al. Community-acquired necrotizing soft tissue infections: a review of 122 cases presenting to a single emergency department over 12 years. J Emerg Med. 2008;34(2):139–46.
24. Lille ST, et al. Necrotizing soft tissue infections: obstacles in diagnosis. J Am Coll Surg. 1996;182(1):7–11.
25. Tillou A, et al. Necrotizing soft tissue infections: improved outcomes with modern care. Am Surg. 2004;70(10):841.
26. McHenry CR, et al. Determinants of mortality for necrotizing soft-tissue infections. Ann Surg. 1995;221(5):558.
27. Dellinger R, et al. Surviving sepsis campaign guidelines committee including the pediatric subgroup surviving sepsis campaign: international guidelines for management of severe sepsis and septic shock: 2012. Crit Care Med. 2013;41(2):580–637.
28. Keung EZ, et al. Immunocompromised status in patients with necrotizing soft-tissue infection. JAMA Surg. 2013;148(5):419–26.
29. Anaya DA, et al. Predictors of mortality and limb loss in necrotizing soft tissue infections. Arch Surg. 2005;140(2):151–7.
30. Wall DB, et al. A simple model to help distinguish necrotizing fasciitis from nonnecrotizing soft tissue infection. J Am Coll Surg. 2000;191(3):227–31.
31. Wong C-H, et al. The LRINEC (Laboratory Risk Indicator for Necrotizing Fasciitis) score: a tool for distinguishing necrotizing fasciitis from other soft tissue infections*. Crit Care Med. 2004;32(7):1535–41.
32. Swain R, et al. A five-year review of necrotising fasciitis in a tertiary referral unit. Ann R Coll Surg Engl. 2013;95(1):57.
33. Latifi R, et al. The roles of early surgery and comorbid conditions on outcomes of severe necrotizing soft-tissue infections. Eur J Trauma Emerg Surg. 2019;45:919–26.
34. George ME, et al. Hyperbaric oxygen does not improve outcome in patients with necrotizing soft tissue infection. Surg Infect. 2009;10(1):21–8.
35. Boccola MA, et al. Risk factors and outcomes for anastomotic leakage in colorectal surgery: a single-institution analysis of 1576 patients. World J Surg. 2011;35(1):186–95.
36. Huh JW, Kim HR, Kim YJ. Anastomotic leakage after laparoscopic resection of rectal cancer: the impact of fibrin glue. Am J Surg. 2010;199(4):435–41.
37. Phitayakorn R, et al. Standardized algorithms for management of anastomotic leaks and related abdominal and pelvic abscesses after colorectal surgery. World J Surg. 2008;32(6):1147–56.
38. Hyman N, et al. Anastomotic leaks after intestinal anastomosis: it's later than you think. Ann Surg. 2007;245(2):254–8.
39. Renner P, et al. Intestinal ischemia: current treatment concepts. Langenbeck's Arch Surg. 2011;396(1):3–11.
40. Wyers MC. Acute mesenteric ischemia: diagnostic approach and surgical treatment. In: Seminars in vascular surgery. Elsevier; 2010.
41. Gaujoux S, et al. Ischemic complications after pancreaticoduodenectomy: incidence, prevention, and management. Ann Surg. 2009;249(1):111–7.
42. Loh AYH, et al. Short and long term outcomes of laparoscopic fenestrating or reconstituting subtotal cholecystectomy versus laparoscopic total cholecystectomy in the management of acute cholecystitis. HPB (Oxford). 2022;24(5):691–9.
43. Buhavac M, Elsaadi A, Dissanaike S. The bad gallbladder. Surg Clin NAm. 2021;101(6):1053–65.
44. Okumura K, et al. Direct Peritoneal Resuscitation (DPR) improves Acute Physiology and Chronic Health Evaluation (APACHE) IV and acute physiology score when used in damage control laparotomies: prospective cohort study on 37 patients. Surgical Technology International; 2022. p. 41.
45. Ashfaq A, et al. The difficult gall bladder: outcomes following laparoscopic cholecystectomy and the need for open conversion. Am J Surg. 2016;212(6):1261–4.
46. Purzner RH, et al. Safe laparoscopic subtotal cholecystectomy in the face of severe inflammation in the cystohepatic triangle: a retrospective review and proposed management strategy for the difficult gallbladder. Can J Surg. 2019;62(6):402–11.
47. Yokoe M, et al. Tokyo guidelines 2018: diagnostic criteria and severity grading of acute cholecystitis (with videos). J Hepatobiliary Pancreat Sci. 2018;25(1):41–54.
48. Mayumi T, et al. Tokyo guidelines 2018: management bundles for acute cholangitis and cholecystitis. J Hepatobiliary Pancreat Sci. 2018;25(1):96–100.
49. Pardo Aranda F, et al. Indocyanine green (ICG) fluorescent cholangiography in laparoscopic cholecystectomy: simplifying time and dose. Dig Liver Dis. 2023;55(2):249–53.
50. Dip F, et al. Does near-infrared fluorescent cholangiography with indocyanine green reduce bile duct injuries and conversions to open surgery during laparoscopic or robotic cholecystectomy? – a meta-analysis. Surgery. 2021;169(4):859–67.
51. de Angelis N, et al. Robotic surgery in emergency setting: 2021 WSES position paper. World J Emerg Surg. 2022;17(1):4.
52. Kubat E, et al. Urgent and elective robotic single-site cholecystectomy: analysis and learning curve of 150 consecutive cases. J Laparoendosc Adv Surg Tech A. 2016;26(3):185–91.
53. Waqar SH, et al. Frequency and risk factors for wound dehiscence: burst abdomen in midline laparotomies. J Ayub Med Coll Abbottabad. 2005;17(4)

54. Denys A, et al. Management of abdominal wound dehiscence: update of the literature and meta-analysis. Hernia. 2021;25(2):449–62.
55. Lengyel BI, et al. Laparoscopic cholecystectomy after a quarter century: why do we still convert? Surg Endosc. 2012;26(2):508–13.
56. Gillespie BM, et al. Incidence of wound dehiscence in patients undergoing laparoscopy or laparotomy- a systematic review and meta-analysis. J Wound Care. 2023;32(8)
57. Eke N, Jebbin NJ. Abdominal wound dehiscence a review. Int Surg J. 2006;91(5)
58. Deerenberg EB, et al. Small bites versus large bites for closure of abdominal midline incisions (STITCH): a double-blind, multicentre, randomised controlled trial. Lancet. 2015;386(10000):1254–60.
59. Lopez-Cano M, et al. EHS clinical guidelines on the management of the abdominal wall in the context of the open or burst abdomen. Hernia. 2018;22(6):921–39.
60. Jensen TK, Gogenur I, Tolstrup MB. Standardized surgical primary repair for burst abdomen reduces the risk of fascial redehiscence. Ann Surg. 2021;274(6):e1115–8.
61. Latifi R. Ventral hernia should be treated surgically and no one should die from it. Surg Technol Int. 2021;39:204–5. https://doi.org/10.52198/21.STI.39.HR1513. PMID: 34816420.
62. Yeh DD, Alam HB. Hernia emergencies. Surg Clin North Am. 2014;94(1):97–130.
63. Parker SG, et al. Identifying predictors of ventral hernia recurrence: systematic review and meta-analysis. BJS Open. 2021;5(2)
64. Hernandez A, Petersen R. Laparoscopic ventral hernia repair. Surg Clin North Am. 2023;103(5):947–60.
65. Petro CC, Melland-Smith M. Open complex abdominal wall reconstruction. Surg Clin North Am. 2023;103(5):961–76.

12 Surgical Decision-Making in Damage Control Surgery: A System-Based Approach

Rifat Latifi and Ruben Peralta

Introduction

Damage control concepts and techniques have been part of clinical armamentarium in trauma and emergency surgery for decades. In recent years, the damage control concept has expanded to other surgical disciplines: emergency neurosurgery, orthopedics, thoracic, vascular, plastic, and other surgical fields. Damage control surgery (DCS) is characterized by abbreviated surgical procedure and termination of the surgical intervention once the bleeding and contamination have been controlled followed by continuous resuscitation and definitive management, once the patient's physiology improves, or when other injuries take priority. It is a staged approach to take in consideration the physiological reserve of the patient, and it is designed to avoid or treat the lethal triad of hypothermia, acidosis, and coagulopathy. In addition, most recently, the so-called lethal diamond have been described and include trauma induced hypocalcemia along with hypothermia, acidosis, and coagulopathy, as an important post-severe trauma syndrome [1, 2].

By addressing critical issues first in a staged approach, DCS can improve outcomes and increase the likelihood of successful long-term recovery for patients with life-threatening injuries.

The decision-making process in DCS is complex and, however, requires solid knowledge of physiology of the patient as well the associated injuries or comorbid disease. In recent years DCS is being augmented with other procedures such as embolization and temporary mobilization for severe bone fractures, such as pelvis and long bones, and finally, DCS in the abdomen is being subsequently treated with direct peritoneal resuscitation [3–5].

Traditionally, the common surgical practice included the completion of the operation without many regards of the physiological condition of the patient. This concept, however, has changed dramatically in recent decades. Pioneered by trauma surgeons, where DCS was first reported, now it has expanded to many more clinical fields and surgical disciplines. Therefore, multiple strategies were developed to avoid this dilemma.

While the damage control surgery (DCS) has become popular in the last few decades, this is not a new concept. Historically the management of devastating abdominal injuries has been documented by the work of others, but the most well-known surgeon is Dr. Pringle, who described the

R. Latifi (✉)
Department of Surgery, The University of Arizona, Tucson, AZ, USA

Tucson Medical Center, Department of Surgery, Tucson, AZ, USA
e-mail: Latifi@surgery.arizona.edu

R. Peralta
Department of Surgery, Trauma Surgery Section, Hamad General Hospital, Doha, Qatar

Universidad Nacional Pedro Henriquez Urena, Santo Domingo, Dominican Republic

R. Latifi (ed.), *Surgical Decision-Making*, https://doi.org/10.1007/978-3-031-67391-7_12

use of packs and digital compression of the portal triad in large liver injuries more than a century ago [6]. Ogilvie, on the other hand, during World War II, described the use of abbreviated laparotomy and open-abdomen technique in severely injured patients [7]. Lucas and Ledgerwood reported the management of liver injuries with temporary perihepatic packings in 1976 [8]. *Stone* described the modern concept of abbreviated laparotomy in 1983. Hemorrhage was controlled by tamponade; bowel injuries were resected, noncritical injured vessels were ligated, and bilio-pancreatic injuries were drained [9]. Later, these patients underwent definitive repairs. The term "damage control" was popularized by *Rotondo* et al. in the 1990s [10], while at the University of Pennsylvania and has become a powerful and useful technique in the management of severely injured patients, since then. The concept of DCS generally consists of five stages, starting with (1) recognizing the indication and timing of DCS, (2) abbreviated operation, (3) Continue resuscitation in the intensive care unit, (4) return to the operating for re-evaluation, and finally (5) completion of the definitive procedure.

Hemostatic Resuscitation: Damage Control Resuscitation (DCR)

DCR consists of utilization of resuscitation strategies that attempt to limit secondary blood loss and prevent the development of coagulopathy. It should start immediately during patient initial evaluation and should continue through the entire resuscitation phase. The principles of DCR are in consonant with damage control surgery. Use of this approach should start with control of bleeding, use of blood products, early activation of the massive transfusion protocol (MTP), and hemostatic agents [11–17].

DCR has been demonstrated to improve mortality, facilitate earlier abdominal closure, decrease healthcare costs, and decrease length of stay [11, 14, 18–21]. Difficult and challenging clinical scenarios are patients with severe Traumatic Brain Injuries (TBI) and associated hemorrhagic shock due to other injuries. A prolonged hypotension should be avoided by utilization of aggressive resuscitation maneuvers with blood products and the temporary addition of vasopressors while bleeding is controlled. In that way we address one of the two main quality indicators in the management of severe TBI: hypotension and hypoxia.

The resuscitation continues during the initial evaluation and management, intraoperatively, and following termination of DCS or abbreviated surgery. This includes resuscitation with intravenous fluids and early administration of blood products and prevention of and correction of the lethal diamond [1, 2]. It is important to emphasize that for major bleeding trauma patients, we recommend aggressive resuscitation with the immediate use of blood products [14, 22]. Warm room and airway circuit and warmer device should be applied to each trauma in the trauma room, operating room, and ICU. A level I rewarmer device is useful at this time where all fluids and blood products should be infused warmed to the patient. In rare cases, continuous arteriovenous rewarming, a technique that permits rapid rewarming of hypothermic patients without requiring cardiopulmonary bypass or heparinization in severely hypothermic patients, is described [23, 24].

Damage control resuscitation (DCR) in brief consists of the following: (1) avoiding or minimizing crystalloid resuscitation and (2) treatment of acidosis that requires optimization of oxygen delivery by providing optimizing cardiac output, hemoglobin, and oxygen saturation. Acute traumatic coagulopathy is a frequent occurrence in severely injured patients [25]. It is corrected by aggressive blood product replacement with fresh frozen plasma, platelets, calcium replacement, fibrinogen concentrate, and/or cryoprecipitate or by the use of low-titer whole blood [22, 26, 27].

Hemostatic adjuvants that have shown effective in the correction of acquired coagulopathy of trauma are tranexamic acid (TXA) [28–31]. We recommend the use of the use of TXA in bleeding trauma patients, and it is part of our MTPs. Prothrombin complex concentrates (PCCs) have been used in selected bleeding patients to correct warfarin, Direct Oral Anticoagulants (DOACS), and clinical conditions associated with elevated

INR especially in bleeding patients and patients with documented bleeding in head CT, but clinical data have failed to demonstrate decreased mortality [32, 33].

Most recently, the Prothrombin Concentrate Complex in Patients With Acute Hemorrhage Following Severe Trauma (PROCOAG)-randomized superiority clinical trial failed to demonstrated reduction of 24-hour blood products but showed an increase in thromboembolic events with the use of 4F-PCC [34]. Recombinant factor VIIa has been shown to reduce the transfusion requirement, but its use is no longer considered part of MTP [35–37].

Indications and Timing of Damage Control

Overall, the primary indication for DCS in the operating room is to rapidly stabilize and manage patients with severe injuries or trauma that require immediate intervention to control bleeding and contamination; prevent further damage, such in case of vascular injuries; and support their overall recovery. Below are some of the situations where damage control surgery (DCS) in the operating room is indicated:

1. *Hemodynamic instability:* Patients who are in shock or have unstable blood pressure due to severe trauma or injuries may require DCS to quickly control bleeding and stabilize their condition.
2. *Extensive soft tissue damage:* Severe injuries to the abdomen or other regions of the body that involve significant soft tissue damage may necessitate DCS to address and repair the damage in a staged approach.
3. *Multiple or complex injuries:* Patients with multiple or complex injuries, such as extensive organ damage, fractures, or significant blood loss, may benefit from DCS to prioritize and address the most life-threatening injuries first.
4. *Intra-abdominal hemorrhage:* Patients with severe internal bleeding within the abdominal cavity may require DCS to locate and control the source of bleeding, often through packing, application of vascular shunt, or temporary closures to stabilize the patient before definitive repair.
5. *Acute abdominal compartment syndrome:* Patients who develop acute abdominal compartment syndrome, a condition characterized by increased pressure within the abdominal cavity that can compromise blood flow to organs, may need DCS to reduce pressure and prevent further damage.
6. *Inability to complete definitive surgery*: In some cases, the extent of a patient's injuries or their unstable condition may prevent the surgical team from completing all necessary repairs in one surgery. DCS allows for the initial stabilization of the patient before further definitive surgeries can be performed.
7. *Prolonged surgery time*: If a surgical procedure is expected to be lengthy or complex, DCS may be used to address immediate life-threatening issues and stabilize the patient before completing the full surgery in a staged approach.

When a surgeon is operating in a patient with hemodynamic instability, hypothermia (<35^0 C), coagulopathy, severe metabolic acidosis (pH < 7.2 or base deficit >8), hypocalcemia, multiple injuries, massive transfusion requirements (>10 units packed red blood cells), and long operative time (>90 minutes) for trauma or emergency, he or she should thing of abbreviating the procedure [13, 14].

System-Based Damage Control Surgery

Although, as stated earlier, DCS was initiated in austere conditions, such as wars and major liver trauma, the benefits of abbreviated surgery have become known in other disciplines and have expanded to emergency general surgery, neurosurgery, orthopedics, thoracic, vascular, and other surgical fields. In the following sections, we will describe DCS in several compartments and surgical conditions.

Damage Control in Neurosurgery

Craniectomy for Trauma

Unilateral (Fig. 12.1) or bilateral craniectomy, also known as decompressive craniectomy (DC), is performed by removing temporarily portion of the skull to relieve pressure on the brain and has become frequent procedure both in civilian and military trauma [38, 39]. Although this procedure is typically performed in cases of severe traumatic brain injury, stroke, brain swelling, or other conditions that result in significantly increased intracranial pressure (ICP), it remains controversial as to the long-term outcomes. A recent study included three trials with a total of 590 participants, including children, adults, and adolescents from multiple countries. The trials compared decompressive craniectomy (DC) combined with standard care, such as induced barbiturate coma or brain cooling, to standard care alone. The trials assessed outcomes up to 6 months after injury, with one study also measuring outcomes at 12 and 24 months. Results showed that DC slightly reduced the risk of death at 6 months and 12 months, with high-quality evidence supporting a reduction in mortality rates. In terms of neurological outcomes, the data was presented in various ways to contextualize clinical decision-making. Results for death or vegetative status versus other outcomes varied between studies, with one study favoring DC. The risk of death or vegetative state was reduced at 12 months with DC compared to standard care. Assessing unfavorable outcomes using different scales showed mixed results at 6 months but indicated a clear benefit of DC at 12 months.

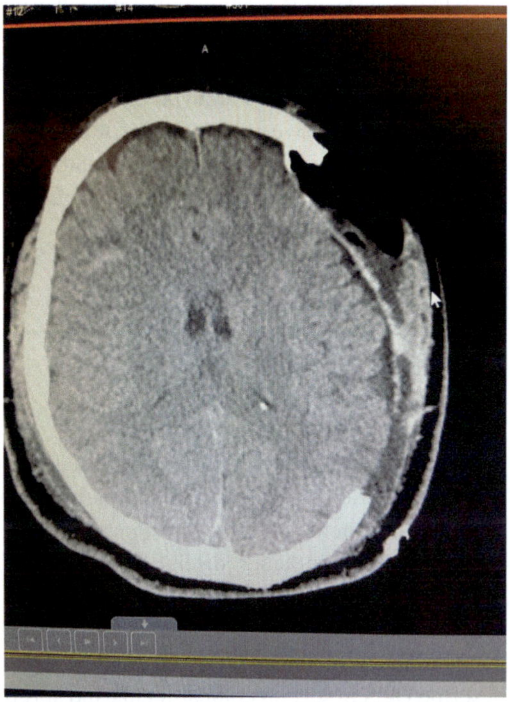

Fig. 12.1 Craniectomy for severe head injury

In terms of reducing intracranial pressure (ICP), the evidence suggests that DC was superior to standard care in reducing ICP within 48 hours. However, data on adverse events were challenging to interpret due to high mortality rates and difficulties in distinguishing treatment-related adverse events from natural disease progression. Generally, there is low-quality evidence suggesting that surgical patients had a higher risk of adverse events.

Bilateral craniectomy may be considered when a patient's condition is critical and there is extensive brain swelling or pressure on both sides of the brain. The decision to perform bilateral craniectomy is based on the patient's clinical status, neurological examination findings, imaging studies, and the severity of the intracranial pressure. In some cases, unilateral craniectomy (removal of only one side of the skull) may be initially performed, and if there is inadequate relief of intracranial pressure or ongoing brain swelling on the contralateral side, bilateral craniectomy may be indicated.

The goal of bilateral craniectomy is to prevent further damage to the brain, improve cerebral perfusion, and reduce the risk of complications such as herniation. By removing portions of the skull on both sides, bilateral craniectomy allows the brain to expand and accommodate swelling, ultimately improving outcomes and reducing the risk of long-term neurological deficits.

Overall, bilateral craniectomy is typically performed in cases of severe intracranial pressure and brain swelling where unilateral craniectomy alone may not provide sufficient decompression or relief. The decision to perform this procedure is individualized based on the specific clinical presentation and needs of each patient, with the primary goal of preserving brain function and optimizing recovery [40].

Damage Control in Thoracic Trauma

Significantly less frequently, DC is done in isolated chest injuries, with exception for a short period of DC during emergency resuscitative thoracotomy, clamping the pulmonary hilum, or twisting the lung along its hilar axis to stop bleeding from the pulmonary parenchyma [41–43]. DCS in thoracic trauma is frequently performed mostly by trauma surgeons, but not as often as DCL. Damage control surgery in thoracic trauma (DCTS) is indicated in cases of severe chest trauma with significant physiological exhaustion, non-compressible torso hemorrhage, multiple bleeding sources, high injury scores, or impending physiological deterioration, and it is performed alone or in combinations with damage control laparotomy (Figs. 12.2 and 12.3). The primary goal is to stabilize the patient rapidly, control bleeding, and minimize complications through lung-sparing techniques, repair of vascular structures, and intrathoracic packing. The decision to perform DCTS considers the urgency of bleeding control, available resources, and the expertise of the surgical team to optimize patient outcomes in complex thoracic injuries. In a recent publication, combining 14 studies with a total of 211 patients, the authors reported that, intrathoracic packing was used in 131 trauma patients, most commonly used to arrest persistent coagulopathic bleeding or oozing either from raw surfaces or requiring additional repairs in conjunction with other operative techniques. Pneumonectomy was a deadly intervention; however, one study reported survivors when pneumonectomy was deferred [44]. The intrathoracic packing is commonly utilized in conjunction with other operative interventions such as cardiography, vein ligation, and arterial repair to manage severe chest trauma effectively. The findings suggest that intrathoracic packing serves as a valuable

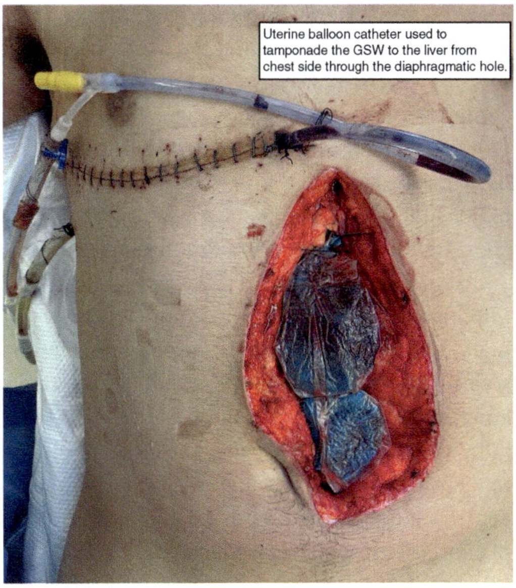

Fig. 12.2 Chest and abdominal damage control surgery post GSW to right thoraco-abdominal injuries. Uterine balloon catheter used to tamponade the GSW to the liver from chest side through the diaphragmatic hole

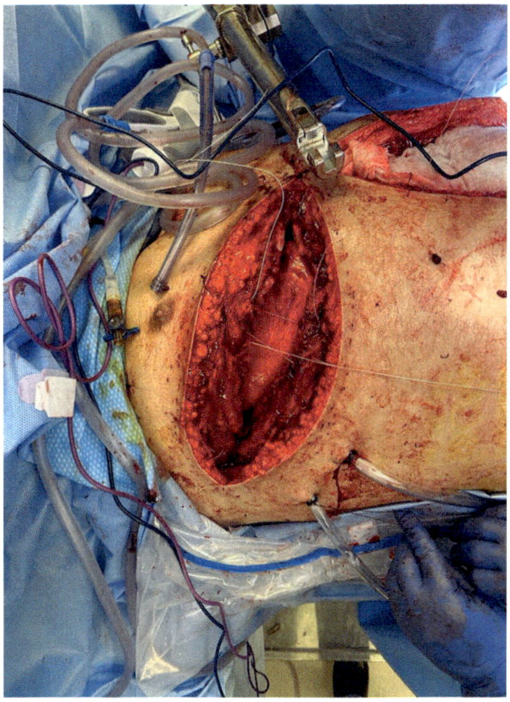

Fig. 12.3 Definitive closure post damage control thoracotomy

tool in controlling hemorrhage from raw surfaces or repaired structures within the chest, highlighting its significance in scenarios of non-compressible torso hemorrhage and severe thoracic trauma. In our experience chest DCS is used rarely and mostly in cases where there is major injury to ribs and chest wall, or degloving chest injuries, with or without lung injury.

Additionally, this review underscores the importance of lung-sparing techniques as the primary treatment option whenever feasible, emphasizing the significance of rapid hemorrhage control in improving patient outcomes. Mortality rates varied significantly across studies included in the review, prompting the call for larger multicenter studies to provide more precise estimates of mortality in patients undergoing intrathoracic packing during DCTS. The study also discusses the detrimental impact of pneumonectomy on mortality rates, advocating for avoiding this aggressive procedure during the index operation and instead recommending measures like leaving a hilar clamp in place for physiological resuscitation before potential lung resection at a later time.

In another review paper of 7 studies that reported 130 DC operations, a gauze packing with temporary closure of the skin with suture was the most frequently reported form of closure. The overall survival rate for the seven studies was 67%. Survival rates ranged from 42 to 77%. Average injury severity score was 30, and 64% of injuries were penetrating in nature. The most common complications included infections (57%: pneumonia, empyema, wound infection, bacteremia), respiratory failure (21%), ARDS (8%), and renal failure (18%) [45].

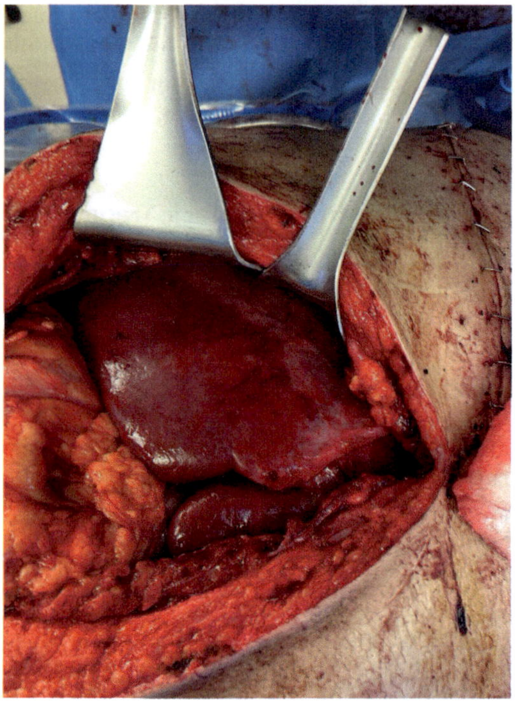

Fig. 12.4 Demonstration of liver ischemia post embolization same patient as in Fig. 12.2

Damage Control Laparotomy

While DCS may be performed in any part of the body from craniectomies to orthopedic injuries, it is most commonly done in abdominal trauma both penetrating and blunt. In general, it is most frequently done in liver injuries and vascular injuries [9, 10]. Initial hemorrhagic control is achieved by packing of the liver; and most vascular injuries can be treated by packing, simple ligation or temporary intraluminal shunts [13, 14] (Figs. 12.2 and 12.4). Hollow viscus injuries are treated by resection of affected areas; and anastomosis is postponed until the patient is stabilized [46]. The majority of biliary-pancreatic injuries can be treated with closed suction drainage [47]. Pre-peritoneal packing in some centers gained popularity in recent years and is performed when there is significant pelvic fracture with hemodynamic instability requiring an operation and embolization [48]. Another historical indication of DC use is the inability to close the abdomen, in order to avoid abdominal compartment syndrome due to massive fluid resuscitation (Figs. 12.5 and 12.6). By using hemostatic resuscitation instead of massive crystalloid resuscitation, the need for leaving the abdomen open has decreased significantly, and thus DC, once overused, is being used less [49]. Other new techniques in management of trauma patient that have become more popular are permissive hypotension whenever clinical

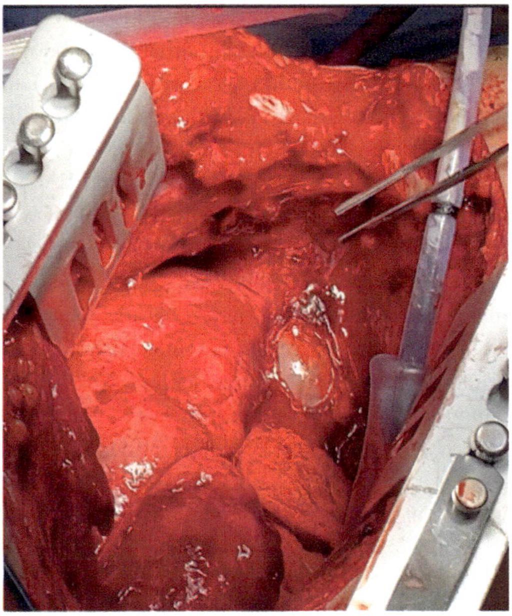

Fig. 12.5 Demonstration of missing piece of pericardium and cardiac contusion from GSW

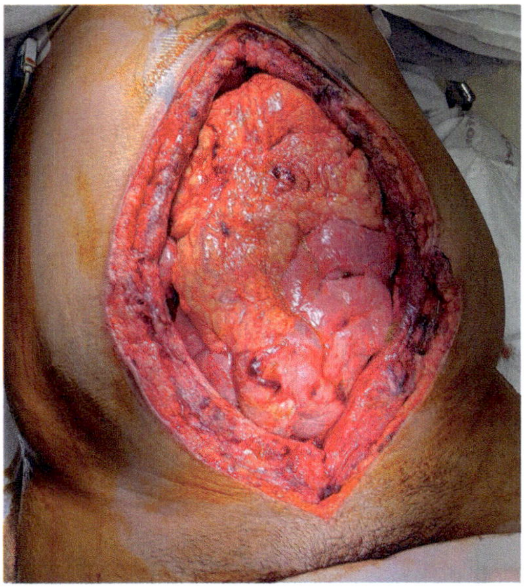

Fig. 12.6 Young male post DCS and temporary abdominal closure, who eviscerated his abdominal content, due to lack of deep sedation, requiring unplanned trip to the operating room

conditions permit. Occasionally, in major torso injuries, one has to pack the chest wall temporarily due to massive rib fractures associated with chest wall soft tissue destruction.

Other compartments where DC may be done are extremity soft tissue injuries, particularly associated with vascular injuries, requiring revascularization; the concept will be addressed in the Damage Control in Orthopedic Trauma section of this chapter.

Damage Control in Vascular Surgery: Abdomen and Beyond

The most commonly used damage control interventions in major vascular injuries are the following: temporary intravascular shunt (TIVS), where the operating surgeon can place shunts in patients with complex vascular injuries in the neck (carotid shunts), chest (aorta, subclavian, innominate or axially artery), abdomen (any major artery or vein), and extremities (particularly femoral arteries), until vascular anastomosis or definitive reconstruction procedure when the patient has reach a more reasonable hemodynamic stability [50]. Most recently, the use of resuscitative endovascular balloon occlusion of the aorta (REBOA) has emerged as promising alternative to packing in the setting of severe ongoing noncompressible major torso hemorrhage [51–55].

Damage Control in Orthopedic Trauma

The damage control orthopedic (DCO) concept refers to the initial rapid skeletal stabilization with external fixation, followed by intramedullary nailing after the systemic inflammatory response has subsided [56–62]. External fixation is also used in open-book pelvic fractures and helps limit venous bleeding. Arterial bleeding is treated by angiographic embolization. External fixation and temporary soft tissue coverage in open fractures are the standard of treatment in critically ill trauma patients. Fasciotomy is performed in vascular injuries and in ischemia reperfusion injuries [63].

Definitive (Injury Repair) Operation

After stabilization and the restoration of the physiological reserve, the patient is returned to the operating room for definitive management. Studies have shown that when patients are returned earlier than 72 hours, they have a lower rate of morbidity and mortality, compared with patients who return later [64]. As trauma and acute care surgeons, in our practice, we return the patient to the operating room within 12–36 hours. One cannot, however, wait for complete normalization of all resuscitative indicators before returning to the OR, as there may be a missed injury that is causing the patient not have normalize the physiological parameters, in the phase of ongoing resuscitation.

During the definitive procedure, a complete exploration is performed, packs are removed, and bleeding sites are controlled. This procedure in fact can be called tertiary operative survey. Small bowel continuity is restored, and patients with colonic injuries are treated with stoma or repair. Closing the abdominal fascia is considered at this time if the patient's clinical condition allows. Other important elements that need to be considered at the stage are long-term nutritional access, completing orthopedic repairs and even potential for tracheostomies, if one suspects long hospitalization or long ICU stay.

Management of Open Abdominal Wound and Definitive Abdominal Closure

Staged abdominal reconstruction has three main functions: washout to reduce contamination, debridement of devitalized tissue, and appropriate reconstruction. This is usually done after correction of the physiological derangement or within 36 hours and helps improve the outcomes in severe injuries. A preoperative patient optimization conduced to an ideal setting for reconstruction (optimal nutritional status, resolution of sepsis, correction of acidosis, hypocalcemia, hypothermia, and coagulopathy). Delaying primary fascial closure is considered according to abdomen condition (edema, viability) [64–66]. The surgical decision-making process on abdominal wall reconstruction has been addressed in more details in Chap. 11. In this section we will describe temporal abdominal closure (TAC). Most commonly, the so-called poor man VAC is used. As stated above, in our practice, if we expect to bring the patient back to the operating room within 12 to 36 hours, we do not use VAC; instead we use the poor man technique. On occasion, the intestines are so swollen, or there is continuation of intra-abdominal pathology (such as pancreatitis) that we are unable to close the fascia at all. In the past we used the technique that uses temporary vicryl mesh, followed by wound VAC and eventually skin graft, with delayed reconstruction. Today, any patient that undergoes DCL will be placed on direct peritoneal resuscitation [4, 5] (Fig. 12.7).

Postoperatively, patients should have good pain control (epidural anesthesia or patient control analgesia), antibiotic treatment until packs are removed, appropriate nutrition, and deep venous thrombosis prophylaxis. The wound should be inspected daily and the drains left in place until

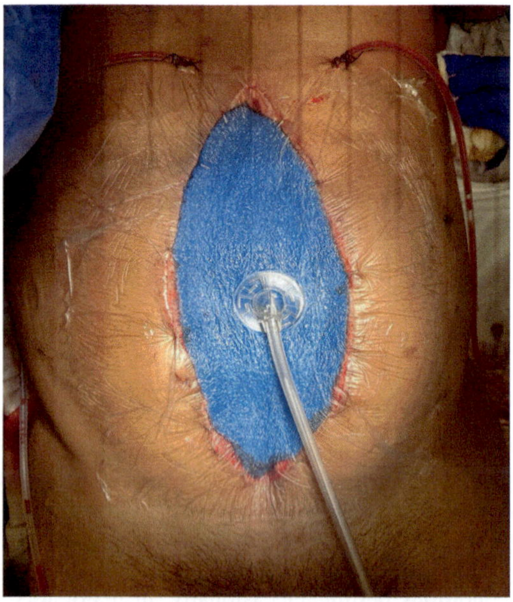

Fig. 12.7 Initiation of Direct Peritoneal Resuscitation using 2 # 19 French catheters for infusion of 2,5% dialysate solution, and Ab Thera Wound VAC

there is minimum drainage. Since the publication of the first edition of this book, definitive abdominal wall closure has evolved into early stage. Latifi's group has reported definitive closure in the acute settings [67]. In this study they compared the outcomes of patients undergoing early complex abdominal wall reconstruction (e-CAWR) in acute settings versus those undergoing delayed complex abdominal wall reconstruction (d-CAWR). Of the 236 patients who underwent CAWR with biological mesh, 79 (33.5%) had e-CAWR. There were 45 males (57%) and 34 females (43%) in the e-CAWR group. The ASA scores of IV and V and Ventral Hernia Working Group (VHWG) grades III and IV were significantly more frequent in the e-CAWR group compared with the d-CAWR one. Postoperatively, the incidence of surgical site occurrence, Clavien-Dindo complications, comprehensive complication index, unplanned reoperations, and mortality were similar between the two groups. Backward linear regression model showed that the timing of CAWR ($\beta = -11.29$, $p < 0.0001$), ASA ($\beta = 3.98$, $p = 0.006$), VHWG classification ($\beta = 3.62$, $p = 0.015$), drug abuse ($\beta = 13.47$, $p = 0.009$), and two comorbidities of cirrhosis ($\beta = 12.34$, $p = 0.001$) and malignancy ($\beta = 7.91$, $p = 0.008$) were the significant predictors of the hospital length of stay left in the model. They concluded that early CAWR led to shorter hospital length of stay compared with d-CAWR in multivariable regression model [67].

Damage Control for Abdominal Catastrophes and Sepsis

Patients with a septic abdomen have similar management focuses as the damage control trauma patient; however, the sequence differs. A longer initial resuscitation phase is used in the septic abdomen. The operative goal at the initial laparotomy is control of the infectious source. In general a temporary abdominal closure is used at the end of the initial laparotomy. A second resuscitative phase is then performed in the ICU in preparation for further surgery. If control of the septic source is not done, then subsequent interventions are required. Common complications include enterocutaneous fistula and intra-abdominal infections (tertiary peritonitis) [68]. In the most recent paper, ten international trauma, acute care, and vascular and endovascular surgery experts reviewed current literature and important concepts of open abdomen. The authors provide an evidence-informed, expert, comprehensive narrative review of the open abdomen and evaluate indications for its use and effectiveness and safety of the above components of open-abdomen management. The comprehensive and up-to-date review focuses on the most common open-abdomen scenarios that a practicing clinician will encounter in his career in the field of general surgery, trauma, acute care surgery, and vascular surgery from perioperative resuscitation strategies to the management of the hostile abdomen with complex enterocutaneous fistulas. They expand in the management description on how to tackle abdominal wall reconstruction from techniques and mesh selections to recovery and follow-up [69].

Complications associated with damage control can be classified as local (abscess, fistula, and intestinal necrosis) or systemic complications (ARDS and MOF). They are also divided into early (missed injuries, infections, and compartment syndrome) and late (fistula, dehiscence).

Several studies have shown improved outcomes since the widespread institution of damage control techniques [70, 71].

Summary

In summary, damage control surgery (DCS) is a staged approach to severely injured patients. Initially, life-threatening injuries are managed rapidly with appropriate abbreviated procedures and aggressive resuscitation. The patient is then stabilized in the ICU. Later, definitive surgical management is performed. This strategy is beneficial and results in improved outcomes. This approach is still evolving, and many studies are done to implement it as a standard management approach to trauma patients. It requires a multidisciplinary team to achieve better outcomes.

References

1. Ditzel RM, Anderson JL, Eisenhart WJ, Rankin CJ, DeFeo DR, Oak S, Siegler J, et al. J Trauma Acute Care Surg. 2020;88(3):434–9. https://doi.org/10.1097/TA.0000000000002570.
2. Napolitano LM. Hemostatic defects in massive transfusion: an update and treatment recommendations. Exp Rev Hematol. 2021;14(2):219–39. https://doi.org/10.1080/17474086.2021.1858788.
3. Smith JW, Neal Garrison R, Matheson PJ, Harbrecht BG, Benns MV, Franklin GA, Miller KR, Bozeman MC, David RJ. Adjunctive treatment of abdominal catastrophes and sepsis with direct peritoneal resuscitation: indications for use in acute care surgery. J Trauma Acute Care Surg. 2014;77(3):393–8. https://doi.org/10.1097/TA.0000000000000393; discussion 398–9. PMID: 25159241.
4. McGuirk M, Kajmolli A, Gachabayov M, Haider A, Bronstein M, Spatz D, Gwardshaladse C, Latifi R. Use of direct peritoneal resuscitation for intra-abdominal catastrophes: a technical note. Surg Technol Int. 2020;28(37):127–31. PMID: 33245138.
5. Okumura K, Latifi R, Smiley A, Lee JS, Shnaydman I, Zangbar B, Bronstein M, Con J, Prabhakaran K, Rhee P, Klein J, Shivaraj K, Klein MD, Miller DM. Direct peritoneal resuscitation (DPR) improves acute physiology and chronic health evaluation (APACHE) IV and acute physiology score when used in damage control laparotomies: prospective cohort study on 37 patients. Surg Technol Int. 2022;41:sti41/1620. https://doi.org/10.52198/22.STI.41.GS1620. Epub ahead of print. PMID: 36041078.
6. Pringle J. Notes on the arrest of hepatic hemorrhage due to trauma. Ann Surg. 1908;48:541–9.
7. Ogilvie WH. The late complications of abdominal war-wounds. Lancet. 1940;2:253–6.
8. Lucas CE, Ledgerwood AM. Prospective evaluation of hemostatic techniques for liver injuries. J Trauma. 1976;16(6):442–51.
9. Stone HH, Strom PR, Mullins RJ. Management of the major coagulopathy with onset during laparotomy. Ann Surg. 1983;197(5):532–5.
10. Rotondo MF, Schwab W, McGonigal MD, et al. Damage control: an approach for improved survival in exsanguinating penetrating abdominal injury. J Trauma. 1993;35(3):375–83.
11. Cannon JW, Khan MA, Raja AS, et al. Damage control resuscitation in patients with severe traumatic hemorrhage: a practice management guideline from the Eastern Association for the Surgery of Trauma. J Trauma Acute Care Surg. 2017;82:605–17.
12. Leibner E, Andreae M, Galvagno SM, Scalea T. Damage control resuscitation. Clin Exp. Emerg Med. 2020;7(1):5–13. https://doi.org/10.15441/ceem.19.089. Epub 2020 Mar 31. PMID: 32252128; PMCID: PMC7141982.
13. Roberts DJ, Bobrovitz N, Zygun DA. Indications for use of thoracic, abdominal, pelvic, and vascular damage control interventions in trauma patients: a content analysis and expert appropriateness rating study. J Trauma Acute Care Surg. 2015;9(4):568–79. https://doi.org/10.1097/TA.0000000000000821.
14. Peralta R, Vijay A, El-Menyar A, et al. Trauma resuscitation requiring massive transfusion: a descriptive analysis of the role of ratio and time. World J Emerg Surg. 2015;10:36. https://doi.org/10.1186/s13017-015-0028-3. eCollection 2015.
15. El-Menyar A, Sathian B, Wahlen BM, Abdelrahman H, Peralta R, Al-Thani H, Rizoli S. Prehospital administration of tranexamic acid in trauma patients: A 1: 1 matched comparative study from a level 1 trauma center. Am J Emerg Med. 2020;38(2):266–71.
16. Asensio JA, Dabestani PJ, Kessler JJ, Miljkovic SS, Peralta R, Lim R, Galvagno S, Cancio L. Exsanguination: reliable models to indicate damage control. In: Asensio JA, Meredith JW, editors. Current therapy of trauma and surgical critical care. 3rd ed. Elsevier; 2023. p. 456–463.e1. https://doi.org/10.1016/B978-0-323-69787-3.00075-7. ISBN 9780323697873.
17. Consunji R, Elseed A, El-Menyar A, Sathian B, Rizoli S, Al-Thani H, Peralta R. The effect of massive transfusion protocol implementation on the survival of trauma patients: a systematic review and meta-analysis. Blood Transfus. 2020;18(6):434–45. https://doi.org/10.2450/2020.0065-20. Epub 2020 Sep 18. PMID: 32955420; PMCID: PMC7605882.
18. Joseph B, Azim A, Zangbar B, et al. Improving mortality in trauma laparotomy through the evolution of damage control resuscitation: analysis of 1,030 consecutive trauma laparotomies. J Trauma Acute Care Surg. 2017;82:328–33.
19. Duchesne JC, Kimonis K, Marr AB, et al. Damage control resuscitation in combination with damage control laparotomy: a survival advantage. J Trauma. 2010;69:46–52.
20. Cannon JW. Hemorrhagic shock. N Engl J Med. 2018;378:370–9.
21. Leibner E, Andreae M, Galvagno SM Jr, Scalea T. Damage control resuscitation. Clin Exp Emerg Med. 2020;7(1):5–13.
22. Rossaint R, Afshari A, Bouillon B, Cerny V, Cimpoesu D, Curry N, Duranteau J, Filipescu D, Grottke O, Grønlykke L, Harrois A, Hunt BJ, Kaserer A, Komadina R, Madsen MH, Maegele M, Mora L, Riddez L, Romero CS, Samama CM, Vincent JL, Wiberg S, Spahn DR. The European guideline on management of major bleeding and coagulopathy following trauma: sixth edition. Crit Care. 2023;27(1):80. https://doi.org/10.1186/s13054-023-04327-7. PMID: 36859355; PMCID: PMC9977110.
23. Gentilello LM, Rifley WJ. Continuous arteriovenous rewarming: report of a new technique for treating hypothermia. J Trauma. 1991;31:1151–4.
24. Gentilello LM, Cobean RA, Offner PJ, et al. Continuous arteriovenous rewarming: rapid reversal of hypothermia in critically ill patients. J Trauma. 1992;32(3):316–27.
25. Brohi K, Singh J, Heron M, et al. Acute traumatic coagulopathy. J Trauma. 2003;54(6):1127–30.
26. Peralta R, Al Thani H, Rizoli S. Coagulopathy in the surgical patient: trauma-induced and drug-

induced coagulopathies. Curr Opin Crit Care. 2019;25(6):668–74.
27. Peralta R, Vijay A, El-Menyar A, Consunji R, Afifi I, Mahmood I, Asim M, Latifi R, Al-Thani H. Early high ratio platelet transfusion in trauma resuscitation and its outcomes. Int J Crit Illn Inj Sci. 2016;6(4):188–93. https://doi.org/10.4103/2229-5151.195448. PubMed PMID: 28149824; PubMed Central PMCID: PMC5225762.
28. CRASH-2 trial collaborators. Effect of tranexamic acid on death, vascular occlusive events, and blood transfusion in trauma patients with significant haemorrhage (CRASH-2): a randomized, placebo-controlled trial. Lancet. 2010;376(9734):22–32. https://doi.org/10.1016/S0140-6736(10)60835.5. Epub 2010 Jun 14.
29. Roberts I, Shakur-Still H, Aeron-Thomas A, Beaumont D, Belli A, Brenner A, Cargill M, Chaudhri R, Douglas N, Frimley L, et al. Tranexamic acid to reduce head injury death in people with traumatic brain injury: the CRASH-3 international RCT. Health Technol Assess. 2021;25(26):1–76. https://doi.org/10.3310/hta25260.
30. Song JX, Wu JX, Zhong H, Chen W, Zheng JC. Therapeutic efficacy of tranexamic acid on traumatic brain injury: a systematic review and meta-analysis. Scand J Trauma Resusc Emerg Med. 2024;32(1):18. https://doi.org/10.1186/s13049-024-01188-z. PMID: 38454455; PMCID: PMC10921791.
31. El-Menyar A, Sathian B, Wahlen BM, Abdelrahman H, Peralta R, Al-Thani H, Rizoli S. Prehospital administration of tranexamic acid in trauma patients: A 1:1 matched comparative study from a level 1 trauma center. Am J Emerg Med. 2019; https://doi.org/10.1016/j.ajem.2019.04.051. ISSN 0735-6757.
32. Al-Majzoub O, Rybak E, Reardon DP, Krause P, Connors JM. Evaluation of warfarin reversal with 4-facto prothrombin complex concentrate compared to 3-factor prothrombin complex concentrate at a tertiary academic medical center. J Emerg Med. 2015:Pii:s0736-4679(15)00799-4. https://doi.org/10.1016/j.jemermed.2015.07.024.
33. Hannadjas I, James A, Davenport R, et al. Prothrombin complex concentrate (PCC) for treatment of trauma-induced coagulopathy: systematic review and meta-analyses. Crit Care. 2023;27:422. https://doi.org/10.1186/s13054-023-04688-z.
34. Bouzat P, Charbit J, Abback P, et al. Efficacy and safety of early administration of 4-factor prothrombin complex concentrate in patients with trauma at risk of massive transfusion: the PROCOAG randomized clinical trial. JAMA. 2023;329(16):1367–75. https://doi.org/10.1001/jama.2023.4080.
35. Schreiber MA, Holcomb JB, Hedner U, et al. The effect of recombinant factor VIIa on coagulopathic pigs with grade V liver injuries. J Trauma. 2002;53:252–9.
36. Martinowitz U, Kenet G, Segal E, et al. Recombinant activated factor VII for adjunctive hemorrhage control in trauma. J Trauma. 2001;51:431–9.
37. Knudson MM, Cohen MJ, Reidy R, Jaeger S, Bacchetti P, Jin C, Wade CE, Holcomb JB. Trauma, transfusions, and use of recombinant factor VIIa: a multicenter case registry report of 380 patients from the Western Trauma Association. J Am Coll Surg. 2011;212(1):87–95. https://doi.org/10.1016/j.jamcollsurg.2010.08.020. Epub 2010 Nov 5. PMID: 21115374.
38. Rubiano AM, Maldonado M, Montenegro J, Restrepo CM, Khan AA, Monteiro R, Faleiro RM, Carreño JN, Amorim R, Paiva W, Muñoz E, Paranhos J, Soto A, Armonda R, Rosenfeld JV. The evolving concept of damage control in neurotrauma: application of military protocols in civilian settings with limited resources. World Neurosurg. 2019;125:e82–93. https://doi.org/10.1016/j.wneu.2019.01.005. Epub 2019 Jan 16. PMID: 30659971.
39. Manet R, Joubert C, Balanca B, Taverna XJ, Monneuse O, David JS, Dagain A. Neuro damage control: current concept and civilian applications. Neurochirurgie. 2023;69(6):101505. https://doi.org/10.1016/j.neuchi.2023.101505. Epub 2023 Oct 8. PMID: 37806039.
40. Sahuquillo J, Dennis JA. Decompressive craniectomy for the treatment of high intracranial pressure in closed traumatic brain injury. Cochrane Database Syst Rev. 2019;12(12):CD003983. https://doi.org/10.1002/14651858.CD003983.pub3. PMID: 31887790; PMCID: PMC6953357.
41. Caceres M, Buechter KJ, Tillou A, Shih JA, Liu D, Steeb G. Thoracic packing for uncontrolled bleeding in penetrating thoracic injuries. South Med J. 2004;97(7):637Y641.
42. Moriwaki Y, Toyoda H, Harunari N, Iwashita M, Kosuge T, Arata S, Suzuki N. Gauze packing as damage control for uncontrollable haemorrhage in severe thoracic trauma. Ann R Coll Surg Engl. 2013;95(1):20Y25.
43. Rizzo AG, Sample GA. Thoracic compartment syndrome secondary to a thoracic procedure: a case report. Chest. 2003;124(3):1164Y1168.
44. Manzano-Nunez R, Chica J, Gómez A, Naranjo MP, Chaves H, Muñoz LE, Rengifo JE, Caicedo-Holguin I, Puyana JC, García AF. The tenets of intrathoracic packing during damage control thoracic surgery for trauma patients: a systematic review. Eur J Trauma Emerg Surg. 2021;47(2):423–34. https://doi.org/10.1007/s00068-020-01428-8. Epub 2020 Jun 28. PMID: 32594214.
45. Douglas A 2nd, Puzio T, Murphy P, Menard L, Meagher AD. Damage control thoracotomy: a systematic review of techniques and outcomes. Injury. 2021;52(5):1123–7. https://doi.org/10.1016/j.injury.2020.12.020. Epub 2020 Dec 30. PMID: 33386155.
46. Mahmood I, Mustafa F, Younis B, Ahmed K, El-Menyar A, Asim M, Al-Hassani A, Peralta R, Al-Thani H. Postoperative complications of intestinal anastomosis after blunt abdominal trauma. Eur J Trauma Emerg Surg. 2018; https://doi.org/10.1007/s00068-018-1013-9. [Epub ahead of print] PubMed PMID: 30251153.

47. Burch JM, Ortiz VB, Richardson RJ, et al. Abbreviated laparotomy and planned reoperation for critically injured patients. Ann Surg. 1992;215(5):476–84.
48. Cullinane DC, Schiller HJ, Zielinski MD, Bilaniuk JW, Collier BR, Como J, Holevar M, Sabater EA, Sems SA, Vassy WM, et al. Eastern Association for the Surgery of Trauma practice management guidelines for hemorrhage in pelvic fracture – update and systematic review. J Trauma. 2011;71(6):1850Y1868.
49. Mahmood I, Mahmood S, Parchani A, Kumar S, El-Menyar A, Zarour A, Al-Thani H, Latifi R. Intra-abdominal hypertension in the current era of modern trauma resuscitation. ANZ J Surg. 2014;84(3):166–71. https://doi.org/10.1111/ans.12169. Epub 2013 Apr 9. PMID: 23574113.
50. Davis TP, Feliciano DV, Rozycki GS, et al. Results with abdominal vascular trauma in the modern era. Am Surg. 2001;67:565–70.
51. Stannard A, Eliason JL, Rasmussen TE. Resuscitative endovascular balloon occlusion of the aorta (REBOA) as an adjunct for hemorrhagic shock. J Trauma. 2011;71:1869–72.
52. Morrison JJ, Ross JD, Houston R, Watson JDB, Sokol KK, Rasmussen TE. Use of Resuscitative endovascular balloon occlusion of the aorta (REBOA) in a highly lethal model of non-compressible torso hemorrhage. Shock. 2014;41:130–7.
53. Morrison JJ, Percival TJ, Markov NP, Villamaria C, Scott DJ, Saches KA, Spencer JR, Rasmussen TE. Aortic balloon occlusion is effective in controlling pelvic hemorrhage. J Surg Res. 2012;177:341–7.
54. Brenner M, Moore L, Dubose J, Tyson G, McNutt M, Albarado R, Holcomb JB, Scalea TM, Rasmussen TE. A clinical series of resuscitative endovascular balloon occlusion of the aorta for hemorrhage control and resuscitation. J Trauma Acute Care Surg. 2013;75:506–5011.
55. Morrison JJ, Ross JD, Rasmussen TE, et al. Resuscitative endovascular balloon occlusion of the aorta: A gap analysis of severely injured UK combat casualties. Shock. 2014;41:388–93.
56. Scalea TM, Boswell SA, Scott JD, et al. External fixation as a bridge to intramedullary nailing for patients with multiple injuries and with femur fractures: damage control orthopedics. J Trauma. 2000;48(4):613–21.
57. Balogh ZJ, Reumann MK, Gruen RL, et al. Advances and future directions for management of trauma patients with musculoskeletal injuries. Lancet. 2012;380(9847):1109–19.
58. Pape HC, Tornetta P 3rd, Tarkin I, et al. Timing of fracture fixation in multitrauma patients: the role of early total care and damage control surgery. J Am Acad Orthop Surg. 2009;17:541–9.
59. Shapiro MB, Jenkins DH, Schwab CW, Rotondo MF. Damage control: collective review. J Trauma-Injury Infect Critical Care. 2000;49(5):969–78.
60. LichteP KP, Dombroski D, Pape HC. Damage control orthopedics: current evidence. Curr Opin Crit Care. 2012;18(6):647–50. https://doi.org/10.1097/MCC.0b013e328359fd57.
61. Pfeifer R, Kalbas Y, Coimbra R, Leenen L, Komadina R, Hildebrand F, Halvachizadeh S, Akhtar M, Peralta R, Fattori L, Mariani D. Indications and interventions of damage control orthopedic surgeries: an expert opinion survey. Eur J Trauma Emerg Surg. 2021;47:2081–92.
62. Enninghorst N, Peralta R, Yoshino O, et al. Physiological assessment of the polytrauma patient: initial and secondary surgeries. Eur J Trauma Emerg Surg. 2011;37:559–66. https://doi.org/10.1007/s00068-011-0161-y.
63. Porter JM, Ivatury RR, Nassoura ZE. Extending the horizons of "damage control" in unstable trauma patients beyond the abdomen and gastrointestinal tract. J Trauma. 1997;42:559–61.
64. Abikhaled JA, Granchi TS, Wall MJ, et al. Prolonged abdominal packing is associated with increased morbidity and mortality. Am Surg. 1997;63(12):1109–13.
65. Diaz JJ Jr, Cullinane DC, Dutton WD, Jerome R, Bagdonas R, Bilaniuk JW, Collier BR, Como JJ, Cumming J, Griffen M, Gunter OL, Kirby J, Lottenburg L, Mowery N, Riordan WP Jr, Martin N, Platz J, Stassen N, Winston ES. The management of the open abdomen in trauma and emergency general surgery: part 1-damage control. J Trauma. 2010;68(6):1425–38. https://doi.org/10.1097/TA.0b013e3181da0da5.
66. Peralta R, Latifi R. Perioperative surgical consideration of patient undergoing abdominal wall reconstruction. R. In: Latifi R, editor. Surgery of complex abdominal wall defects. New York: Springer; 2013. p. 173–7.
67. Gogna S, Latifi R, Choi J, Con J, Prabhakaran K, Anderson PL, Policastro AJ, Klein J, Samson DJ, Smiley A, Rhee P. Early versus delayed complex abdominal wall reconstruction with biologic mesh following damage-control surgery. J Trauma Acute Care Surg. 2021;90(3):527–34. https://doi.org/10.1097/TA.0000000000003011. PMID: 33507024.
68. Waibel BH, Rotondo M. Damage control for intra-abdominal sepsis. https://doi.org/10.1016/j.suc.2012.01.006.
69. Roberts DJ, Leppäniemi A, Tolonen M, Mentula P, Björck M, Kirkpatrick AW, Sugrue M, Pereira BM, Petersson U, Coccolini F, Latifi R. The open abdomen in trauma, acute care, and vascular and endovascular surgery: comprehensive, expert, narrative review. BJS Open. 2023;7(5):zrad084. https://doi.org/10.1093/bjsopen/zrad084. PMID: 37882630; PMCID: PMC10601091.
70. Johnson JW, Gracias VH, Schwab CW, et al. Evolution in damage control for exsanguinating penetrating abdominal injury. J Trauma. 2001;51(2):261–71.
71. Chovanes J, Cannon JW, Nunez TC. The evolution of damage control surgery. https://doi.org/10.1016/j.suc.2012.04.002.

13 Surgical Decision-Making Process and Definitive Abdominal Wall Reconstruction: An Update

Ruben Peralta and Rifat Latifi

Introduction

Reconstruction of complex abdominal wall defects and recreating functional abdominal wall represent major challenges, often requiring surgical creativity and a strategy that involves different aspects of care along the various stages of treatment [1]. These challenges need to be understood primarily by the surgeon but by the patient as well. The issues range from defining the anatomy at hand and the pathology to understanding the impact of the clinical condition, physiology, nutritional status, and wound care. Redefining the anatomy and physiology, timing the definitive surgery, executing perfectly the operative plan, making intraoperative decisions that are often considered "outside surgical dogma or box," long-term follow-up, and ensuring full recovery of the patient to normal functional status are all basic requirements for every one of these cases. One very important factor is the dedication of the surgeon to these patients and to their surgical problems, and these operations cannot and should not to be performed by an "itinerary surgeon."

The management of these patients should be approached in a stepwise fashion, ensuring that each phase is truly understood by the surgeon, as well as by the patient and their family. There are systematic reviews and meta-analysis as well as several surgical societies' guidelines addressing this complex clinical entity [2–7], but while there is always room for a creative surgical approach, disciplined protocols and a well-planned surgical strategy, particularly in patients with abdominal wall defects complicated by fistulas or stomas, make the intraoperative management process easier and may improve postoperative outcomes. Such a strategy has been described in a six-step strategy for management of enterocutaneous fistulas (ECFs), known as "SOWATS" (S, sepsis control; O, nutrition optimization; W, wound care; T, timing; A, anatomy; and S, surgery) [8]. Use of this approach on 79 patients led to spontaneous closure in 23 (29%) patients after a median period of 39 (range 7–163) days. Forty-nine patients required operative repair after median period of 101 (range 7–374) days; closure was achieved in 47 (96%) patients. The reported mortality was 10% during the study period, although in a separate publication, the authors reported that 44/135 or 32.5% of patients died [9]. While this strategy is applicable in the acute setting, it does not address important aspects of the man-

R. Peralta
Department of Surgery, Trauma Surgery Section, Hamad General Hospital, Doha, Qatar

Universidad Nacional Pedro Henriquez Urena, Santo Domingo, Dominican Republic

R. Latifi (✉)
Department of Surgery, The University of Arizona, Tucson, AZ, USA

Tucson Medical Center, Department of Surgery, Tucson, AZ, USA
e-mail: Latifi@surgery.arizona.edu

R. Latifi (ed.), *Surgical Decision-Making*, https://doi.org/10.1007/978-3-031-67391-7_13

agement of these patients as part of the continuum of care. Initial diagnosis, the immediate postoperative period, postoperative care following definitive surgery, and finally long-term follow-up are all equally important to consider. To address these aspects, Latifi et al. have expanded the six-step strategy to nine steps and call it "ISOWATS PL" [10] where I, identification and diagnosis of the postoperative fistula; S, sepsis and source control; O, optimization of nutrition; W, providing and ensuring wound care; A, redefining the anatomy and understanding the pathology at hand; T, timing of definitive surgery and/or takedown of fistulas; S, definitive surgery and surgical creativity; P, postoperative care; and L, long-term follow-up. We adhere to the "ISOWATS PL" strategy as much as possible, although we sometimes cannot strictly follow all nine steps in certain patients, as some often require emergency surgery. In this chapter, we will discuss the decision-making process for parts of our nine-step approach, which deal with timing of the surgery, and the methods and techniques used to reconstruct the complex abdominal wall defects.

Timing to Definitive Repair

We have previously described that the decision if and when to reoperate on patients with complex abdominal wall defects should be individualized and represents one of the most important steps in the surgical management of these patients [10]. The timing can divided in the acute setting, that is, post-damage control surgery, or electively. In both phases, we base this decision to perform complex abdominal wall reconstruction (CAWR) on many factors, particularly on the comorbid diseases and on the anatomy of the surgical problem. In addition to considering the clinical status and physiology of the patient, one has to remember that these large defects can be functionally devastating and lead to further weight gain and more problems and potentially may lead to major morbidity and or death. If patients have serious comorbid diseases such as super obesity with BMI >40 or higher or a BMI of 35 or higher and are experiencing obesity-related health conditions, severe heart disease, high-grade liver cirrhosis (decompensated cirrhosis), or lung disease (dependent upon oxygen therapy at home), even though they do not have symptoms of obstructions, one should carefully evaluate the decision of whether to operate, except in situations involving intestinal obstruction not responding to conservative treatment. While not all surgeons agree, at times the strategy for these patients should be "more is less," and in our opinion the definitive surgery is the only choice and should be performed. We prefer to operate earlier rather than later, assuming that the patient is not prohibitively at high risk for major complications from anesthesia alone.

While timing when to repair large abdominal wall hernias is less debatable [11–13], operating on fistulas and knowing how long a surgeon should wait until takedown is more contentious. Delaying surgery anywhere from 12 to 36 months to improve the outcomes in patients with ECF has been suggested [2, 3, 14], although prolonging surgery for longer than 1 year following ECF diagnosis doubles the risk of postoperative refistulization [15], and waiting longer than 36 weeks increases the reported risk for fistula recurrence by five times [16]. There are no solid data to inform such decisions, and thus the individual patient's condition is the main factor that should be used as a guide.

Surgical Approach and Technique

Once the decision to operate has been made jointly by the patient and the surgeon, deciding on the definitive reconstruction technique is the next most important challenge. Most patients who have previously undergone large abdominal surgeries have a midline abdominal incision, so their lateral abdominal wall may be free of scars

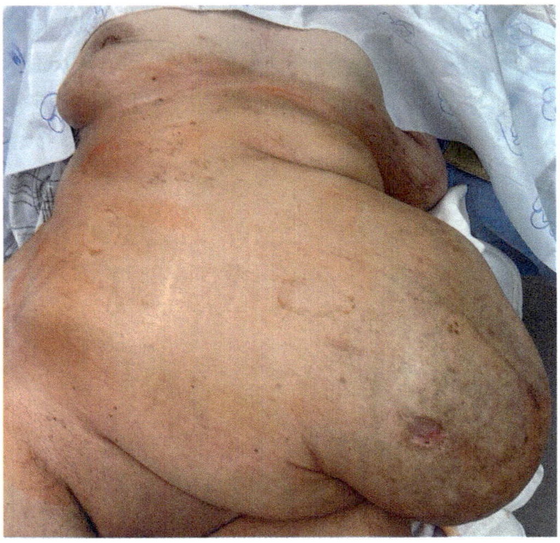

Fig. 13.1 A. A 54-year-old-female with large "asymptomatic" abdominal wall hernia, with the majority of small and large bowels in the hernia on the left side who underwent bilateral amputation for severe peripheral vascular disease, and was unable to mobilized herself to the wheelchair. (** All figures are courtesy of Rifat Latifi, MD)

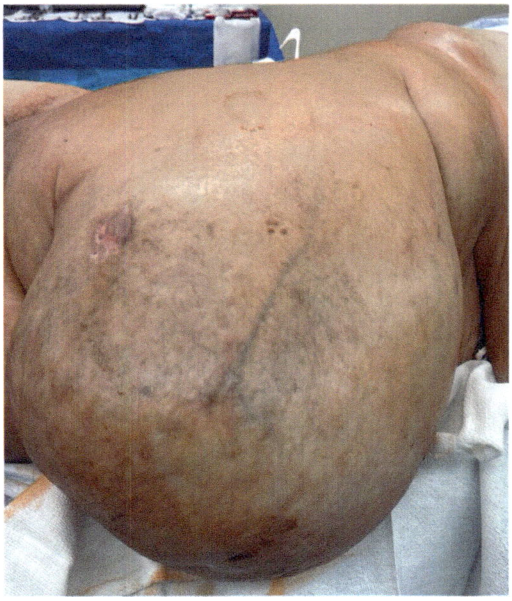

Fig. 13.2 Another view of a large left sided hernia. (** All figures are courtesy of Rifat Latifi, MD)

and defects, thereby providing a well-vascularized soft tissue donor site. There are a number of exceptions, however, especially when the patient has had any lateral incision (open appendectomy, open cholecystectomy) or stomas due to intra-abdominal catastrophe with sepsis and or fistulas, when adhesions can be a very challenging problem. Every hernia needs to be repaired, unless contraindicated, as they do not become smaller and eventually will have complications, but particularly the giant hernia with loss of abdominal domain (Figs. 13.1, 13.2, 13.3 and 13.4), the abdominal wall can be anatomically restored with minimal tension and without compromising the integrity of the abdominal muscles, vessels, and nerves. The surgical goals are to establish gastrointestinal (GI) tract continuity; obtain full closure of the abdominal wall; avoid the postoperative abdominal compartment syndrome; minimize the formation or recurrence of fistulas, hernias, and wound infections; and strive to restore the patient's functionality. In patients with frozen abdomen, or when a split-thickness skin graft (STSG) exists, dealing with adhesions, resecting fistulas, and performing the anastomo-

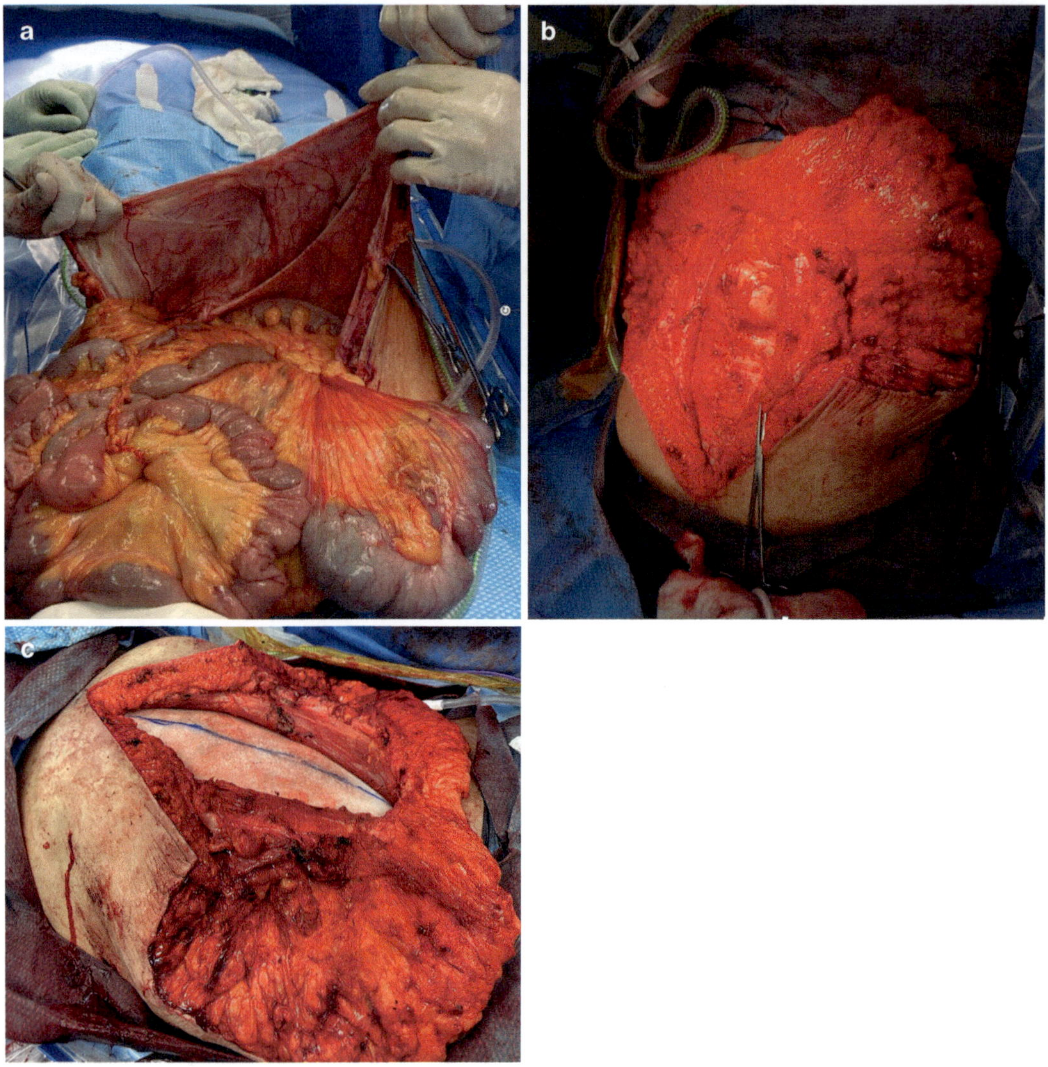

Fig. 13.3 (**a**–**c**). (**a**) Intraoperative view of case in Figs. 13.1 and 13.2 demonstrating large multiple pockets of hernia; (**b**). Post closure of posterior component release with posterior rectus sheet closure; (**c**) Placement of biologic mesh in the retro-rectus position (Strattice™). (** All figures are courtesy of Rifat Latifi, MD)

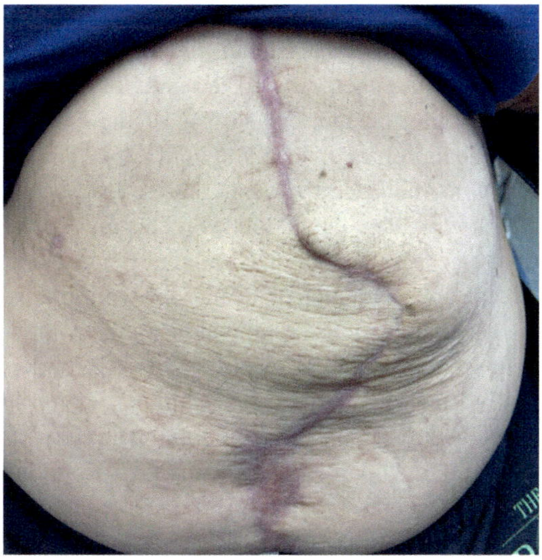

Fig. 13.4 Six-months post-operative view of the patient in Fig. 13.1, 13.2 and 13.3. (** All figures are courtesy of Rifat Latifi, MD)

sis requires experience, and even entering the abdomen may prove challenging.

Definitive Abdominal Wall Reconstruction

Creating a new abdominal wall may represent a serious surgical challenge, and both the surgeon and the patient should be prepared for a lengthy procedure (i.e., entering the abdomen, lysis of adhesions, resecting the fistulas, and performing the anastomosis). Some authors have suggested that reconstruction should be performed by combining expertise with other surgeons [17]; this created a multidisciplinary team that is much preferred for centers of excellence. On occasions we have used the principle of damage control on demand, returning the next day for definitive surgery. We find this approach a very useful technique to completely reinspect the anastomoses, enterotomies (if any caused), or ensuring that there are no missed enterotomies, and or any bleeding from retroperitoneum, before performing the final closure. We use intraoperative indocyanine green (ICG) if there is any question of viability of both flaps and for evaluation of the viability of the intestine anastomosis [18].

If native tissue can be used without undue tension, then it should be utilized. If that is not possible, a synthetic or biologic prosthesis can be used instead. In most patients, some sort of combination of reconstruction techniques will be needed. If the midline tissue cannot be easily approximated, or if mesh reinforcement is needed (as it is in almost all abdominal wall defects larger than 6 cm), then other techniques must be considered. For example, if midline tissue cannot be easily approximated, in order to avoid undue tension on the tissue and postoperative compartment syndrome, the lateral components, bilaterally, need to be released and a neo-abdominal wall created. Tissue transposition of myocutaneous flaps through lateral component separation is the procedure of choice [19, 20]. Component separation results in medial advancement of intact rectus myofascial units bilaterally, enabling the closure of defects of up to 10 cm in the upper abdomen, 20 cm in the mid-abdomen, and 6–8 cm in the lower abdomen. The component separation technique is based on an enlargement of the abdominal wall surface by separating and advancing the muscular layers. Some form of component separation, alone or in combination with other adjunct procedures, has become common practice. For smaller hernias preoperative administration of botulinum toxin A (BTA). However, the evidence is considered weak since the literature is based on small number of patients and a large heterogeneity concerning study design [21–24]. In our experience, however, the injection of BTA preoperatively did not improve closure at all.

Other methods can be used to reconstruct the abdominal wall defect complex defects such as local advancement or regional flaps, distant flaps, or combined flap and mesh; however, which technique is used will depend on the pathology at hand and the experience and practice of the surgeon and or institution. Closure of extensive upper midline abdominal wall and thoracoabdominal defects, particularly subxiphoid large defects in patients post-heart transplant initially treated with left ventricular assist device (LVAD), represents a very challenging problem, but with surgical creativity a single-stage reconstructive solution is the best option available.

Timing of the procedure depends on the preoperative evaluation, the physiological condition of the patient, and the anatomical condition of the tissues. The presence of the so-called pinch sign (i.e., easy retraction of the skin or skin graft over the defect) is a good indicator that the adhesions are subsiding and that it is appropriate to schedule the abdominal reconstruction. In our experience, the optimal time for abdominal wall reconstruction is 6–12 months after the first procedure (when adhesions are less prominent).

The Component Separation Techniques

Two component separation techniques with some modifications have been described. The reader is advised to dive deeper in each of these techniques elsewhere. Briefly, during the anterior component separation (ACS) technique for abdominal wall reconstruction (Fig. 13.5), the anterior abdominal skin flaps are developed and dissected out laterally from the chest wall to the anterior superior spine, and then the aponeurosis of the external oblique muscle is divided longitudinally 2 cm laterally to the lateral edge of the rectus sheath, which will allow the mobilized rectus myofascial component to be mobilized medially and facilitate the approximation of the midline with sutures.

There are various modifications of the component separation procedures [3, 4, 25–33]. A minimally invasive surgical technique can be employed [34–37], but in our opinion and experience, this technique can be employed in highly selected patients. Other tissue transfer techniques have been utilized and described as well. Vascularized flaps provide autologous tissue coverage and help avoid the use of foreign material. In general, pedicle flaps are an alternative option for small defect repair. Free flaps cover large thoracoabdominal wall defects in a single-stage reconstructive procedure; however, they are complex procedures and require institutional expertise [3–7, 38–49].

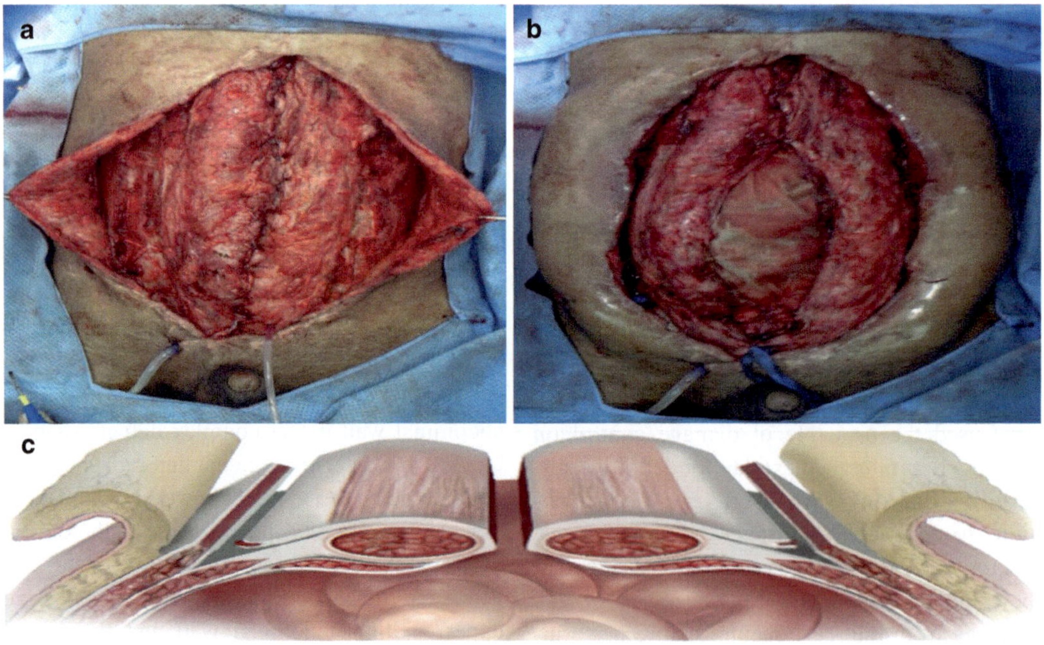

Fig. 13.5 (**a**–**c**). An Illustration of Anterior Component Separation: (**a**) ACS in a young male who sustained severe multiple abdominal injury; (**b**) Temporary closure for the same patient in whom we performed damage closure on demand using Vicryl mesh; (**c**) Illustration of ACS. (** All figures are courtesy of Rifat Latifi, MD)

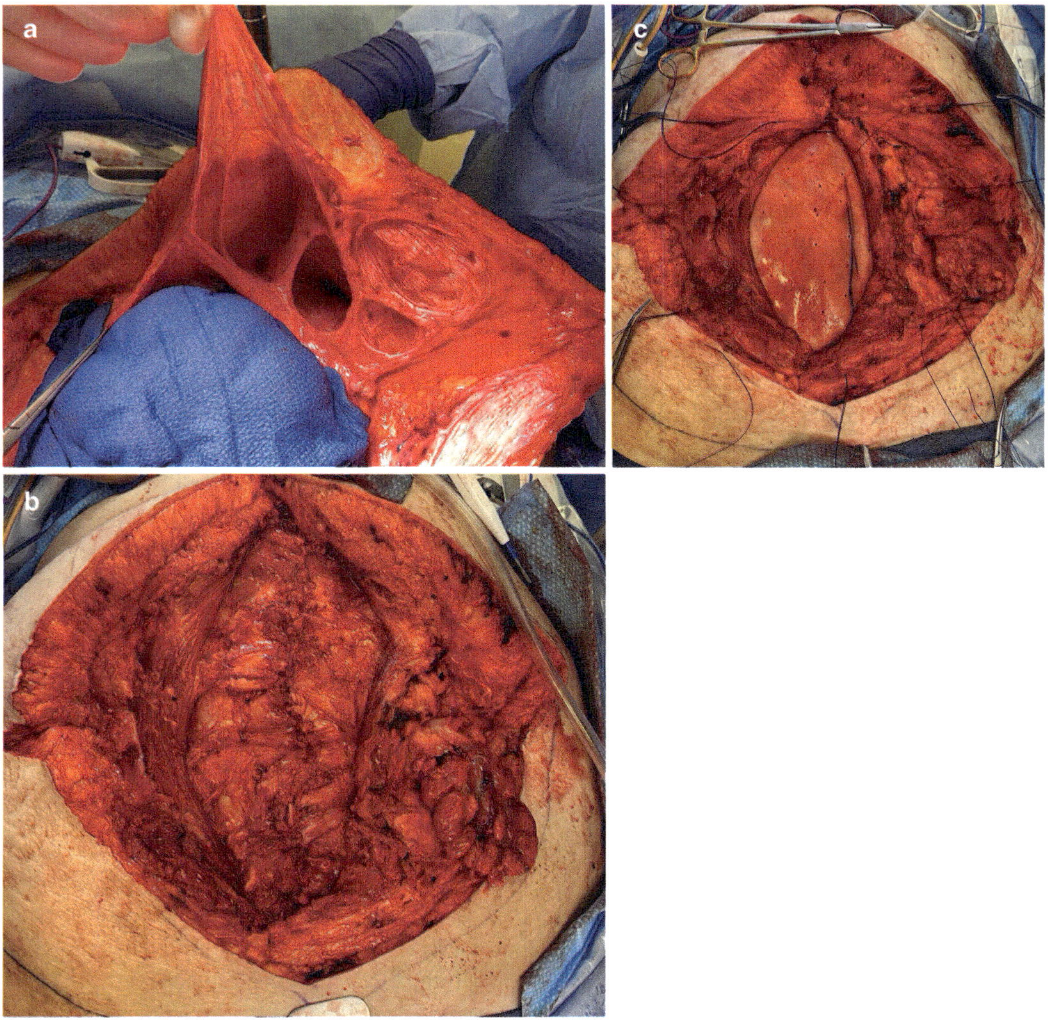

Fig. 13.6 (a–c). Posterior Component Separation in a patient with complex multi-abdominal wall hernias. (**a**) Multiple hernia sacs. (**b**) Release and closure of posterior rectus sheet. (**c**) Closure of abdominal wall over the Strattice ™ mesh, after the mesh was fixed transfascialy and two large drains (Blake #19 Fr) were placed. (** All figures are courtesy of Rifat Latifi, MD)

In our practice we have almost entirely have abended ACS and have replaced with posterior component separation (PCS) (Fig. 13.6a, b, c, d) with or without a TAR, unless we are forced to combine both techniques in complex cases.

The placement of synthetic or biologic graft is recommended even if you perform component release [50]. The question of whether the mesh should be biologic or synthetic mesh depends mostly on its availability and patient's clinical profile abdominal infection risk, although deciding how and where to place the mesh should be given special consideration. Deciding between the three most common techniques used to place a mesh during abdominal wall reconstruction (i.e., onlay, underlay, and interposition or bridge placement) depends on the surgeon's expertise and the clinical status of the patient, as well as the presence of the abdominal wall. For most of our patients who experienced major abdominal wound contamination in the past or at the time of reconstruction, we prefer biologic mesh, although the data to support this decision, while intuitive, are not solid. Each of these techniques has their own pros and cons and should be used based one's surgical expertise and patient selection.

Onlay Placement

From a technique standpoint, onlay placement is the easiest way to situate the mesh. When the abdominal wall edges are easily approximated, free of defects and contamination, there is no contraindication to using synthetic mesh. In these situations, with synthetic mesh, preference should be given to the onlay placement technique, although there is concern for higher risk of seroma formation. There is always a small risk of wound infection, and one needs to remove the mesh if it gets infected, but currently this is a standard of care. The key element of this approach is fixing the mesh both laterally and over the edge of the midline. We prefer fixing the mesh to the fascia using absorbable sutures (Vicryl 2.0 or 3.0), either interrupted or continuous. The main objective is to re-establish closure, and the primary author uses three or four large, closed-suction drains (19 French) under the subcutaneous tissue and keeps the drains in until the individual drain output is less than 25 ml over 24 hours.

Underlay Placement

Underlay graft placement, as demonstrated in Fig. 13.6, has now become the main technique in all high-risk and complex ventral hernia defect reconstructions. It is more involved, but once it is mastered and perfected, it does not add significant operative time, and results are excellent. Although it is believed that that underlay graft placement is associated with lower incidence of seroma, in our practice the determining factor is the thickness of the pannus over the fascia. For this reason, we prefer to combine panniculectomy and abdominoplasty with CAWR in patients with large pannus. The decision to perform underlay technique is an important one and should be done after freeing the abdominal wall entirely from any adhesions, as far laterally as possible both posteriorly (using posterior component separation-PCS) or anteriorly (using anterior component separation-ACS release technique). The mesh can be placed under rectus muscles, after releasing the posterior rectus sheet, with or without transverse abdominis release (TAR). Most PCS are combined with some form of TAR [51, 52].

Placement of the interrupted sutures should ensure complete stretching of the mesh once sutures are tight. Sutures are placed using the "parachuting" technique under direct vision at all times. The direct-vision parachuting technique minimizes the potential for bowel injury during fixing of graft on the abdominal wall. When lateral component release is used, sutures in the anterior abdominal wall are placed as far laterally as possible and must include the medial edge of the external oblique fascia. Doing so prevents bulging laterally at the release component site, which the patient might think the bulging is a new hernia. It is important to ensure that sutures are close enough to each other to prevent intestinal herniation between the sutures. A number of techniques of "underlay" placement have been described, including retro-rectus and sublay, as well as release of posterior aspect of the rectus. If the peritoneum is intact and not violated from stoma placement of other reason, retro-rectus and pre-peritoneum mesh placement may have advantages [36].

While retromuscular mesh repair has gained popularity, a number of associated complications have been reported, including surgical-site infections (SSIs) in 19.6% of cases, and the overall recurrence rate was 16.9%. In one study, the highest rate of recurrence (25%) occurred when hernia was repaired with biologic mesh, followed by synthetic mesh (16.2%), and bioabsorbable mesh (17.1%). The lightweight mesh use was associated with 22.9% vs mid-weight mesh (10.6%) ($p = 0.045$). The only predictor of recurrence was the presence of an SSI (OR 3.1, 95% CI 1.5–6.3; $p < 0.01$). Similarly, after multivariate analysis, diabetes, hernia width > 20 cm, and use of biologic mesh were statistically associated with the development of a surgical-site occurrence (SSO) ($p < 0.05$). Notably, the mere presence of contamination was not independently associated with wound morbidity ($p = 0.11$). SSO and SSI rates anticipated by a recent risk prediction model were 50–80% and 17–83%, respectively, compared with our actual rates of 20–46% and 7–32% [53]. We believe that PCS or placement of the mesh in retromuscular space is the technique of choice and should be employed as often as possible.

Bridge Mesh Placement

In patients with a major loss of abdominal wall domain, approximating the medial edges of the abdominal wall may be impossible, despite performing bilateral anterior or posterior compartment release. In this situation, the only remaining option is to use mesh as a bridge, but patients should be advised that there is high likelihood of hernia recurrence and/or wall laxity that will mimic hernia. The suture bites are placed at least 2 or 3 cm into the muscles and fascia. One should avoid tacking the mesh on the edge of the fascia, given the risk of herniation or suture failure. If at all possible, the "bridge" should be covered with native skin and subcutaneous tissue. However, when mesh is used as a bridge and there is no skin or subcutaneous tissue to cover the mesh, then the use of a wound vacuum-assisted closure (VAC) with continuous irrigation is very useful to keep the mesh moist and to speed up the process of granulation for later skin grafting. Based on the extent of the operation and dissection, the postoperative course can be quite complicated. Wound infection, necrosis of mucocutaneous flaps, seroma, and long-term open wounds are common, and the patient should be prepared for these possibilities in advance. We encourage to establish a multidisciplinary enhanced recovery program after abdominal wall reconstruction which have been demonstrated to reduce the length of hospital stay [36]. In cases of large hernia, such are those defects post damage control surgery, if there is a post operative wound dehiscence (Fig. 13.7), there is a need for multiple return to operating room and creativity. In these cases we prefer closure by using re-enforcement with biologic mesh that in fact it is a form of bridge (Fig. 13.8a, b, c, d, e). All patients who have dehiscence or necrosis of the postoperative period need to return at once to the operating (OR), and a multistep approach needs to be instituted to close the abdomen, in order to prevent fistula and long hospitalization.

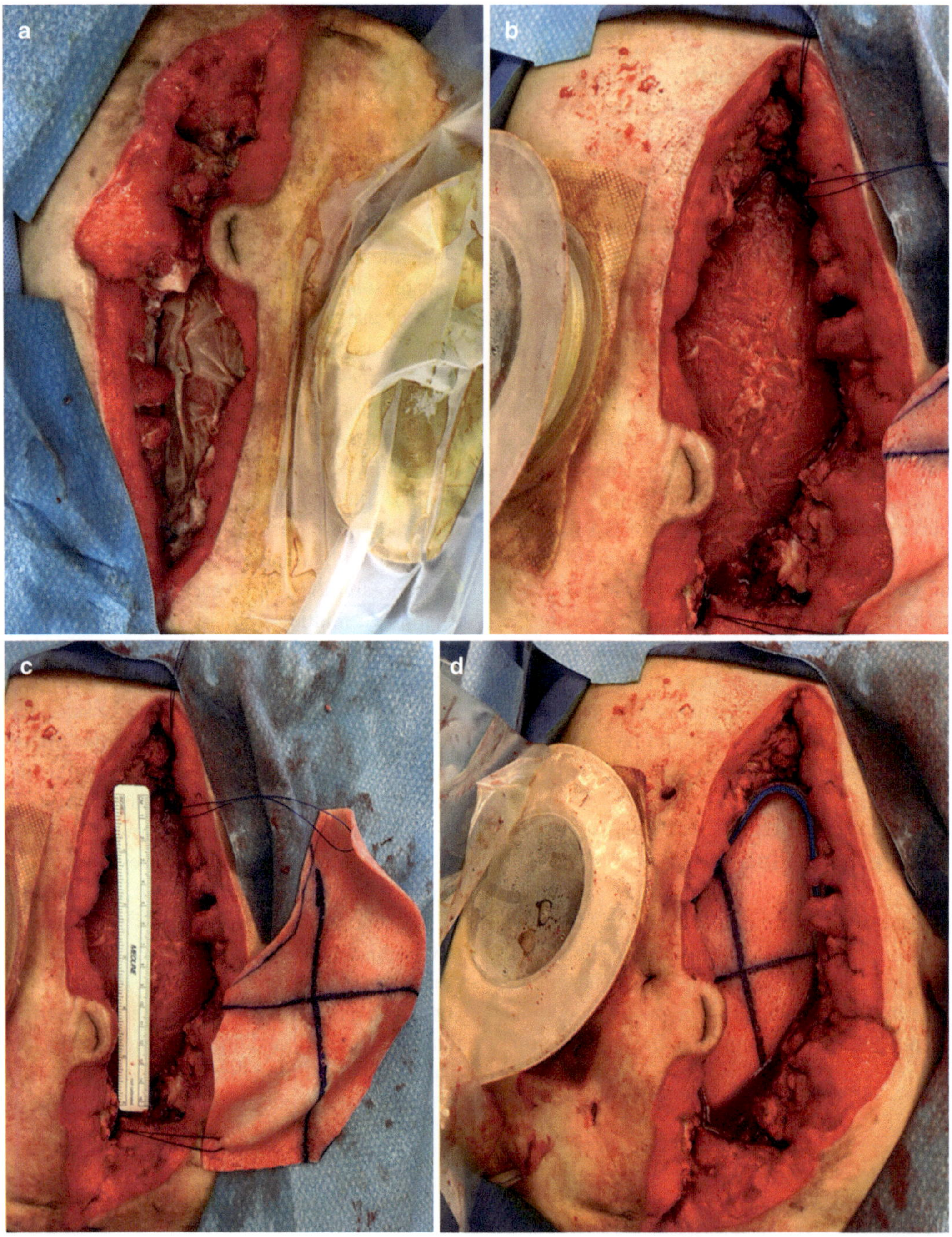

Fig. 13.7 (**a–d**). A 45 year old female with intra-abdominal catastrophe secondary to perforated sigmoid colon due to diverticulitis, underwent multiple trips to the operating room, post DCS, before she was eventually closed. (**a**) Patient who underwent DCS, eventually closure primarily, followed by dehiscence and DCS. (**b**) Same patient as in Fig. 13.7a, now with frozen abdomen. (**c**) Due to frozen abdomen, and inability to perform posterior component release, we decided to "parashoot" the biologic mesh for re-enforcement. (**d**) Final placement of Strattice™ (biologic mesh), that was followed by "en-mass" closure. (Fig. 13.8e). (** All figures are courtesy of Rifat Latifi, MD)

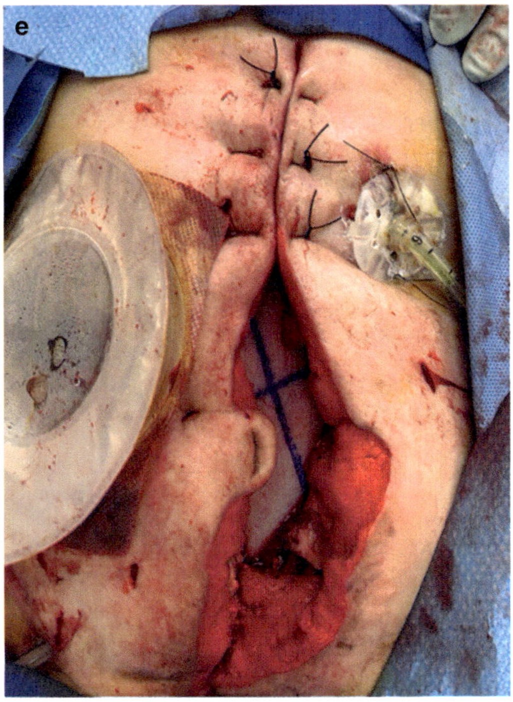

Fig. 13.8 En masse closure of abdominal wall tissue in patient Fig. 13.7. (**e**) En masse closure of abdominal wall tissue. (** All figures are courtesy of Rifat Latifi, MD)

Summary

The reconstruction of complex abdominal wall defects continues to evolve and still poses a major challenge for the clinical surgeon. Successful abdominal wall reconstruction relies primarily on good judgment, careful perioperative preparation, expertise in performing the surgical technique, and close follow-up. The physiology of the patient, defect size, its location, and level of contamination are considerations that influence the type of repair of abdominal wall defects and kind of mesh used [54].

References

1. Higa G, Latifi R. A difficult abdomen: clinical course-based management. In: Surgery of complex abdominal wall defects. Springer; 2013. p. 47–58.
2. Sava J, Alam HB, Vercruysse G, et al. Western Trauma Association Critical Decisions in Trauma Committee. Western Trauma Association critical decisions in trauma: Management of the open abdomen after damage control surgery. J Trauma Acute Care Surg. 2019;87(5):1232–8. https://doi.org/10.1097/TA.0000000000002389. PMID: 31205219.
3. Roberts DJ, Leppäniemi A, Tolonen M, Mentula P, Björck M, Kirkpatrick AW, Sugrue M, Pereira BM, Petersson U, Coccolini F, Latifi R. The open abdomen in trauma, acute care, and vascular and endovascular surgery: comprehensive, expert, narrative review. BJS Open. 2023;7(5):zrad084. https://doi.org/10.1093/bjsopen/zrad084. PMID: 37882630; PMCID: PMC10601091.
4. Diaz JJ Jr, et al. Eastern Association for the Surgery of Trauma: a review of the management of the open abdomen—part 2 "management of the open abdomen". J Trauma Acute Care Surg. 2011;71(2):502–12.
5. Atema JJ, Gans SL, Boermeester MA. Systematic review and meta-analysis of the open abdomen and temporary abdominal closure techniques in non-trauma patients. World J Surg. 2015;39(4):912–25. https://doi.org/10.1007/s00268-014-2883-6. PMID: 25446477.
6. Mahoney EJ, Bugaev N, Appelbaum R, Goldenberg-Sandau A, Baltazar GA, Posluszny J, Dultz L, Kartiko S, Kasotakis G, Como J, Klein E. Management of the open abdomen: a systematic review with meta-analysis and practice management guideline from the Eastern Association for the Surgery of Trauma. J Trauma Acute Care Surg. 2022;93(3):e110–8. https://doi.org/10.1097/TA.0000000000003683. Epub 2022 May 12. PMID: 35546420.
7. Coccolini F, Roberts D, Ansaloni L, et al. The open abdomen in trauma and non-trauma patients: WSES guidelines. World J Emerg Surg. 2018;13:7. https://doi.org/10.1186/s13017-018-0167-4.
8. Visschers RG, et al. Guided treatment improves outcome of patients with enterocutaneous fistulas. World J Surg. 2012;36(10):2341–8.
9. Visschers R, et al. Health-related quality of life in patients treated for enterocutaneous fistula. Br J Surg. 2008;95(10):1280–6.
10. Latifi R, Peralta R, Al H. Thani, abdominal wall reconstruction in patients with an open abdomen and enterocutaneous fistulas: a nine-step treatment strategy. In: Surgery of complex abdominal wall defects. Springer; 2013. p. 133–46.
11. Rohrich RJ, et al. An algorithm for abdominal wall reconstruction. Plastic Reconstruct Surg. 2000;105(1):202–16.
12. Sukkar SM, et al. Challenging abdominal wall defects. Am J Surg. 2001;181(2):115–21.
13. Lowe JB. Updated algorithm for abdominal wall reconstruction. Clin Plastic Surg. 2006;33(2):225–40.
14. Lynch AC, et al. Clinical outcome and factors predictive of recurrence after enterocutaneous fistula surgery. Anna Surg. 2004;240(5):825.

15. Owen RM, et al. Definitive surgical treatment of enterocutaneous fistula: outcomes of a 23-year experience. JAMA Surg. 2013;148(2):118–26.
16. Brenner M, et al. Risk factors for recurrence after repair of enterocutaneous fistula. Arch Surg. 2009;144(6):500–5.
17. Leppäniemi A, Tukiainen E. Reconstruction of complex abdominal wall defects. Scand J Surg. 2013;102(1):14–9.
18. Abdelrahman H, El-Menyar A, Peralta R, Al-Thani H. Application of indocyanine green in surgery: a review of current evidence and implementation in trauma patients. World J Gastrointest Surg. 2023;15(5):757–75. https://doi.org/10.4240/wjgs.v15.i5.757. PMID: 37342859; PMCID: PMC10277941.
19. Albanese A. Eventracion mediana xifoumbilical gigante: metodo para su tratamiento. Rev Asoc Med Argent. 1951;65(709–710):376–8.
20. Ramirez OM, Ruas E, Dellon AL. "Components separation" method for closure of abdominal-wall defects: an anatomic and clinical study. Plast Reconstr Surg. 1990;86(3):519–26.
21. Soltanizadeh S, Helgstrand F, Jorgensen LN. Botulinum toxin A as an adjunct to abdominal wall reconstruction for incisional hernia. Plastic Reconstruct Surg—Global Open. 2017;5(6):e1358. https://doi.org/10.1097/GOX.0000000000001358.
22. Elstner KE, Read JW, Saunders J, Cosman PH, Rodriguez-Acevedo O, Jacombs ASW, Martins RT, Ibrahim N. Selective muscle botulinum toxin A component paralysis in complex ventral hernia repair. Hernia. 2020;24(2):287–93. https://doi.org/10.1007/s10029-019-01939-3. Epub 2019 Apr 4.
23. Timmer AS, Ibrahim F, Claessen JJM, Aehling CJ, Kemper TCPM, Rutten MVH, Boermeester MA. Comparison of two versus three bilateral botulinum toxin injections prior to abdominal wall reconstruction. J Abdom Wall Surg. 2023;2:11382. https://doi.org/10.3389/jaws.2023.11382.
24. Deerenberg EB, Elhage SA, Shao JM, Lopez R, Raible RJ, Kercher KW, Colavita PD, Augenstein VA, Heniford BT. The effects of preoperative botulinum toxin a injection on abdominal wall reconstruction. J Surg Res. 2021;260:251–8. https://doi.org/10.1016/j.jss.2020.10.028. Epub 2020 Dec 23.
25. Tashkandi A, Bueno-Lledó J, Durtette-Guzylack J, Cayeux A, Bukhari R, Rhaeim R, et al. Adjunct botox to preoperative progressive pneumoperitoneum for incisional hernia with loss of domain: no additional effect but may improve outcomes. Hernia. 2021. https://doi.org/10.1007/s10029-021-02387-8.
26. de Vries Reilingh TS, et al. Repair of giant midline abdominal wall hernias: "components separation technique" versus prosthetic repair. World J Surg. 2007;31(4):756–63.
27. Latifi R, Turégano F. Current management of enterocutaneous fistulas. Eur J Trauma Emerg Surg. 2011;37(3):207–8.
28. Leppäniemi A. The hostile abdomen—a systematic approach to a complex problem. Scand J Surg. 2008;97(3):218–9.
29. Vargo D. Component separation in the management of the difficult abdominal wall. Am J Surg. 2004;188(6):633–7.
30. Fabian TC, et al. Planned ventral hernia. Staged management for acute abdominal wall defects. Ann Surg. 1994;219(6):643.
31. Kushimoto S, et al. Usefulness of the bilateral anterior rectus abdominis sheath turnover flap method for early fascial closure in patients requiring open abdominal management. World J Surg. 2007;31(1):2–8.
32. Sailes FC, et al. Synthetic and biological mesh in component separation: a 10-year single institution review. Ann Plast Surg. 2010;64(5):696–8.
33. Espinosa-de-los-Monteros A, et al. Components-separation technique for closure of transverse non-midline abdominal wall incisional hernia. J Plast Reconstr Aesthet Surg. 2011;64(2):264–7.
34. Harth KC, Rosen MJ. Endoscopic versus open component separation in complex abdominal wall reconstruction. Am J Surg. 2010;199(3):342–7.
35. Ghali S, Turza KC, Baumann DP, Butler CE. Minimally invasive component separation results in fewer wound-healing complications than open component separation for large ventral hernia repairs. J Am Coll Surg. 2012;214(6):981–9. https://doi.org/10.1016/j.jamcollsurg.2012.02.017. Epub 2012 Apr 21. PMID: 22521439; PMCID: PMC3889113.
36. Switzer NJ, Dykstra MA, Gill RS, Lim S, Lester E, de Gara C, Shi X, Birch DW, Karmali S. Endoscopic versus open component separation: systematic review and meta-analysis. Surg Endosc. 2015;29(4):787–95. https://doi.org/10.1007/s00464-014-3741-1. Epub 2014 Jul 25.
37. Butler CE, Campbell KT. Minimally invasive component separation with inlay bioprosthetic mesh (MICSIB) for complex abdominal wall reconstruction. Plast Reconstr Surg. 2011;128:698–709.
38. den Hartog D, et al. Open surgical procedures for incisional hernias. The Cochrane Library. 2008.
39. Muramatsu K, Ihara K, Taguchi T. Selection of myocutaneous flaps for reconstruction following oncologic resection of sarcoma. Ann Plast Surg. 2010;64(3):307–10.
40. Servant JM, et al. Reconstruction of large thoracoabdominal defects using two-stage free tissue transfers and prosthetic materials. J Plast Reconstr Aesthet Surg. 2006;59(4):360–5.
41. Erni D, Harder Y. The dissection of the rectus abdominis myocutaneous flap with complete preser-

vation of the anterior rectus sheath. Br J Plast Surg. 2003;56(4):395–400.
42. Fulda GJ, Khan SU, Zabel DD. Special issues in plastic and reconstructive surgery. Crit Care Clin. 2003;19(1):91–108.
43. Arnez Z, et al. Breast reconstruction using the free superficial inferior epigastric artery (SIEA) flap. Br J Plast Surg. 1999;52(4):276–9.
44. Wei CY, et al. The versatility of free rectus femoris muscle flap: an alternative flap. Microsurgery. 1995;16(10):698–703.
45. Hill HL, Nahai F, Vasconez LO. The tensor fascia lata myocutaneous free flap. Plast Reconstr Surg. 1978;61(4):517–22.
46. Nahai F, Hill LH, Hester RT. Experiences with the tensor fascia lata flap. Plast Reconstr Surg. 1979;63(6):788–99.
47. Wong C-H, et al. Reconstruction of complex abdominal wall defects with free flaps: indications and clinical outcome. Plast Reconstr Surg. 2009;124(2):500–9.
48. Tukiainen E, Leppäniemi A. Reconstruction of extensive abdominal wall defects with microvascular tensor fasciae latae flap. Br J Surg. 2011;98(6):880–4.
49. Björck M, et al. Classification—important step to improve management of patients with an open abdomen. World J Surg. 2009;33(6):1154–7.
50. Richmond B, et al. Component separation with porcine acellular dermal reinforcement is superior to traditional bridged mesh repairs in the open repair of significant midline ventral hernia defects. Am Surg. 2014;80(8):725–31.
51. Novitsky YW, Elliott HL, Orenstein SB, Rosen MJ. Transversus abdominis muscle release: a novel approach to posterior component separation during complex abdominal wall reconstruction. Am J Surg. 2012;204:709–16.
52. Novitsky YW, Fayezizadeh M, Majumder A, Neupane R, Elliott HL, Orenstein SB. Outcomes of posterior component separation with transversus abdominis muscle release and synthetic mesh sublay reinforcement. Ann Surg. 2016;264:226–32.
53. Cobb WS, et al. Open retromuscular mesh repair of complex incisional hernia: predictors of wound events and recurrence. J Am Coll Surg. 2015;220(4):606–13.
54. Rosen MJ, Krpata DM, Petro CC, et al. Biologic vs synthetic mesh for single-stage repair of contaminated ventral hernias: a randomized clinical trial. JAMA Surg. 2022;157(4):293–301. https://doi.org/10.1001/jamasurg.2021.6902.

Surgical Decision-Making in Difficult Situations in Pediatric Surgery

14

B. S. Ratta, Geeta Kekre, Dhananjay Vaze, and Kshama Kulkarni

Introduction

Pediatric surgery encompasses a wide array of clinical scenarios, each presenting unique challenges and complexities. Within this specialized field, surgical decision-making in difficult situations demands a nuanced and comprehensive approach. To illustrate the intricacies of surgical decision-making in pediatric cases, we will explore the diverse use cases spanning congenital anomalies, trauma, oncology, and other complex conditions. These use cases showcase the multifaceted nature of surgical decision-making in pediatric surgery, emphasizing the need for meticulous evaluation, collaboration, and ethical considerations in managing challenging scenarios.

Decision-making is a complex process, and surgical decision-making is no exception to the rule. It is not only complex to start with but needs refinement, adjustments, and reconsideration till the desired results are achieved. It is a process that happens at subconscious and conscious/intellectual levels. These two levels can't be visualized as water-tight compartments but need to be perceived as a continuum. An expert surgeon confidently and repeatedly works through these levels to review, reanalyze, and reassess their own decisions to achieve the desired result.

Pediatric surgeons are tasked with making decisions that not only address immediate concerns but also consider the evolving needs of children as they grow. Congenital anomalies, growth-related changes, and the need for minimally invasive yet effective interventions are just a few of the challenges that make pediatric surgery distinct.

In the pediatric population, "surrogate decision-makers" are often required for the consenting process to help understand the underlying pathology. This is especially important in some life-threatening emergencies like inhaled foreign bodies and midgut volvulus. In developing countries, it is a social emergency to assign sex for the upbringing of a child born with ambiguous genitalia.

The challenges one faces when operating on a child may be medical as well as socioeconomic. In pediatric practice, one is likely to encounter children with associated genetic syndromes or multiple congenital anomalies. Resources for such patients are often limited. Equipment of the appropriate dimensions and expertise in ancillary services may not readily be available. Nevertheless, judicious utilization of available

B. S. Ratta (✉) · G. Kekre
Department of Pediatric Surgery, Ruby Hall Clinic, Pune, India

D. Vaze
Department of Pediatric Surgery, DY Patil Medical College, Pune, India

K. Kulkarni
Department of Pediatric Surgery, Surya Hospital, Pune, India

R. Latifi (ed.), *Surgical Decision-Making*, https://doi.org/10.1007/978-3-031-67391-7_14

resources could make the difference between morbidity (or even mortality) and a healthy life with normal life expectancy for these children.

The Medically Complex Pediatric Surgical Patient

It is not uncommon to be faced with a surgical problem in a pediatric patient who suffers from a genetic, chromosomal, or metabolic syndrome. Ideally, such patients should be cared for at specialized centers with dedicated multidisciplinary pediatric teams. However, it is not rare for such children to present in an emergency at the healthcare facility nearest to them.

Assessing a syndromic child in an emergency requires a calm and patient approach. A detailed history from the parent or caregiver when available will provide valuable information that can help a surgeon understand the signs exhibited by the child. For example, a child with a neurological condition presents with what might be appendicitis but may not cry out loud even when in agony. A caregiver will be able to point out grimaces and facial expressions of pain. Children with special needs may be difficult to soothe and cajole, making it challenging to pick up signs such as guarding and rebound tenderness.

Anesthesia risks require due consideration when treating such children. It is always advisable to have pediatric intensive care available at the same center where the surgery is being performed. Difficult airway, poor muscle tone, and altered metabolism greatly increase the risks of general anesthesia. Post-operative care, wound care, analgesia, and drug therapy all must be tailored keeping in mind the child's physical and mental status.

Pediatric Surgical Emergencies in the Resource-Limited Setting

A time-sensitive emergency in a pediatric patient needs to be handled with prudence. Utilization of resources, especially diagnostic, must be optimized to provide the best patient outcomes. Resources such as time, imaging modalities, ancillary services, finances, intensive care, etc. may all be in short supply. The astute surgeon must decide on the need for surgery, plan for the surgical process, and execute the surgery while keeping the patients' interests in mind.

Testicular Torsion

A common example of a time-sensitive pediatric emergency is testicular torsion. One may not have a sonologist on hand to demonstrate the lack of testicular blood flow, but a sound clinical evaluation and a high index of suspicion should enable the surgeon to establish the diagnosis. A reasonable surgeon may decide to explore the scrotum rather than wait for imaging when the index of suspicion is high.

Midgut Volvulus

Another example of a surgical emergency that may not allow the luxury of detailed imaging is midgut volvulus in the newborn. One may have little more than an X-ray and a clinical picture of bilious vomiting in the infant, with sonographic assessment either unavailable or not possible at the given moment. It may be better in that scenario to operate right away than to wait and run the risk of compromised bowel vascularity.

Trauma

The most limited resource while dealing with pediatric trauma is time. Surgical decisions in pediatric trauma must be guided above all by the patient's clinical picture. There is no benefit to rushing a hypovolemic, hypothermic child into a CT scanner before adequate fluid resuscitation is done. Point-of-care ultrasound to detect free fluid in the abdomen and the thorax when available can guide management. A detailed ultrasound study is seldom required. Lack of response to fluid resuscitation in a child with abdominal or thoracic trauma should prompt surgical exploration rather than further imaging. A thorough clinical assessment, including a log roll and a per rectal examination, and a clear picture of the mechanism of injury (when available) go a long way in guiding surgical management. Bear in mind that blood pressure is an unreliable indicator of volume status in the pediatric patient. A decision on nonoperative management of solid organ injury will depend on the availability of intensive monitoring and a well-staffed 24-hour operating suite. In the absence of these, one must choose between transferring the patient to a center with these facilities or exploring the abdomen upfront.

Ileocolic Intussusception

The management of ileocolic intussusception is evolving toward nonoperative reduction. However, there are multiple caveats to this statement. Nonoperative reduction is best suited to ileocolic intussusception in a child between 6 months and 18 months of age. Outside this age group, nonoperative reduction must be approached with caution. The likelihood of a pathological lead point including a malignancy such as lymphoma being the cause of intussusception is high outside this age group. Even in the absence of a pathological lead point, nonoperative reduction is less likely to be successful in an intussusception older than 48 hours or in a distended abdomen. Obvious intestinal obstruction is a contraindication for nonoperative reduction. When attempting nonoperative reduction, the operating room must be ready for an emergency exploration. Intestinal perforation is a common and dreaded complication of nonoperative reduction necessitating immediate exploration.

Factors Contributing to Surgical Decision-Making in Difficult Situations

1. Clinical complexity in pediatric surgical patients often presents with complex clinical conditions such as congenital anomalies, tumors, or traumatic injuries. These complex cases require thorough evaluation and careful consideration of treatment options.
2. Anatomical variations in children's anatomy can differ significantly from that of adults posing challenges for surgical planning and execution. Anatomical variations in pediatric patients can impact the choice of surgical approach and techniques.
3. Physiological considerations such as the impact of surgery on growth and development, as well as the unique metabolic and nutritional needs of pediatric patients, must be factored into surgical decision-making.
4. Ethical and legal considerations in surgically treated pediatric patients often involve complex ethical and legal considerations such as the need for parental consent, the best interests of the child, and the potential long-term implications of surgical interventions.

Strategies for Surgical Decision-Making in Difficult Situations

1. Multidisciplinary approach: in difficult surgical cases involving a multidisciplinary team of pediatric surgeons, pediatric anesthesiologists, intensivists, and other specialists can provide comprehensive insights and expertise. Collaboration among team members can help in formulating the most appropriate treatment plan.
2. Shared decision-making: engaging parents or guardians in shared decision-making processes is essential in pediatric surgical care providing families with comprehensive information regarding the surgical options, potential risks, and expected outcomes allows families for more informed decision-making.
3. Advanced imaging and technology: utilizing advanced imaging modalities such as MRI, CT, and 3D modeling can aid in preoperative planning and intraoperative decision-making. These technologies provide detailed anatomical information allowing for precise surgical interventions.

4. Ethical consultation: in complex cases with ethical dilemmas, involving an ethics committee or consultant can offer valuable insights and guidance in navigating the ethical considerations surrounding surgical decision-making.
5. Simulation and rehearsal: in some complex pediatric surgical cases, especially those involving rare anatomical anomalies or challenging procedures, simulation and rehearsal of the surgical approach can be invaluable. This can help anticipate potential complications and refine the surgical plan.

Use Cases

Use Case 1: Neonatal Abdominal Catastrophes

Surgical decision-making in neonatal abdominal catastrophes involves complex considerations due to the delicate nature of neonatal patients and the potential severity of abdominal conditions. Neonatal abdominal catastrophes may include conditions such as intestinal obstruction, necrotizing enterocolitis, gastroschisis, omphalocele, and other congenital anomalies.

A surgeon called to the neonatal intensive care unit (NICU) to evaluate and plan treatment for a newborn baby with a surgical emergency must make some crucial decisions. When is the best time to operate the baby? What is the best surgery to perform in the given circumstances? Must this be a staged surgery? It is important to keep in mind that neonates have limited to no reserve, are highly susceptible to sepsis, and present a formidable anesthesiology challenge.

Anorectal Malformations

Anorectal malformations (ARMs) require immediate attention in the newborn period. If neglected, a neonate with an ARM will develop overt features of intestinal obstruction which can be life-threatening. Feeding must be held off until the malformation has been assessed and a decision on surgery has been made. Examination and investigation for associated cardiac, spinal, and renal defects and VACTERL-H association must be complete. A prone cross-table X-ray film helps to identify the level of the malformation.

Broadly speaking, all malformations other than vestibular fistula in girls and some types of perineal fistula in boys require a staged approach. The first step is to construct a suitable colostomy to provide an outlet for stool. This colostomy must be constructed keeping in mind the subsequent surgery. An adequate length of colon distal to the ostomy must be preserved to allow pull-through at a later date. Accordingly, the surgeon must construct a high sigmoid divided colostomy. In some cases, particularly in high lesions and in the pouch colon, it may be more prudent to construct a right transverse colostomy. However, children do not tolerate proximal bowel diversions as well as adults do. They are especially susceptible to dehydration, malnutrition, anemia, and prolapse with ileostomies and poorly constructed transverse colostomies.

A perineal or a vestibular fistula may be adequate to allow decompression of the bowel of a breastfed infant. In such cases, surgery can be deferred until the child can undergo a primary reconstruction. Where facilities are available, primary reconstruction can be done in the first 72 hours of life while the baby is still in the NICU. However, at most centers, it is still standard practice to perform the reconstruction once the child has demonstrated satisfactory weight gain. Home rectal washouts are administered in the interim to ensure that the bowel remains decompressed.

Esophageal Atresia with or Without Tracheo-esophageal Fistula

A potentially life-threatening anomaly, esophageal atresia, calls for vigilance and promptness in surgical decision-making. The clear priorities are to prevent aspiration and to establish a conduit for feeding. Rapid evaluation for associated cardiac anomalies and the VACTERL-H association is imperative before intervention. The presence of a right-sided aortic arch as detected by 2D echo has a bearing on the operative approach.

Surgery is usually deferred until the first 24 hours of life have passed. An X-ray taken after this interval is a more reliable indicator of whether or not a tracheo-esophageal fistula is present. Until surgery is possible, the lungs must be protected from aspiration pneumonitis by thorough oral suctioning and use of a Replogle tube. Reflux of secretions from the stomach into the lungs via the tracheo-esophageal fistula must be prevented by appropriate positioning. If the child has to be transferred to another center for surgery, suctioning must continue during transport.

If an X-ray taken after 16 to 24 hours of birth shows no abdominal gas shadows, it is unlikely that a fistula between the esophagus and the trachea exists. In that case, one may forego thoracic exploration in the newborn period and simply construct a cervical esophagostomy and a feeding gastrostomy, with the understanding that the child will require gastroesophageal replacement at a later date.

If a fistula is found to be present, it must be ligated through a thoracic approach. One must be careful to identify the fistula correctly because it is easy to mistake the left bronchus or the aorta for the fistula in such a tiny thoracic cavity. Moreover, either or both of the proximal and distal esophageal pouches may be communicating with the trachea in which case both connections need to be ligated. The surgical approach is usually through the right hemithorax, hence the significance of identifying a right-sided aortic arch by looking for it on 2D echo.

Once the fistula has been ligated, a careful attempt must be made to establish esophageal continuity by a primary anastomosis. Care must be taken to avoid overzealous dissection and mobilization which can jeopardize the vascularity of the esophageal segments. A wide, oblong anastomosis is performed to minimize anastomotic stricture. Anti-reflux medication must be administered postoperatively. The child must be monitored for any signs of anastomotic disruption.

If a primary anastomosis is not possible, or a major anastomotic leak has developed, then a cervical esophagostomy with a feeding gastrostomy must be performed. If an anastomosis looks tenuous at the time of surgery, it is advisable to convert to a cervical esophagostomy with a feeding gastrostomy, as an anastomotic leak into the mediastinum can cause a newborn to deteriorate rapidly.

Myelomeningocele

Open neural tube defects are a direct portal for infection to the central nervous system (CNS). Moreover, they carry the risk of traumatic rupture and fatal coning in that event. It is for this reason that the defect must be closed within the first few days of birth. A ventriculoperitoneal shunt is more often than not inserted during the same surgery. Emphasis is placed on maintaining asepsis and protecting the defect with sterile nonadhesive and nonirritant dressings until surgery can be performed. Cultures are obtained from the exposed neural placode to document sterility or contamination. The motor and sensory deficit must be well documented before closure. Although closure is not expected to improve neurological deficits, care must be taken not to worsen it. Parental counseling regarding bowel and bladder management must begin at the time of diagnosis.

Intestinal Atresia

Intestinal atresia poses a surgical challenge due to the wide discrepancy between the proximal and distal bowel. The intestine proximal to the site of atresia may be many times the diameter of the distal unused intestine making end-to-end anastomosis difficult. Moreover, the ectatic proximal intestine is often hypoperistaltic, leading to stasis and increasing the risk of recurrent obstruction or anastomotic leak. The ectasia may extend over a great length of the proximal intestine; therefore resection of the dilated bowel is not always a practical solution. Tapering or plication of the proximal bowel may be done with the attendant risk of a leak from the extended suture line or obstruction from the plicated bowel. Multiple atresias are often encountered, and multiple anastomoses may be performed in these cases. The goal is to preserve as much bowel as possible, prevent short bowel syndrome, and minimize the need for parenteral nutrition. Of course, this may be easier said than done. Multiple intestinal atresias and apple peel defects of the mesentery often leave the surgeon with little choice. It is necessary in those cases to work closely with the neonatologist to establish parenteral nutrition as well as enteral feeding.

Gastroschisis and Ruptured Omphalocele

An abdominal catastrophe such as a ruptured omphalocele or a gastroschisis can be alarming at first, but a calm and measured approach is necessary in both situations. The first priority of the treating team is to prevent sepsis, hypothermia, and dehydration. Where feasible, immediate reduction can be achieved in the obstetric operating room provided the center is equipped for intensive monitoring of abdominal compartment syndrome. Where immediate or primary closure is not possible or carries a high risk of abdominal compartment syndrome, a sterile silastic silo bag must be applied. In case the child must be transported to another facility, care must be taken not to injure or aggravate the inflammation of the bowel. The infant may be wrapped in a sterile plastic sheet to prevent loss of fluid and heat as well as to prevent contamination of the exposed bowel. Delayed closure can then be undertaken at a well-equipped facility. During closure, the surgeon needs to keep an eye on lower limb perfusion and ventilatory pressures. Decreased lower limb perfusion which can be identified by the use of a saturation probe on the foot and increased ventilatory pressure requirements to deliver tidal volume indicate raised intra-abdominal pressure. The surgeon may in this case opt to create a ventral hernia by closing the skin and without closing the fascia. Alternatively, lateral release incisions may be placed on the skin and fascia. Gastroschisis is often associated with intestinal atresia. However, exposure to amniotic fluid in utero renders the bowel edematous and inflamed, unsuitable for resection and anastomosis. Therefore, it may be necessary to re-operate on the patient for an atresia a few days after closure. The child will require parenteral nutrition in the interim.

Complicated Appendicitis (Abscess or Phlegmon Formation)

A lack of physiologic and immunologic reserve, a small abdominal cavity allowing an intra-abdominal infection to easily spread, a relatively small omentum that cannot wall off an infection, and a thin-walled appendix in young age group increase the morbidity and mortality for appendicitis. Neonatal and infant perforation rates are high; hence tailoring of surgical recommendations is needed. This is because many times the leucocyte counts may remain normal and the appendix may not be visualized or only mildly enlarged on ultrasonography in this age group.

Patients with imaging consistent with perforated appendicitis with an associated large phlegmon or abscess may be managed nonoperatively with intravenous (IV) antibiotics, with percutaneous drainage of abscesses if technically feasible. Alternatively, appendectomy may be appropriate management in the hands of a skilled provider if available. For patients managed nonoperatively for their appendiceal abscess, the routine practice is to do an interval laparoscopic appendectomy; however, there are data to support that patients do not require standard "interval appendectomy" 6 weeks following resolution; these cases should be individualized based on the shared decision between the parents of the child and the surgeon.

Complicated Inguinal Hernias

Any infant who has an inguinal hernia risks having their bowels becoming incarcerated and, in severe cases, strangulated. Most inguinal hernias are asymptomatic, and corrective surgery is advised early to avoid complications. Manual reduction of the incarcerated hernia is tried initially, and if successful, the child is posted for definitive repair in the next 24 to 48 hours. If the incarcerated inguinal hernia is left unreduced, these infants progress rapidly to strangulation. However, in children with an incarcerated inguinal hernia, reduction should be performed only if there is no evidence of obstruction, shock, or peritonitis from the gangrenous bowel. Early reduction aims to prevent bowel necrosis, decrease the likelihood of testicular atrophy, and stabilize the patient.

If the incarcerated hernia cannot be reduced, or if the infant is suspected of having a strangulated inguinal hernia, then an emergency exploration is advised.

Inhaled Foreign Bodies

This is very common especially in the age group of 1 to 3 years, as toddlers are inquisitive and may ingest or inhale foreign bodies, with or without the knowledge of their caretaker. This may result in acute respiratory distress causing immediate airway compromise and the need for urgent investigation. Many times these objects are radiolucent and may not be picked up in radiographs. However, if there is an unexplained acute respiratory deterioration in a toddler with lung collapse or overinflation, emergency bronchoscopic assessment and removal of the foreign body are life-saving measures and ensure good short- and long-term prognosis.

However, if a pediatric bronchoscope is not available or pediatric surgical expertise is not available, then as a temporizing measure, the foreign body can be advanced post carina to tide over the crisis and stabilize the patient from respiratory distress.

Ambiguous Genitalia

The birth of a baby with ambiguous genitalia presents a psychosocial emergency for the parents. Although immediate surgical intervention is usually not required, a thorough physical examination and appropriate investigation help to assign a gender at birth. A multidisciplinary team involving a pediatric surgeon, a neonatologist, an endocrinologist, a geneticist, and a psychologist is required. The prevailing cultural environment and the existing law of the land need to be taken into consideration when caring for such babies. The age at surgery and the choice of surgery to be performed depend on multiple genetic, anatomic, psychological, and even medicolegal factors. Such decisions must be made jointly by the multidisciplinary team in the best interest of the child.

When faced with a neonate presenting with an abdominal catastrophe, several key factors are taken into account when making surgical decisions:

1. Clinical Assessment: The neonate's clinical condition and stability are the primary concern. Initial assessments include vital signs, physical examination, and laboratory tests to evaluate the severity of the condition and any associated systemic disturbances.
2. Imaging Studies: Diagnostic imaging, particularly ultrasound and radiographic studies, may be used to assess the nature and extent of the abdominal pathology. These imaging studies can provide valuable information about the location and severity of the issue, aiding in surgical planning.
3. Consultation and Multidisciplinary Approach: Neonatal abdominal catastrophes often benefit from a multidisciplinary approach involving neonatologists, pediatric surgeons, radiologists, and other specialists. Collaboration ensures comprehensive evaluation and the development of a well-rounded treatment plan.
4. Stabilization: If the neonate's condition is unstable, initial measures may include resuscitation, correction of fluid and electrolyte imbalances, and addressing any associated systemic complications to optimize the patient's condition for surgery.
5. Assessment of Surgical Feasibility: The surgical team evaluates the feasibility of intervention based on the specific pathology. Factors such as the presence of bowel ischemia, perforation, and associated congenital anomalies are carefully considered.
6. Timing of Surgery: Timing is critical in neonatal abdominal catastrophes. Expedited surgical intervention may be necessary in cases of intestinal perforation, necrotizing enterocolitis, or strangulated hernias to prevent further deterioration. In other cases, surgical timing may depend on the neonate's stability and the need for preoperative optimization.

7. Surgical Technique: The choice of surgical technique is influenced by the underlying pathology. For example, in the case of gastroschisis or omphalocele, the goals include a gentle reduction of bowel contents and closure of the abdominal wall defect. In conditions such as necrotizing enterocolitis or intestinal atresia, the surgical approach may involve resection of necrotic bowel segments and anastomoses.
8. Postoperative Care Planning: Anticipating the postoperative needs of the neonate is crucial. This includes considerations such as ongoing monitoring, nutritional support, wound care, and potential long-term complications or squeal of the surgical intervention.
9. Family Communication and Informed Consent: Open communication with the family is vital. The surgical team should provide clear and empathetic explanations of the condition, the proposed surgical intervention, and the potential outcomes. Informed consent, acknowledging the risks and benefits of surgery, is an essential part of the decision-making process.
10. Ethical Considerations: In some instances, complex ethical considerations may arise, especially in situations where the prognosis is poor and the potential for long-term morbidity is high. The involvement of an ethics committee or consultant may be necessary to navigate these challenging scenarios. Ultimately, surgical decision-making in neonatal abdominal catastrophes must be holistic.

Use Case 2: Rare Renal Tumors

Surgical decision-making for rare renal tumors in children involves a multidisciplinary approach and careful consideration of several factors specific to the type of tumor. Rare renal tumors in children may include conditions such as Wilms' tumor, clear cell sarcoma, malignant rhomboid tumor, renal cell carcinoma, and others.

Here is how surgical decision-making may be approached in the context of rare renal tumors in children:

1. Diagnostic Evaluation: As with any surgical decision-making process, a thorough diagnostic evaluation is crucial. Imaging studies, such as ultrasound, CT scans, and MRI, help in characterizing the tumor size, location, and extent of local invasion. Biopsy may be considered in cases of diagnostic uncertainty.
2. Tumor Biology and Aggressiveness: Understanding the specific biology and aggressiveness of the rare renal tumor is paramount. Some tumors may be more aggressive and require more immediate surgical intervention, while others may necessitate a more nuanced approach based on their behavior and potential for metastasis.
3. Staging and Risk Stratification: Tumor staging and risk stratification play vital roles in determining the appropriate surgical approach. The extent of local disease, involvement of regional lymph nodes, and presence of distant metastases are key considerations in the overall treatment plan.
4. Evaluation of Metastatic Disease: In some cases of rare renal tumors, the presence of metastatic disease may significantly influence the surgical approach. This evaluation may involve additional imaging and, in some cases, a biopsy of suspected metastatic lesions.
5. Nephrectomy vs. Nephron-Sparing Surgery: The decision between nephrectomy and nephron-sparing surgery depends on the tumor's size, location, and the child's overall renal function. Preservation of renal function is a crucial consideration, especially in cases where the tumor is amenable to partial resection, especially in bilateral cases.
6. Surgical Approach and Extent of Resection: The choice of surgical approach, including open, laparoscopic, or robotic-assisted techniques, is influenced by the tumor's characteristics and the child's anatomy. For

aggressive tumors, achieving clear margins while minimizing the risk of tumor spillage is essential.

7. Lymph Node Assessment: In cases where regional lymph node involvement is a concern, the surgical team may consider lymph node sampling or dissection to accurately stage the disease and guide adjuvant treatment decisions.
8. Role of Adjuvant Therapy: Surgical decision-making also encompasses considerations regarding the potential role of adjuvant therapy, such as chemotherapy or radiation, following surgical resection. The surgical team collaborates closely with medical and radiation oncologists to plan a comprehensive treatment strategy.
9. Long-Term Functional and Oncologic Outcomes: Anticipating the long-term functional and oncologic outcomes is critical. Close follow-up, monitoring for potential late effects of treatment, and ongoing surveillance for disease recurrence are integral components of the overall surgical decision-making process.
10. Psychosocial Support and Family Involvement: The surgical team works closely with the child and family, providing comprehensive psychosocial support and ensuring that the family is actively involved in shared decision-making throughout the treatment journey.
11. Research and Clinical Trials: In the context of rare renal tumors, consideration of participation in clinical trials and research protocols may influence surgical decision-making. Access to novel therapies and a deeper understanding of the underlying tumor biology can be facilitated through participation in collaborative research efforts.

Surgical decision-making in the context of rare renal tumors in children requires a tailored, patient-centered approach that accounts for the specific tumor biology, risk stratification, and the child's long-term well-being. Collaboration among pediatric surgeons, urologic oncologists, pediatric oncologists, and other specialists is essential for optimizing treatment outcomes and ensuring comprehensive care for these complex and challenging conditions.

Use Case 3: Pediatric Traumatic Amputations

Pediatric traumatic amputations present unique challenges in surgical decision-making and management. When addressing pediatric traumatic amputations, several key considerations come into play:

1. Extent and Type of Amputation: The specific type and level of traumatic amputation significantly influence surgical decision-making. Whether it involves partial foot amputation, below-knee amputation, above-knee amputation, or upper extremity amputation, the anatomical site and tissue viability guide the surgical approach.
2. Vascular and Soft Tissue Assessment: Vascular and soft tissue assessment is critical to determine the adequacy of blood supply and tissue viability in the residual limb. Reconstructive options, including replantation, revision amputation, and tissue coverage procedures, depend on the condition of the residual limb and the child's overall vascular status.
3. Replantation Considerations: In cases of traumatic amputation, particularly in upper extremity injuries, it is advisable to evaluate replantation. Factors such as the mechanism of injury, ischemia time, and the presence of associated injuries are carefully considered while evaluating replantation.
4. Multidisciplinary Team Collaboration: Surgical decision-making for pediatric traumatic amputations involves multidisciplinary collaboration with orthopedic, plastic, reconstructive, and vascular surgeons and therapists to address the complex functional and psychosocial needs of the child.
5. Bone and Joint Integrity: The preservation of bone and joint integrity is an essential consideration, particularly for growing children.

Limb-length inequalities, joint stability, and long-term functional outcomes are carefully evaluated when planning surgical interventions, such as revision amputation or reconstructive procedures.

6. Functional Rehabilitation Potential: Assessing the child's potential for functional rehabilitation and prosthetic fitting plays a crucial role in surgical decision-making. Preservation of length, functional muscle units, and sensation in the residual limb are important for optimizing prosthetic outcomes and long-term functional independence.
7. Psychosocial and Developmental Impact: Recognizing the psychosocial and developmental impact of traumatic amputations on children is integral to surgical decision-making. Involving child life specialists, psychologists, and social workers is critical in addressing the emotional and developmental needs of the child and family throughout the treatment.
8. Prosthetic Considerations: Anticipating the child's prosthetic needs and preferences influences surgical decision-making. Creating a residual limb that is well-suited for prosthetic fitting and incorporating the child's input in the decision-making process is essential for optimizing postamputation quality of life.
9. Long-Term Follow-Up and Support: Surgical decision-making for pediatric traumatic amputations encompasses long-term follow-up and support. Monitoring for complications, addressing the child's growth-related needs, and providing ongoing psychosocial support are integral components of postamputation care.
10. Patient and Family-Centered Care: It is important to engage the child and family in shared decision-making. This helps in addressing their concerns and providing comprehensive education about the surgical options. This helps in managing expectations of outcomes. It is crucial to ensure patient and family-centered care throughout the treatment process.
11. Research and Innovation: Embracing ongoing research and innovation in the field of pediatric traumatic amputations influences surgical decision-making. Access to novel technologies, prosthetic advancements, and participation in clinical trials contribute to advancing the care and outcomes for pediatric amputees. Surgical decision-making for pediatric traumatic amputations requires a comprehensive and individualized approach that considers the child's unique physiological, anatomical, developmental, and psychosocial needs. Collaboration among multidisciplinary teams, active involvement of the child and family, and a focus on long-term functional and psychosocial outcomes are fundamental in addressing the complexities of pediatric traumatic amputations.

Use Case 4: Difficult Situations in Pediatric Urology Arise When Dealing with Complex Conditions That Require Surgical Intervention

Several key difficult situations in pediatric urology, along with their associated challenges in surgical decision-making, include the following:

1. Multifactorial Genitourinary Anomalies:
   (a) Challenge: Children with multiple genitourinary anomalies present a complex surgical challenge due to the need for comprehensive and integrated treatment plans.
   (b) Surgical Decision-Making: Such cases involve a multidisciplinary team approach, considering the overall impact on genitourinary function, potential long-term complications, and the need for staged procedures.
2. Rare Congenital Anomalies:
   (a) Challenge: cloacal exstrophy or persistent cloaca presents unique challenges due to the scarcity of experience with similar cases and limited evidence-based guidelines.

   (b) Surgical Decision-Making: Rare congenital anomalies require a highly individualized approach, with innovation, adaptation of surgical techniques, and close collaboration with a network of specialized experts in the field.
3. Bladder Exstrophy and Epispadias Complex:
   (a) Challenge: This condition involves significant surgical and reconstructive challenge, impacting both anatomical and psychological aspects.
   (b) Surgical Decision-Making: The multidisciplinary team plays a critical role in decision-making, considering not only the surgical aspects but also the potential long-term impact on urinary continence, sexual function, and psychosocial well-being.
4. Intraoperative Complications:
   (a) Challenge: Unforeseen intraoperative complications, such as vascular injury or inadequate tissue viability, can significantly affect the surgical plan and the long-term outcome.
   (b) Surgical Decision-Making: Real-time decisions in response to intraoperative complications require alternative surgical approaches, extended procedures, and prompt communication with the medical team to reduce potential adverse effects.
5. Neurogenic Bladder Dysfunction:
   (a) Challenge: This condition involves balancing the need for bladder drainage and preservation of renal function, often complicated by associated neurological issues.
   (b) Surgical Decision-Making: Regarding operative interventions or conservative management, it involves careful consideration of the child's neurological status, renal function, potential for bladder reconstruction, and long-term impact on quality of life.

Complex Congenital Anomalies

Children with complex or rare congenital anomalies, such as craniofacial malformations, congenital diaphragmatic hernia, or imperforate anus, present intricate surgical challenges. Decision-making involves the coordination of multidisciplinary teams, including pediatric surgeons, neonatologists, anesthesiologists, geneticists, and other specialists, to create comprehensive treatment plans tailored to the individual child's needs.

Surgical decision-making in these cases requires considering long-term functional and cosmetic outcomes, the potential for staged interventions, and careful management of perioperative risks.

These diverse use cases reflect the breadth of challenges encountered in pediatric surgical decision-making, emphasizing the need for expertise, collaboration, and ethical considerations in optimizing outcomes for pediatric patients across the spectrum of complex clinical scenarios.

In conclusion, the use cases discussed exemplify the intricate nature of surgical decision-making in pediatric cases, emphasizing the crucial role of comprehensive assessment, multidisciplinary collaboration, ethical considerations, and optimizing outcomes for young patients. The challenges presented in these scenarios span a spectrum of congenital anomalies, oncological conditions, traumatic injuries, and complex surgical pathologies, highlighting the diverse and ever-evolving landscape of pediatric surgical care.

One resounding theme across these use cases is the imperative of meticulous preoperative evaluation, advanced imaging, and detailed surgical planning to address the unique anatomical considerations and physiological fragility of pediatric patients. Understanding the intricacies of neonatal and pediatric physiology is essential in navigating complex surgical interventions ensuring optimal outcomes while minimizing the risk of complication.

Furthermore, these use cases emphasize the importance of multidisciplinary collaboration, wherein pediatric surgeons work closely with pediatric anesthesiologists, neonatologists, pediatric oncologists, pediatric intensivists, and other sub-specialists to formulate comprehensive treatment plans. The synergy between surgical expertise and multidisciplinary input is fundamental in addressing the holistic needs of pediatric patients, particularly in cases involving complex congenital anomalies, oncological resection, and long-term surgical management.

Ethical considerations permeate every aspect of pediatric surgical decision-making, encompassing discussions on informed consent, family-centered care, and the pursuit of patient-centered outcomes. The ethical dimensions of pediatric surgery are particularly pronounced in cases involving rare congenital anomalies, end-of-life decision-making, and complex surgical interventions with the potential for long-term impact on a child's quality of life.

Moreover, these use cases shed light on the evolving landscape of pediatric surgical innovations, including minimally invasive techniques, advancements in neonatal surgical care, and the integration of cutting-edge technologies into pediatric surgical practice. As the field of pediatric surgery continues to progress, embracing these innovations while upholding the highest standards of safety and efficacy becomes paramount in ensuring the best possible outcomes for young patients.

The cases highlighted in this discussion also showcase the significance of ongoing research, education, and training in pediatric surgical decision-making. Continuous efforts to advance the understanding of pediatric surgical pathologies, refine surgical techniques, and disseminate best practices are vital in equipping pediatric surgeons with the knowledge and skills necessary to navigate the complexities of challenging clinical scenarios.

Finally, these use cases serve as a testament to the resilience and unwavering dedication of surgical teams in confronting the most formidable challenges in caring for pediatric patients. The commitment to optimizing long-term quality of life, providing compassionate family-centered care, and pushing the boundaries of surgical innovation exemplifies the extraordinary pursuit of excellence in pediatric surgery.

Suggested Readings

Almond PS, et al. Principles and practice of pediatric surgery. Lippincott Williams & Wilkins; 2012.

Caty MG, Azizkhan RG, Lillehei CW. Pediatric surgery. 2-volume set. Saunders; 2011.

Holcomb GW, et al. Ashcraft's pediatric surgery. 6th ed. Elsevier; 2019.

Hollier L, Schwartz MR, Caldamone A, editors. Pediatric surgery. 7th ed. Elsevier; 2020.

Karp N. Ethical decision making in pediatric surgical practice. Oxford University Press; 2021.

Levitt MA, Peña A. Handbook of pediatric surgical patient care. Springer; 2017.

Mattei P. Pediatric surgical decision making. In: Pediatric surgery. Cham: Springer; 2019.

Oldham KT, Colombani PM, Foglia RP. Surgery of infants and children: scientific principles and practice. 7th ed. Elsevier; 2012.

St. Peter SD, Snyder CL, Ostlie DJ. Textbook of pediatric surgical oncology. Springer; 2018.

Zamzow E. Core curriculum for neonatal intensive care nursing. Elsevier Health Sciences; 2018.

15 Surgical Decision-Making: Melanoma

Rondi Kauffmann and Cameron Schlegel

Introduction

The care of the melanoma patient has evolved considerably over the last 10 years. Improvements in systemic therapies have paved the way for discussions about whether and when to de-escalate surgical intervention. Single-agent and dual-agent immunotherapies are widely used in the adjuvant setting and have a high response rate and good long-term survival [1]. The development of targeted therapies for patients with tumors exhibiting specific mutations offers yet another strategy to downstage locally advanced disease or improve survival in patients with metastatic disease [2, 3]. As systemic therapies have improved long-term survival in patients with melanoma, the complexity around surgical decision-making has increased. Surgical excision of localized and locoregional disease remains the optimal strategy for cure, and resection of metastatic disease has a growing role in select patients. Against this backdrop, the experience, judgment, and decision-making of the surgeon play a pivotal role in the multidisciplinary care of the patient with melanoma.

R. Kauffmann (✉) · C. Schlegel
Division of Surgical Oncology and Endocrine Surgery, Vanderbilt University Medical Center, Nashville, TN, USA
e-mail: rondi.kauffmann@vumc.org; cameron.schlegel@vumc.org

Preoperative Decision-Making

The Role of Sentinel Lymph Node Biopsy

Immunotherapy has revolutionized the way melanoma is treated. Its role in the perioperative setting is rapidly evolving and thus must be considered in operative planning. Ipilimumab is a human antibody against CTLA 4 that improves overall survival in Stage III high-risk melanoma patients and is the first approved immunotherapy for melanoma [4]. Subsequently, multiple other agents have been found to improve recurrence-free survival for Stage III/IV melanoma patients, including PD-1 inhibitors nivolumab (approved in 2017) and pembrolizumab (approved in 2019), as well as BRAF/MEK-targeted therapy (dabrafenib and trametinib, approved in 2018) [5–7].

With data supporting the role of immunotherapy in advanced-stage melanoma, natural questions have arisen to its role in earlier-stage melanoma patients. Patients with Stage IIB/C disease have similar prevalence to those patients with Stage III disease but a greater risk of recurrence and melanoma-specific death when compared to Stage IIIA patients, closely mirroring the trajectory of Stage IIIB patients [8, 9]. Keynote 716 was published in 2022 and evaluated the role of immunotherapy in patients with Stage IIB/C disease. The addition of adjuvant pembrolizumab significantly reduced the risk of disease or death in Stage IIB/C patients when

R. Latifi (ed.), *Surgical Decision-Making*, https://doi.org/10.1007/978-3-031-67391-7_15

compared to placebo alone [9]. CheckMate 76K was published shortly thereafter, demonstrating improvement in recurrence-free survival with nivolumab adjuvant treatment in Stage IIB/C patients, with a 58% reduction in risk of death or disease recurrence in patients treated with nivolumab vs placebo [10].

Given the potential role of immunotherapy in earlier, non-lymph node-positive disease, the role of sentinel lymph node biopsy in these patients with thicker melanomas has been called to question and remains under active discussion [11]. Arguments in favor of sentinel lymph node biopsy include its prognostic impact, locoregional control, adjuvant therapy options, and consideration of immunotherapy tolerance. Thus, all patients should be discussed and considered by a multidisciplinary team.

Sentinel lymph node biopsies may significantly inform patient conversation and potential immunotherapy decisions. In a recent paper using SEER data to model estimated 5-year melanoma-specific risk, the inclusion of sentinel lymph node biopsy in Stage IIB/C melanoma patients improved adjuvant therapy decision-making [12]. When considering adjuvant therapy, certain agents, specifically BRAF/MEK inhibitors, remain approved only for Stage III disease, and thus completion of lymph node staging in this patient population remains crucial [7].

Patient factors, including their ability to undergo surgical therapy and subsequent immunotherapy, must be considered in a multidisciplinary discussion prior to proceeding with surgical therapy. Lymph node biopsy is often performed under general anesthesia and adds time to the procedure, particularly in high-risk or elderly patients. In addition, there is a range of tolerance of immunotherapy depending on agent(s) and duration, with grades 3 and 4 adverse events ranging from 10% to 16% in the previous quoted Stage IIB/C data [9, 10]. Multi-disciplinary discussion prior to operative intervention is important, and consideration of sentinel lymph onde biopsy may be adjusted by patient frailty, co-morbidities that may predict poor systemic therapy tolerance, or those who are not interested in systemic therapy. Improvement in locoregional control is an additional consideration, particularly in patients who may not be candidates for further systemic therapy.

Options for the Bad Operative Candidate

A diagnosis of cancer in an elderly patient presents a unique challenge to the surgeon. Not only do patients in this population have a higher likelihood of presenting with multiple other comorbid medical conditions that render them more fragile and complex, but they are also more likely to have lower health literacy and higher rates of depression [13]. Discussions regarding quality of life and not just quantity of life should be a priority for all patients who are faced with undergoing cancer treatment but are particularly important for elderly patients for whom life expectancy at baseline is shorter than their younger counterparts. Goals of care including cure, minimizing toxicities, and feeling well enough to participate in activities of daily living (ADLs) should be defined early [14, 15]. In some cases, this discussion may lead to a decision for nonoperative management, or less aggressive surgical management. For patients who are poor operative candidates or wish to avoid surgery for other reasons and have early-stage melanoma (melanoma in situ or T1aN0 invasive), data supports the use of Mohs micrographic surgery as an alternative to standard wide local excision with a slight survival advantage for Mohs micrographic surgery in a retrospective study using the National Database [16]. Older patients often have less physiologic reserve and can be expected to respond to surgery differently than younger patients and require longer recovery time. Thus, while standard of care stipulates the performance of sentinel node biopsy for invasive melanomas >1.01 mm in depth, the surgeon should carefully consider the risks and benefits of sentinel node biopsy in elderly patients with melanoma. It has been observed that sentinel node involvement by melanoma is less common in elderly patients, even those with thick melanomas, which may be due to atrophy of dermal lymphatic channels in

Table 15.1 For older adults, geriatric assessment reduces cancer treatment side effects

Components of a geriatric assessment	
Domain	Example
Physical performance	·Assess balance, gait speed, and strength
Functional status	·Assess difficulty with activities such as bathing, dressing, and eating
Comorbidities	·Assess the presence of other illnesses, as well as hearing and visual impairments
Cognition	·Assess orientation, memory, and concentration
Nutrition	·Assess weight and change in weight over 6 months
Social support	·Assess the presence of social support in activities of daily living when needed
Polypharmacy	·Assess the number of regularly scheduled medications and high-risk medications
Psychological status	·Assess depression and anxiety

Was originally published by the National Cancer Institute (https://www.cancer.gov/news-events/cancer-currents-blog/2021/cancer-geriatric-assessment-fewer-side-effects)

older patients [17]. Assessment of overall patient condition relative to comorbidities using a health measurement tool such as the Karnofsky performance status can help the surgeon decide whether performance of sentinel node biopsy, which usually requires spinal or general anesthesia, is worth the additional surgical and anesthetic risk relative to primary wide local excision alone [18]. It is interesting to note that the pivotal trial upon which the use of sentinel node biopsy is based (MSLT-1) excluded patients aged >75 years [19]. Despite this, other studies have shown the utility and feasibility in elderly patients [20]. For elderly patients who proceed with surgery, careful planning to minimize time in the hospital, addressing the risk of sundowning, ease of transportation burdens, and ensuring adequate assistance postoperatively are vital [14].

Upon initial pre-surgical evaluation of an elderly patient with melanoma, it is important to assess the chronologic vs. physiologic age of the patient. Recognizing that age is just a number and a healthy 85-year-old may tolerate surgery and systemic therapy better than a 55-year-old with multiple comorbidities, this preoperative evaluation provides important information about comorbidities, medication use, and ability to perform activities of daily living. In the adjuvant setting, an ongoing multidisciplinary discussion about treatment plans is imperative. Many clinical trials exclude patients with significant comorbidities or older age [21]. Because elderly patients with cancer are also more likely to have accumulated comorbidities, the optimal doses of treatments or expected side effects are not necessarily known in this population [22]. Results from a clinical trial showed that use of a formal geriatric assessment is an important component of multidisciplinary cancer treatment planning [23]. This is a health measurement tool for elderly patients, which provides clinicians with information that can be used to guide treatment choices for elderly patients with advanced cancer. In that trial, patients whose care was informed by the geriatric assessment experienced fewer side effects of treatment and were less likely to experience falls during the course of their cancer treatment. While there were no differences in survival between the intervention and nonintervention arms, the reduced side effects and risk of falls would be expected to be associated with improved quality of life. While the tool was evaluated in the context of a medical oncology treatment plan, it has clear utility for surgeons as well. The components of the geriatric assessment are shown below, with the full assessment accessible in the publication of the original trial (Table 15.1) [23].

Intraoperative Challenges

The Non-mapping Sentinel Lymph Node

The use of dual tracer technique has significantly improved the accuracy and consistency of sentinel lymph node biopsies. Success rates of lymphoscintigraphy to identify sentinel lymph nodes is estimated to be around 95% [19, 24]. This is higher in patients with extremity melanomas

(95.3% in the axilla, 99.3% in the groin) but significantly lower for mapping of the head and neck, with rates of sentinel node identification as low as 84.5% [19]. A variety of factors should be considered when this is encountered.

One variable is the frequency and volume of lymphoscintigrams performed at an institution. Like many procedures, these injections and mapping come with a learning curve, with significant improvements in accuracy with increasing volumes. Morton et al. found the rate of false negatives was 10.3% during their first 25 cases, falling to 5.2% afterward [19]. Ensuring adequate training and volume to improve lymphoscintigram accuracy should be considered when planning these cases.

Despite adequate training, we know that the surgeon will encounter scenarios where no sentinel lymph node is identified on initial lymphoscintigram. SPECT/CT has been shown to increase the identification of sentinel lymph nodes, with detection rates by SPECT/CT averaging 98.28%, compared to 95% for planar lymphoscintigraphy [24]. Additional nodal basins are identified by SPECT/CT in 17.87–38.1% of patients compared to planar lymphoscintigraphy alone [24, 25]. Surgeons also felt that the addition of SPECT/CT changed the location and shortened the length of incision in 16–81% and 6–45% of patients, respectively [25]. While time and resources must also be considered when ordering these preoperative tests, if access to a SPECT/CT is available, it may significantly increase node identification and can be of particular use for head and neck melanomas.

Melanoma staging and previous perioperative treatment discussions must also be taken into account when no sentinel lymph node is identified. In patients with Stage IIB/C tumors where immunotherapy may already play a role in perioperative treatment, as previously discussed, consideration of medical oncology referral if not already complete, staging imaging, and close surveillance should be considered. All patients should undergo close lymph node basin monitoring, and integrating ultrasound surveillance in non-mapping patients should be considered on a case-by-case basis.

Challenges in Melanoma Excision: The Closure

While much of our consideration of melanoma excision focuses on the removal and margin status of the melanoma itself, equally important and complex is the consideration of closure. While one should try to anticipate challenges with closure as often as possible preoperatively with a multidisciplinary team, intraoperative situations arise in which previous closure plans must change based on tissue and size of defect.

Janis et al. described the concept of a reconstructive ladder (Fig. 15.1). Rather than a specific sequence of closure options, this provides a framework to review the possibilities surgeons may consider when faced with a challenging closure [26, 27]. If primary closure cannot be achieved, a temporary wound dressing or permanent secondary intention closure may be an option. Considerations should include whether wound contracture will cause significant morbidity or movement limitations, as in adjacent or overlying a joint, as well as scarring and long-term cosmesis. Delayed reconstruction, in any form, is an option when the surgeon finds themselves without reconstructive help and may be a preferred option for certain melanomas to confirm clearance of margins. This is particularly true for locally recurrent or thicker lesions, melanoma in situ with ill-defined borders, and desmoplastic melanomas at higher risk of positive margins [27].

Skin grafts are an excellent option for reconstruction to allow for easy surveillance without significant tissue rearrangement. Split-thickness skin grafts (STSG) are shallow skin harvests that can be meshed and placed in a variety of locations. In some locations such as over joints where primary closure may appear possible, if this significantly limited the mobility of a joint, grafts may be another option to consider. Full-thickness skin grafts are alternatives to split-thickness, including the entirety of the dermis down to subcutaneous tissues. These grafts undergoing less secondary contraction compared to STSG but have a higher risk of complete or partial failure [28].

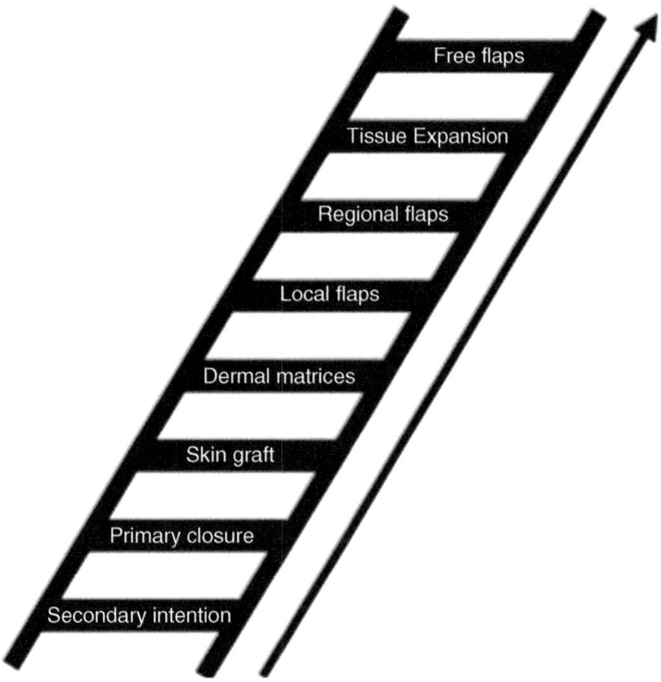

Fig. 15.1 Reconstructive ladder from Gimenez et al. [27], adapted from Janis et al. [26]

Local, regional, and free flaps are alternative options that maintain their own blood supply and may be ideal for poorly vascularized tissue [27]. If the surgeon anticipates a flap may be required, it is important to avoid local beveling or thinning of the surrounding tissue which is vital to flap perfusion. In addition, significant rotational flaps may make it challenging for the surgeon in the future if they must readdress either a positive margin or attempt lymph node mapping.

Challenging Referrals

Sentinel Node Biopsy After Previous Excision

Invasive melanoma can pose a clinical diagnostic challenge, particularly since it can appear similar to benign skin processes or be amelanotic. The melanoma surgeon is periodically confronted with a patient who underwent an excision of a presumed benign skin lesion in an outpatient clinic with pathology revealing a "surprise" melanoma on final pathologic assessment. Re-excision of such lesions to obtain adequate skin margins is challenging when the orientation of the scar is sub-optimal or subsequent excision will require a more complex reconstruction such as split-thickness skin graft or local flap due to the location of the original incision. Even more challenging from a surgical decision-making perspective is when to perform sentinel node biopsy at the time of re-excision in the setting of previous excision. There is some controversy in this area, with experts disagreeing on accuracy and acceptable false-negative rate of sentinel node biopsy for previous excision. If previous excision did not involve extensive undermining or complex rotational flap reconstruction, then sentinel node biopsy performed concurrently with the definitive wide local excision has been shown to result in an acceptable rate of identification of the draining nodal basin and false-negative rate less than 10% [29, 30]. However, in patients with previous complex rotation flap reconstruction, sentinel node biopsy results in higher false-negative rates, and we would generally not attempt sentinel node biopsy, preferring instead to surveil the expected draining nodal basins every 3 months with nodal basin ultrasound [31].

Resection of Metastatic Disease

As systemic therapies for melanoma have improved, the number of patients living with metastatic disease has similarly increased. Hence, surgeons are increasingly being asked to evaluate patients for resection of metastatic disease. Number and location of metastases, response to previous treatments, mutational status, and disease-free interval are important points of consideration. Such decisions are best made in the context of a multidisciplinary tumor board discussion, in which representatives from medical oncology, surgical oncology, pathology, radiology, and radiation oncology are present to render their opinions. Prior to surgical resection, consideration should be given to the use of neoadjuvant immunotherapy, whether alone or in combination, or BRAF/MEK-targeted therapies for patients with actionable melanoma mutations [32]. Such therapies have been shown to be associated with associated with improved event-free survival when followed by adjuvant therapy [33]. The surgeon considering metastasectomy must carefully select patients offered surgery. In the era of modern systemic treatment, resection of metastatic disease is associated with improved overall survival, particularly for patients with metastatic disease to the gastrointestinal tract who undergo curative surgical resection [34]. Surgical resection thereby remains an important component of multidisciplinary melanoma care in the era of effective immunotherapy and targeted systemic therapies.

References

1. Larkin J, Chiarion-Sileni V, Gonzalez R, et al. Five-year survival with combined nivolumab and ipilimumab in advanced melanoma. N Engl J Med. 2019;381:1535–46.
2. Rogala P, Czarnecka AM, Cybulska-Stopa B, et al. Long-term outcomes of targeted therapy after first-line immunotherapy in BRAF-mutated advanced cutaneous melanoma patients—real-world evidence. J Clin Med. 2022;11(8):2239.
3. Schummer P, Schilling B, Gesierich A. Long-term outcomes in BRAF-mutated melanoma treated with combined targeted therapy or immune checkpoint blockade: are we approaching a true cure? Am J Clin Dermatol. 2020;21(4):493–504.
4. Eggermont AMM, Chiarion-Sileni V, Grob JJ, et al. Prolonged survival in stage III melanoma with ipilimumab adjuvant therapy. N Engl J Med. 2016;375:1845–55.
5. Weber J, Mandala M, Del Vecchio M, et al. Adjuvant nivolumab versus ipilimumab in resected stage III or IV melanoma. N Engl J Med. 2017;377:1824–35.
6. Eggermont AMM, Blank CU, Mandala M, et al. Adjuvant pembrolizumab versus placebo in resected stage III melanoma. N Engl J Med. 2018;378:1789–801.
7. Long GV, Hauschild A, Santinami M, et al. Adjuvant dabrafenib plus trametinib in stage III *BRAF*-mutated melanoma. N Engl J Med. 2017;377:1813–23.
8. Poklepovic AS, Luke JJ. Considering adjuvant therapy for stage II melanoma. Cancer. 2020;126:1166–74.
9. Luke JJ, Ascierto PA, Carlino MS, Gershenwald JE, Grob J-J, Hauschild A, Kirkwood JM, Long GV, Mohr P, Robert C, et al. KEYNOTE-716: Phase III study of adjuvant pembrolizumab versus placebo in resected high-risk stage II melanoma. Future Oncol. 2020;16:4429–38. https://doi.org/10.2217/fon-2019-0666.
10. Kirkwood JM, Del Vecchio M, Weber J, Hoeller C, Grob JJ, Mohr P, Loquai C, Dutriaux C, Chiarion-Sileni V, Mackiewicz J, Rutkowski P, Arenberger P, Quereux G, Meniawy TM, Ascierto PA, Menzies AM, Durani P, Lobo M, Campigotto F, Gastman B, Long GV. Adjuvant nivolumab in resected stage IIB/C melanoma: primary results from the randomized, phase 3 CheckMate 76K trial. Nat Med. 2023;29(11):2835–43. https://doi.org/10.1038/s41591-023-02583-2. Epub 2023 Oct 16. Erratum in: Nat Med. 2023 Nov 3;: PMID: 37845511; PMCID: PMC10667090.
11. Rutkowski P, Kosela-Paterczyk H. Perioperative therapy in melanoma: several questions still remain. Ann Surg Oncol. 2023;30:2365–567.
12. Sharon CE, Straker RJ 3rd, Gimotty PA, Chu EY, Mitchell TC, Miura JT, Marchetti MA, Bartlett EK, Karakousis GC. Sentinel lymph node biopsy status improves adjuvant therapy decision-making in patients with clinical stage IIB/C melanoma: a population-based analysis. J Am Acad Dermatol. 2022;88:802. https://doi.org/10.1016/j.jaad.2022.11.033.
13. Estape T. Cancer in the elderly: challenges and barriers. Asia Pac J Oncol Nurs. 2018;5:40–2.
14. https://www.cancer.net/navigating-cancer-care/adults-65/cancer-care-decisions-older-adults. Accessed 08 Dec 2023.
15. DuMontier C, Loh KP, Soto-Perez-de-Celis E, Dale W. Decision making in older adults with cancer. ASCO. 2021;39(19):2164–75.
16. Ceraghlou S, Christensen SR, Agogo GO, Girardi M. Comparison of survival after Mohs micrographic surgery vs wide margin excision for early-stage invasive melanoma. JAMA Dermatol. 2019;155(11):1252–9.

17. Balch CM, Soong SJ, Gersehnwald JE, et al. Prognostic factors analysis of 17,600 melanoma patients: validation of the American Joint Committee on Cancer melanoma staging system. J Clin Oncol. 2001;19:3622–34.
18. Moreno-Ramirez D, Terjera-Vaquerizo A, Mendonca FI, Ojedi-Vila T, Ferrandiz L. Making decisions on sentinel lymph node biopsy for malignant melanoma: prioritization of determinants using a decision tree. J Eur Acad Dermatology Venereol. 2017;31:e247–9.
19. Morton DL, Cochran AJ, Thompson JF, et al. Sentinel node biopsy for early-stage melanoma: Accuracy and morbidity in MSLT-I, an international multicenter trial. Ann Surg. 2005;242:302–13.
20. Koskivuo I, Hernberg M, Vihinen P, et al. Sentinel lymph node biopsy and survival in elderly patients with cutaneous melanoma. Br J Surg. 2011;98:1400–7.
21. The Lancet Healthy Longevity Editorial Series. Older patients with cancer: evidence-based care needs evidence. The Lancet. 2021;2(11):e678.
22. National Cancer Institute, News and Events, Cancer Blog. https://www.cancer.gov/news-events/cancer-currents-blog/2021/cancer-geriatric-assessment-fewer-side-effects. Accessed 08 Dec 2023.
23. Mohile SG, Mohamed MR, Xu H, et al. Evaluation of geriatric assessment and management on the toxic effects of cancer treatment (GAP70+): a cluster-randomised study. Lancet. 2021;398(10314):1894–904.
24. Quartuccio N, Garau LM, Arnone A, Pappalardo M, Rubello D, Arnone G, Manca G. Comparison of ^{99m}Tc-labeled colloid SPECT/CT and planar lymphoscintigraphy in sentinel lymph node detection in patients with melanoma: a meta-analysis. J Clin Med. 2020;9(6):1680. https://doi.org/10.3390/jcm9061680. PMID: 32498217; PMCID: PMC7356992.
25. Trinh BB, Chapman BC, Gleisner A, Kwak JJ, Morgan R, McCarter MD, Gajdos C, Kounalakis N. SPECT/CT adds distinct lymph node basins and influences radiologic findings and surgical approach for sentinel lymph node biopsy in head and neck melanoma. Ann Surg Oncol. 2018;25(6):1716–22. https://doi.org/10.1245/s10434-017-6298-0. Epub 2018 Jan 12
26. Janis JE, Kwon RK, Attinger CE. The new reconstructive ladder: modifications to the traditional model. Plast Reconstr Surg. 2011;127(Suppl 1):205s–12s.
27. Gimenez AR, Winocour SJ, Chu CK. Reconstructive techniques in melanoma for the surgical oncologist. Surg Oncol Clin N Am. 2020;29:349–67.
28. Adams DC, Ramsey ML. Grafts in dermatologic surgery: review and update on full- and split-thickness skin grafts, free cartilage grafts, and composite grafts. Dermatologic Surg. 2005;31(8 Pt 2):1055–67.
29. Gannon CJ, Rousseau DL, Ross MI, et al. Accuracy of lymphatic mapping and sentinel lymph node biopsy after previous wide local excision in patients with primary melanoma. Cancer. 2006;107(11):2647–52.
30. McCready DR, Ghazarian DM, Hershkop MS, et al. Sentinel lymph-node biopsy after previous wide local excision for melanoma. J Can Chirurgie. 2001;44(6):432–4.
31. Faries MB, Thompson JF, Cochran AJ, et al. Completion dissection or observation for sentinel-node metastasis in melanoma. N Engl J Med. 2017;376:2211–22.
32. Menzies AM, Amaria RN, Roseman EA, et al. Pathological response and survival with neoadjuvant therapy in melanoma: a pooled analysis from the International Neoadjuvant Melanoma Consortium (INMC). Nat Med. 2021;27(2):301–9.
33. Amaria RN, Prieto PA, Tetzlaff MT, et al. Neoadjuvant plus adjuvant dabrafenib and trametinib versus standard of care in patients with high-risk, surgically resectable melanoma: a single-centre, open-label, randomized, phase 2 trial. Lancet. 2018;19:181–93.
34. Deutsch GB, Flaherty DC, Kirchoff DD, et al. Association of surgical treatment, systemic therapy, and survival in patients with abdominal visceral melanoma metastases, 1965–2014 relevance of surgical cure in the era of modern systemic therapy. JAMA Surg. 2017;152(7):672–8.

Surgical Decision-Making in Post-Bariatric Complications

16

Tricia Kim, Daniel Jo, Jonathan Giannone, and Ashutosh Kaul

Bariatric surgery procedures, while providing significant benefits, do bring along with them potential complications that all surgeons must be well versed in. These complications can range from perioperative issues to long-term significant nutritional deficiencies [2, 3]. When problems happen after bariatric surgery, preexisting comorbidities and the specific surgical technique employed, can make management challenging for even the most skilled surgeons.

Our objective is to provide recommendations for the management of common technical complications that may arise after bariatric surgery. Postoperative problems like venous thromboembolism, management of weight regain, or dietary deficiencies will not be discussed in this chapter.

Laparoscopic Banding

Band Slippage

Band slippage is described as a prolapse of the stomach wall through the gastric band, which commonly occurs anteriorly or posteriorly reflecting the path in which the stomach herniates through the band [4]. An anterior slip occurs with downward migration of the band, causing the anterior wall of the stomach to shift upwards. A posterior slip is associated with herniating of the posterior wall of the stomach through the band.

Patients may present with abdominal pain, early satiety or food intolerance, nausea/emesis, and acid reflux. If there is suspicion that a band has slipped, confirmation may be obtained by an upright plain film or upper gastrointestinal (GI) series.

A tailored approach is usually needed for the treatment of a slipped gastric band, depending on the patient's symptoms and the extent of the slip. In cases of mild slippage without significant symptoms, deflating the band may be the initial step in relieving pressure on the stomach followed by close observation for any symptom improvement or further deterioration.

Slippage with severe symptoms not relieved by band deflation requires urgent surgical intervention [5]. Without revision or removal of the gastric band, complications including erosion, obstruction, and perforation may occur. We recommend laparoscopic approach with low threshold for removal of the gastric band. It is advisable to wait for any swelling and irritation to go down if revisional surgery is planned at the same time as the slipped band is removed. We begin by removing the access port with a transverse incision and then paying careful attention to evaluate the port and tubing for breaks. The tubing is cut just distal to the connection to the port and the

T. Kim · D. Jo · J. Giannone · A. Kaul (✉)
Department of Surgery, Westchester Medical Center, Valhalla, NY, USA
e-mail: jonathan.giannone@wmchealth.org; ashutosh.kaul@wmchealth.org

R. Latifi (ed.), *Surgical Decision-Making*, https://doi.org/10.1007/978-3-031-67391-7_16

specimen is sent for pathology. The abdomen is insufflated and 5-mm ports are placed through the prior laparoscopic scars with an upsized 12-mm port for band extraction. Adhesions are lysed, and once the gastric band is identified, fibrous adhesions on the band are dissected free using an energy device. The band is unbuckled and removed from around the stomach. It is then extracted from the 12-mm port, examined for any bilious staining that would suggest an erosion, and then sent to pathology. In severe band slips, if removal of the band relieves the obstruction, we prefer not to take down the gastrogastric plication as the tissue may be friable.

Pouch Enlargement

Pouch enlargement refers to the dilation or expansion of the stomach pouch and will typically occur if the band is too tight or the patient overeats. Patients may present with similar symptoms as band slippage. Management involves radiological assessment, band adjustment, fluid removal from the port, and surgical revision including possible band removal and dietary counseling. An enlarged gastric pouch may also cause significant gastroesophageal reflux disease (GERD). Managing this condition starts with medical optimization through GERD-specific medications. If symptoms persist or in severe cases, adjusting the gastric band to alleviate pressure or completely removing the band may be necessary for relief and to prevent further complications. These patients will need monitoring which includes periodic surveillance with an upper endoscopy to assess the condition of the esophagus and stomach.

Band Erosion/Perforation

Band erosion is a serious complication where the band migrates into the gastric lumen. This can be caused by various factors including material of the band itself, excessive filling of the band, slippage, pouch dilation, infection, and injury to the gastric wall during implantation [6]. Risks of band erosion are also increased in patients using nonsteroidal anti-inflammatory drugs (NSAIDs), smoking, and alcohol abuse [7]. In the event of complete erosion, there is a risk that the band can migrate distally potentially leading to an intestinal obstruction.

Patients may present with similar symptoms as those seen in band slippage. Additionally, they may also present with signs of an acute abdomen or peritonitis which could stem from a gastric perforation as a result of the band erosion. An upper endoscopy can diagnose erosion as the band will be visualized protruding into the gastric lumen. When the band migrates further, an abdominal CT can be useful in determining the location and extent of any resulting obstruction.

The treatment of gastric band erosion typically involves the surgical removal of the eroded band. Most of the time, this can be done laparoscopically, but depending on the severity of the erosion and any related problems, an endoscopic approach or even open treatment may be needed. After the band is removed, the stomach tissue is allowed to heal. In cases where band erosion has resulted in a significant residual defect, the surgical approach may include using surrounding omentum to patch it and placement of a drain.

Port Complications

Complications such as pain or tenderness at port site, infection, disruption, leakage, tubing problems, skin erosion, and rotation/flip can occur. Port site infections typically occur in the early postoperative period and present with cellulitis or abscess and require prompt medical attention, antibiotics, and surgical interventions including incision and drainage. Infection at the port site months after placement necessitates a thorough evaluation to rule out possible band erosion as erosion can sometimes manifest as infection at the port or along the subcutaneous tubing. Tube malfunctions are usually not emergencies, but they typically necessitate surgical intervention to replace the tubing. Port rotation or migration may additionally also require surgery to correct the issue.

Laparoscopic Sleeve Gastrectomy

Bleeding

Post-sleeve gastrectomy bleeding can originate from several sites including the staple line, short gastric vessels, trocar incision points, or due to accidental injury to the liver or spleen. Prompt management of bleeding is critical, and its incidence has been reported to be between 1.2% and 5.6% after sleeve gastrectomies [23]. This chapter will specifically concentrate on the bleeding associated with the staple line and its management strategies.

If bleeding is detected from the staple line intraoperatively, the area should be reinforced with either clips or sutures to prevent further complications. Postoperative bleeding may manifest through symptoms of nausea with or without hematemesis, melena, hematochezia, or abdominal pain. Hemodynamic instability or transfusion requirements of two or more units of packed red blood cells within 24 hours are usual indicators for surgical re-exploration. It is important to stabilize the patient with intravenous (IV) fluid resuscitation and Foley catheter placement. Anticoagulation should ideally be discontinued, and administration of reversal agents should be considered. Stable patients with a suspected intraluminal staple line bleed may undergo urgent upper endoscopy to identify and control the source of bleeding.

Interventions during endoscopy might include the application of clips, thermal coagulation, or injection of epinephrine. An experienced endoscopist should do the endoscopy with little insufflation to minimize any potential strain on the staple line. To confirm the existence of a hematoma in stable patients with suspected intra-abdominal bleeding, a CT scan can be a useful diagnostic tool.

Numerous surgical techniques have been suggested to decrease staple line bleeding, including choosing the correct height of the staple, applying precompression prior to staple firing, utilizing buttressing material, oversewing the staple line, and application of fibrin sealants. An intraoperative protocol was found to be helpful in detecting silent bleeds, and it involved increasing the systolic blood pressure above 140 mm Hg while concurrently decreasing intra-abdominal insufflation pressure below 10 mm Hg prior to closure. Implementing this protocol had been associated with a decrease in postoperative bleeding complication [8, 9].

To minimize significant bleeding during sleeve gastrectomies, we employ staple line reinforcement in our practice. Excellent hemostasis should be achieved before completing the procedure. At the conclusion of the surgery, we also advise applying topical fibrin sealant along the staple line, if necessary.

Late bleeding more than 3 months postoperative is typically due to ulcers, gastritis, or malignancy and should subsequently be diagnosed with upper endoscopy and imaging modalities.

Leak

One of the most concerning complications following sleeve gastrectomy is a staple line leak with a reported incidence ranging between 0 and 7% [10].

The approach to addressing leaks is nuanced and depends on a variety of factors including the underlying cause of the leak—whether it's mechanical, technical, or due to compromised blood flow (ischemia)—as well as the clinical presentation, which may range from subclinical (asymptomatic) to clinical (symptomatic). The timing of the leak's discovery also influences management, with early and delayed leaks potentially requiring different treatment protocol [11].

Leak after sleeve gastrectomy can have multifactorial causes which include either patient-related, technical, or physiological causes. Many preexisting conditions like diabetes, renal failure, and use of steroids may impair wound healing increasing risk of leak. Technical factors implicated include inappropriate staple selection, poor surgical technique, and inadequate staple line reinforcement.

Avoiding bunching of tissue, stapling slightly away from the gastroesophageal junction, and use of staple line reinforcement may decrease the risk of leak. Most commonly, leaks occur at the proximal portion of the staple line just below the esophagogastric junction. Some reasons proposed for the higher leak in this location include the tenuous arterial supply in that area, increased pressure proximal to the incisura, and decreased tissue thickness [11–13].

Clinical signs suggestive of a leak include tachycardia (heart rate ≥ 120 beats/min), fever of ≥38 °C, and abdominal pain or back pain. Leaks are categorized based on the time of occurrence postoperatively: early leaks occur 1–3 days postoperatively, and delayed leaks are diagnosed after 1 week [14, 15]. They are diagnosed through a combination of clinical presentation, laboratory tests, and radiological imaging. Laboratory findings such as elevated white blood cell count, C-reactive protein levels, and lactic acid can also indicate a leak. Radiological imaging play a crucial role, and CT with IV and oral (water-soluble) contrasted study in the stable patient can reveal an intra-abdominal collection and extravasation of contrast. Additionally, an upper GI study can also reveal a leak. Leaks may also be subclinical with contained leakage adjacent to the staple line that may be managed conservatively with adequate nutrition (enteral or parenteral) with or without interventional radiology (IR) drainage. When imaging cannot rule out a leak but there is a high index of suspicion, a diagnostic laparoscopy is warranted in symptomatic patients.

Patients with an uncontained leak should undergo emergent operative exploration, and consideration should be given to strategic drain placement and feeding access via nasojejunal tube or jejunostomy tubes. Jejunostomy tube is particularly recommended if delayed healing is expected. Initial management should include IV fluid resuscitation, initiation of broad-spectrum antibiotics, and implementation of NPO (nil per os, or nothing by mouth). Primary repair is seldom feasible in these cases, and usually surgeons perform patch omentoplasty to cover the leak site and appropriate drain placement.

Delayed leaks are preferentially treated conservatively with initiation of targeted antibiotic therapy, IR, or endoscopic drainage of fluid collection, making patients NPO with nutrition support. Endoscopic interventions are often used and include placement of stents (self-expanding metal stents, partially covered self-expanding metal stents, covered self-expanding plastic stents) [16]. Other techniques that include endoscopic vacuum-assisted closure (EVAC) and percutaneous transesophageal gastro-tubing (PTEG) have also been reported [19–21]. Late leaks are in some centers treated with covered stents for about 6 weeks. After this period the leak is then reassessed using endoscopic methods. If healing is satisfactory, the stent is removed, and the previously leaking site may then be secured further if needed with endoclips, fibrin sealants, or even endoscopic suturing. Stent migration represents a notable complication, occurring 16.9–59% of the time [17]. Stent migration can be reduced by fixation with endoscopic clips or sutures. Post-stenting, patients may experience side effects including nausea, emesis, drooling, early satiety, and retrosternal discomfort [18].

Chronic leaks may be challenging to treat and the leaks persisting after 12 weeks or more of non-operative management may necessitate conversion to a Roux-en-Y (RNY) gastric bypass, RNY esophago-gastrojejunostomy, or fistula-jejunostomy.

The treatment algorithm commonly followed for gastric sleeve leaks in a hemodynamically stable patient is source control (i.e., IR drainage vs laparoscopic drainage) and subsequent endoluminal stent placement. Septic or unstable patients may need immediate operative intervention with washout, drain placement, and consideration for nutritional support.

Stenosis

Stenosis after a sleeve gastrectomy, which is narrowing in the sleeve, has a reported incidence of 0.6–4.5% [22]. Usually, stenosis occurs at the level of the incisura and proper selection of bougie size and beginning of stapling at adequate distance from the pylorus on the antrum can minimize these complications. A twist or kink in the sleeve anatomy can also cause a functional stenosis.

Symptoms of stenosis usually include food intolerance, progressive dysphagia, regurgitation, and drooling. An upper GI series can assess the anatomy of the sleeve, and an upper endoscopy is helpful for both diagnosing the area of stenosis and offer therapeutic options. Initially managing stenosis after sleeve gastrectomy often entails period of observation and careful monitoring. Majority of stenosis respond well to nonsurgical approaches including endoscopic balloon dilations, which has shown to have 76% efficacy [24]. For severe or refractory cases, surgical revision to gastric bypass is considered the definitive treatment option.

Acid Reflux

Gastroesophageal reflux disease (GERD) is associated with morbid obesity. Research to date presents conflicting evidence regarding the impact of sleeve gastrectomy on GERD, with some studies showing an increase in GERD after sleeve while others suggest a decrease [23]. Morbidly obese patients with significant preoperative reflux are counseled to consider a Roux-en-Y (RNY) gastric bypass which has been shown to significantly improve or even resolve GERD symptoms [25]. After sleeve gastrectomy, patients experiencing persistent GERD symptoms are typically prescribed proton pump inhibitors (PPIs) for at least 12 weeks. Continued or worsening symptoms are an indication to proceed with further work-up including upper endoscopy to check for anatomical issues like hiatal hernia, along with pH monitoring to assess reflux severity. Should symptoms persist despite conservative measures, we discuss the possibility of conversion to an RNY gastric bypass as a revisional surgical option.

Gastric Bypass

Intro

The gastric bypass, pioneered by Dr. Mason and Ito in the 1960s, has remained a staple in bariatric surgery due to its effectiveness. The introduction of minimally invasive surgical techniques in the 1990s further boosted its popularity. The RNY gastric bypass stands out as the most commonly used technique because of its extensive use and well-documented outcomes [1].

The most common RNY configuration of the gastric bypass consists of the creation of a small gastric pouch (with a volume of ~30 mL), connected to a 150 cm alimentary or "Roux" limb that is then joined to a ~ 50 cm biliary limb in a "Y" configuration leading to a common channel. The resultant weight loss from this procedure is attributed to several factors: restricted caloric intake, reduced nutrient absorption, and alterations in hormones and behavior, all contributing to significant and sustained weight reduction and improvements in obesity-related health conditions [3]. Postoperatively, patients usually experience rapid weight loss with about half of the weight loss occurring in the first 6 months after surgery and continuing up to 18–24 months after surgery [26].

The gastric bypass can be performed in either the open fashion or using minimally invasive techniques including laparoscopic or robotic approaches with relatively low morbidity and mortality [27–30]. Minimally invasive surgical techniques are usually associated with shorter hospital stays, reduced postoperative pain, fewer pulmonary complications, wound complications, and better cosmesis [29, 30]. The laparoscopic RNY gastric bypass, despite its advantages, is a technically challenging surgery with a steep learning curve. No matter the surgical approach taken, gastric bypass can result in complications which can pose management conundrums [30]. Surgeons need to be proficient in promptly recognizing and treating complications after gastric bypass surgery as delays might have grave consequences. The complications will be categorized into early and late stages, with an emphasis on those that occur most frequently in general surgical practice.

Early Complications

Early complications of gastric bypass surgery usually occur within hours or the first few days after surgery; however, there have been documented reports of occurrences up to 2 months after surgery [31].

Bleeding

Postoperative hemorrhage following gastric bypass is reported with a frequency ranging from 0.3% to 4.4% [32, 34, 35, 40]. Most bleeding episodes (70%) occur in the early postoperative period, which is within the first 30 days following surgery [34]. The bleeding generally comes from intraperitoneal or intraluminal sites, the most frequent being the anastomoses at the gastrojejunostomy (GJ) and jejunojejunostomy (JJ) sites. Other rarer sites include the gastric remnant and from the site of complications like gastric fistulae and perforations. Factors that increase the risk of bleeding include a history of previous surgeries and presence of type 2 diabetes [33, 35].

When patients experience postoperative hemorrhage after gastric bypass surgery, the diagnosis and identification of the bleeding source depend heavily on the early clinical presentation. Melena or hematochezia is a sign of an intraluminal hemorrhage and can reveal information about the location and speed of the bleed (proximal versus distal in the gastrointestinal system). It's important to remember that the lack of rectal bleeding does not rule out an intraluminal source; on the other hand, signs like increased abdominal circumference, new abdominal bulge development, and widespread abdominal pain may correspond to an intraperitoneal bleeding. Though they are rare, shock symptoms including pallor, diaphoresis, tachycardia, and hypotension usually indicate significant bleeding.

It is critical to take into account a number of factors during the initial assessment of a patient who has bleeding after gastric bypass surgery. These include the patient's current medications (NSAIDs, anticoagulants, acid suppressive therapy), the length of time the symptoms have been present, the time since surgery, and any previous endoscopy or surgical reports.

The strategy in controlling postoperative hemorrhage after gastric bypass surgery is complicated and depends on several factors. Intraluminal bleeding in the early postoperative phase is commonly caused by GJ anastomosis and tends to resolve spontaneously. According to data from a single-center study of early postoperative bleeding after laparoscopic gastric bypass, more than 90% of bleeding events were managed without the need for invasive procedures [35]. For hemodynamically stable patients with a hemoglobin drop of less than 2 g/dL and no indication of continuous bleeding, therapy normally consists of close monitoring, discontinuing oral intake (bowel rest), and administering acid-suppressive medicine. Acid suppression is typically maintained for 30 days with a plan to perform an endoscopic examination during that time frame if bleeding persists. For more severe bleeding, therapeutic strategies are tailored based on the precise location of the hemorrhage.

Given a patient's altered surgical anatomy after gastric bypass surgery, localizing the source of bleeding can be a diagnostic challenge. Intraluminal bleeding after gastric bypass surgery usually occurs at the GJ anastomosis, the staple line of the pouch or excluded stomach, or the JJ anastomosis. In the setting of more brisk bleeding with hemodynamic instability, CT angiography can be helpful in localizing the source of bleeding from both intraperitoneal and intraluminal sources and can help guide the therapeutic approach. However, bleeding is typically slower and intraluminal with no significant changes in patient hemodynamics. In these scenarios, upper endoscopy has dual roles in diagnosis and treatment, and it is frequently the preferred diagnostic modality. Endoscopic intervention should be considered for severe bleeding indicated by a hemoglobin loss of more than 2 g/dL, hemodynamic instability, or repeated bleeding events when conservative therapy has been unsuccessfully tried [36]. Endoscopic therapy for intraluminal bleeding is effective even within the first 48 hours after surgery with success rates approaching 90% [37].

Despite its effectiveness, upper endoscopy has limitations, namely, the ability to evaluate and treat only the proximal gastric pouch and GJ anastomosis. For bleeding at the more distal JJ anastomosis, laparoscopic-assisted endoscopy or surgical revision of the JJ anastomosis should be considered.In some instances, angiography and subsequent embolization are used as part of the therapeutic plan. In our experience, angiographic embolization is employed as a last resort if endoscopic procedures fail to control bleeding in patients with significant perioperative risks. Surgical intervention becomes imperative when bleeding is unresponsive to endoscopic or radiological interventions.

For intraperitoneal bleeding, surgeons should maintain a low threshold for abdominal exploration to ascertain the source. Intraperitoneal hemorrhage may originate from various locations including the mesentery, omentum, spleen, liver, or trocar insertion sites.

Late postoperative bleeding, which happens more than 30 days after surgery, is a rare occurrence, but it has been observed as late as 25 years after the initial bariatric surgery [32]. Late bleeding following gastric bypass surgery can be due to severe gastritis, marginal ulcers at the anastomosis, fistula formation, or ulcerations within the gastric pouch, residual stomach, or duodenum [33]. To effectively control late postoperative bleeding, the cause needs to be precisely localized, which often requires a collaborative approach from a multidisciplinary team that includes surgical, gastroenterological, and interventional radiology services. Prevention strategies ought to stress the avoidance of ulcer-inducing agents such as NSAIDs, corticosteroids, tobacco, and immunosuppressive medications whenever possible. Additionally, the patient should be stabilized as soon as possible and transferred to a higher-level tertiary or quaternary care center for specialized treatment if necessary.

Leak

Leaks after gastric bypass surgery are a particularly alarming complication due to their quick onset and potentially serious consequences. The incidence of leaks following laparoscopic gastric bypass ranges from 1% to 6% with these complications often appearing during the first 10 days after surgery [38]. Surgeons must maintain a high level of suspicion for leaks following gastric bypass as the typical indications of peritonitis can be obscured by obese patients' body habitus. Tachycardia, fever, and tachypnea are the symptoms that are most indicative of a leak and have the highest predictive sensitivity.

The prevention of subsequent problems resulting from anastomotic leakage is contingent upon early detection and timely intervention. These leaks can be identified by diagnostic imaging techniques such as upper gastrointestinal fluoroscopy or CT scans with oral contrast. It's important to keep in mind, however, that this kind of imaging shouldn't postpone the necessary leak management. Often the quickest and most accurate way to identify and treat is to perform operative exploration especially if clinical evaluation suggests a significant leak with clinical deterioration. This approach ensures timely resolution and may enhance patient outcomes.

Management of an anastomotic leak usually requires surgical intervention to wash out the contaminants, provide drainage, and establish feeding access. Nonoperative management is an exception and is usually reserved for those rare instances where a minor leak is evident on imaging and the patient presents with minimal symptoms and minor laboratory abnormalities. Even in those cases, patients must be monitored closely with a low threshold for operative exploration if there is any clinical decline.

When clinical signs such as tachycardia, abdominal pain, or tachypnea suggest a leak, immediate surgical exploration is usually indicated. When an adept surgical team is available, starting with a laparoscopic approach may be appropriate, but there should be a low threshold to convert to an open procedure if necessary to ensure proper exposure and washout. The primary goal in managing a leak is to control contamination, which is often achieved through vigorous irrigation and adequate drainage. With sufficient drainage and nutritional support, most small leaks will heal spontaneously. Intra-abdominal drains are maintained, and output is monitored as oral intake is gradually increased. Drains are usually removed when output falls below 20–30 mL.

If high drain output persists after 2–4 weeks, further investigations may be needed. It is our usual practice to wait longer than 6 weeks before considering further surgical intervention to ensure that the fluid collection is adequately contained and the patient's nutritional status is optimized. Both elements are important before any revisional surgery.

In the event of an early anastomotic leak identified during exploration, full revision of the anastomosis is rarely recommended. Attempting primary suture repair is often not beneficial as inflamed tissues may not reliably retain sutures. Instead, utilizing omental or serosal patches can be effective in sealing small to moderate leaks, especially when combined with sufficient drainage.

The decision to redo a surgical anastomosis may be necessary under certain conditions, such as extensive necrosis of the anastomosis or ongoing ischemia at the anastomotic site [39]. It is usually appropriate to stage any reconstruction to optimize care, address complications systematically, and improve outcomes in these complex scenarios. If an anastomosis has questionable perfusion in the setting of a leak, intraoperative Doppler ultrasound, indocyanine green (ICG) fluorescence or SPY technology can be used as adjuncts to evaluate perfusion of the tissue. In cases where complex reconstruction appears likely, the best course of action is to stabilize the patient with wide drainage to minimize ongoing contamination and transfer to a specialized tertiary center with expertise in revisional bariatric surgery and higher level of care.

Due consideration should also be made to establish feeding access during the operative exploration of anastomotic leaks. Indications for initiating enteral nutrition include expected inability to consume food for more than 2 weeks, inability to restore intestinal continuity during surgery, and critically ill patients facing extended hospitalizations. It is also recommended for the treatment and prevention of malnutrition and nutritional deficiencies. The location of the tube placement should be individualized to the patient with the aim of maximizing nutrient absorption and avoiding leakage exacerbation or contact with the leak. Feeding tubes can be placed into the excluded stomach, the roux limb distal to the GJ anastomosis, or the common channel distal to the JJ anastomosis.

Beyond establishing enteral access, feeding tubes can be strategically positioned into an anastomotic defect to serve as external drainage and create a controlled fistula, facilitating the healing of anastomotic leaks by secondary intention. Concurrently, intra-abdominal drains are typically placed adjacent to the feeding tube to help reduce further contamination. This method of intraluminal drainage is also beneficial for intestinal decompression in cases where prolonged postoperative intestinal dysmotility is anticipated. This procedure has the protective effect of reducing high intraluminal pressures and preventing retrograde pressure build-up, which could otherwise compromise the integrity of proximal anastomoses.

Inaccurate Construction

Misconstruction of the RNY configuration, termed a Roux-en-O, is rare and an underreported outcome of bariatric surgery with potentially devastating consequences for patients [42]. Improper construction occurs when the biliopancreatic limb is mistakenly anastomosed to the gastric pouch resulting in a closed "O" loop (Fig. 16.1). Patients typically present with abdominal pain, biliary emesis, esophagitis, severe dehydration, and nutritional malnutrition. The nonspecific nature of these symptoms along with altered surgical anatomy can pose diagnostic challenges and often delay diagnosis [43]. Diagnostic tools such as endoscopy, CT with contrast, and swallow studies may fail to identify the incorrect configuration especially when intestinal dilation masks the actual pathology [44]. Indicators on CT scans suggesting a Roux-en-O configuration include dilation of the proximal small bowel between the gastric pouch and gastric remnant with decompressed distal small bowel and colon. Notably, the hepatobiliary iminodiacetic acid (HIDA) scan aids in the diagnosis of this misconfiguration when the radiotracer moves into the duodenum and then backflows into the esophagus [40, 41]. Once a diagnosis has been confirmed, surgery is often required to correct the anatomy.

In certain cases, patients with a misconstructed Roux-en-O can exhibit symptoms similar to those with an internal hernia or bowel obstruction. Under these circumstances, it is critical to

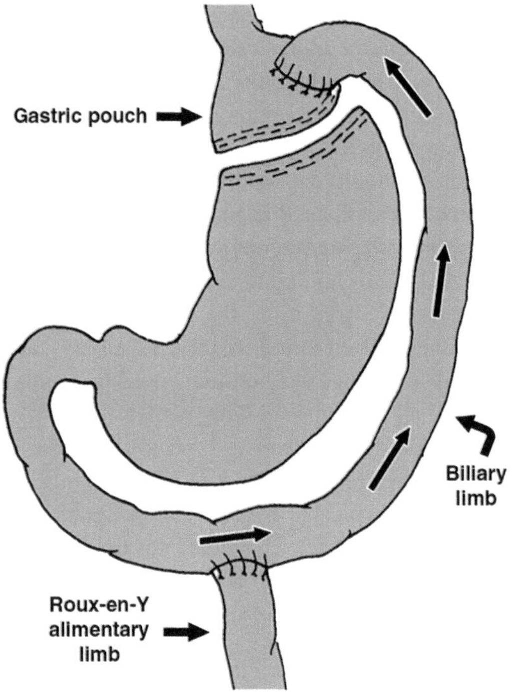

Fig. 16.1 Roux-en-O configuration [43]

take the patient to the operating room where the diagnosis is often made during surgery. These surgical procedures can be complicated due to the presence of significant scar tissue from previous surgeries and the modified anatomy. When navigating a surgical field that has been previously altered and may be incorrectly constructed, we recommend starting exploration from regions of known anatomy. Typically, this involves locating the terminal ileum and tracing the bowel in reverse to clarify the anatomical layout. To accurately trace the intestine in a retrograde manner, it may be necessary to perform lysis of adhesions. Both the GJ and JJ anastomoses must be clearly identified, along with the bowel segment connecting them, to accurately diagnose the blind "O" loop.

After pinpointing the misconstructed area, it is helpful to label the proximal Roux limb using sutures, clips, or a penrose drain to secure the limb's proper alignment. With the Roux limb and the biliary limb correctly identified, the GJ and JJ anastomoses can be resected and new connections established in the correct RNY configuration. If a segmental bowel resection is required for any reason during the operation, it is important to ensure the bowel is re-anastomosed in an isoperistaltic orientation [43].

Late Complications

Small Bowel Obstruction

Small bowel obstruction is a notable risk following gastric bypass surgery. Early postoperative obstructions, typically within the initial month, are usually attributed to technical issues during surgery. Conversely, obstructions that develop later can arise anytime post-surgery with a reported occurrence of 1–5% within a 68-month timeframe [45]. Late-stage obstructions can originate from various complications, including internal hernias, adhesive disease, jejunojejunostomy stenosis or kinking, incisional hernias, intussusceptions, and bezoars [47].

The clinical presentation of these obstructions varies based on their location and severity. In the event of complete obstruction of alimentary or common limbs, patients may experience significant symptoms such as nausea, vomiting, abdominal swelling, bloating, pain, electrolyte imbalances, dehydration, and a rapid heartbeat. However, partial or intermittent obstructions often result in subtler symptoms like recurring mild abdominal pain, sometimes following meals, difficulty with oral intake, or an inability to gain weight. Blockages in the biliopancreatic limb following RNY gastric bypass often present subtly with central upper abdominal pain or a persistent sensation of fullness in the left upper abdomen, occasionally accompanied by unexplained hiccoughs and tachycardia. Shoulder pain may also arise from diaphragmatic irritation due to an enlarged stomach. Elevated serum amylase and lipase could indicate chronic obstruction, though classic symptoms like nausea, vomiting, and obstipation might be absent, posing diagnostic challenges. Prompt recognition and medical attention for these symptoms post-surgery are crucial for avoiding severe complications.

Diagnosing obstructions can be challenging. They can be identified with an upper gastrointestinal series or a CT scan, but imaging is not always conclusive. Notably, CT scans have a false-negative rate of up to 20% for detecting internal hernias or similar causes of obstruction post-gastric bypass [40]. Due to the varied symptoms and the diagnostic limitations of standard imaging, having a low index of suspicion is essential when evaluating post-gastric bypass patients presenting with nonspecific abdominal pain, swelling, and poor dietary intake. In such cases, maintaining a low threshold for performing diagnostic laparoscopy is crucial to determine the exact cause of the obstruction.

After gastric bypass surgery, intestinal obstructions are frequently caused by internal hernias [39, 40]. These hernias arise when the intestine protrudes through a defect often due to a gap in the mesentery created during surgery. A RNY gastric bypass can be performed using either an antecolic or retrocolic fashion, and understanding the positioning of the Roux limb relative to the transverse colon is crucial. The retrocolic approach involves creating a window through the transverse mesocolon for the Roux limb to pass beneath the transverse colon, leading to three potential hernia sites: the transverse mesocolon defect, the site of the jejunojejunostomy, and the Petersen defect, which is the space between the Roux limb and the transverse mesocolon. In contrast, the antecolic approach positions the Roux limb anterior to the transverse colon resulting in two potential hernia sites at the jejunojejunostomy and the Petersen defect. Knowledge of these potential hernia sites is invaluable during surgery for effectively identifying and managing an internal hernia.

The initial goal during operative exploration is to carefully trace the small bowel from the terminal ileum toward the ligament of Treitz in a retrograde fashion. This approach not only helps in reducing an internal hernia but also allows for the assessment of potential ischemia along the bowel.

The focus then shifts to investigating potential sites of mesenteric defects at all potential sites depending on roux limb configuration. In a retrocolic configuration, the Roux limb will traverse through the transverse mesocolon—the size of the defect in the transverse mesocolon should be big enough to allow only the Roux limb and its mesentery to traverse through the defect. If a mesenteric defect is found at any location, the defect(s) should be sutured to prevent future internal herniations. If an internal hernia has been ruled out and no mesenteric defect is found, the bowel should again be traced in its entirety from the terminal ileum up to the jejunojejunostomy, ligament of Treitz, and gastrojejunostomy carefully lysing adhesions between bowel, omentum, abdominal wall, and solid organs.

An additional, albeit less common, cause of obstruction to consider is a jejunal intussusception, which typically involves the retrograde prolapse of the common channel into the Roux or biliopancreatic limb and is estimated to occur in 0.1% to 0.3% of cases [46]. Management options include reduction of the intussusception, reduction followed by enteropexy, or a complete overhaul of the jejunojejunostomy. Despite various interventions, recurrence is a possibility, and currently, there is insufficient evidence to declare one treatment method superior to another.

After surgery or revision for RNY configurations, nasogastric tube decompression is debated especially as it only provides limited relief to biliopancreatic limb and gastric remnant. If the gastric remnant needs decompression, a gastrostomy tube insertion is often performed. Nasogastric tube insertion in the immediate postoperative period should be done with care or even under fluoroscopic guidance to avoid injury to the gastrojejunal anastomosis.

Stenosis

Stenosis at the anastomoses usually presents gradually. GJ anastomosis narrowing has been reported to occur in 3–20% cases while JJ strictures are less common [48]. Presenting symptoms are typically increasing difficulty in swallowing, epigastric discomfort, retching, and vomiting. Stenosis at the GJ anastomosis is often due to GERD or marginal ulcers. Other contributing factors include the patient's age, compromised blood flow to the anastomosis, and technical aspects including size of the GJ anastomosis and technique of creating the anastomoses [48, 49].

The diagnosis and management of GJ anastomosis stenosis are predominantly endoscopic. GJ stenosis is defined endoscopically as any opening with a diameter < 10 mm in size [49]. Endoscopic management using either balloon or bougie dilation aims to stretch the GJ anastomosis to a diameter of ~12–15 mm. Success and reduction of symptoms can occur in up to 90% of patients following endoscopic dilation of GJ anastomosis within 6 months [50]. Repeated endoscopic dilations can be performed safely for symptomatic relief or if stricture recurs with no set limit on the number of procedures. Nonetheless, it is important to take into account the possibility of a perforation with repeated dilations. Balancing symptom relief of anastomotic strictures with the risk of weight regain is crucial as over-dilation may compromise the restrictive benefit of the gastric bypass leading to increased calorie intake and possible weight regain. Therefore, it's recommended to avoid dilating the GJ anastomosis beyond a diameter of 20 mm.

Rarely, if endoscopic management is unsuccessful in treating anastomotic strictures, surgical revision may be necessary. Revisional operations may be complicated by scar tissue and ideally referred to high-volume centers experienced in revisional surgery.

Fistula

Fistula is an uncommon complication following gastric bypass surgery occurring in about 1–2% of patients. A gastrogastric fistula is an abnormal opening between the newly created gastric pouch and the gastric remnant. This communication allows content to leak to the excluded stomach leading to complications such as reflux, inadequate weight loss, or other GI issues. Surgical technique advancements and improved stapling technology have reduced its incidence, but complications remain serious [51].

A gastrogastric fistula should be considered in the differential diagnosis of patients presenting with abdominal discomfort after gastric bypass. These may be identified in upper GI radiographic studies, and an upper GI endoscopy usually provides conclusive proof.

Gastrogastric fistula can be managed medically, endoscopically, or surgically. Given the high association of gastrogastric fistula with marginal ulcers, the initial step in management is to start with antacid treatment with proton pump inhibitors and sucralfate [52]. Smaller fistulas may heal with medical therapy alone, and if symptoms are alleviated with medical management, more invasive treatments may be avoided. Endoscopic techniques for fistula closure have recently been used with varying success rates and generally have lower complications and morbidity compared to surgery. Surgical repair tends to provide higher odds of success for larger fistulas and greater weight loss. Indications for surgical revision include refractory ulcers, significant pain, weight loss, failure, or weight regain after RNY gastric bypass surgery. Surgical repair can be challenging and usually entails identification and division of the fistulous communication. Revision may include remnant, gastrectomy with fistula excision, GJ anastomosis revision, or a combination of both procedures.

References

1. Faria GR. A brief history of bariatric surgery. Porto Biomed J [Internet]. 2017;2(3):90–2. Available from: https://www.sciencedirect.com/science/article/pii/S2444866416300186
2. Mason EE, Ito C. Gastric bypass in obesity. Surg Clin N Am. 1967;47(6):1345–51.
3. MacDonald KG, Long SD, Swanson MS, Brown BM, Morris P, Lynis Dohm G, et al. The gastric bypass operation reduces the progression and mortality of non-insulin-dependent diabetes mellitus. J Gastrointest Surg [Internet]. 1997;1(3):213–20. Available from: https://www.sciencedirect.com/science/article/abs/pii/S1091255X97801126?via%3Dihub
4. Eid I. Complications associated with adjustable gastric banding for morbid obesity: a surgeon's guide. Can J Surg. 2011;54(1):61–6.
5. Egberts K, Brown WA, O'Brien PE. Systematic review of erosion after laparoscopic adjustable gastric banding. Obes Surg. 2011;21(8):1272–9.
6. Singhal R, Bryant C, Kitchen M, Khan KS, Deeks J, Guo B, et al. Band slippage and erosion after laparo-

scopic gastric banding: a meta-analysis. Surg Endosc. 2010;24(12):2980–6.
7. Moser F, Gorodner MV, Galvani CA, Baptista M, Chretien C, Horgan S. Pouch enlargement and band slippage: two different entities. Surg Endosc. 2006;20(7):1021–9.
8. De Angelis F, Abdelgawad M, Rizzello M, Mattia C, Silecchia G. Perioperative hemorrhagic complications after laparoscopic sleeve gastrectomy: four-year experience of a bariatric center of excellence. Surg Endosc. 2016;31(9):3547–51.
9. Park JY. Diagnosis and management of postoperative complications after sleeve gastrectomy. J Metab Bariatric Surg. 2022;11(1):1.
10. Aurora AR, Khaitan L, Saber AA. Sleeve gastrectomy and the risk of leak: a systematic analysis of 4,888 patients. Surg Endosc. 2011;26(6):1509–15.
11. Rached AA. Gastric leaks post sleeve gastrectomy: review of its prevention and management. World J Gastroenterol [Internet]. 2014;20(38):13904. Available from: https://dx.doi.org/10.3748%2Fwjg.v20.i38.13904
12. Berger ER, Clements RH, Morton JM, Huffman KM, Wolfe BM, Nguyen NT, et al. The impact of different surgical techniques on outcomes in laparoscopic sleeve gastrectomies: the first report from the metabolic and bariatric surgery accreditation and quality improvement program (MBSAQIP). Ann Surg [Internet]. 2016;264(3):464–73. Available from: https://journals.lww.com/annalsofsurgery/pages/articleviewer.aspx?year=2016&issue=09000&article=00009&type=Fulltext
13. Bhojwani R, Jain N, Mahawar K. Leaks after sleeve gastrectomy—a narrative review. J Bariatric Surg. 2022;1(1):2.
14. Csendes A, Braghetto I, León P, Burgos AM. Management of Leaks after laparoscopic sleeve gastrectomy in patients with obesity. J Gastrointest Surg. 2010;14(9):1343–8.
15. Rosenthal RJ. International sleeve gastrectomy expert panel consensus statement: best practice guidelines based on experience of >12,000 cases. Surg Obes Relat Dis. 2012 Jan;8(1):8–19.
16. Walsh C, Karmali S. Endoscopic management of bariatric complications: a review and update. World J Gastrointest Endosc. 2015;7(5):518.
17. Mathus-Vliegen EMH. The cooperation between endoscopists and surgeons in treating complications of bariatric surgery. Best Pract Res Clin Gastroenterol. 2014 Aug;28(4):703–25.
18. Alanezi H, Alshehri A, Alrobiea A, Yoo MW. The causes, prevention, and management of gastric leakage after laparoscopic sleeve gastrectomy: a review article. J Metab Bariatric Surg. 2019;8(2):28–33.
19. Mann C, Berlth F, Tagkalos E, Hadzijusufovic E, Lang H, Grimminger P. Endoscopic management of complications—endovacuum for management of anastomotic leakages: a narrative review. Ann Esophagus. 2022;1(5):15.
20. Oshiro T, Saiki A, Suzuki J, Satoh A, Kitahara T, Kadoya K, et al. Percutaneous transesophageal gastro-tubing for management of gastric leakage after sleeve gastrectomy. Obes Surg. 2014;24(9):1576–80.
21. Archid R, Wichmann D, Klingert W, Nadiradze G, Hönes F, Archid N, et al. Endoscopic vacuum therapy for staple line leaks after sleeve gastrectomy. Obes Surg. 2019;30(4):1310–5.
22. Rebibo L, Hakim S, Abdennaceur Dhahri T, Yzet DR, Régimbeau J-M. Gastric stenosis after laparoscopic sleeve gastrectomy: diagnosis and management. Obes Surg. 2015;26(5):995–1001.
23. Laffin M, Chau J, Gill RS, Birch DW, Karmali S. Sleeve gastrectomy and gastroesophageal reflux disease. J Obes. 2013;2013:1–6.
24. Chang SH, Popov VB, Thompson CC. Endoscopic balloon dilation for treatment of sleeve gastrectomy stenosis: a systematic review and meta-analysis. Gastrointest Endosc. 2020;91(5):989–1002.e4.
25. Peterli R, Wölnerhanssen BK, Peters T, Vetter D, Kröll D, Borbély Y, et al. Effect of laparoscopic sleeve gastrectomy vs laparoscopic Roux-en-Y gastric bypass on weight loss in patients with morbid obesity. JAMA [Internet]. 2018;319(3):255. Available from: https://jamanetwork.com/journals/jama/fullarticle/2669728
26. Sugerman HJ, Starkey JV, Birkenhauer R. A randomized prospective trial of gastric bypass versus vertical banded gastroplasty for morbid obesity and their effects on sweets versus non-sweets eaters. Ann Surg. 1987 Jun;205(6):613–24.
27. Wittgrove AC, Clark GW, Tremblay LJ. Laparoscopic gastric bypass, Roux-en-Y: preliminary report of five cases. Obes Surg. 1994;4(4):353–7.
28. Higa KD, Ho T, Boone KB. Laparoscopic Roux-en-Y gastric bypass: technique and 3-year follow-up. J Laparoendosc Adv Surg Techs. 2001 Dec;11(6):377–82.
29. Nguyen NT, Goldman C, Rosenquist CJ, Arango A, Cole CJ, Lee SJ, et al. Laparoscopic versus open gastric bypass: a randomized study of outcomes, quality of life, and costs. Ann Surg. 2001 Sep;234(3):279–91.
30. Luján JA, Frutos MD, Hernández Q, Liron R, Cuenca JR, Valero G, et al. Laparoscopic versus open gastric bypass in the treatment of morbid obesity. Ann Surg. 2004;239(4):433–7.
31. Podnos YD. Complications after laparoscopic gastric bypass. Arch Surg. 2003;138(9):957.
32. Rabl C, Peeva S, Prado K, James AW, Rogers SJ, Posselt A, et al. Early and late abdominal bleeding after Roux-en-Y gastric bypass: sources and tailored therapeutic strategies. Obes Surg [Internet]. 2011;21(4):413–20. Available from: https://cbc.org.br/wp-content/uploads/2013/07/01042011-ObS.pdf
33. Gupta A, Shah MM, Kalaskar SN, Kroh M. Late postoperative bleeding after Roux-en-Y gastric bypass: management and review of literature. BMJ Case Rep [Internet]. 2018;11(1):e226271. Available from: https://pubmed.ncbi.nlm.nih.gov/30567217/

34. Heneghan HM, Meron-Eldar S, Yenumula P, Rogula T, Brethauer SA, Schauer PR. Incidence and management of bleeding complications after gastric bypass surgery in the morbidly obese. Surg Obes Rel Dis: Official J Am Soc Bariatric Surg [Internet]. 2012;8(6):729–35. Available from: https://pubmed.ncbi.nlm.nih.gov/21798818/
35. Pereira A, Santos RF, Costa-Pinho A, Silva A, Nogueiro J, Carneiro S, et al. Early postoperative bleeding after laparoscopic Roux-En-Y gastric bypass: a single center analysis. Obes Surg. 2022;32(6):1902–8.
36. García-García ML, Martín-Lorenzo JG, Torralba-Martínez JA, Lirón-Ruiz R, Miguel Perelló J, Flores Pastor B, et al. Emergency endoscopy for gastrointestinal bleeding after bariatric surgery. Therap Algor Cirugia Espanola [Internet]. 2015;93(2):97–104. Available from: https://pubmed.ncbi.nlm.nih.gov/25438773/
37. Valli PV, Gubler C. Review article including treatment algorithm: endoscopic treatment of luminal complications after bariatric surgery. Clin Obes. 2017;7(2):115–22.
38. Kassir R, Debs T, Blanc P, Gugenheim J, Ben Amor I, Boutet C, et al. Complications of bariatric surgery: presentation and emergency management. Int J Surg. 2016;27:77–81.
39. Bell BJ, Bour ES, Scott JD, Cobb WS, Carbonell AM. Management of complications after laparoscopic Roux-en-Y gastric bypass. Minerva Chirurgica [Internet]. 2009 64(3):265–276. Available from: https://pubmed.ncbi.nlm.nih.gov/19536052/
40. Acquafresca PA, Palermo M, Rogula T, Duza GE. SERRA E. Early surgical complications after gastric by-pass: a literature review. ABCD Arquivos Brasileiros de Cirurgia Digestiva (São Paulo) [Internet]. 2015;28(1):74–80. Available from: https://www.scielo.br/j/abcd/a/FCzqwMgvd5jSVwcxcr4XFwx/?lang=pt&format=pdf
41. Gupta V, Umapathy L, Gulati A, Singh G. "O" configuration of biliary-enteric drainage: a preventable surgical error. Indian J Surg. 2015;77(S1):156–8.
42. De Rosa E, De R, Caprio D, Rd B, De Caprio C, Moretto C, et al. Clinics in surgery a rare cause of severe protein-energy malnutrition following bariatric surgery. OPEN ACCESS Citation: A Rare Cause of Severe Protein-Energy. 2018, 3:2232. Available from: https://www.clinicsinsurgery.com/open-access/a--rare-cause-of-severe-protein-energy-malnutrition-following-bariatric-surgery-3654.pdf
43. Mitchell MT, Gasparaitis AE, Alverdy JC. Imaging findings in Roux-en-O and other misconstructions: rare but serious complications of Roux-en-Y gastric bypass surgery. Am J Roentgenol. 2008;190(2):367–73.
44. Bigolin AV, Iaroseski J, Rodrigues AP, De Lima JNC. Roux-en-O: how it happens and how to fix it. Obes Surg. 2021;32(1):223–4.
45. Harakeh A, Kallies KJ, Borgert AJ, Kothari SN. Bowel obstruction rates in antecolic/antegastric versus retrocolic/retrogastric Roux limb gastric bypass: a meta-analysis. Surg Obes Relat Dis. 2016;12(1):194–8.
46. Singla S, Guenthart BA, May L, Gaughan J, Meilahn JE. Intussusception after laparoscopic gastric bypass surgery: an underrecognized complication. Mini Invasive Surg. 2012;2012:1–8.
47. Koppman JS, Li C, Gandsas A. Small bowel obstruction after laparoscopic Roux-en-Y gastric bypass: a review of 9,527 patients. J Am Coll Surg [Internet]. 2008;206(3):571–84. Available from: https://pubmed.ncbi.nlm.nih.gov/18308230/
48. De Simone B, Chouillard E, Ramos AC, Donatelli G, Pintar T, Gupta R, et al. Operative management of acute abdomen after bariatric surgery in the emergency setting: the OBA guidelines. World J Emerg Surg. 2022;17(1):51.
49. Blackstone RP, Rivera LA. Predicting stricture in morbidly obese patients undergoing laparoscopic Roux-en-Y Gastric Bypass: a logistic regression analysis. J Gastrointest Surg. 2007;11(4):403–9.
50. Kumbhari V, le Roux CW, Cohen RV. Endoscopic evaluation and management of late complications after bariatric surgery: a narrative review. Obes Surg. 2021;31(10):4624–33.
51. Carrodeguas L, Szomstein S, Soto F, Whipple O, Simpfendorfer C, Gonzalvo JP, et al. Management of gastrogastric fistulas after divided Roux-en-Y gastric bypass surgery for morbid obesity: analysis of 1292 consecutive patients and review of literature. Surg Obes Relat Dis. 2005 Sep;1(5):467–74.
52. Dolan RD, Jirapinyo P, Maahs ED, Thompson CC. Endoscopic closure versus surgical revision in the management of gastro-gastric fistula following Roux-en-Y gastric bypass. Endosc Int Open [Internet]. 2023;11(6):E629–34. Available from: https://pubmed.ncbi.nlm.nih.gov/37397860/

17 Surgical Decision-Making in Hepatobiliary and Pancreatic Surgery

Beatriz Chumbinho, Pedro Custódio, Mafalda Sobral, and Hugo Pinto Marques

Introduction

During the past decades, liver and pancreatic surgery have witnessed countless and tremendous changes, leading to disruptive innovations and continuous improvements regarding safety, rapidity, precision, and overall efficiency of surgical procedures [1].

HPB surgery has long been recognized as one of the most challenging fields in general abdominal surgery because of its anatomical complexity, diversity of presentations, and historically high morbidity rates [2].

Nonetheless, it is also one of the most interesting, dynamic, and rapidly evolving surgical areas, especially since the widespread introduction of minimally invasive surgery in this field. Newly discovered systemic therapeutic regimens continuously stretch the limits of surgical resectability. The modern "bridging therapies," on which intervention radiology is of solemn importance, extend the possibility of cure for a greater number of patients. Transplant oncology is also seeing exponential growth.

Given the multiple surgical and concomitant systemic therapeutic options, it is impossible for the surgeon to be the only participant in decision-making – multidisciplinary team (MDT) meetings have long been standard of care, in many instances with the surgeon at the center of the decision-making process.

In this stimulating field, it is important to understand and aid surgeons in their decision-making. However, the literature on surgeons' decision-making is scarce – it concentrates on the preoperative stages of diagnosis and treatment planning, especially on investigative pathways and algorithms of care. Regarding intraoperative decision, information is even rarer, with some studies on intraoperative decisions which focus mainly on the technical aspects of surgical procedures or on the surgeon's physiology [3].

This review will focus on the various stages of surgical decision-making in HPB, as well as specific problems encountered in each stage.

Multidisciplinary Team Meeting

Role of Radiology

One of the fundamental elements for a successful multidisciplinary decision is the presence of experienced diagnostic and interventional radiologists.

No decision should be made without a thorough revision of the available imaging of every clinical case. Every MDT meeting must have experienced radiologists, both proficient in

B. Chumbinho · P. Custódio · M. Sobral · H. P. Marques (✉)
Hepato-Biliary-Pancreatic and Transplantation Centre, Curry Cabral Hospital/Local Health Unit of São José, and NOVA Medical School, Lisbon, Portugal
e-mail: pedrocustodio@campus.ul.pt

R. Latifi (ed.), *Surgical Decision-Making*, https://doi.org/10.1007/978-3-031-67391-7_17

diagnostic and interventional radiology. This allows to provide a fair number of options for patients who are not candidates for surgical resection, those who need reduction of their tumoral burden and those whose best treatment will solely depend on local-regional and systemic therapies.

Since the implementation of angiography, where notorious advances in diagnosis where possible, intervention radiology has seen significant growth. With hybrid systems, combining angiography and computer tomography, it is possible to overlay previously obtained images onto real-time fluoroscopic images. New software allows for a 3D reconstruction, obtaining a "navigation route" for the lesions to be treated. The development of locoregional ablation techniques, such as radiofrequency and microwave ablation, can now offer a therapeutic alternative in patients with oncologic disease. In patients with refractory portal hypertension, transjugular portosystemic shunt (TIPSS) is an important tool in treating bleeding from esophageal varices or bridging in liver transplantation. In patients with insufficient liver volume, portal or hepatic vein embolization, or both, can increase the volume of the functional remnant liver allowing for safe surgery.

With the above procedures described, many pathologies may fall into the scope of interventional radiology or surgery, depending on the multidisciplinary team meeting decision. Namely, patients with hepatocellular carcinoma (HCC), depending on size and location (among other factors), can be candidates for liver transplantation, surgical resection, microwave ablation, or chemoembolization, among many other options.

Role of Pathology

Accurate pathological classification and understanding of the molecular pathogenesis of liver tumors are essential for correct patient management and prognosis [4]. Molecular discoveries have illumined our understanding of the underlying basis of many types of tumors, including primary liver neoplasms [5].

Particularly in the case of hepatocellular carcinoma (HCC), in recent years a series of molecular changes have been discovered which, in connection to specific clinical and pathological features, have led to a proposed new subtype classification. This is of the utmost importance as oftentimes a subset of HCC patients present with advanced inoperable tumors that rely on systemic approaches. In cholangiocarcinoma, classification has evolved from being based purely on biliary tree location to several pathological subsets (mass performing/periductal infiltrating/intraductal; large/small duct; well/moderately/poorly differentiated). As in other tumors, genetic mutation screening has gained traction, with the identification of several poor prognosis mutations [6]. Liquid biopsies identify circulating tumor cells, cell-free nucleic acids, and secreted proteins. Unlike tissue biopsy, liquid biopsy is generally less intrusive, less costly, and safer. There is an increased interest in novel biomarkers from liquid biopsies to guide the diagnosis and treatment of many tumors, such as HCC and cholangiocarcinoma [4, 6].

Role of Oncology

Traditionally, there have been few effective options for the systemic treatment of primary liver, bile duct, and pancreatic malignancies. Recent advances on immunotherapy and tumor-directed therapies have allowed for better patient survival in the palliative setting, as well as the development of more effective adjuvant and possibly even neoadjuvant agents. Current agents used in advanced/metastatic hepatocellular carcinoma include immune checkpoint inhibitors, antiangiogenic agents, chimeric antigen receptor (CAR)-T cell therapy, and small molecule inhibitors (such as PD-1; PD-L1). The combination of immunotherapy and liver-directed therapy is a promising approach that integrates two distinct strategies to improve outcomes in HCC. Combining these approaches can potentially synergize their effects and improve overall treatment outcomes [7].

Also, in cholangiocarcinoma, improved understanding of the molecular pathogenesis has allowed for development of targeted therapies. Both in intrahepatic and perihilar cholangiocarcinoma, tumor-directed therapies have been increasingly used in the clinical trial setting [8] with promising results. Ongoing research also focuses on the role of gut microbiota imbalances in the pathogenesis of cholangiocarcinoma, which has led to several clinical trials studying the impact of probiotics in its treatment. Patients with colorectal liver metastases have an unquestionably unique disease biology among those with stage 4 cancers. The efforts to understand these exceptional responders have led to numerous novel scientific discoveries and to the evolution of clinical paradigms. Current areas of interested in these patients include ablative therapies, hepatic arterial infusion, transarterial therapies, and stereotactic body radiation therapy, either as an adjunctive to resection or as isolated therapy [9]. A dedicated team of medical oncologists is therefore essential to the multidisciplinary decision-making in hepato-pancreatic-biliary (HBP) surgery, both in the perioperative setting and in advanced disease stages.

Role of Gastroenterology

Gastroenterologists and hepatologists are pivotal for decision-making in multidisciplinary discussion of HPB patients. They provide insightful inputs on the clinical aspects of these patients and optimization of the medical treatment, as well as in assessing candidacy of a patient for surgery. A good knowledge of the intricacies of the overall clinical status of these patients plays a fundamental role in evaluating the best timing for a successful handling of surgical aggression. This is also true for the postoperative period, where gastroenterologists' contribution is also extremely valuable in optimizing postresection liver function and managing eventual complications.

An experienced gastroenterologist is also skilled in endoscopic procedures, which come in handy when considering which therapeutical option is best suited for a patient. Gastroenterology has evolved throughout the years. Since the first endoscopic retrograde cholangiopancreatography (ERCP), in 1968, until the present time, a shift was observed, now serving not only as a diagnostic tool but allowing the treatment of several conditions. From the simplest cases of choledocholithiasis to pancreatic head cancer, ERCP grants optimization of bile duct drainage, permitting borderline patients to complete neoadjuvant treatment before resection. All of the patients discussed on multidisciplinary meeting may benefit from a gastroenterologist's perspective [10].

Many other medical specialties, such as radiotherapy, nuclear medicine, anesthesiology, intensive care medicine, and others should be part of an MDT. Likewise, nonmedical healthcare professionals such as nurses, physiotherapists, pharmacists, and nutritionists, should also participate in MDT meetings. More than a multidisciplinary discussion, participating of a multidisciplinary *team* allows for better communication, assuring better ability to adapt to unforeseen clinical scenarios. Some studies have also proposed that working in a multidisciplinary setting raises the number of patients who are eligible for resection [11, 12] and therefore not considered palliative [13].

Stages of Surgical Decision in Hepato-Biliary-Pancreatic Surgery

Preoperative

Preoperative decision in hepato-biliary-pancreatic surgery (HBP) is a dynamic and multidisciplinary process that evolves several key factors. Correct and complete patient and pathology assessment is key and should be performed thoroughly through history, physical examination, and evaluation of analytic and imagological workup. There are however some key components that are specific to HBP surgery.

In liver surgery, for example, the assessment of lesion and consequent extent of resection must consider the future liver remnant (FLR), considering both volume and function. This double evaluation has become essential in surgical decision-making in modern hepatic surgery. Diagnostic and therapeutic interventional radiologic procedures play an essential role, through the increasing use of portal vein embolization and liver venous deprivation. Control volumetry imaging following these procedures allows for better preoperative planning.

In pancreatic surgery, namely, in tumors of the head and neck of the pancreas, an efficient biliary drainage should be guaranteed to reduce postoperative morbidity. This may imply an endoscopic retrograde cholangiopancreatography (ERCP) to ensure safer bilirubin levels.

In the HBP field, it is mandatory that oncological cases are performed by an experienced team, in referral, high-volume centers. If left untreated, one certainly should expect rapid disease progression, as well as severe impairment in functional status and quality of life, even in young patients. On the other hand, the surgical aggressiveness of resections in HBP surgery emphasizes the need for a holistic patient preoperative evaluation. Staging should be complete and functional status should be assessed. Preoperative evaluation from an anesthesiologist is important for patient selection and preoperative optimization allowing for better outcomes. Clearly, in some patients the best course of action may be not to operate. Social and community support is critical, especially if substance addiction plays a major role in patient pathophysiology.

Preoperative discussion is always performed in a MDT setting, with the participation of surgeons, medical oncologists, pathologists, diagnostic radiologists, interventional radiologists, anesthesiologists, intensive care specialists, gastroenterologists, endocrinologists, psychiatrists, psychologists, nurses, physical therapists, and other medical and nonmedical staff. In HBP surgery, there are some technical aspects that should be addressed by experienced surgeons: some patients may require anatomical resections or not; two-stage surgery may be needed; a reverse, "liver first" approach might be an option; there may be a need for biliary or vascular resection; and the approach, whether open, laparoscopic, or robotic should be decided.

Shared decision-making (SDM) has been gaining attention in recent years. SDM is characterized by active, bidirectional communication between healthcare professionals and patients, in order to make (treatment) decisions together [14]. In addition, SDM leads to improved patient outcomes, in particular less decisional conflict and potentially even reduced healthcare costs [14]. A recent study comparing patient and surgeons' perspective on SDM was performed in the setting of both benign and malignant liver pathology. This showed that SDM had room to improve in both situations, although it was lower in the benign tumor population.

HBP surgeons possess multiple tools at their disposal, which should be used not only to plan the surgical intervention adequately but also to minimize the number of intraoperative decisions, which are subject to several more biases.

Intraoperative

Despite the progress in diagnostic methods, there are still circumstances in which the surgical team is forced to decide on critical aspects of the procedure "on the go." This may occur either because of a change in patients' pathology or physiology or because of an intraoperative complication.

A key aspect of intraoperative decision is the understanding that HBP oncological pathology is rapidly progressing, which means that preoperative scans – albeit recent – are frequently outdated by the time of surgery. To help overcome this problem, liver surgeons are trained in intraoperative ultrasound (IOUS), to better evaluate the size and location of lesions, which is not unusual to lead to a total modification of the planned resection strategy. But much more information may be extracted from IOUS, as it allows the recognition of the patient's real anatomy and its variations, helps to establish resection planes, sets the boundaries for resection assuring a safe margin, and targets lesions for intraoperative locoregional therapy if needed. HBP surgeons must be flexible and adapt to these technical modifications, while still considering every aspect discussed in the preoperative setting.

An experienced anesthesiology team is of uttermost importance. Communication during surgery is fundamental for surgical success. Major or complex HBP surgeries can cause great hemodynamic instability, and dialog between surgeons and anesthesiologists is pivotal to reduce morbidity and mortality risk in order to maximize the chances of cure. One example of this setting is the patient's fluid balance as it can severely change the course of the procedure.

Intraoperative complications impose definite decisions under pressure, which can dramatically impact the surgeon. HBP surgery presents a broad spectrum of potential complications due to the complexity of the resections, presence of anatomical variations, and technical challenges which are frequently caused by advanced tumors. These complications range from major life-threatening bleeding, which must be dealt with immediately, to less urgent although no less severe, irreversible ductal injuries which may hinder future surgical reconstruction.

The importance of a well-trained and well-prepared team cannot be stressed enough. Fellows should be taught to perform surgical techniques in the same manner, increasing reproducibility throughout the entire team. The epitome of intraoperative decision-making process is perhaps liver transplant surgery, where all the previously mentioned aspects are part of the regular practice. Even the most technically competent surgeon can be lost without a cooperating team, reinforcing the need for high-volume centers in the HBP pathology treatment.

Postoperative

The immediate postoperative period is frequently the most critical for patients, their relatives, and even the surgeon. Advanced HBP surgery requires a dedicated intensive care unit and team, equipped with state-of-the-art monitoring and organ support. These complex procedures can severely impact hemodynamic and metabolic stability, which must be rapidly and efficiently reversed in order to decrease patient morbidity and mortality and improve overall outcomes. In recent years, procedure-specific postoperative protocols have been shown to improve patient outcomes [15] and are in place in most high-volume centers, to aid the surgical team and decrease variability in postoperative decision-making.

During the postoperative period, the surgical team must closely monitor patients' status in order to rapidly act if there are changes in the normal postoperative course. In case of clinical deterioration, surgeons must decide on which pathway to take, aided by adequate complementary diagnostic exams. Often the most difficult decisions for the HBP surgeon are not when a life-threatening complication occurs, and decision-making is particularly hard in patients who are still stable but gradually worsen. One must bear in mind the avoidance of futility without compromising patient treatment.

In the event of a surgical complication, a multidisciplinary step-up approach is usually used, i.e., endovascular embolization in the case of major bleeding, percutaneous or endoscopic drainage for intra-abdominal collections after liver and pancreatic surgery, stent placement for bile leaks, etc. In modern HBP surgery, re-intervention is often the last resort in the management of surgical complications. In pancreatic surgery, in particular, difficult decisions must be made regarding patient's gradual deterioration, with refractory intra-abdominal collections and peritonitis in the setting of clinically relevant pancreatic fistula. In this case re-intervention can be the last resort although not guaranteed to immediately improve patients' status. Immediate postoperative surgeons must overcome their wishful thinking and critically evaluate patient's status to reduce failure-to-rescue in these procedures.

Surgical treatment, however, is not finished when the patient is discharged home after a successful surgery. Outpatient follow-up is increasingly more important given the shortening admission times in minimally invasive surgery. Close monitoring and patient education are warranted to rapidly detect complications and act accordingly.

In oncological patients, subsequent management is decided in MDT meeting setting as it might be necessary to undergo systemic therapy. This decision is not always straightforward and can be hindered by patient status following HBP surgery. On the other hand, the long-term survival in non-oncological patients also holds its own challenges. For example, bile duct reconstructive procedures can cause bile congestion, with anastomotic stenosis and secondary biliary cirrhosis. In these patients a long time follow-up should be implemented.

Practical Examples of Multidisciplinary Decision-Making in HBP Surgery

Case 1

A 42-year-old female, with no relevant medical history, was referred to our center due to obstructive jaundice with a total bilirubin of 9 mg/dL and a Ca 19.9 of 25 u/mL. A CT scan was performed (as shown in Fig. 17.1) and suggested a Klatskin tumor type IIIb.

A percutaneous cholangiogram was performed, and an external biliary stent was placed to optimize biliary drainage (Fig. 17.2). Biopsies of the bile duct were compatible with cholangiocarcinoma.

The case was discussed in our MDT meeting, and a robotic left hepatectomy extended to segments I and V was planned. Here, we present the most important steps of the surgical procedure:

1. Lymphadenectomy of stations 7, 8a, 8p, 12, and 13a was performed.
2. Identification of right hepatic artery coming from the superior mesenteric artery (Fig. 17.3).
3. Identification and ligation of the left branch of the portal vein (Fig. 17.4).
4. Parenchyma is divided after indocyanine green injection, ensuring good vascularization.

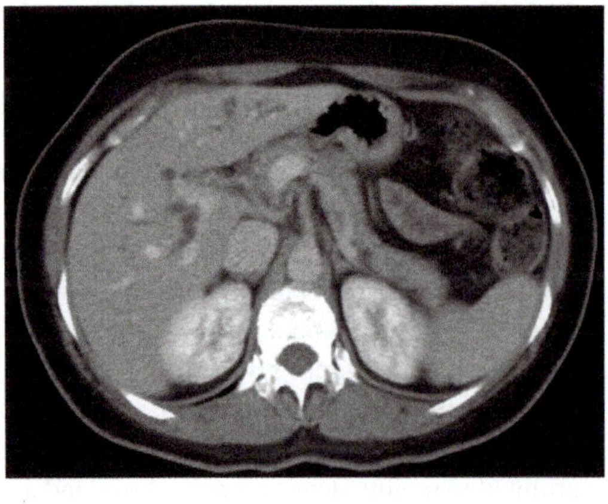

Fig. 17.1 CT scan showing Klatskin tumor type IIIb

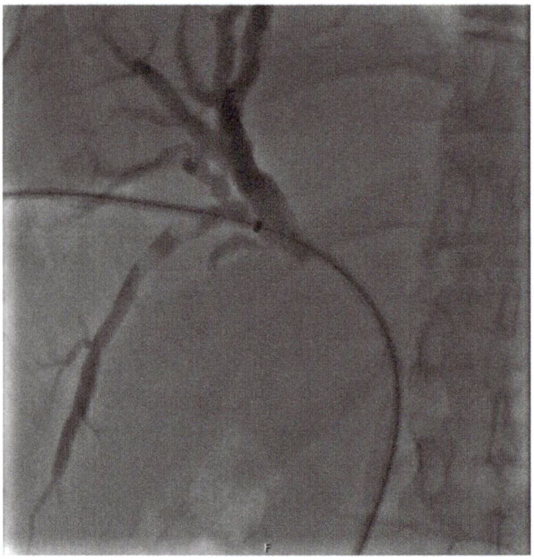

Fig. 17.2 Placement of an external biliary drainage using percutaneous cholangiography

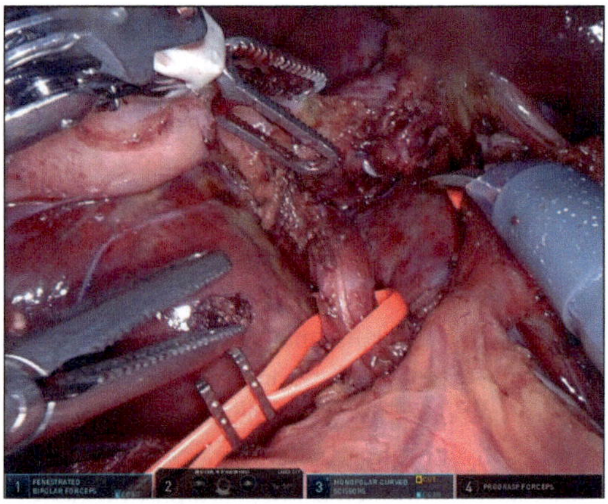

Fig. 17.3 Identification of median hepatic artery

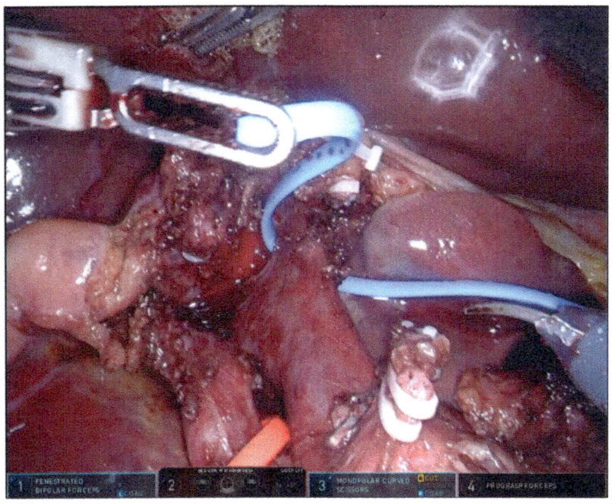

Fig. 17.4 Identification of the left branch of the portal vein

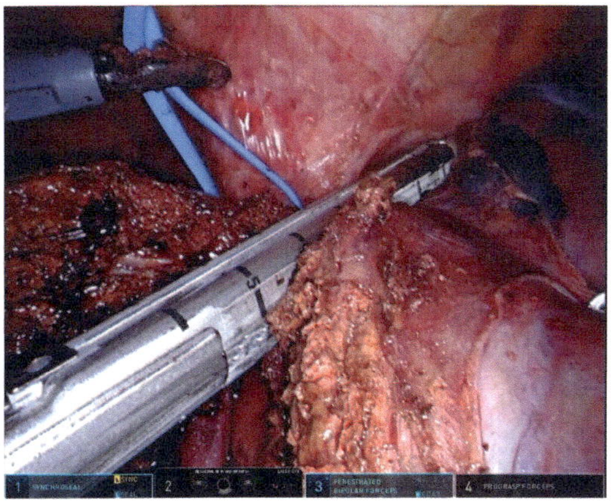

Fig. 17.5 Ligation of the left hepatic vein and remaining right liver parenchyma

5. Identification of proximal right biliary duct that is sent to frozen section analysis.
6. Identification and ligation of left hepatic vein (Fig. 17.5) and removal of the specimen (left extended hemihepatectomy and bile duct).
7. Hepaticojejunostomy for the right bile ducts using 5/0 PDS.

Case 2

Male, 73 years old, presented with six synchronous right liver metastases (biggest lesion was 69 mm) in the context of ascending colon cancer,

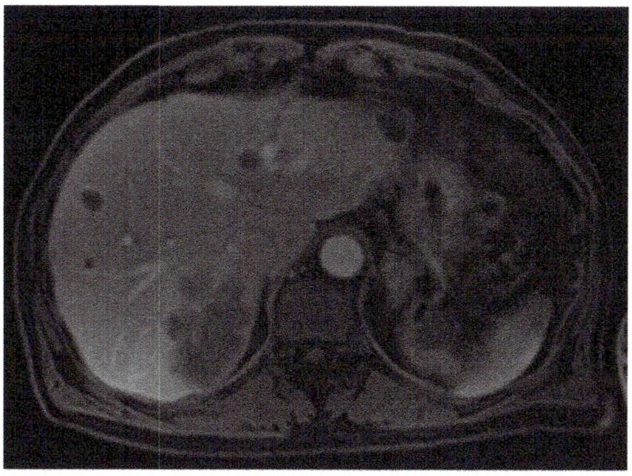

Fig. 17.6 Synchronous CLRM in right hemi liver. The left hemiliver presents several cysts

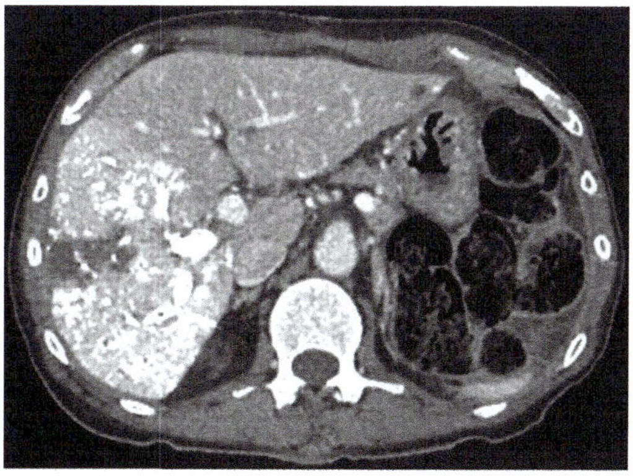

Fig. 17.7 Liver imaging post-right portal vein embolization

previously submitted to right colectomy (Fig. 17.6). Due to high tumor burden on the right liver, it was decided on our MDT meeting that the patient should be submitted to a right hepatectomy although due to insufficient liver volume, a right portal vein embolization had to be done before liver resection. The volumetry imaging after embolization revealed a future liver remnant (FLR) of 47% (Figs. 17.7 and 17.8), and a right hemihepatectomy was performed.

Case 3

A male, 83 years old, with a personal history of rheumatoid arthritis, presented with obstructive jaundice. Imaging showed a bile duct stone and a

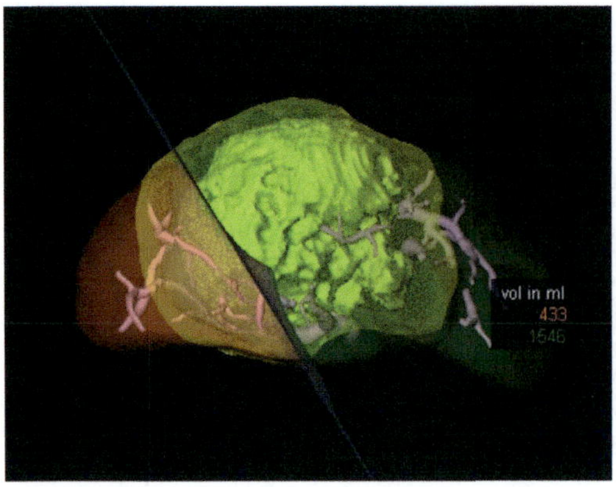

Fig. 17.8 Liver imaging post-right portal vein embolization

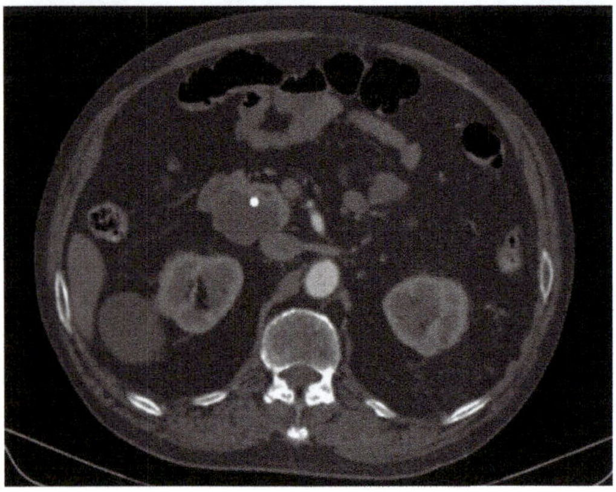

Fig. 17.9 Cystic lesion in pancreatic head

cystic lesion of the pancreatic head (45 mm) (Fig. 17.9). After ERCP with clearance of the bile duct and stent placement, it was decided that the patient should be monitored in outpatient appointments. During this follow-up period, a fine-needle aspiration (FNA) biopsy was performed. The biopsy revealed a mucinous neoplasm. In the following 2 months, the patient presented again with obstructive jaundice which was attributed to the presence of the mucinous lesion. He was again discussed in our MDT meeting, and it was decided to perform a Whipple procedure.

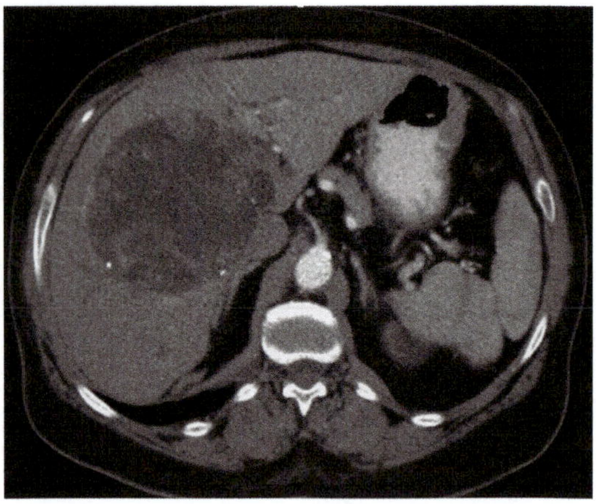

Fig. 17.10 Central cystic mass with enhancing solid components

Case 4

A female, 74 years old, with a personal history of hypertension presented with iron deficiency anemia. A CT scan was performed which showed a central liver mass encompassing segments IV, V, and VIII, with approximately 11x9 cm, with cystic areas and solid components (Fig. 17.10), highly suggestive of biliary cystic tumor.

In our MDT discussion, it was decided that the patient should be submitted to a right trisectionectomy with previous right portal vein embolization due to insufficient liver volume. A left biliary drainage was also performed as the patient developed obstructive jaundice.

Intraoperatively, we became aware of probable insufficient liver volume and invasion of the left portal vein. We were forced to alter our initial strategy and performed an associating liver partition and portal vein ligation for staged hepatectomy (ALPPS) procedure, with reconstruction of the left portal vein to the main trunk (Figs. 17.8 and 17.9).

The postoperative period was uneventful and volumetry imaging at 1-week post-op revealed a FLR of 32%. The patient was then submitted to completion of the ALPPS procedure with a right trisectionectomy 2 weeks following the first surgery (Figs.17.11, 17.12, 17.13 and 17.14).

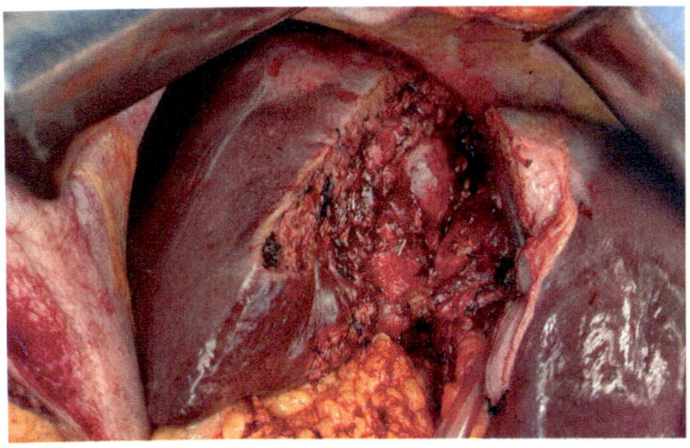

Fig. 17.11 Liver hepatotomy during the first procedure

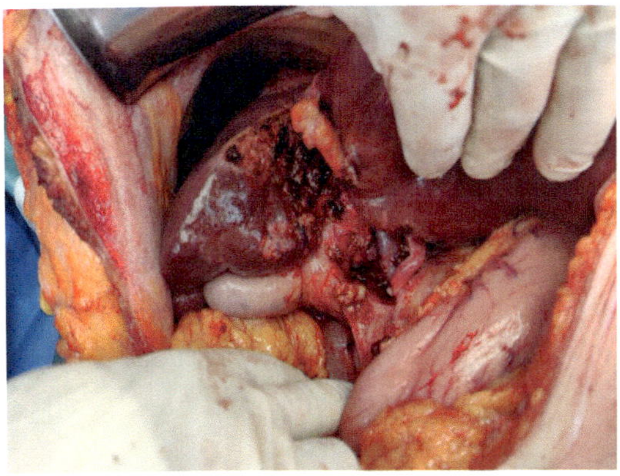

Fig. 17.12 ALPPS stage 1 with reconstruction of the left portal vein

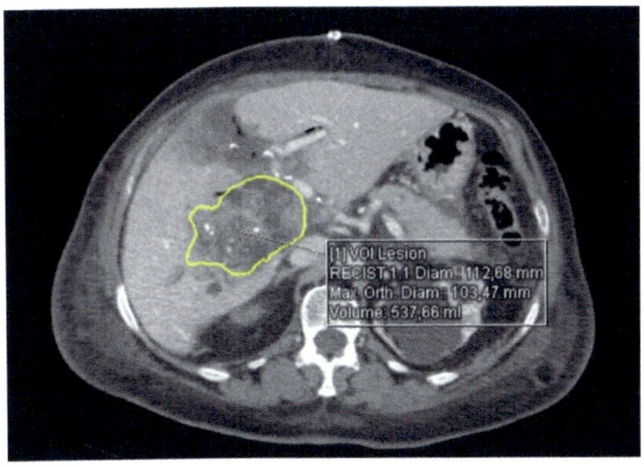

Fig. 17.13 Liver volumetry at 1 week post-op

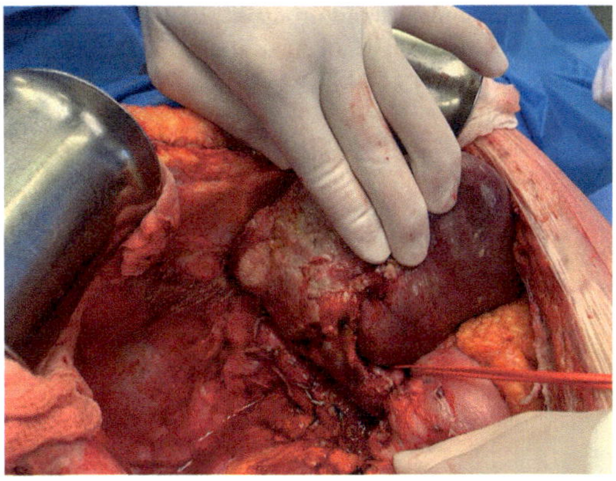

Fig. 17.14 Completion of right trisectionectomy (ALPPS stage 2)

References

1. Pioneers in laparoscopic hepato-biliary-pancreatic surgery. Miyasaka, Yoshihiro. 2018, J Hepato-Biliary-Pancreatic Sci, pp. 109–114.
2. Delpero, Jacques Belghiti e Jean Robert. Blumgart's Surgery of the Liver, Biliary Tract and Pancreas. s.l. : Elsevier, 2023. 0323697844.
3. Flin, Rhona. How do surgeons make intraoperative decisions? 2007, Jun.
4. Advances in histological and molecular classification of hepatocellular carcinoma. Choi, Joon Hyuk. s.l. : Biomedicines. 2023;11(9):2582.
5. How molecular discoveries have changed liver tumor pathology: a brief review. Taheri, Negar. s.l. : Arch Pathol Lab Med. 2023.
6. Cholangiocarcinoma: recent advances in molecular pathobiology and therapeutic approaches. Khosla, Divya. s.l. : Cancers. 2024;16(4):801.
7. Advances in Immunotherapy for Hepatocellular Carcinoma (HCC). Bicer, Fuat. s.l. : Cur Oncol. 2023;30 (11):9789-9812.
8. Advances in the management of cholangiocarcinoma. Zori, Andreas G. s.l. : World J Hepatol. 2021;13(9):1003–1018.
9. Updated management of colorectal cancer liver metastases: scientific advances driving modern therapeutic innovations. Patel, Ranish. 6, s.l. : Cell Mol Gastroenterol Hepatol. 2023;16:881–894.
10. Setup of multidisciplinary team discussions for patients with cholangiocarcinoma: current practice

and recommendations from the European Network for the Study of Cholangiocarcinoma (ENS-CCA). Casadio, M. 1, s.l. : ESMO Open, 2022;7.
11. The impact of a hepatobiliary multidisciplinary team assessment in patients with colorectal cancer liver metastases: a population-based study. Engstrand, Jennie. 9, s.l. : Oncologist. 2017;22:1067–1074.
12. Effect of specialist decision-making on treatment strategies for colorectal liver metastases. Jones, R P. 9, s.l. : Br J Surg. 2012; 99:1263–1269.
13. A 10-year study of outcome following hepatic resection for colorectal liver metastases – the effect of evaluation in a multidisciplinary team setting. Lordan, J.T. 3, s.l. : Eur J Surg Oncol. 2009;35:302–306.
14. Current level of shared decision-making in hepatobiliary surgical oncology (SAPACHA). Haaft, Britte H.E.A. ten. s.l. : HBP, 2024;26.
15. Enhanced recovery following liver surgery: a systematic review and meta-analysis. Hughes MJ, McNally S, Wigmore SJ. s.l. : HPB (Oxford), 2014;16:699–706.

Decision-Making in Hepatobiliary and Pancreatic Surgery: Acute Care Surgeon's Perspective

18

Thav Thambi-Pillai, J. M. Guido, Stephanie Y. Hung, and Hassan Turaihi

Introduction

Being a competent acute care surgeon is a challenging job as one needs to be a master of many areas. There is nothing more daunting than being confident in managing hepatobiliary pathology especially trauma related to this part of the body.

For ease of discussion, we have detailed the chapter under the following four topics:

1. Management of acute pancreatitis
2. Approach to difficult gallbladder
3. Surgical techniques for managing pancreatic trauma
4. Management of liver trauma

Acute Pancreatitis

Acute pancreatitis (AP) is one of the most common gastrointestinal conditions encountered in the United States, resulting in ER visits of 13.5 per 10,000 persons with an annual estimated admission incidence of 13–40 per 100,000 persons [1]. Admission rates for acute pancreatitis have steadily risen over the last 2 decades [2]. While mortality overall from acute pancreatitis is low at 1%, complicated pancreatitis can result in mortality more than 20% of the time [1]. Morbidity and associated cost can be significant, with estimates of as high as 2.69 billion dollars per year being spent on management of AP.

AP occurs after the pancreas sustains an acute injury to the acinar cells, causing pancreatic inflammation. This injury triggers activation of digestive enzymes, the kinin system, and complement cascade resulting in pancreatic parenchyma autodigestion. Pancreatic duct obstruction, commonly seen with gallstone pancreatitis, is the most common cause of acinar damage with alcohol remaining the second leading cause of AP [2, 3]. The severity of AP is thought to be correlated with degree of apoptosis from cellular necrosis. The early phase of AP occurs during the first week of disease resulting in a systemic inflammatory response (SIRS). The late phase persists beyond 1 week, lasting for 4 weeks to months, and is frequently marked by persistent organ dysfunction and complications [3].

Diagnosis

Acute pancreatitis is commonly characterized by both the revised Atlanta criteria (RAC). The RAC require 2 or more of the following to diagnose acute pancreatitis: epigastric abdominal pain; serum lipase and/or amylase greater than three times the upper limit of normal; evidence of acute

T. Thambi-Pillai (✉) · J. M. Guido · S. Y. Hung
H. Turaihi
Department of Surgery, University of South Dakota Sanford School of Medicine, Sioux Falls, SD, USA
e-mail: Thavam.Thambi-Pillai@SanfordHealth.org; Jenny.Guido@SanfordHealth.org; Hassan.Turaihi@SanfordHealth.org

R. Latifi (ed.), *Surgical Decision-Making*, https://doi.org/10.1007/978-3-031-67391-7_18

pancreatitis on imaging (ultrasound, contrast-enhanced computed tomography, or magnetic resonance imaging) [1, 3].

The RAC grades AP severity by presentation and duration of organ failure in presence of local symptoms. Mild AP is present in patients without organ failure or local complications. Moderately severe AP occurs in patients with transient organ failure (less than 48-hour duration) and/or local complications. Severe AP occurs in patients with organ failure persisting beyond 48 hours with or without local complications [2]. About 80% of patients will develop mild to moderately severe disease with anticipated discharge within 1 week of hospitalization, 20% will develop severe disease with protracted clinical course that can extend over weeks to months [2].

The RAC then uses morphologic types to characterize acute pancreatitis either into interstitial edematous AP or necrotizing pancreatitis (NP). Interstitial edematous pancreatitis (IEP) is characterized by edema and inflammation of the pancreatic parenchyma and peripancreatic tissues. IEP occurs 85% of the time with acute pancreatitis with a mortality rate of 3% [1]. NP occurs when this process progresses to peripancreatic or pancreatic tissue death. Necrotizing AP constitutes approximately 15% of AP cases that accounts for a mortality of 17%. Mortality then rises to 30% if pancreatic necrosis becomes infected [1]. Both forms of pancreatitis can be associated with the development local complications of fluid collections [2].

Peripancreatic collections are further classified by timing of onset to predict associated morbidity. IEP-associated fluid collections are present for less than 4 weeks and are characterized by a homogenous collection found adjacent to normal fascial planes without associated necrosis. These tend to be un-encapsulated collections. After 4 weeks, fluid collections are then named pseudocysts and appear as an encapsulated, usually homogenous, fluid collections without solid components. Encapsulated fluid collections in NP may be sterile or exhibit gas formation on imaging to suggest underlying infectious process. These fluid collections are then termed walled off necrosis (WON) [3].

Several different classification systems can assist in determining appropriate initial level of care and guide ongoing clinical management based on predicted severity of disease. Given the variability and clinical course of AP, prognostic indicators for AP are set by several systems including the Ranson criteria, Acute Physiology and Chronic Health Evaluation II (APACHE II) classification system, and more recently the bedside index for severity and acute pancreatitis (BISAP) score. Initial assessment should include assessment of the following risk factors that can predict severe course: age greater than 60 years, BMI greater than 30, chronic alcohol use, preexistent comorbidities, presence of SIRS, laboratory markers consistent with hypovolemia, and presence of chest X-ray infiltrates or effusions [2].

Initial Management of Acute Pancreatitis

For patients admitted with AP, treatment focuses primarily on the acute symptoms. Consideration for ICU admission should occur in patients with severe pancreatitis and signs of inflammatory response or organ failure [3]. Pain control, fluid resuscitation, and optimal nutrition remain the initial tenets of management. Goal-directed fluid resuscitation should address improvement in urine output and vital signs to maximize improvement in end-organ perfusion. More recent literature supports fluid resuscitation with lactated Ringer's solution compared to normal saline to reduce risk of developing SIRS at 24 hours. Caution should be undertaken to avoid fluid overload, particularly in patients with pre-existing heart failure or renal disease [1, 2].

Prophylactic antibiotic use has not demonstrated a mortality benefit or reduction in the development of pancreatic infection in NP in randomized controlled studies [1]. Broad-spectrum antibiotics with pancreatic penetration that cover both aerobic and anaerobic Gram-negative and Gram-positive microorganisms should only be prescribed if infected necrosis is confirmed or strongly suspected [4].

Optimization of nutritional support is critical for patients with AP, given hypermetabolism, metabolic derangements, negative nitrogen balance, and inflammatory response found in this condition. Historically, initiation of enteral nutrition was delayed in order to provide pancreatic rest [1]. Current evaluation of existing literature supports early use of enteral nutrition.

Patients receiving early enteral nutrition exhibit decreases in multiple organ failure, systemic infection, and even mortality. Importantly, it is not necessary to wait until the patient's pain is resolved prior to resuming enteral feeding in AP. The most recent guidelines of the American Gastroenterological Association recommend initiating enteral feeding within 24–72 hours of admission. Patients who tolerate oral nutrition should have a low fat or solid diet. If the patient is unable to tolerate enteral nutrition within 72 hours of admission, nasal enteral feeding via nasogastric or nasojejunal access should be initiated. If patients cannot tolerate enteral feeding due to obstruction, paralytic ileus, or other causes, parenteral nutrition should be started within 72 hours. Patients with evidence of steatorrhea or malabsorption should be evaluated for exocrine pancreatic insufficiency and if present semielemental formulas should be considered for nutritional support [1, 2, 5–7].

Surgical Treatment of Acute Pancreatitis

Patients with severe AP often receive aggressive fluid resuscitation and may develop intra-abdominal hypertension requiring decompression. Intra-abdominal hypertension (IAH) can occur early in severe AP secondary to pancreatic inflammatory processes coupled with aggressive fluid resuscitation. The incidence of IAH can be as high as 60-80%. IAH may be rapidly transformed into abdominal compartment syndrome (ACS) secondary to increasing intra-abdominal inflammation, capillary leakage, and visceral edema causing progressive ascites. ACS is diagnosed when intra-abdominal pressures are greater than 20 mmHg and new onset organ dysfunction occurs. Medical therapy is used first line to manage IAH via nasogastric decompression, percutaneous drainage of ascitic fluid, and neuromuscular blockade if indicated. If patients fail to respond to these nonoperative measures and clinically deteriorate, they will require surgical decompression. Management of surgical decompression is performed most commonly via midline laparotomy, consideration of a subcostal approach can be undertaken [3].

Gallstone pancreatitis

Biliary pancreatitis is a frequent consult for the acute care surgeon. Early cholecystectomy after gallstone pancreatitis is completed to prevent complications of recurrent pancreatitis (8%) and readmission (20%) associated with delayed cholecystectomy [1]. Biliary pancreatitis can recur up to 33% of patients when cholecystectomy is not performed [8].

The gallstone PANC randomized controlled trial evaluated patients with mild gallstone pancreatitis undergoing cholecystectomy within 24hrs of admission(early) vs those undergoing cholecystectomy after clinical resolution of symptoms (control group). Significant reduction in length of stay (LOS) and health system costs without increase in major complication or worsening in quality of life were reported. There was a noted increase in minor complications and more readmissions that occurred in the early cholecystectomy group compared to the control group [9]. The Poncho (Same Admission versus Interval Cholecystectomy for Mild Gallstone Pancreatitis) multicenter randomized control trial demonstrated that cholecystectomy during index admission, versus delayed cholecystectomy, reduced the rate of recurrent gallstone-related complications in patients with mild gallstone pancreatitis [8]. Further, current AGA guidelines recommend cholecystectomy during index admission, particularly in patients with mild AP [1].

Current literature overall seems to support early cholecystectomy with intraoperative cholangiogram during the same admission for mild gallstone pancreatitis but question remains regarding timing for cholecystectomy in patients with moderately severe acute biliary pancreatitis. The few small retrospective studies in the literature demonstrate conflicting data. A more recent study using data from the MANCTRA-1 (Compliance With Evidence-Based Clinical Guidelines in the Management of Acute Biliary Pancreatitis) data set examined whether early cholecystectomy (within 14 days of hospital admission) versus delayed cholecystectomy (after 14 days of hospital admission) led to changes in mortality or postoperative complications in patient with moderate or severe biliary pancreatitis. Biliary pancreatitis was classified using the RAC. Patients with moderately severe biliary pancreatitis experienced increased postoperative morbidity and mortality after early cholecystectomy across all groups. ASA score, age, severe complications of biliary pancreatitis requiring surgical intervention, and absence of bile duct clearance by ERCP were all risk factors identified to be associated with morbidity and mortality in these patients. While the risk of gallstone-related events progressively increase if cholecystectomy is not performed for biliary pancreatitis, timing of surgical intervention must be balanced with the understanding that patients undergoing early cholecystectomy experience increase in postoperative complications and even mortality [8]. For patients with severe AP or those with peripancreatic collections, consideration for delaying early cholecystectomy should occur [4]. Consideration should also be given to evaluation with contrast-enhanced CT or MRI for peripancreatic fluid collections prior to cholecystectomy in this population [4]. Further studies are needed to determine optimal timing in this patient subgroup of AP.

Some patients cannot tolerate cholecystectomy during same admission for AP. Patients with clinical findings suspicious for ongoing biliary obstruction including symptoms of ascending cholangitis, choledocholithiasis, and total bilirubin greater than 4 mg/dL should be considered for ERCP. ERCP should additionally be considered in patients who are poor surgical candidates, in those that require biliary decompression to prevent recurrent AP [3]. If cholecystectomy cannot be completed during admission, patients ideally should still undergo delayed cholecystectomy within 2–4 weeks after discharge if deemed medically fit to minimize risk of recurrent gallstone pancreatitis.

Gallstone pancreatitis is commonly self-limiting, but in the setting of NP with associated peripancreatic fluid collections, timing of cholecystectomy is challenging. Historically, cholecystectomy was postponed until resolution of fluid collections; for 6 weeks after development of pancreatic fluid collections; and/or general improvement of local and systemic inflammation. The Dutch pancreatitis group evaluated optimal timing of cholecystectomy for necrotizing biliary pancreatitis and demonstrated that the risk of recurrent AP and biliary events increased when cholecystectomy is delayed more than 8 weeks after discharge. It is notable that timing of cholecystectomy did not increase operative complications and this study, but early cholecystectomy was associated with an increase in conversion to an open technique [10].

Management of Peripancreatic Fluid Collections

Peripancreatic fluid collections in interstitial edematous AP are classified by timing of development. Prior to 4–6 weeks after episode of AP, these collections tend to remain asymptomatic and resolve within 1–2 weeks. Generally, less than 20% of the time these collections will persist for more than 4 weeks to form an encapsulated pseudocyst [1]. Between 5 and 15% of patients with AP will develop a pseudocyst. Asymptomatic collections, less than 50 mm in diameter, can be monitored serially with ultrasound or contrast-enhanced CT imaging [4]. As up to 70% of pseudocysts resolve without intervention, intervention should be considered for patients developing symptoms associated with their pseudocyst, infection of the pseudocyst, or pseudocyst enlarging to greater than 6 cm [3]. Patients may present with symptoms secondary to mass effect including nausea and vomiting, early satiety, and abdominal pain.

The treatment of choice for noninfected pancreatic pseudocysts is drainage via either transpapillary or transmural endoscopic approach. If the pseudocyst is in direct approximation with the gastric or duodenal wall, transmural drainage is completed. Transpapillary drainage is first-line treatment if the pseudocyst comes into direct contact with the pancreatic duct. Pseudocyst gastrostomy can be performed for pseudocysts directly adjacent to the posterior wall of the stomach. Pseudocysts that are smaller than 4 cm in size and are located in the head or uncinate process of the pancreas can be approached by pseudocyst duodenostomy [3].

Percutaneous drainage of pseudocyst is typically not recommended given the high risk of associated complications including need for repeat intervention, increased length of stay, increased risk of pancreatic fistula, and morbidity and mortality. This treatment modality should be considered in patients with infected pseudocysts without pancreatic obstruction or large pseudocysts that are poor candidates for other interventions [1].

Pancreatic walled off necrosis (WON) occurs relatively late, usually 3–5 weeks after onset of AP. Asymptomatic WON does not mandate intervention and can resolve spontaneously; however, symptomatic WON generally requires intervention. Secondary infection and pancreatic necrosis result in increased morbidity and mortality for patients, thus necrotic tissue should be removed to prevent septic complications. Most commonly, WON is treated with percutaneous drainage or endoscopic drainage, reserving surgical drainage for failure of one of the two previous modalities [4].

In general, invasive intervention on NP fluid collection should be postponed until at least 4 weeks after initial presentation, even if percutaneous drains are placed, sooner collection should be allowed to wall off and mature prior to any further necrosectomy. The POINTER trial evaluated patients that underwent immediate drainage and antibiotic use versus immediate antibiotic use and delayed drainage of infected pancreatic necrosis. This trial did not demonstrate any difference in complications between the two groups, but demonstrated that 39% of patients in the delayed intervention group were successfully treated with antibiotics alone and required less necrosectomy procedures (51% in the early group versus 22% in the delayed group) [3, 11].

Necrotizing Pancreatitis and Treatment Modalities

Pancreatic and peripancreatic necrosis are serious complications of AP with secondary infection of necrotic tissue remaining a leading cause of mortality in patients with NP. Contrast-enhanced CT is the preferred imaging modality for diagnosis of NP as it can identify the presence of gas in the necrotic collection. Magnetic resonance imaging may be used, but is less sensitive than CT. Diagnosis of infected necrosis is based on imaging findings in conjunction with clinical criteria including rising serum inflammatory markers and fever [12]. Historically, open surgical necrosectomy was the treatment of choice for managing infected pancreatic necrosis. Minimally invasive procedures, such as the step-up approach, hybrid techniques, and endoscopic approaches to debridement have become increasingly popular recently.

Patients that develop walled off pancreatic necrosis (WOPN) after AP can be considered for endoscopic necrosectomy. During endoscopic necrosectomy, the endoscope advanced to the level of the duodenum or stomach at the point where necrotic tissue can be visualized adjacent to the viscera. Transgastric or transduodenal access is made, allowing for guidewire to be inserted and coiled into the necrotic cavity. Serial dilation occurs to dilate the wall of the stomach or duodenum to at least 15 mm, and the stent is inserted across the length of the opening to the point of the necrotic cavity [3]. The endoscopist may choose to use a plastic double-pigtail stent, a self-expandable metal stent (SEMS) or a lumen-apposing metal stents (LAMS). The metal stents are larger in diameter and provide access for potential subsequent debridement. LAMS are designed to be delivered via a single step delivery platform resulting in shorter intervention time.

Retrospective studies, as well as more recent randomized clinical trial, have mixed results regarding efficacy and complications between the 2 metal stent types, and more research is needed to determine optimum stent type [12].

The Panter trial from the Dutch pancreatitis group introduced a minimally invasive step-up approach to the management of necrotizing pancreatitis. The step-up approach has 3 components. Initially, delaying timing for intervention allows for encapsulation of the pancreatic collection and WOPN to optimize conditions for intervention. Next, use of a percutaneous or endoscopic transgastric catheter is used to drain the collection. After patients show clinical improvement, debridement is required either via endoscopic or surgical necrosectomy. Patients should be reevaluated approximately 72 hours in between steps, allowing for the least invasive treatment approach possible with progressively invasive procedures added to treat infected pancreatic necrosis [13, 14]. The step-up approach to pancreatic debridement decreased the incidence of new multi-system organ failure from 40 to 12% compared with laparotomy. The PENGUIN trial demonstrated a reduced rate of pancreatic fistulas, no occurrence of new onset multi-system organ failure, and reduced inflammatory markers in patients in the endoscopic arm as opposed to the surgical necrosectomy group. The TENSION trial did not demonstrate significant difference in mortality or major morbidity in patients undergoing an endoscopic versus surgical step-up approach. However, fewer pancreatic fistulas, shorter length of stay, and decreased overall mean cost were noted in the endoscopic step-up approach. The MISER trial compared an endoscopic step-up approach to minimally invasive surgery. There were no differences in mortality rates among groups, but patients in the endoscopic approach were again less likely to develop either enterocutaneous or pancreaticocutaneous fistulas, had a lower rate of complications, lower rate of SIRS, lower cost, and less disease-related adverse effects than those in the surgical group [12].

Ultimately both endoscopic and surgical step-up approaches to pancreatic debridement are very effective. The endoscopic approach may be superior in reducing major complications including pancreaticocutaneous fistulas, cost, length of stay, and increased quality of life with infected pancreatic necrosis. However, the surgical step-up approach may be superior to the endoscopic approach in reduction of mortality and major complications. While consensus varies, it seems reasonable that endoscopic approach should be considered first in patients with infected pancreatic necrosis [4].

Minimally invasive methods for debridement of infected NP are increasingly utilized. Techniques include minimal access retroperitoneal pancreatic necrosectomy (MARPN) and video-assisted retroperitoneal debridement (VARD). The MARPN procedure begins with placement of the 12 French catheter via CT guidance by interventional radiology. This access tract is serially dilated up to 30 French during the minimally invasive procedure so a rigid nephroscope can be advanced, serving as a visualization instrument and working channel for necrosectomy. An irrigation drainage system for continuous lavage is placed at the end of the procedure and lavage continues at the bedside. MARPN can be performed multiple times until clinical improvement is noted. The VARD is a hybrid of the manual and laparoscopic necrosectomy. A left flank subcostal incision is made allowing for direct manual debridement followed by laparoscopic inspection and debridement with laparoscopic instruments of the tissue cavity. Continuous lavage access is obtained to allow for ongoing debridement [12].

Failure in minimally invasive treatment modalities may lead to need for pancreatic open necrosectomy. Pancreatic necrosectomy is performed through an open midline laparotomy or subcostal laparotomy, and access is gained to the area of pancreatic necrosis after dissection of the gastrocolic ligament. Manual dissection and debridement are completed, followed by lavage. Open surgical necrosectomy can be performed with open packing with reevaluation of the cavity serially approximately every 48 hours until the abdomen can be closed after inserting drains. Alternatively, closed packing is performed when multiple drains are placed in the residual cavity after necrosectomy, the abdomen is closed, and continuous lavage is performed via dual-lumen saline slumps and silicone rubber tubes to allow inflow and outflow of the lavage irrigant. Planned repeat laparotomy provides continuous removal of necrotic tissue over the upcoming days [12]. Open necrosectomy can be complicated by difficulty in access to infected collections, need for large laparotomy incision, hernia complications, and possibility of enterocutaneous fistula formation [3]. Open surgical necrosectomy for acute pancreatitis historically was associated with elevated mortality rates as high as 50% or greater. More recent studies demonstrate improvement in mortality between 11 and 23% with complication rates remaining high between 64 and 73%. Minimally invasive procedures remain better tolerated than open necrosectomy procedures, resulted in decreased postoperative multi-system organ failure and improvement in treatment success rates [12]. Consideration of laparotomy and open necrosectomy should be delayed for as long as possible or avoided to decrease morbidity and mortality rates [4]. Practice patterns remain variable but approaches starting with conservative measures followed by endoscopic drainage or percutaneous drainage, then minimally invasive procedures produce superior outcomes to traditional open necrosectomy for patients with infected pancreatic necrosis [4]. Despite significant increases in morbidity and even mortality with open necrosectomy, surgeons still need to remain comfortable with this techniques for patients who fail treatment with more minimally invasive modalities.

We believe that the care needs to be individualized to each patient based on the clinical situation and local expertise available based on above guidelines. In our experience, surgical necrosectomy requires less reoperations compared to endoscopic or percutaneous approach but needs to be weighed against patient's operative risk and complication rate.

Hemorrhagic Complications

Acute upper gastrointestinal bleeding can be common in AP and frequently results from stress ulcers, peptic ulcer disease, or hemorrhagic gastroduodenitis. Rarely, massive hemorrhage occurs into the gastrointestinal tract or abdominal cavity. Erosion of the splenic artery, pancreaticoduodenal, and gastroduodenal arteries can lead to rupture or pseudoaneurysm formation. The splenic artery is most commonly affected. Pseudoaneurysm should be suspected if patients have repeated episodes of gastrointestinal bleeding, bloating, or increasing abdominal pain (associated with a pulsatile mass). If patients develop severe and life-threatening bleeding, arteriography with embolization of the bleeding vessel can be effective, otherwise emergent exploratory laparotomy is required [4].

Difficult Gallbladder

Cholecystectomy is one of the most common surgical procedures performed in the United States with about 300,000 cholecystectomies performed annually [15]. Despite the commonality of this procedure, it can easily become one of the most frustrating procedures performed even for the most seasoned surgeon. Management of the difficult gallbladder is a controversial topic, and there are multiple ways and opinions as to how best deal with this situation. The goal of this section is to provide insight into recognizing characteristics of a difficult gallbladder and safely dealing with technically difficult cholecystectomies and any postoperative complications that may arise.

Preoperative Considerations-The 3P's: Patient, Physician, and Pathophysiology

Making the decision on whether or not to proceed with cholecystectomy can be a difficult one. Factors that play into a difficult cholecystectomy can be categorized into the 3P's: the patient, the physician, and the pathology.

Patient characteristics that contribute to a more difficult gallbladder include previous abdominal surgeries, cirrhosis, advanced age greater than 65, and pregnancy [16, 17]. Physician experience also plays a role in whether or not a cholecystectomy will be difficult. Undoubtedly, what is considered a difficult gallbladder will vary significant from a newly minted attending compared to a surgeon ready for retirement. Despite the amount of experience one has, in the setting of a difficult gallbladder, a surgeon should seek help or guidance if there are any concerns about how to proceed.

The pathophysiology of the disease will be the most critical in defining the difficulty of the surgery. The degree of inflammation encounter is the foremost contributor to the difficulty of the surgery. Indicators of the severity of inflammation can be seen in lab work and on imaging. The Tokyo Guidelines characterize moderate acute cholecystitis as inflammation for more than 72 hours, leukocytosis greater than 18k, and signs of significant local inflammation such as gangrene or emphysema [18]. Severe acute cholecystitis is cholecystitis with end-organ dysfunction secondary to sepsis. Chronic cholecystitis, especially with greater than 10 episodes of biliary colic and signs of a retracted gallbladder on ultrasound are also red flags. Furthermore, previous attempts at cholecystectomy as well as previous percutaneous drainage tubes make subsequent dissection more difficult.

By recognizing these warning signs of a difficult gallbladder, a surgeon can best prepare themselves and the patient for possible outcomes. It is imperative that while obtaining informed consent, the patient is prepared to expect a possible bailout procedure and the subsequent complications that may arise from them.

The Pregnant Patient

Nonoperative management of symptomatic gallbladder disease has a high risk of recurrence, with the highest risk if diagnosed in the first trimester. If the disease remains uncomplicated, rates of preterm labor and abortion are similar for operative and medical management. However, up to 50% of patients with recurrent symptoms require hospitalization and about 23% of these patients went on to develop acute cholecystitis, cholangitis, or gallstone pancreatitis. Preterm labor and fetal loss resulted in 20% and 10–60% of cases, respectively, depending on severity of disease [19]. No significant increased risk of premature labor and maternal or fetal complications have been observed in pregnant women undergoing lap cholecystectomy versus the general obstetric population. Given the low risk of surgery to the mother and fetus, all pregnant women regardless of trimester should be considered for lap cholecystectomy for biliary disease. Women past their first trimester should be placed in the left lateral decubitus position to improve cardiac output and venous return. Subcostal entry via Hasson or Veress needle is recommended, and insufflation should be kept between 10 and 15 mmHg. It is highly recommended that obstetric services be available in the facility where the procedure is being performed.

Cholecystectomy in Cirrhotic Patients

Patients with cirrhosis pose a unique set of challenges due to portal hypertension, coagulopathy, ascites, and hepatic insufficiency. As a first step, it is important to evaluate the MELD (Model for End-stage Liver Disease) score and Child-Pugh (CPT) classification. Generally, MELD score predicted postoperative morbidity better than CPT classification. The published literature shows that cholecystectomy is safe in patients with MELD <13 or Child A or B classification. Laparoscopic cholecystectomy can be safely performed in a tertiary care center with expertise in caring for patients with end-stage liver disease. Further details are beyond the scope of this chapter.

Choledocholithiasis

When considering taking the patient to the operating room for cholecystectomy, not only do surgeons need to consider the severity and timing of intervention but also other confounders such as common bile duct stones, that would limit the ability for care at one's home institution. This is especially true for community surgeons who do not have ready access to MRCP or ERCP especially on the weekends or have the equipment or comfort level to explore the common bile duct. This oftentimes will sway the decision if the patient stays or gets transferred.

Four risks factors have been identified by the AGSE for choledocholithiasis. These being dilated common bile duct, total bilirubin >1.7, presence of common bile duct stone on ultrasound, and acute cholangitis. MRCP/EUS or IOC are recommended if there is 1 risk factor present. There is greater than 50% chance if 2 or more of these risk factors are present and the duct should be evaluated preoperative with ERCP or intraoperative intervention. Without any of these risk factors, there is less than 10% chance of choledocholithiasis [20].

If a stone is found intraoperatively, clearance of the duct can be attempted by first trying to flush the stone or administering 1 gram of glucagon. Depending on the surgeon's experience, a laparoscopic transcystic vs transcholedochal common bile duct exploration can be performed. If a duct exploration is not possible, postoperative ERCP is a reasonable option however it is recommended that the cystic stump be generously controlled with an additional endoloop or extra clips. Leaving a drain by the cystic duct stump in order to control for a possible bile leak secondary to stump blowout is also recommended.

Timing of Cholecystectomy

In the idea world, all patients would present for cholecystectomy within 72 hours of onset of disease. Intervention within the first 72 hours is aided by having a plane in between the liver and gallbladder secondary to edema. Furthermore, early intervention has been shown to decrease length of stay, costs, bile leak rates, and conversion rates to open if intervened on within 24 hours of admission [21]. However, oftentimes this is not the case and surgeons must consider the risks versus benefits of surgical intervention. After 72 hours, it is not uncommon to find that the plane has fibrosed, making the dissection even more difficult, especially in the setting of an intrahepatic gallbladder. Historically, most surgeons have opted to wait 6 weeks post onset of disease to try and reduce the amount of inflammation as much as possible to make dissection easier. Caution must be taken in this scenario as there can be a failure rate of up to 20% with medical management of cholecystitis [22]. Of note, studies have shown that there is no difference in conversion rate, morbidity, or mortality if a cholecystectomy is pursued with the 72-hour window, in between, or beyond the 6-week waiting period.

In the case of patients that are too sick to tolerate surgical intervention bridging with a cholecystostomy tube is a reasonable therapy until the patient is well enough for surgical intervention. Prior to cholecystectomy, cholangiogram can be performed to see if the cystic duct is patent as a measure of residual inflammation and also gives the surgeon a chance to delineate out the anatomy further. If a patient chooses to not undergo surgery, the cholecystostomy tube can be removed however they must be cautioned that recurrent cholecystitis can occur again especially if they have gallstones. It is preferable that the cholecystostomy tube remains in place until surgery can be performed.

In especially frail patients who will probably never be surgically be optimized, cholecystostomy tubes can be left in place with occasional exchanges and capped. Should they develop another bout of cholecystitis, the drain can be placed to gravity.

Intraoperative Conduct

No matter what technology or technique is applied in performing a cholecystectomy, the tenants of a safe cholecystectomy must be followed. The hepatocystic triangle must be adequately cleared, and the cystic plate should be exposed by

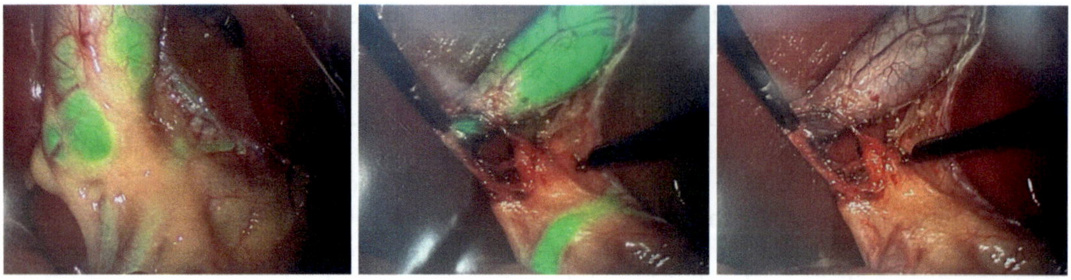

Fig. 18.1 The first photo shows ICG view clearly highlighting the gallbladder, cystic duct, and the common bile duct. Second photo shows the critical view of safety (CVS) on ICG mode, and third photo same CVS on normal laparoscopic view

dissecting out the lower third of the gallbladder. Two and only two structures should be seen entering the gallbladder. The critical view of safety (CVS) must be obtained prior to transection of structures [23]. If there are any doubts about the anatomy, a cholangiogram or use of indocyanine green (ICG) fluoroscopy can be performed to help delineate out biliary anatomy. We use 0.625 mg IV in the preoperative area. Rouviere's sulcus which is the cleft of the liver running anterior to segment 1 of the liver can be a helpful landmark intraoperatively. This line of demarcation separates the cystic duct and artery superiorly and common bile duct inferiorly. In the case of severe inflammation or fibrosis in which the critical view cannot be found, the surgeon must be prepared to utilize bail out procedures in order to avoid dreaded bile duct injuries. Options for bail out include subtotal reconstituting cholecystectomy, fenestrated cholecystectomy, or surgical drainage of the gallbladder (Fig. 18.1).

With a subtotal fenestrated approach, the anterior wall of the gallbladder is resected, and gallstones are removed. The cystic duct may or may not be ligated during the procedure. With this approach, there is a higher chance of bile leak and a drain should be left close to the gallbladder remnant. If a persistent bile leak is still observed 3–5 days after surgery, the drain should be placed to gravity until resolution of the leak which should self-resolve in several weeks or the patient can be referred for ERCP. Typically, a drain output of 200 mls or less per day will resolve within 2 weeks.

In a reconstituting cholecystectomy approach, the gallbladder remnant is sutured closed after removal gallstones. The rates of bile leakage are less with this technique; however, there is a greater risk of recurrent gallbladder disease.

It is imperative that if bleeding is encountered during dissection that endoclips are not fired haphazardly. Placing pressure using a Kitner or using small strips of surgicel can be used to slow or stop the bleeding. Beware of Moynihan's hump which is a tortuous right hepatic artery that approaches very close to the gallbladder and cystic duct. It occurs in 3–16% of cases and is more likely to be seen in cirrhotic patients. In these patients, the cystic artery can be very short and sometimes there will not be a true main cystic artery coming off but many small offshoots. The right hepatic artery can be mistaken for the cystic artery and ligated by mistake, or even worse torn. Ductal injuries are oftentimes preceded by vascular injuries and if significant bleeding is encountered, the surgeon should consider converting to a "dome down" technique versus open cholecystectomy.

Common Bile Duct Injury

Despite best efforts, common bile duct injuries still do occur. A majority of the time this is due to surgeon disorientation and misinterpretation of aberrant anatomy as "normal." Only 3% of the time are injuries due to departing from orthodox operative strategy or sloppy dissection. Generous use of cholangiography can help reorient the surgeon. Of note, cholangiography will not prevent a bile duct injury but will help to recognize an injury sooner. If a bile duct transection is discovered intraoperatively, the surgeon should remember these three words: stop, drop, and roll. Stoppage of the surgery is needed as this has now become a highly emotional situation. Dropping the instruments and also allow the heart rate to slow down will allow you to make a more rational decision. Finally, roll the care of the patient to another surgeon, ideally a hepatobiliary surgeon at a tertiary care center. Studies have shown that attempts by the index surgeon to repair the injury resulted in an extremely low success rate and significantly increased length of stay compared to repairs performed by a hepatobiliary surgeon at a tertiary care center.

In closing, recognizing a difficult gallbladder preoperatively and planning subsequent intraoperative conduct with possible bailout techniques are important. Being able to recognize when and where to stop prior to biliary injury is key. And above all, do not be afraid to ask for help.

Pancreatic Trauma

Pancreatic trauma is a rare but complex and challenging medical condition encountered by the acute care surgeon. The pancreas is located deep within the retroperitoneum overlying the aorta in the upper abdomen and is divided into three-thirds in relation to the superior mesenteric vessels, it is surrounded by vitals structures oriented horizontally in the upper abdomen. It has a rich and extensive blood supply which makes hemorrhage from this area difficult to control with simple suture ligation. Estimates for the incidence of pancreatic injury range from 0.2% to 12% of abdominal traumas; blunt trauma accounts for the mechanism most frequently encountered and to a lesser extent in penetrating trauma due to the fatal nature of these penetrating injuries. Early recognition and management of such injuries are paramount to avoid the dreaded implications of missed injury.

Pancreatic injury is rarely an isolated injury; it can result from various mechanisms. Due to the sometimes subtle presentation of pancreatic injury, the trauma surgeon should have a high index of suspicion-based mechanism. Incidents, such as blunt trauma due to a forceful impact on the upper abdomen, are commonly seen in car accidents, falls, or physical assaults and from penetrating trauma such as stab or gunshot wounds which can directly damage the pancreas.

Mortality of pancreatic injury is in the range of 10–12%, morbidities can be up to 60%. The key predictor of outcome is the integrity of the pancreatic duct.

Early death is usually from the associated injuries. It is estimated that 40% of cases are associated with vascular, liver, or stomach injuries. Mortality is proportional to the number of injured organs. When pancreatic injury is left untreated, the mortality can be as high as 50–90%. Survivors likely will have chronic pain, pancreatitis, and pseudocysts.

Clinical signs and symptoms are non-specific and may include abdominal pain, nausea, vomiting, and epigastric tenderness. The biochemical marker may aid in establishing the diagnosis if used alone; serum amylase is neither sufficiently sensitive nor specific for the diagnosis of pancreatic injury in a report by Takashima et al., 83% of patients with pancreatic injury showed elevated serum amylase levels at least 3 h after the initial trauma; however, the levels did not correlate with injury severity. Serum amylase is not specific to pancreas injury and will also be elevated in hemorrhagic shock, and other internal organ injuries such as the liver, bowel, and ovaries. In suspected traumatic pancreatic injury, serial serum amylase measurements are recommended. A normal level has a high negative predictive value.

Imaging studies such as CT scans or MRIs help assess the extent and nature of the injury. Thin slices CT scan is considered the gold standard to diagnose pancreatic injury with sensitivity and specificity in the range of 80–90%. Signs of injury include intrapancreatic split, complete transection, or an enhanced pancreas with an unenhanced hematoma.

Pancreatic injury on occasion can be difficult to detect on a CT scan obtained in the trauma bay and may take time to develop. The trauma surgeon should consider repeating the CT scan if there is a high index of suspicion for pancreatic injury particularly when the patient develops unexplained or worsening abdominal pain or upward trending serum amylase.

ERCP and MRI don't play a significant role in the acute trauma setting. However, stable trauma patients may add more information regarding the integrity of the pancreatic duct.

Intraoperatively, if pancreatic injury is suspected, the pancreas should be evaluated by opening the lesser sac and visually assessing the gland, liberal kocherization of the duodenum can facilitate exposure of the pancreatic head. The tail of the pancreas can be assessed by mobilizing the spleen from the lateral attachments and lifting the pancreas from the retroperitoneal attachments. Hematoma involving the pancreas needs exploration to ensure adequate visualization of the gland. Complete transection of the gland or laceration greater than 50% carries a high risk of pancreatic duct disruption [24].

The patient's hemodynamic stability and any further potentially fatal injuries should be taken into consideration by the trauma surgeon. Damage control by widely draining the lesser sac is a bailout maneuver with an acceptable outcome.

Another tool in the armamentarium of the trauma surgeon is intraoperative cholangiography. This tool can be useful for assessing pancreatic ductal disruption. The technique involves surgical removal of the gallbladder and accessing the cystic duct. inject contrast under fluoroscopic visualization. If the pancreatic duct is not visualized, 2mg of IV morphine can induce spasm of the sphincter and facilitate a pancreatogram.

The American Association for the Surgery of Trauma (AAST) published a grading system classification system for pancreatic injury:

- Grade I: Hematoma with minor contusion or superficial laceration without duct injury
- Grade II: Major contusion or laceration without duct injury
- Grade III: Distal transection or deep parenchymal injury with duct injury
- Grade IV: Proximal transection or deep parenchymal injury involving the ampulla (and/or intrapancreatic common bile duct)
- Grade V: Massive disruption of the pancreatic head ("shattered pancreas")

Grades I and II do not involve the duct and are considered low-grade injuries. Grades III, IV, and V involve the duct and constitute high-grade injuries. With this system, typically, higher-grade injuries correlate with higher mortality and complications.

Fortunately, the majority of traumatic pancreatic injuries are mild contusions that will resolve with conservative measures and supportive care. On the other hand, severe lacerations or complete organ destruction (high-grade III–IV) blunt pancreatic injuries or involvement of the main pancreatic duct will require immediate surgical intervention to repair the damage, remove dead tissue, or, in extreme cases, partial or complete removal of the pancreas.

Surgical Options

Surgical treatment for pancreatic injuries demands a tailored approach, considering the specific injury, the patient's condition, and the aim to restore both the organ's function and the patient's overall health. Advancements in surgical techniques and postoperative care continue to improve outcomes, making surgical intervention more effective and safer for individuals facing pancreatic trauma.

1. Observation and Nonoperative Management:
    - Contusions or minor injuries (grade I/II pancreatic injuries): Mild injuries often don't require surgical intervention. Close monitoring in a hospital setting with supportive care, pain management, and ensuring proper healing might suffice.
    - If there is concern for pancreatic duct disruption, studies like ERCP or MRCP could considered as it may change the grade of

the injury and therefore the recommended treatment plan. The use of octreotide is controversial. Somatostatin analogues have been used by many surgeons in an attempt to reduce post-pancreatectomy fistula. In elective pancreatic resection, pasireotide, a longer-acting somatostatin analogue, has been shown to reduce postoperative pancreatic fistula [25]. This analogue has not been studied in the trauma patient population. Guidelines from the Eastern Association for the Surgery of Trauma recommend against the routine use of octreotide for postoperative prophylaxis related to traumatic pancreatic injuries to prevent fistula.

2. Distal Pancreatectomy
   - Severe Injuries: If the injury affects the tail or body of the pancreas extensively, distal pancreatectomy of the damaged portion might be necessary. Splenic preservation in trauma situations can be technically challenging and is more time-consuming than a distal pancreatectomy for this reason most adult and pediatric surgeons favor distal pancreatectomy and splenectomy and closure of the proximal stump to minimize bleeding and operative time. There are different techniques for closing the pancreatic stump, none is proven to be superior in minimizing post-pancreatectomy fistula. Stapler closure and handsewn closure of the pancreatic stump are the standard methods described in the literature, other studies have shown a lower incidence of post-pancreatectomy fistula when the main pancreatic duct is identified and clipped [26].
   - Post-splenectomy vaccination in the trauma patient population is recommended during the patient's hospital admission. The lifetime risk of overwhelming post-splenectomy infection is approximately 5% for patients who receive splenectomy for hematologic disorders and significantly lower for trauma patients (Fig. 18.2) [27].

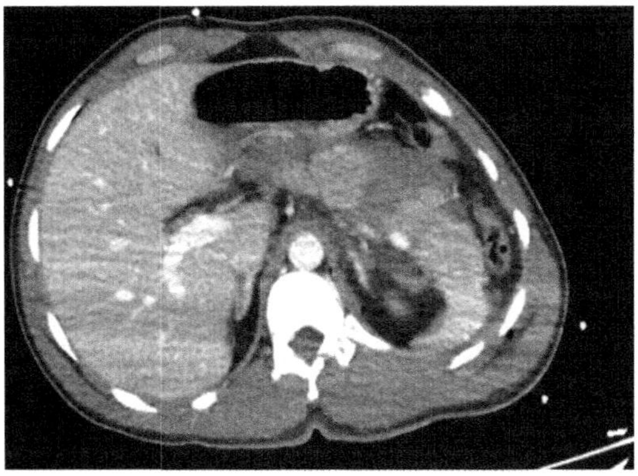

Fig. 18.2 CT scan of the abdomen with IV contrast demonstrating hematoma and disruption of the pancreatic body. The patient was managed with distal pancreatectomy with splenic preservation

3. Pancreaticoduodenectomy (Whipple Procedure):
   - Complex injuries: Severe trauma to the head of the pancreas or duodenum is the most challenging situation faced by the trauma surgeon and may necessitate a Whipple procedure. In hemodynamically unstable patients, staging the resection and reconstruction can be done to minimize operative time and anesthesia exposure. Whipple procedure should be carried out within 24–48 hours following the patient's presentation to reduce the risk of traumatic pancreatitis which will complicate the surgical resection. In unstable patients, the surgeon may opt for hemorrhage control, wide external drainage to manage fluid collections or leaks, and utilize postoperatively MRCP to evaluate the status of the pancreatic duct, followed by ERCP and stenting if a main pancreatic duct injury is identified. Sharpe et Al published their data on managing 87 patients with proximal pancreatic injuries by closed suction drainage, in this group there were seven fistulas (8.1%) and five abscesses (5.7%), and no pancreatic-related mortality suggesting the majority of these complex injuries can be managed by widely draining the lesser sac. The downside to such an

approach is the risk of developing chronic grade b pancreatic fistula which will result in a long hospital course and the need for multiple interventions [28].

Post-Surgical Care

Pancreatic trauma can lead to complications, such as infections, pancreatic insufficiency, bleeding, pancreatic fistulas, and in severe cases death. By far pancreatic fistula is the most common complication encountered, fortunately majority will resolve spontaneously.

Postoperative hemorrhage is a serious complication of pancreatic trauma. Although the mechanism remains unknown, it is thought to be associated with pancreatic fistulas and intraperitoneal abscesses.

Aggressive management of pancreatic fistula, early detection of infection, and ensuring adequate nutrition are vital for successful outcomes. Dietary adjustments or enzyme replacements might be necessary.

Management of this complex patient population usually requires a dedicated multidisciplinary team. The prognosis of such injuries varies depending on the extent of the injury, the promptness of treatment, and the patient's overall health.

Surgical treatment for pancreatic injuries demands a tailored approach, considering the specific injury, the patient's condition, and the aim to restore both the organ's function and the patient's overall health. Advancements in surgical techniques and postoperative care continue to improve outcomes, making surgical intervention more effective and safer for individuals with pancreatic trauma.

Liver Trauma

Liver is the most commonly injured abdominal organ following a blunt trauma. Liver is a highly vascular organ with dual blood supply with difficult to access venous drainage. Fortunately, majority of the liver injuries are minor and heal with nonoperative management. About 1 in 7 hepatic injuries require operative intervention [29].

Liver injury should be suspected when there is blunt or penetrative trauma to the right upper quadrant or right chest especially lower chest. In a stable patient, CT scan with IV contrast is the best way to evaluate the extent of livery injury.

Hepatic Injury Grading

The American Association for the Surgery of Trauma (AAST) is the most commonly used classification system, and it grades based on the extent of hematoma and depth of laceration/parenchymal disruption.

The imaging criteria of the AAST grades of hepatic injury are as follows:

Grade I: Subcapsular hematoma <10 percent surface area. Parenchymal laceration <1 cm in depth.

Grade II: Subcapsular hematoma 10–50 percent surface area; intraparenchymal hematoma <10 cm in diameter. Laceration: 1–3 cm parenchymal depth and ≤10 cm in length.

Grade III: Subcapsular hematoma >50 percent of surface area; ruptured subcapsular or parenchymal hematoma. Intraparenchymal hematoma >10 cm. Laceration >3 cm in depth. Any injury in the presence of a liver vascular injury or active bleeding contained within liver parenchyma.

Grade IV: Parenchymal disruption involving 25–75% of a hepatic lobe. Active bleeding extending beyond the liver parenchyma into the peritoneum.

Grade V: Parenchymal disruption of >75 percent of a hepatic lobe. Juxta hepatic venous injury to include retro hepatic vena cava and central major hepatic veins.

Management Options

The management approach to liver injuries depends on:

1. Hemodynamic status of the trauma patient
2. Presence of other injuries
3. Overall patient condition and comorbidities
4. Grade of liver injury

Typically, grades 1–3 hepatic injuries can be managed nonoperatively. An area of active bleeding within the liver in a stable patient, it can be managed with angioembolization with low morbidity and mortality. If the patient develops fever, abdominal pain or jaundice, development of (infected) biloma, or abscess should be suspected. Abscess may be managed with percutaneous drainage and antibiotics. Bile leak is best managed by ERCP with sphincterotomy and biliary stenting when indicated.

Patients with blunt trauma who are hemodynamically unstable with positive FAST should be taken to OR. Same is true with penetrative trauma patients where extrahepatic injuries are suspected. Surgical management of liver injury is challenging even in experienced hands. It is imperative that operative surgeon is familiar with both extra- and intra-hepatic liver anatomy.

The goal of the operation is to control bleeding which can be achieved through following means based on the extent of the injury:

1. Perihepatic packing is the first step in liver hemostasis and provides opportunity for resuscitation to be caught up.
2. Exposure is key which can be achieved with appropriate generous incision and a good retraction system (Thompson or Bookwalter).
3. Taking down the ligaments (falciform, triangular, and coronary ligaments) help with decreasing tension and traction injury and improves exposure.
4. Simple bleeding can be controlled by monopolar electrocautery in high setting (coagulation >80) on spray mode. If available, more advanced energy sources such as argon beam coagulator or bipolar radiofrequency energy source (Aquamantys bipolar sealer).
5. There are multiple topical hemostatic agents available in the market. For severe bleeding, authors prefer absorbable fibrin sealant patch (Evarrest).
6. Separated liver edges can be brought together using #1 chromic catgut suture on a blunt-tip needle in horizontal mattress fashion.
7. If bleeding continues, consider Pringle maneuver with direct liver suturing and omental packing possibly selective vessel ligation.
8. If liver debridement/resection is needed, it is better to wait until take back/second look surgery.
9. Juxta hepatic venous injuries are difficult to manage and good to get early involvement of a transplant/HPB surgeon. Packing followed by endovascular stenting, atriocaval shunts, venovenous bypass, and total vascular exclusion are potential methods but due to the nature of the injury, the mortality remains very high. Hepatic avulsion is a nonsurvivable injury.

Conclusion

Being an acute care surgeon at a busy hospital is truly a humbling experience despite years of experience. There is no substitute to a well-oiled system and team work. Having standardized guidelines and protocols and following them would help decrease variability and hence, improve quality. Regular multidisciplinary trauma and surgical morbidity and mortality conferences with frank and professional discussions with colleagues would help improve the knowledge of the team and subsequently, the patient outcomes.

References

1. Palumbo R, Schuster KM. Contemporary management of acute pancreatitis: What you need to know. J Trauma Acute Care Surg. 2024;96(1):156–65. https://doi.org/10.1097/TA.0000000000004143.
2. Mederos MA, Reber HA, Girgis MD. Acute pancreatitis: a review. JAMA. 2021;325(4):382–90. https://doi.org/10.1001/jama.2020.20317.
3. Ashraf H, Colombo JP, Marcucci V, Rhoton J, Olowoyo O. A clinical overview of acute and chronic pancreatitis: the medical and surgical management. Cureus. 2021;13(11):e19764. https://doi.org/10.7759/cureus.19764.

4. Zerem E, Kurtcehajic A, Kunosić S, Zerem Malkočević D, Zerem O. Current trends in acute pancreatitis: diagnostic and therapeutic challenges. World J Gastroenterol. 2023;29(18):2747–63. https://doi.org/10.3748/wjg.v29.i18.2747.
5. Petrov MS, Kukosh MV, Emelyanov NV. A randomized controlled trial of enteral versus parenteral feeding in patients with predicted severe acute pancreatitis shows a significant reduction in mortality and in infected pancreatic complications with total enteral nutrition. Dig Surg. 2006;23:336–44. discussion 44-5. 28.
6. Wu XM, Ji KQ, Wang HY, Li GF, Zang B, Chen WM. Total enteral nutrition in prevention of pancreatic necrotic infection in severe acute pancreatitis. Pancreas. 2010;39:248–51.
7. Poropat G, Giljaca V, Hauser G, Stimac D. Enteral nutrition formulations for acute pancreatitis. Cochrane Database Syst Rev. 2015;3:CD010605.
8. Di Martino M, Ielpo B, Pata F, Pellino G, Di Saverio S, Catena F, De Simone B, Coccolini F, Sartelli M, Damaskos D, Mole D, Murzi V, Leppaniemi A, Pisanu A, Podda M, MANCTRA-1 Collaborative Group. Timing of cholecystectomy after moderate and severe acute biliary pancreatitis. JAMA Surg. 2023;158(10):e233660. https://doi.org/10.1001/jamasurg.2023.3660.
9. Isbell KD, Wei S, Dodwad SM, Avritscher EB, Mueck KM, Bernardi K, Hatton GE, Liang MK, Ko TC, Kao LS. Impact of early cholecystectomy on the cost of treating mild gallstone pancreatitis: gallstone PANC trial. J Am Coll Surg. 2021;233(4):517–525.e1. https://doi.org/10.1016/j.jamcollsurg.2021.06.023.
10. Hallensleben ND, Timmerhuis HC, Hollemans RA, Pocornie S, van Grinsven J, van Brunschot S, et al. Optimal timing of cholecystectomy after necrotising biliary pancreatitis. Gut. 2022;71:974–82.
11. Boxhoorn L, van Dijk SM, van Grinsven J, Verdonk RC, Boermeester MA, Bollen TL, et al. Immediate versus postponed intervention for infected necrotizing pancreatitis. N Engl J Med. 2021;385:1372–81.
12. Purschke B, Bolm L, Meyer MN, Sato H. Interventional strategies in infected necrotizing pancreatitis: indications, timing, and outcomes. World J Gastroenterol. 2022;28(27):3383–97. https://doi.org/10.3748/wjg.v28.i27.3383.
13. Besselink MG, van Santvoort HC, Nieuwenhuijs VB, Boermeester MA, Bollen TL, Buskens E, et al. Minimally invasive 'step-up approach' versus maximal necrosectomy in patients with acute necrotising pancreatitis (PANTER trial): design and rationale of a randomised controlled multicenter trial [ISRCTN13975868]. BMC Surg. 2006;6:6.
14. van Santvoort HC, Besselink MG, Bakker OJ, Hofker HS, Boermeester MA, Dejong CH, et al. A step-up approach or open necrosectomy for necrotizing pancreatitis. N Engl J Med. 2010;362:1491–502.
15. Hassler KR, Collins JT, Philip K, et al. Laparoscopic cholecystectomy. [Updated 2023 Jan 23]. In: StatPearls [Internet]. Treasure Island (FL): StatPearls Publishing; 2023 Jan. Available from: https://www.ncbi.nlm.nih.gov/books/NBK448145/
16. Hussain, Abdulzahra FRCS, FICMS, D.S. Difficult laparoscopic cholecystectomy: current evidence and strategies of management. Surg Laparoscopy Endoscopy Percutaneous Tech;21(4):211–217, August 2011. https://doi.org/10.1097/SLE.0b013e318220f1b1.
17. Bourgouin S, Mancini J, Monchal T, Calvary R, Bordes J, Balandraud P. How to predict difficult laparoscopic cholecystectomy? Proposal for a simple preoperative scoring system. Am J Surg. 2016;212(5):873–81. https://doi.org/10.1016/j.amjsurg.2016.04.003. Epub 2016 Jun 1.
18. Yokoe M, Hata J, Takada T, Strasberg SM, Asbun HJ, Wakabayashi G, Kozaka K, Endo I, Deziel DJ, Miura F, Okamoto K, Hwang TL, Huang WS, Ker CG, Chen MF, Han HS, Yoon YS, Choi IS, Yoon DS, Noguchi Y, Shikata S, Ukai T, Higuchi R, Gabata T, Mori Y, Iwashita Y, Hibi T, Jagannath P, Jonas E, Liau KH, Dervenis C, Gouma DJ, Cherqui D, Belli G, Garden OJ, Giménez ME, de Santibañes E, Suzuki K, Umezawa A, Supe AN, Pitt HA, Singh H, Chan ACW, Lau WY, Teoh AYB, Honda G, Sugioka A, Asai K, Gomi H, Itoi T, Kiriyama S, Yoshida M, Mayumi T, Matsumura N, Tokumura H, Kitano S, Hirata K, Inui K, Sumiyama Y, Yamamoto M. Tokyo guidelines 2018: diagnostic criteria and severity grading of acute cholecystitis (with videos). J Hepatobiliary Pancreat Sci. 2018;25(1):41–54. https://doi.org/10.1002/jhbp.515. Epub 2018 Jan 9.
19. Pearl JP, Price RR, Tonkin AE, Richardson WS, Stefanidis D. SAGES guidelines for the use of laparoscopy during pregnancy. Surg Endosc. 2017;31(10):3767–82. https://doi.org/10.1007/s00464-017-5637-3. Epub 2017 Jun 22.
20. ASGE Standards of Practice Committee, Buxbaum JL, Abbas Fehmi SM, Sultan S, Fishman DS, Qumseya BJ, Cortessis VK, Schilperoort H, Kysh L, Matsuoka L, Yachimski P, Agrawal D, Gurudu SR, Jamil LH, Jue TL, Khashab MA, Law JK, Lee JK, Naveed M, Sawhney MS, Thosani N, Yang J, Wani SB. ASGE guideline on the role of endoscopy in the evaluation and management of choledocholithiasis. Gastrointest Endosc. 2019;89(6):1075–1105.e15. https://doi.org/10.1016/j.gie.2018.10.001. Epub 2019 Apr 9. PMID: 30979521; PMCID: PMC8594622.
21. Kirkendoll SD, Kelly E, Kramer K, Alouidor R, Winston E, Putnam T, Ryb G, Jabbour N, Perez Coulter A, Kamine T. Optimal timing of cholecystectomy for acute cholecystitis: a retrospective cohort study. Cureus. 2022;14(8):e28548. https://doi.org/10.7759/cureus.28548. PMID: 36185866; PMCID: PMC9519057.
22. Popowicz A, Enochsson L, Sandblom G. Timing of Elective Cholecystectomy After Acute Cholecystitis: A Population-based Register Study. World J Surg. 2023;47(1):152–61. https://doi.org/10.1007/s00268-

022-06772-x. Epub 2022 Oct 24. PMID: 36280615; PMCID: PMC9726773.

23. Strasberg SM, Brunt LM. Rationale and use of the critical view of safety in laparoscopic cholecystectomy. J Am Coll Surg. 2010;211(1):132–8. https://doi.org/10.1016/j.jamcollsurg.2010.02.053. Epub 2010 May 26. Ahmed O, Walsh TN. Surgical Trainee Experience with Open Cholecystectomy and the Dunning-Kruger Effect. J Surg Educ. 2020 Sep-Oct;77(5):1076–1081. https://doi.org/10.1016/j.jsurg.2020.03.025. Epub 2020 May 1. PMID: 32362558.
24. Heitsch RC, Knutson CO, Fulton RL, Jones CE. Delineation of critical factors in the treatment of pancreatic trauma. Surgery. 1976;80:523–9.
25. Allen PJ, Gönen M, Brennan MF, Bucknor AA, Robinson LM, Pappas MM, Carlucci KE, D'Angelica MI, DeMatteo RP, Kingham TP, Fong Y, Jarnagin WR. Pasireotide for postoperative pancreatic fistula. N Engl J Med. 2014;370(21):2014–22. https://doi.org/10.1056/NEJMoa1313688. Erratum in: N Engl J Med. 2014 Jul 3; 371(1):94.
26. Papoulas M, Kontis E, Hadjicosta O, Pinsker N, Heaton N, Menon KV. A novel technique for pancreatic stump closure: clip ligation of the duct and associated suturing of pancreas. Cureus. 2020;12(3):e7414. https://doi.org/10.7759/cureus.7414. 32337138; PMCID: PMC7182156.
27. Cullingford GL, Watkins DN, Watts AD, Mallon DF. Severe late postsplenectomy infection. Br J Surg. 1991;78(6):716–21. https://doi.org/10.1002/bjs.1800780626.
28. Sharpe JP, Magnotti LJ, Weinberg JA, Zarzaur BL, Stickley SM, Scott SE, Fabian TC, Croce MA. Impact of a defined management algorithm on outcome after traumatic pancreatic injury. J Trauma Acute Care Surg. 2012;72(1):100–5. https://doi.org/10.1097/TA.0b013e318241f09d.
29. Malhotra AK, Fabian TC, Croce MA, et al. Blunt hepatic injury: a paradigm shift from operative to nonoperative management in the 1990s. Ann Surg. 2000;231:804.

Ethical Issues in Surgical Decision-making

19

Alberto R. Ferreres

Introduction

In an isolated fashion someone invading other's body_, surgery may be considered a felony. In order a surgical procedure be considered a therapeutic intervention and thus be justified, it must comply with two requisites: the indication of the surgical procedure and the patient's informed consent. The concept of value may have different meanings to the participants of the health care alliance, which include clinicians, surgeons, and the patient and his or her relatives. For the patient, value may represent the equation between the perceived benefits of surgery versus the costs of treatment, not only on a financial basis. This value may include, among other factors, the tolerance of risk and/or uncertainty, the fear of surgery, the tolerance of pain, the length of disability and possible sequelae, the preferred lifestyle, the requirements and needs for peace of mind, and the wellness for living the rest of their life.

Surgery possesses five unique characteristics that set it apart from any other medical field [1]:

- Surgery harms before it heals
- Surgery penetrates the patient's body and thus is highly invasive. According to Judge Benjamin Cardozo in Schloendorff v Society of New York Hospitals (1914): "A surgeon who performs an operation without the patient's consent commits an assault"
- Surgery is fallible, that means that surgery is prone to human error
- Surgical decision-making is performed many times under circumstances of uncertainty
- Surgery is likely to incur in risks, accidents, complications, and sequelae

Every time a surgeon and his or her patient are confronted to a surgical operative decision, they will encounter 2 kinds of determinations to take: the first one is related to *How to treat?* questions, which is a matter of medical science, knowledge, and expertise, and secondly, decisions about *Why to treat?*, linked to surgical ethics grounds.

The art and science of decision-making rest on six basic pillars [2]:

i. Information: when the availability of data is better, the surgeon is in a better position to define a strategy, but this circumstance is not the usual one encountered in clinical practice, since uncertainty is a constant factor.
ii. Knowledge, both the theoretical and practical aspects are valuable assets.
iii. Expertise, based on previous exposure to similar circumstances.

A. R. Ferreres (✉)
School of Medical Sciences, University of Buenos Aires, Buenos Aires, Argentina

Hospital de Clínicas "José de San Martín" University of Buenos Aires, Buenos Aires, Argentina

University of Washington, Seattle, WA, USA
e-mail: aferreres@hospitaldeclinicas.uba.ar; aferre17@uw.edu

R. Latifi (ed.), *Surgical Decision-Making*, https://doi.org/10.1007/978-3-031-67391-7_19

iv. Intuition, which is a characteristic of the "master" surgeon.
v. Assessment, which consists in the evaluation of each of the elements of the decision.
vi. Judgment, combining information, knowledge, expertise, and assessment.

The Decision-Making Process

As in most medical fields, decision-making in general surgery is performed many times under conditions of uncertainty and is characterized by the following features, no matter how urgent the decision or life-threatening is the condition [3]:

- Uncertainty about the medical condition of the patient as well as to the extent and compromise of the disease. Example I: Although a patient may have in-depth studies with 3-D image reconstruction of liver metastases, intraoperative ultrasound may prove different findings and thus change the course of the procedure. Example II: operating a 45-year old lady with gallbladder stones and cholestasis with dilatation of the CBD and finding a mass in the head of the pancreas and not a CBD stone.
- There is usually a set of well-defined strategies from which to choose, according to the evidence and practice guidelines.
- Uncertainty regarding the future consequences of the action which is going to be undertaken. Will the patient survive the operation? Is the risk of surgical morbidity and mortality worth taking in order to relieve the symptoms of the disease?
- A set of preferences held by the decision-maker (the surgeon) which has to be accepted by the patient and applied to the possible and different accounts. It is worth mentioning that during the surgical procedure, the surgeon should bear in mind the patient's choices or advance directives, the exception being an intraoperative accident or unexpected findings, which may impose a deferral in the final therapeutic decision.
- One or even more constraints may limit the set of possible alternatives, in particular the condition of the patient under general anesthesia, time of the procedure, and unexpected situations.
- The most important point is that the decision must be taken ("the surgeon decides") since delaying it or preserving the "status quo" is in itself a decision with its pertinent consequences.

- There are different stages for decision-making in the field of surgery:

  a. In the preoperative period, while the surgical indication should be grounded and needs to be discussed, in elective or emergency situations.
  b. During the intraoperative period, when the patient is usually under general anesthesia and unable, of course, to participate in any decision. It is mandatory that the surgeon should make the best decisions on behalf of the patient, following previous discussions, shared decisions, guidelines, suggestions, expectations, and postoperative lifestyle. Nonetheless, most times all the possible alternatives regarding unexpected findings or intraoperative situations may not have been discussed in-depth with the patient or his/her surrogates.
  c. During the postoperative course, regarding the early diagnosis and adequate management of complications and the requirement of extraordinary methodologies or resources.
  d. During the follow-up period, preventing unnecessary studies or procedures to search for eventual issues, tumor recurrences, or sequelae.
  e. End-of-life issues, trying to prevent futile treatments [4].

Successful decision-making in surgery is achieved through the integration of evidence, inference, and experience. These three qualities are necessary for the acquisition of knowledge and its application in clinical practice and problem-resolving. The elements of knowledge are complex and include intuition and obedience to the teaching of elders. The acronym EIEIO summarizes all the elements of knowledge in clinical surgery, as coined by Marshall: evidence, inference, experience, intuition, and obedience [2]. Inductive reasoning lies at the foundation of evidence-based surgery. It is based upon intervention, observation, and application of the principles of probability, first described by British clergyman and mathematician Thomas Bayes (1701–1761). The strongest evidence is that which arises form the most powerful tool inductive science: the randomized control trial. Inference is probably the most commonly used capacity when performing surgical decisions in individual patients. When a surgeon needs to perform a complex medical decision, there are seldom rigorous and precise data from randomized control trials aiding his or her decision-making process. Even if strong data are available, the surgeon must tailor the obtained results to the specific circumstances of the patient, and this is usually the case in the field of surgery. Nonetheless, the surgeon's level of experience guides his or her decision-making in three broad areas: (a) as an imperfect arbitrator of the published knowledge; (b) the published and generalizable knowledge must be integrated with the particular strengths, limitations, and values of the individual surgeon; and (c) it must be used as a mechanism to fit a therapeutic approach to the particular situation, needs, and values of a particular individual patient

Surgical intuition derives from the integration of prior knowledge, experience, and cognitive skills. It is the characteristic trait of those who we recognize as a master surgeon or an expert. The characterization of expertise is expressed in quick pattern recognition and complicated scripts. Obedience is the uncritical adoption of the counsel of one's teachers and predecessors, often expressed as an aphorism.

Decision-making within the patient–surgeon relationship has different approaches [5]:

1. Paternalistic model: though this model has been very much criticized, it is the one that many times models the relationship between a surgeon and his or her patient. This model usually places the patient in a passive, more vulnerable and thus dependent role vis-à-vis the surgeon as an expert.
2. Informed decision-making model (informed choice): the foundation of this model lies on the information provided by the health agent/provider, so it may be supposed the patient is in a better position to make an informed decision. This is not always the case in the real world of every surgery and in particular, emergencies and trauma care. This model set asides the surgeon from the decision-making process by limiting the role to one of information provider. Besides, most times, the patient, though legally competent, is impaired and cannot make the best decisions regarding his/her welfare, and information asymmetry and understanding is one of its main disadvantages.
3. Professional as an agent model: based on the fiduciary nature of the patient–surgeon relationship, considering the latter will make the best decision on the patient's behalf for the benefit and welfare of the former.
4. Shared decision-making or patient-centered care: the IOM defined this model as "care that is respectful of and responsive to individual patient preferences, needs and values" and ensures that "patient's values guide all clinical decisions." This definition highlights the importance of surgeons and patients working together to produce the best possible outcomes.

On the other hand, the patient–surgeon relationship is built upon trust, so it is preferable to speak about it from a fiduciary viewpoint, not as a contract. As John Gregory (1724–1773) stated, the physician [6] must be in a position to reliably know the patient's interests, should be concerned primarily with protecting and promoting the interests of the patient and only secondarily with protecting and promoting his or her own interests.

The concept of the surgeon as the patient's moral fiduciary can be captured in these considerations:

- The surgeon, whatever his or her field of specialization, should make the protection and promotion of the patient's interest the primary consideration in the surgeon–patient relationship as well in surgical research and education.
- This primary commitment holds self-interest in the background and makes it a systematically secondary consideration.
- Self-interest is thus blunted and not permitted to generate the "vice" of selfishness in the surgeon's professional character, making the fiduciary's role morally demanding.

The patient–surgeon relationship is attained and perfected throughout the process of surgical informed consent, which includes the following elements [7]:

1. Preconditions: competence and voluntary attitude of the patient.
2. Information: disclosure and treatment recommendations by the surgeon and the patient's understanding of the provided information.
3. Consent: decision-making (acceptance or refusal), communication, registration, and the patient's final authorization to proceed.

Since surgeons should in no way offer an "a la carte" menu of surgical options to the disease or pathologic condition encountered by a particular patient, they should not be forced to act contrary to their knowledge, beliefs, standard of care, provided they agree with the generally accepted ones. Decisions in surgical care are increasingly being performed by multidisciplinary teams. However, the decision-making process is not well established and many times, unawareness of the patient's values and preferences, lifestyle, and choices is the rule and consequently the therapeutic decision _though scientifically impeccable_is not always in the patient's best interest [8].

Surgical decision-making in the operating room (OR) is a non-technical skill but it is a must and a requirement: it is definitively related to critical, cognitive, and interpersonal abilities that complement manual dexterity. The surgeon will be confronted by difficult decision-making situations in the OR environment and must be prepared to take the best decisions on behalf of the patient [9]. Surgical procedures are characterized by time constraints, changing goals, increased risks, high uncertainty, unexpected situations, unanticipated troubles, and inadequate data provision [10]. If the operation proceeds without significant problems, there will be no reason to change the course of action. But when confronted with sudden or unexpected situations (bleeding, unexpected findings, increased risks, accidents, technical difficulties, etc.), the surgeon will be forced to change the course of action. The initial step is the situation awareness of a change in the governing conditions, which is closely related to the cognitive monitoring of the developing steps of a surgical procedure. Once the surgeon detects any abnormality in the course and smooth development of events, the second step is the situation assessment, which includes the identification and definition of the problem, the assessment of risk, and the time constraints under which the decision needs to be taken. The strategy of decision-making may take different mechanisms, one or more at a time: intuitive, rule-based, analytical, or creative. The aim is to resolve the situation as soon as possible and with the least amount of collateral harm to the patient (Fig. 19.1).

INTRAOPERATIVE DIFFICULTY OR ADVERSE SITUATION

↓

SITUATION AWARENESS

↓

SITUATION ASSESSMENT

- Identification and definition of the problem
- Evaluation
- Stratification of risk (high, medium, low)
- Time constraints?

↓

DECISION STRATEGY

- Intuitive
- Rule-based
- Analytical
- Creative

↓

DECISION MAKING

↓

ADOPTION OF A COURSE OF ACTION

Fig. 19.1 Intraoperative decision-making steps

Surgical Ethics Tools to Aid in the Decision-Making Process

Surgical ethics is based on the recognition of the rights of patients undergoing or requiring surgical care. An important point is that there is no surgical intervention possible without the presence of, and the active role played by, a surgeon. The surgeon is an essential part of this dyadic relationship, since not a single surgical intervention should not be performed without the presence of a surgeon fully supported by a team of health care professionals in an adequate setting.

The ethical duties of a surgeon stem from these ethical foundations: the surgeons' responsibility to society, to surgery as a whole, and to the self-regulation of the surgical profession; the professional obligation to use the body of scientific knowledge entrusted to surgeons to serve others; and lastly, to the relationship among surgeons, between surgeons and their associations, and between these two and the society to which they belong. The surgeon–patient relationship intertwines the surgeon on one side, who holds the role of "authority" because of training, expertise, wisdom, and judgment; and on the other, the patient, who holds a position of "authority" to consent that upon his or her body an intervention may be performed. This bond is characterized by trust. The concept of the surgeon as a fiduciary of the patient, as mentioned before, lies at the core of Surgical Ethics [11].

All types of surgeons should rely on tools which may assist and provide them with a framework for ethical analysis and help them in the decision-making to help address and manage clinical difficult cases. Firstly, surgeons should be acquainted and familiarized with the ethical principles as collated by Beauchamp and Childress: beneficence, non-maleficence, respect for autonomy, and justice [12]. Beneficence means to do the good for others and refers to the quality of being ready to act or do with a prime consideration of the benefit and blessing for the other. The principle of non-maleficence concerns the duty of not causing harm to others and is represented by the *primum non nocere* dictum. Although it is usually considered the fundamental core of the Hippocratic tradition of medical ethics, it is not present in the Hippocratic Corpus except in the phrase from Epidemics, Book 1, Chapter 2: "At least do no harm." Nonmaleficent actions include not only not generating harm but also not risking its production. The principle of patient autonomy highlights the power and preeminence of each individual to make his or her own decisions with respect to health care and research. The essential requirements are liberty (freedom from any outside influences), authority (sufficiency to do), and intention (willingness to act). The principle of respect for patient autonomy in the health care setting is achieved by the informed consent process, which represents the encounter of two competent sides (patient and physician). The principle of justice derives originally from Aristotle, who defined it as "the rendering to each individual of what is due to him or her." Justice is considered treatment with fairness, equity, and egalitarianism in conflicts among individuals, and recently the concepts of John Rawls have influenced the current concept of justice, trying to solve the questions of distributive justice on the grounds of the greater good.

Mc Cullough et al recommend a four-step approach [13]:

i. Identification of the facts in each case: a full and complete knowledge of all the facts and data of a particular patient as well as diagnostic studies and therapeutic alternatives are the initial requirements for a sound and grounded ethical analysis. Awareness regarding the patient's opinion, preferences, and opinion should be taken into account.
ii. Ethical analysis: this assessment should consider the so-called four appeals. The first one is related to the fiduciary role of the surgeon and the rest refer to the ethical principles of beneficence, respect for autonomy and justice.
    a. Appeal to virtues: in connection to the short- and long-term implications of the surgeon's role as a fiduciary for the patient.
    b. Appeal to consequences: special consideration is given to the risk/benefit equation.
    c. Appeal to rights: the full respect to the patient's positive and negative right is mandatory.
    d. Appeal to justice and fairness: takes into account financial, material, and human resources.
iii. Ethical argument: answers should be given to the following questions: "Are the reasons clearly stated?" "Are there other options that could apply to the case?"
iv. Issues of power and authority: as mentioned before, the surgeon is an authority in view of his or her knowledge, training, wisdom, and expertise while at the same time the patient decides and consents to whatever is to be done or not upon his or her body.

Jonsen and Siegler propose a "four-box model" to aid in solving ethical issues in clinical patient care, which is perfectly suitable to surgical patients. This model links the four ethical principles with the true circumstances of a real clinical situation [14].

1. Medical indications: reflect the principles of beneficence and non-maleficence and refer to the diagnostic and therapeutic options for the treatment and approach of the surgical condition confronted by a patient.
2. Patient preferences: address the principle of respect for autonomy and express the choice of the patient.
3. Quality of life: applies the principles of beneficence, non-maleficence, and respect for autonomy and describes features before and after the surgical intervention.
4. Context features: linked to the principles of justice and fairness, take into account the particular setting and available resources in each particular case.

Many surgeons have encountered or will encounter the following question: "Doctor, if this were you or your relative, what would you do?" This question represents a request for expert advice, a situation a surgeon should not refuse to answer which he or she considers the best option. One of the precautions is that the advice may be based on personal values, which may not be identical or similar to the patient's ones [15]. Surgeons are confronted daily to this question, which may be asked in different situations:

- When the patient is in possession of a great amount of technical information with mortality and outcomes figures, both favorable and/or unfavorable, which may be overwhelming and confusing. In such cases, the patient is trying to convey that he or she is over-informed and not able to make a reasonable choice.
- When the patient is making difficult choices and merely needs support. He or she is really asking, "Doctor, am I making the right choice?"
- When the patient is facing difficult alternatives_usually life or death choices or very different treatment options_ he or she is asking for assistance or for the physician to make the choice.

The question in each of these three situations requires a different answer, but each certainly deserves a reply. The task is to have a clear understanding of what the patient and relatives need and want from the surgeon in charge.

As mentioned, there are three stages in which Surgical Ethics impact the decision-making process:

1. Preoperative or pre-intervention
2. Intraoperative or intra-intervention
3. Postoperative or post-intervention

The first stage is of paramount importance since this is the time-lapse when the surgical indication and the therapeutic decision-making process are thought, proposed, discussed, and accepted. The opposite situation would mean the performance of an unnecessary, useless, ineffective, or discretionary procedure. As mentioned before, a surgical procedure requests a solid and grounded indication and the mandatory informed consent process to justify it, otherwise it should be considered a felony. The determination of the need of an operation or a surgical intervention is done in accordance to the efficacy of the procedure, the nature and stage of the disease, the benefit/ risk ratio, the availability and efficacy of non-operative treatment, the presence of other diseases, conditions, or comorbidities, the appropiateness, the consideration of contextual factors, and most importantly, the patient own values. Among these, the perceived benefits of the surgery or intervention versus the costs, the tolerance of risk, fear of surgery, tolerance of pain/disability, the preferred lifestyle, requirements for peace of mind, and how the patient wants to live the rest of their lifes should be highlighted. Crile made a distinction between appropriate and inappropriate procedures, the latter being classified as: a) operations inappropriate for the disease; b) operations inappropriate for a given patient; and c) operations appropriate for the disease and the patient, but performed by a surgeon who has not been adequately trained. Basically, unnecessary surgery arises from three recognized causes: ignorance, incorrect judgment, or dishonesty, which would encompass incompetence, indifference, or immorality. From these three, the ethical and medico-legal implications of a procedure that is not supported or justified by scientific evidence clearly emerge [8]. It is also important to mention the concept of "time until treatment equipoise" (TUTE) which may be only applied to operations performed purely on prognostic grounds, advising the patient of the relative risks of the two approaches in terms of the time elapsing after an intervention before the risk of the intervention is nullified and reversed by the cumulative risk of conservative management expressed as a single figure (hours, weeks, months, years) [16].

Another important aspect is the use of extraordinary measures (including surgery) in the last stages of life. It is worth remembering the words of John Gregory (1724–1773), the one who transformed medicine from a trade into a profession. He defined Medicine as "The art of preserving health, of prolonging life, of curing disease and of making death more easy." There is generally a contrast in how physicians die and how patients die, being much more invasive and extraordinary in the latter. This brings the concept of futility in surgical treatment and in medicine, which _ according to the Oxford English Dictionary_ can be defined "as serving no useful purpose, completely ineffective or producing no valuable effect." A distinction should be made between effect and benefit, since effective treatments, if not beneficial, should be considered futile as well.

When defining the futility or not of a proposed surgical intervention, the need to achieve a goal of care should be precisely assessed, in particular these three issues: the regain of function, the improvement in the quality of life, and the palliation of symptoms. Most times futility discussions make clear a failure of effective communication between the patient and his/her family and the surgeon/ surgical team. Many times the approach to this issue is incorrect since the question posed is "Do you want everything done?" and the answer is most times "Do everything," but the right answer should be "Do everything, that is reasonable."

Futility should also be considered goal-specific and as such, may be considered physiological, quantitative, or qualitative. Physiological futility is when the proposed intervention cannot physiologically achieve the desired effect and represents the most objective type of futility judgment. Quantitative futility occurs when the proposed intervention is highly unlikely to achieve the desired effect and qualitative futility is when the proposed intervention, if successful, will probably produce such a poor outcome or result in an unacceptable quality of life, that it is deemed best not to attempt it [17]. Aligning therapeutic decisions and their corresponding impact and outcomes with the values and expected wishes of patients is sometimes difficult. The best-case/ worst-case framework popularized by the University of Wisconsin, Madison has been useful as an aid [18].

The patient will be exposed to surgical futility when any surgical treatment is considered:

i. Ineffective: unable to change the natural history of a disease or its trajectory toward death.
ii. Non beneficial: unable to satisfy any good or value.
iii. Disproportionately burdensome to the patient, physically, psychologically, or financially.

Surgical care should not be provided in these circumstances: when it falls apart the limits of professional standard of care, when it is negligent or when it compromises the physician's integrity. And it is mandatory that this surgical care is patient-oriented or patient-centered care meaning "providing care that is respectful of and responsive to individual patient preferences, needs, and values, and ensuring that patient values guide all clinical decisions." Another important aspect of futility is represented by the option of withdrawal or withholding life-sustaining treatments no longer consistent with the goals of supportive care. It represents a difficult topic to discuss prematurely but needs to be done, so as to have a clear and detailed knowledge of the patient's goals, choices, and preferences. Meanwhile the evaluation of effectiveness is best determined by the acting surgeon, the evaluation of benefit is best determined by the patient (what is good for him or her), and the evaluation of burden needs to be assessed by both patient and physician.

In the intraoperative stage, the surgeon should always stand on the side of the informed consent process, in accordance with the patients' wishes, in particular when confronted to unexpected findings or life-threatening complications. During the postoperative stage, the focus will undoubtedly be placed on the early recognition and adequate management of surgical complications. The concept of "failure to rescue," first developed in 1992 by Silber and colleagues, captures the idea that, although not every complication of medical care is preventable, health care systems should be able to rapidly identify and treat complications when they occur [19].

In Table 19.1, we propose a systematic approach for ethical decision-making VITDM, which comprises five steps:

- Verify all the facts and issues pertaining to a particular case, enabling a deep knowledge of the medical/surgical condition, its prognosis, the available evidence for that condition, the

Table 19.1 An ethical decision-making primer—VITDM

1. Verify facts and issues Ethical conflict/dilemma/issues Facts and clinical background Expected outcomes/risks Scientific evidence Patient's preferences and choices	2. Include different perspectives Keep the patient's interests and welfare at the center Engage all interested stakeholders Gather all needed information about values, context, and beliefs Rely on the four ethical principles	
3. Take into consideration Determine therapeutic options Shared- decision with patient Quality of life (QoL) Determine: appropriateness, acceptability, standard of care, values, principles, interests, motivations, biases	4. Define the path When in doubt, stop and reflect Consider other options/ approaches Build a strong case to advocate Choose course of action Operationalize the decision Communication Implementation	5. Monitor outcomes Patient satisfaction Outcomes and consequences Improvement mechanisms

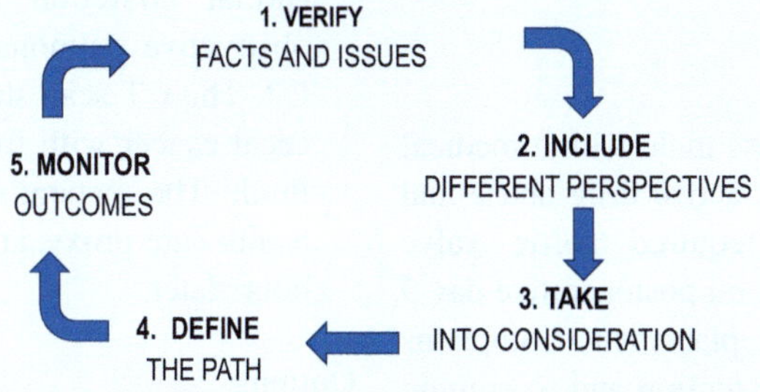

odds of doing vs not doing, the preferences, choices, and decision of the patient as well as perfectly identifying where the ethical conflict resides.

- Include different perspectives, but always keeping the patient's interests and welfare at the center, and relying on the four ethical principles.
- Take into consideration different issues, such as the appropriateness, standard of care, values, beliefs, motivations as well as the future quality of life.
- Define the path, choosing the best decision, taking it down to practice, with adequate and proper communication.
- Monitor the outcomes, mainly the patient's satisfaction and that of their relatives.

Conclusions

Every surgeon, either a trainee or an expert, should be superb in the domain of decision-making. All difficult circumstances in clinical practice should be challenged with a systematic approach and a flawless decision-making strategy, and this process must take into account the preoperative, intraoperative, and postoperative stages, as well as the follow-up period and the last moments of life [20]. The intraoperative decision-making stage is probably the most difficult to perform due to time constraints and unexpected findings. The deep knowledge of the ethical background and framework (VITDM) provides a very useful tool to assist in the decision-making process when challenged with difficult situations in everyday surgical practice worldwide.

- Surgeons must have a clear understanding of the goals of care and patient's values before the therapeutic proposal
- A definition of mutual decision-making should be just that—mutual
- Patients often appreciate appropriate guidance from their surgeon
- Assessing potential harm and interpreting the likelihood of a successful outcome should be performed by an skilled and trained physician
- Surgeons should be trained not only to cure but also to comfort and be knowledgeable

about the goals and ideals of palliative care medicine

- Trust between the patient, the family, and the surgical team is mandatory
- Refraining from an active and operative role also requires skilled communication with a humanistic approach
- Many surgeons lack adequate training in how to discuss this form of patient care
- Conversations should be patient-centered but not patient-driven
- Increased communication leads to greater patient satisfaction and a decrease in futile treatments

Case Discussion #1

- A 54-year-old homeless male with a medical history of intravenous active drug abuse and endocarditis which required aortic valve replacement, currently on postoperative day 9 of a redo aortic valve replacement. Complains of acute abdominal distention and worsening sepsis and the diagnosis is acute mesenteric ischemia due to septic emboli. The patient is under respiratory support, and no presence of relatives, neither advance directives nor health care power of attorney. The prognosis is uncertain, the operation turns in a very high morbidity and mortality, and likely ending in the patient with an ostomy and/or short gut syndrome, circumstances which may be unacceptable to the patient or even very difficult to handle given his homelessness and drug abuse issue. The surgical team also considers topics of unfair discrimination.

Which should be the due course of action?
Options:

1) Seek social service support to aid in the decision
2) Palliative care considering the situation is irreversible
3) Laparotomy, massive bowel resection according to the findings and ileostomy at 50 cm from Treitz ligament and decision of no extraordinary measures
4) Laparotomy, due to the findings of massive small and large bowel ischemia, closure and implementation of palliative measures

Option 4) was performed, and the patient died 5 hours after the operation.

Case Discussion #2

- A 93-year-old lady with Alzheimer's dementia presenting to the emergency department with severe abdominal pain and distention. Medical history including: congestive heart failure with ejection fraction 20% after a myocardial infarction 3 months ago, chronic obstructive pulmonary disease with at-home O2. The CT scan shows a grossly perforated cecal cancer with free intraperitoneal air and fluid. The patient's grand-daughter is her health care proxy, arrives to the ED couple of hours later.

Options:

1) Do you offer a choice between a right hemicolectomy and comfort care?
2) Do you discuss the value of palliative care with the grand-daughter (health care proxy)?
3) Do you admit the patient for emergency surgery and postoperative ICU admission?
4) Do you admit the patient for pain control and comfort measures?

Option 2) was performed, the grand-daughter accepted the proposal of admission for palliative care, the lady passed away the same night of admission.

Case Discussion #3

- A 69-year-old lady with a medical history of a Kausch-Whipple operation for pancreatic head carcinoma 4 years ago. She presents for follow-up consultation with jaundice and abdominal pain, stating she wants "everything" for her treatment, including whatever new or experimental treatments available or under research. Work-up shows an abdominal mass, a recurrence with obstruction of the hepaticojejunostomy, and liver disseminated metastases. A biliary decompressive drainage is placed for relief of symptoms. The patient returns a fortnight later with weight loss, nausea, and vomiting due to a small bowel obstruction related to the above-mentioned mass.

Options:

1) Referral to a hospice institution
2) Surgical exploration and eventual resection with anastomosis or bypass
3) Admission and implementation of ordinary measures for comfort and prevention of pain
4) Ambulatory palliative care

Option 3) was implemented, the lady was in her right mind, decided being admitted and included a DNR order. She died peacefully after four days.

References

1. Ferreres AR. Ethical debate: the ethics of non-performing extended lymphadenectomy in patients with gastrointestinal cancer. World J Surg. 2013;2013(37):1821–8.
2. Marshall JC. Surgical decision-making: integrating evidence, inference and experience. Surg Clin North Am. 2006;86:201–5.
3. Bartlett LM. The teaching of surgical judgment. Am J Surg. 2004;121:220–2.
4. St Martin L, Patel P, Gallinger J, Moulton CA. Teaching the slowing-down moments of operative judgment. Surg Clin North Am. 2012;92:125–35.
5. Barry MJ, Edgman-Levitan S. Shared-decision making: the pinnacle of patient-centered care. N Engl J Med. 2012;366:780–1.
6. McCullough LB. John Gregory's writings on medical ethics and philosophy of medicine. Dordrecht: Kluwer Academic Publishers; 1998.
7. Cainzos MA, Gónzalez-Vinagre S. Informed consent in surgery. World J Surg. 2014;38:1587–93.
8. Ferreres AR. Unnecessary Surgery (Editorial) Cir Esp (Engl Ed) 2023 Dec;101(12):813–815. https://doi.org/10.1016/j.cireng.2023.11.003. Epub 2023 Nov 11.
9. Cristancho SM, Vanstone M, Lingard L et al. When surgeons face intraoperative challenges: a naturalistic model of surgical decision making. Am J Surg 2013: 205-156-162.
10. Flin R, Youngson G, Yule S. How do surgeons make intraoperative decisions? Qual Saf Health Care. 2007;16:235–9.
11. Ferreres AR. The ethical duties and obligations of a surgeon. In: Ferreres AR, Angelos P, Singer EA, editors. Ethical issues in surgical care. Chicago: American College of Surgeons; 2017.
12. Beauchamp TL, Childress JF. Principles of biomedical ethics. New York: Oxford University Press; 1994.
13. McCullough LB, Jones JW, Brody BA. Surgical ethics. New York: Oxford University Press; 1998.
14. Jonsen AR, Siegler M, Winslade WJ. Clinical ethics: a practical approach to clinical decisions in clinical medicine. New York: McGraw Hill; 2010.
15. Kon AA. Answering the question: "doctor, if this were your child, what would you do?". Pediatrics. 2006;118:393–4000.
16. Noorani A, Hippelainen M, Nashef SAM. Time until treatment equipoise: a new concept in surgical decision making. JAMA Surg. 2014;149:109–11.
17. Sokol DK. The slipperiness of futility. BMJ. 2009;338:b 2222. https://doi.org/10.1136/bmj.b2222.
18. Kruser JM, Nabozny MJ, Steffens NM, Brasel KJ, Campbell TC, Gaines ME, Schwarze ML. "Best case/Worst case:" qualitative evaluation of a novel communication tool for difficult in-the-moment surgical decisions. J Am Geriatr Soc. 2015;63:1805–11.
19. Silber JH, Williams SV, Krakauer H, Schwartz. Hospital and patient characteristics associated with death after surgery. A study of adverse occurrence and failure to rescue. Med Care. 1992;30(7):615–29.
20. Binkley CE, Reynolds JM, Shuman A. From the eyeball test to the algorithm-Quality of life, disability status and clinical decision making in surgery. N Engl J Med. 2022;387:1325–8.

Surgical Decision-Making in Emergency Management of Colon and Rectal Malignancies

20

Ryan Bendl and James Clarke

Background

Successful management of colon and rectal cancer typically adheres to protocolized staging and treatment algorithms. Preoperative planning, combined with medical optimization, establishes an ideal scenario to enhance the patient's oncologic outcome. However, many colorectal cancer patients present acutely with obstruction or worse with obstruction and perforation, necessitating swift, life-saving action. In these instances, surgical decision-making is more complex and difficult necessitating often damage control surgery initially. The stakes are high, but preparedness, along with prompt action, are crucial for achieving successful short- and long-term outcomes.

Colorectal cancer ranks as the second leading cause of cancer-related mortality among both men and women worldwide. The American Cancer Society anticipates a staggering number of new cases in 2024, projecting 106,500 cases of colon cancer and 46,220 cases of rectal cancer in the United States alone [1]. Globally, the burden of colorectal cancer is immense, with over 1.1 million newly diagnosed cases of colon cancer and 700,000 cases of rectal cancer reported in 2020 [2].

The lifetime risk of developing colorectal cancer is significant, with men facing a 1 in 23 chance and women a 1 in 25 chance of being diagnosed with the disease. It is estimated to cause approximately 53,000 deaths in 2024 [1]. There is hope however, as the incidence of colorectal cancer has been declining since the mid-1980s, largely attributed to increased screening efforts and lifestyle modifications. Unfortunately, this positive trend has been overshadowed by a concerning rise in colorectal cancer rates among individuals under 55 years old since the mid-1990s, with a 1–2% annual increase noted in both colon and rectal cancers. In response to this trend, the United States Preventive Services Task Force took proactive measures by lowering the screening age from 50 to 45 in their May 2021 update on colorectal cancer screening guidelines [3].

Despite the availability of well-established screening protocols, a significant minority of colorectal cancer patients—ranging from 10 to 30%—present with acute surgical indications such as bleeding, obstruction, or perforation [3]. This acute presentation underscores the critical need for prompt intervention and highlights the importance of preparedness for colorectal surgeons, general surgeons, acute care surgeons, and surgical oncologists.

Patients undergoing emergency surgery for colon cancer exhibit elevated surgical morbidity

R. Bendl (✉)
New York Medical College, Westchester Medical Center, Valhalla, NY, USA
e-mail: Ryan.Bendl@wmchealth.org

J. Clarke
Westchester Medical Center, Valhalla, NY, USA
e-mail: James.Clarke@wmchealth.org

R. Latifi (ed.), *Surgical Decision-Making*, https://doi.org/10.1007/978-3-031-67391-7_20

rates and mortality rates compared with those undergoing elective colon cancer surgery, 64% versus 24% and 34% versus 7%, respectively [4]. Perioperative mortality rate remains notably higher in the emergency operation group, alongside a decreased rate of overall and cancer-specific 5-year survival after curative surgery [5]. These findings emphasize the critical importance of preventive measures and early intervention strategies in managing colon cancer to mitigate the risks associated with emergency surgeries and improve patient outcomes.

By promoting early detection, implementing evidence-based interventions, and providing comprehensive care, we can strive to reduce the burden of this disease and improve outcomes for patients. A comprehensive approach to colorectal cancer surgical emergencies mandates a thorough examination of the abdomen and pelvis, integral to the diagnostic and therapeutic process. Even in cases where no formal resection is planned, obtaining a tissue diagnosis is paramount to inform treatment decisions effectively. Biopsies of any extracolonic or metastatic lesions are imperative for accurate staging and to guide subsequent immunochemical therapies postoperatively.

Given that patients presenting acutely often have not undergone routine colonoscopic evaluation, it is essential to remain vigilant regarding the possibility of synchronous colon cancer, which occurs in approximately 3.5% of patients [6]. In such scenarios, manual palpation of the entire colon becomes indispensable in the emergency setting. Conducting a full colonoscopy may prove challenging, if not impossible, particularly in cases of perforation, obstruction, or significant bleeding. Thus, manual palpation serves as a pragmatic intraoperative necessity for detecting synchronous lesions.

Identification of synchronous lesions necessitates careful consideration of the treatment approach. Depending on the clinical scenario, options may include extended resection, multiple resections, or comprehensive postoperative evaluation to ensure optimal management of both index and synchronous tumors. This proactive approach not only aids in maximizing oncologic outcomes but also minimizes the risk of missed or undertreated disease, ultimately improving patient prognosis.

Patients presenting with symptomatic colon or rectal cancers often exhibit signs of advanced disease, primarily due to the presence of perforation or obstruction. These conditions inherently indicate a more progressed stage of cancer, potentially involving adjacent or distant organs and structures. Achieving an R0 resection, indicating complete removal of the tumor with negative margins, may necessitate extended or multivisceral resections to ensure thorough excision of the malignancy.

To guide surgical decision-making and optimize patient outcomes, the National Comprehensive Cancer Network (NCCN) provides comprehensive guidelines for the management of colorectal cancer patients. These guidelines emphasize the importance of meticulous surgical techniques and thorough pathological examination. Specifically, the NCCN recommends the identification and examination of lymph nodes at the origin of feeding vessels, with a minimum of 12 lymph nodes required to establish the appropriate N stage [7].

In cases where clinically positive lymph nodes are encountered outside of the planned resection field, they should be considered suspicious and subsequently biopsied or removed whenever feasible. Failure to address positive nodes may result in an incomplete (R2) resection, compromising the effectiveness of treatment and potentially impacting long-term outcomes [7]. Therefore, adherence to NCCN guidelines ensures a standardized approach to surgical management, facilitating optimal oncologic control and improving overall patient care.

In addition to ensuring thorough lymphadenectomy, achieving appropriate resection margins is critical in colorectal cancer surgery. The consensus among experts suggests that for most colon and rectal cancer resections, a margin of 5 cm is generally deemed adequate. However, in cases involving very distal rectal cancers, a shorter margin of 2 cm or even 1 cm may suffice [7].

The determination of the optimal resection margin goes beyond mere length considerations. The site of proximal and distal transection is also influenced by factors such as vascular ligation, performed in conjunction with lymphadenectomy. This ensures that the resection encompasses the tumor and its associated lymphatic drainage, thereby reducing the risk of local recurrence and improving oncologic outcomes. By tailoring the resection margins to the specific characteristics of the tumor and its anatomical location, surgeons can achieve maximal tumor clearance while preserving vital structures and function.

The National Comprehensive Cancer Network (NCCN) panel underscores the importance of judiciously considering minimally invasive colectomy, emphasizing the need for surgeons experienced in these techniques. Despite its potential benefits, tumors that present with acute obstruction, perforation, or evident local invasion into surrounding structures are generally not considered appropriate candidates for minimally invasive colon resection. Such cases often necessitate immediate intervention and may pose technical challenges that are better addressed through traditional open surgery.

Furthermore, patients with clinical obstruction or perforation, coupled with additional high-risk features, require comprehensive evaluation and management. Adjuvant treatment strategies play a crucial role in optimizing outcomes for these individuals, and the decision-making process should be guided by the anticipated need for such therapies.

The management of acute surgical rectal cancer emergencies represents a formidable challenge within the realm of colorectal care, particularly with the standardization of preoperative treatment protocols. Neoadjuvant chemotherapy and radiation therapy have emerged as the cornerstone of care for locally advanced rectal cancers, offering a paradigm shift in treatment approaches [8].

This multimodal therapy not only serves to shrink tumor size and reduce the risk of local recurrence but also enhances the feasibility of tumor resection and facilitates sphincter preservation—a critical consideration for maintaining quality of life postoperatively [9]. By addressing the disease burden upfront, neoadjuvant therapy optimizes the surgical landscape, enabling more effective tumor removal and functional outcomes.

Emergent resection of locally advanced rectal cancer without prior multimodal therapy is strongly discouraged as it may compromise the patient's oncologic outcome. The omission of neoadjuvant treatment in such cases can heighten the complexity of surgical intervention, increase the risk of intraoperative complications, and compromise the potential for achieving optimal oncologic control.

In the emergent setting, the primary goal of treatment is to address the immediate physiological insult while also considering long-term oncologic outcomes. Maintaining a delicate balance between managing the acute surgical emergency and optimizing cancer therapy is paramount.

Whenever feasible, efforts should be made to address the cancer concurrently with the acute surgical intervention. This approach not only streamlines patient care but also maximizes the potential for achieving curative outcomes. However, in cases where curative intent is not feasible due to the severity of the emergency or the extent of disease, alternative options must be explored.

In such situations, consideration should be given to future resection or palliative measures aimed at alleviating symptoms and improving quality of life. Additionally, adjunct therapies such as embolization, radiation therapy, and stenting may play a crucial role in temporizing the disease and optimizing the patient's medical condition before definitive surgical or oncologic interventions.

Consultation with interventional radiologists, radiation oncologists, and interventional gastroenterologists is indispensable in navigating these complex scenarios. Their expertise in nonsurgical interventions can offer valuable insights and contribute to the multidisciplinary management of patients with emergent colorectal cancer presentations.

By adopting a holistic approach that integrates surgical, oncologic, and supportive care strategies, healthcare providers can effectively address the emergent needs of patients while safeguarding their long-term oncologic outcomes. Collaboration among diverse medical specialties is essential in ensuring comprehensive and personalized care for individuals facing colorectal cancer emergencies.

Patients undergoing emergent colorectal procedures should be counseled regarding the possibility of a stoma and its implications. While many emergency surgeries occur rapidly, often without planned, formal stoma marking, surgeons should be prepared to mark patients preoperatively to facilitate postoperative care, particularly given the likelihood of subsequent chemotherapy.

In patients with metastatic disease, the primary oncologic goal is to minimize delays in initiating systemic chemotherapy. Intraoperative decision-making regarding stoma creation versus reanastomosis hinges on several factors, including perforation, contamination, size discrepancy, and stool burden. Balancing the risks of anastomotic leak against the potential benefits of preserving bowel continuity is essential.

Anastomotic leak represents a serious complication with profound implications for oncologic outcomes. Studies, such as a Danish nationwide cohort study involving 9,333 patients, have demonstrated the detrimental effects of anastomotic leaks on long-term prognosis [10]. These include increased rates of distal recurrence, long-term mortality, and reduced likelihood of receiving adjuvant chemotherapy, leading to delays in treatment initiation.

Moreover, a larger meta-analysis involving 21 studies and over 21,000 patients corroborated these findings, emphasizing the negative prognostic impact of anastomotic leaks on local recurrence [11]. While their influence on distal recurrence appears less pronounced, the overall message underscores the importance of meticulous surgical technique and postoperative care in minimizing complications and optimizing oncologic outcomes.

In summary, the decision to divert or reanastomose in emergent colorectal procedures must be guided by careful consideration of patient factors, intraoperative findings, and the overarching goal of preserving oncologic integrity. Proactive measures to mitigate the risk of anastomotic leak are crucial for enhancing long-term prognosis and ensuring timely access to adjuvant therapies, ultimately improving patient survival and quality of life.

Additional considerations which need not be done intraoperatively but should be considered early in the perioperative course would include CT scan of the chest to complete the staging workup as well as laboratory CEA level which can be used to assess the patient's disease response postoperatively. The role of circulating tumor DNA in recurrence detection and treatment guidance is yet to be fully established.

Ostomy Surgery

The creation of an intestinal stoma is an essential tool that should remain at the forefront of a surgeon's armamentarium for managing both urgent and non-urgent cases of colon and rectal cancer. While it can serve as a contingency plan in certain situations, the decision to construct a stoma should be considered prior to surgery. Preoperative stoma marking has been linked to decreased occurrences of postoperative and peristomal issues, along with enhancements in patient self-care and overall quality of healthcare. According to a comprehensive review of 10 studies encompassing 2109 patients, preoperative stoma marking was correlated with a reduction in complications such as prolapse, retraction, skin necrosis, and hernias [12].

Technical steps to consider for stoma creation include initially marking the patient's skin. In emergency situations, this is typically performed in the emergency department or preoperative holding area. Ideally, a smooth area with the rectus abdominis muscle should be chosen to ensure proper appliance adherence, avoiding deep skin folds. It is beneficial to examine the patient in lying, sitting, and standing positions. For patients with significant central adiposity, selecting a location in the upper abdomen within their line of sight can facilitate easier self-care [13]. Additionally, marking multiple locations is advisable as intraoperative findings may favor one location over another.

Moreover, there should be a minimum of 2 inches between the edge of the laparotomy incision (if performed) and the intended stoma site. This spacing allows for a secure seal of the stoma appliance to the skin, reducing the risk of leakage and preventing skin necrosis between the incision and the stoma. Practically, authors typically mark all skin creases with the patient sitting and then draw a vertical line 2 inches off the midline.

For non-obese patients, placement is preferably within the ostomy triangle defined by the anterior superior iliac spine, umbilicus, and pubic tubercle. Conversely, in patients with a large pannus, upper abdomen placement is favored.

Following excision of an appropriately sized disc of skin at the designated location, it is important to divide the subcutaneous tissue rather than excising or "coring out" it [14]. A vertical incision of 2–3 cm in the anterior fascia, followed by a perpendicular 1 cm fascial incision, should be made. Subsequently, the rectus muscle should be split in the direction of its fibers, and a major vertical incision in the posterior rectus sheath is warranted. Attention should be paid to ensuring the mesentery of the bowel wall is not twisted during this process.

In obese patients, where passing the bowel wall may pose difficulty, utilizing a surgical glove [15] or wound protector [16] had been described to facilitate easier passage of the bowel through the trephine. In scenarios such as distal obstruction with markedly dilated bowel, an oversized fascial incision may occasionally be necessary. However, this may increase the risk of developing a clinically significant parastomal hernia, thus tightening the fascia once the bowel has been delivered is advisable.

A systematic review and meta-analysis conducted in 2020 examined the efficacy of stoma support devices [17]. The overall incidence of stoma retraction among patients was found to be 2.8%. Interestingly, there was no significant difference in the incidence of retraction between groups that used stoma support rods and those that did not. However, the use of stoma support rods was associated with a notable increase in complications, including stoma necrosis, peristomal dermatitis, and mucocutaneous separation [18].

Regrettably, the average BMI measurement did not account for obese patients, who typically face more complex challenges during stoma creation. This highlights a potential limitation in the study's findings. Moreover, as per the 2022 practice parameters set forth by the American Society of Colon and Rectal Surgery, the routine use of prophylactic mesh to prevent parastomal hernias during stoma creation is no longer recommended [19].

Finally, the authors advocate for visual inspection of the colon, paying careful attention to the cecum, in cases of colonic obstruction. Failure to recognize colonic ischemia through a "blind stoma" may have catastrophic ramifications. Therefore, thorough examination during surgical procedures is paramount to ensure proper diagnosis and treatment.

Colon Cancer

The oncologic resection of colon cancer involves removing both the entire tumor and the lymph node basin draining the tumor. Achieving negative margins is crucial for ensuring a complete oncologic resection [7, 20]. Like rectal cancer, the radial margin holds prognostic significance, as a positive radial margin can lead to higher rates of local recurrence. Traditionally, margins have been described as a 5 cm segment of normal bowel both proximally and distally. This ensures an adequate resection of the mesocolon and adequate removal of the draining lymph nodes. Complete resection of the mesocolon, including the named vessel for the involved colon segment, results in devascularization of the surrounding colon segment harboring the tumor.

The optimal approach in an emergent situation depends on both the patient's condition and the surgeon's expertise and comfort level. Achieving oncologic resection requires ensuring adequate proximal and distal margins of at least 5 cm, along with proper resection of the mesocolon to facilitate lymphadenectomy. An open approach may be necessary if the patient cannot tolerate pneumoperitoneum or if proximal dilation from obstruction hinders abdominal visibility. For unstable patients, an open approach is often preferable as it typically allows for quicker resection and control of contamination or bleeding.

A right colectomy can be performed through an open or minimally invasive approach, usually laparoscopically or robotically, and may involve either a medial or lateral approach. The choice between medial and lateral approaches affects the timing of central artery ligation; it's done before bowel mobilization in the medial approach and typically after mobilization in the lateral approach. In the medial approach, the cecum is elevated toward the right lower quadrant to expose the tethering of the ileocecal artery at its origin. The peritoneum on the mesocolon is then incised, and the ileocolic vessels are isolated while ensuring the identification and protection of the duodenum. Once adequately isolated, the ileocolic artery is ligated at its origin, and the ileocolic pedicle may be ligated at the surgeon's discretion.

Subsequently, the mesocolon is separated from the retroperitoneum, with only the lateral peritoneal and omental attachments remaining. Posterior attachments to the small bowel mesentery are divided to ensure adequate mobility for a tension-free anastomosis. The lateral attachments of the ascending colon are divided towards the hepatic flexure, and the hepaticocolic ligament and hepatic flexure can be mobilized either from the patient's right or by entering the lesser sac at the planned transection site. After complete mobilization, the transverse colon mesentery is divided at the level of the right branch of the middle colic artery, and the small bowel can be divided to the planned proximal margin. The use of a wound protector is recommended to reduce the risk of local recurrence, implantation, and wound infection.

The anastomosis can be performed using either a handsewn or stapled technique, in either an end-to-end or side-to-side configuration. The size discrepancy between the large and small bowel favors a side-to-side anastomosis, which can be done in an isoperistaltic or antiperistaltic fashion. Many surgeons routinely place a "crotch stitch" at the distal corner of the anastomosis to alleviate tension on the staple line.

Open technique in the setting of colorectal oncologic emergency such as perforation, obstruction, or bleeding may provide the most expeditious access to source control for bleeding and perforation and visualization in the setting of a large bowel obstruction. Right colectomy in an open fashion is done through midline laparotomy incision. This also allows a thorough evaluation of the peritoneal cavity.

The lateral approach involves first mobilizing the lateral peritoneal attachments, commonly known as mobilizing the white line of Toldt. The colon and mesocolon are elevated away from the retroperitoneum in the avascular plane. Efforts not to violate the fascia of the mesocolon should be made to ensure its intact excision. The omentum was separated from the transverse colon and once fully mobilized, attention is placed upon the ileocolic pedicle to aid in its identification. Ligation is performed at its origin from the superior mesenteric vessels. The mesentery of the terminal ileum is divided to achieve at least a 5cm margin from the ileocecal valve. The right branch of the middle colic artery is identified by elevating the transverse colon and should be ligated lesions of the right colon. The decision of whether to perform an anastomosis in an oncologic emergency is complex and depends on multiple factors. The patient's overall condition and the degree of abdominal hostility are important considerations. Ileocolonic anastomoses typically have favorable standard leak rates ranging from 1 to 3% [11]. However, creating an ileostomy poses risks for complications such as high output, leakage, prolapse, herniation, mucocutaneous retraction, separation, and ischemia.

In cases of perforation, the morbidity of the septic insult significantly influences short-term outcomes and can also delay the timing of adjuvant therapy, impacting long-term outcomes. Patients may present with either contained or free perforations, both of which result in worse outcomes compared to non-perforated colon cancers. Cheynel et al. compared short- and long-term outcomes for 89 perforated colon cancers and 5462 uncomplicated colon cancers, finding that perforated cancers had higher operative mortality and 5-year local recurrence rates [21]. Surprisingly, the incidence of peritoneal carcinomatosis was twice as high in perforated compared to uncomplicated colon cancers.

In the context of an obstructed right colon mass, the functionality of the ileocecal valve holds significant importance. When dealing with an obstructed right colon cancer and a competent ileocecal valve, special attention should be directed toward the cecum due to the heightened risk of perforation (Fig. 20.1).

However, if the ileocecal valve is incompetent, patients can often be managed temporarily with nasogastric decompression, though eventual intervention becomes necessary.

For unstable patients experiencing colorectal obstruction, perforation, or bleeding, the consideration of damage control surgery arises. The primary objective in such cases is source control, with secondary goals focusing on gastrointestinal reconstruction and delayed abdominal closure, which may be addressed in a subsequent operation. A "second look" operation might be warranted to further address fecal contamination and perform additional washout. Damage control surgery serves to correct acidosis, coagulopathy, and hypothermia before proceeding with definitive surgical management. When a definitive resection isn't immediately feasible due to surgical expertise or other factors, plans for early reintervention should be established.

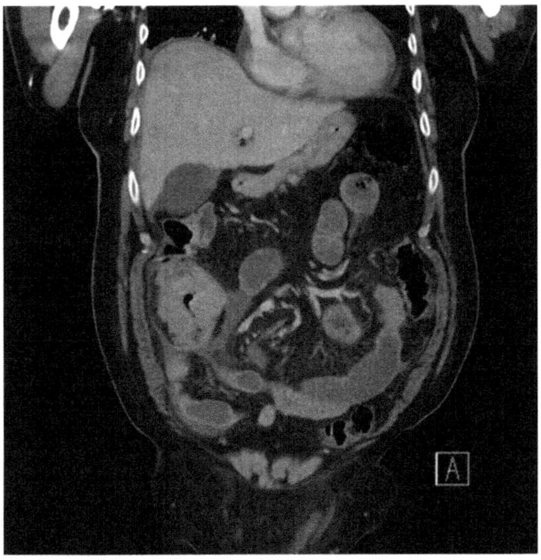

Fig. 20.1 Closed-loop obstruction secondary to obstructing mass of ascending colon with competent ileocecal valve

Various surgical options can be considered for lesions in the transverse colon, including transverse colectomy, extended right or left colectomy, or subtotal colectomy. However, the prevalence of transverse colectomy has been decreasing with the rise of minimally invasive surgery. Additionally, the overall prognosis for transverse colon cancers tends to be less favorable compared to cancers located in other parts of the colon.

In a subtotal colectomy, the right colon and hepatic flexure are mobilized as previously described. The entire lesser sac is opened, and the splenic flexure is mobilized. Ileocolic pedicle ligation is performed, followed by a high ligation of the middle colic artery at its origin from the superior mesenteric artery. The inferior mesenteric vein is isolated and ligated at the inferior border of the pancreas, while preserving the inferior mesenteric artery. Finally, an ileocolic anastomosis is created.

Resection of left-sided colonic malignancies can be approached either medially or laterally. The lateral approach involves mobilizing the sigmoid and descending colon laterally along the white line of Toldt to access the retroperitoneal plane. The colon is then retracted medially to expose the areolar plane between the mesocolon and retroperitoneum. Dissection continues until the sigmoid mesocolon is mobilized to the midline, aiding in the identification of the ureter. Dissection then progresses toward the splenic flexure, with mobilization of the splenic flexure facilitated by posterior mobilization of the mesocolon to the inferior border of the pancreas. Resection of omental adhesions may be neces-

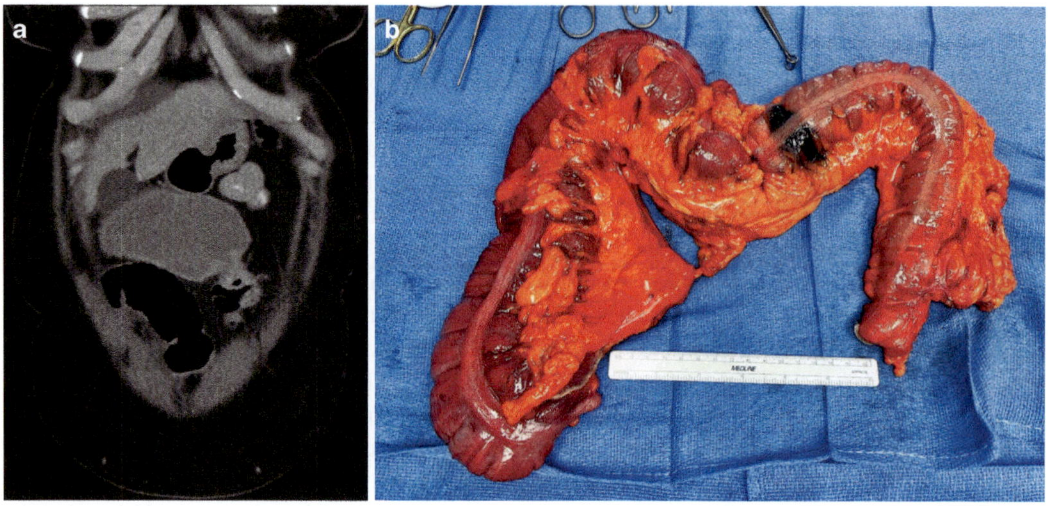

Fig. 20.2 (**a**) Obstructing mid-transverse colon mass, CT image. (**b**) Obstructing mid-transverse colon mass, surgical specimen, high ligation of ileocolic and middle colic vessels

sary to aid in the mobilization of the splenic flexure. The inferior mesenteric artery (IMA) is isolated at its origin from the aorta by creating a window on the superior side of the vessel medial to the inferior mesenteric vein (IMV). The IMA is then ligated after ensuring it has been separated from the left ureter. The IMV can be elevated from the retroperitoneum, isolated, and ligated at the inferior border of the pancreas.

For distal transection, the mesentery is divided at the rectosigmoid junction, identified by the splaying of the tenia. A linear stapler is commonly used for transection of the bowel wall. Careful consideration is given to the creation of an end colostomy, proximal diverting ileostomy, or primary anastomosis. If an anastomosis is fashioned using either a standard transanal end-to-end anastomosis stapler or in a handsewn fashion, a leak test should be performed.

In cases of proximal obstruction, size mismatch can pose challenges. A side-to-end anastomosis can serve as an alternative means for primary anastomosis in such situations. The decision to perform a Hartmann procedure instead of a primary anastomosis should be based on the patient's health, the condition of the bowel, and the level of contamination or inflammation in the pelvis (Fig. 20.2).

A diverting loop ileostomy is warranted to mitigate the potential septic complications of an anastomotic leak in this setting. Deferring primary anastomosis is often the safest option and is generally not criticized.

Rectal Cancer

Managing an acutely complicated rectal cancer is a daunting surgical scenario. The progression and standardization of preoperative staging, strategizing, and multimodal management often necessitate delaying surgical intervention, especially in patients with locally advanced rectal cancer. Even in urgent situations, it is crucial to avoid emergent resection of locally advanced cancers as this could compromise oncological outcomes. Neoadjuvant treatment has now become the gold standard in managing locally advanced rectal malignancies. It not only diminishes tumor size and reduces local recurrence rates but also enhances tumor resection success and sphincter preservation rates (Fig. 20.3) [9].

When faced with an obstructing rectal tumor, diversion is typically the preferred treatment approach. When deciding between an ileostomy and a loop colostomy, several factors need consid-

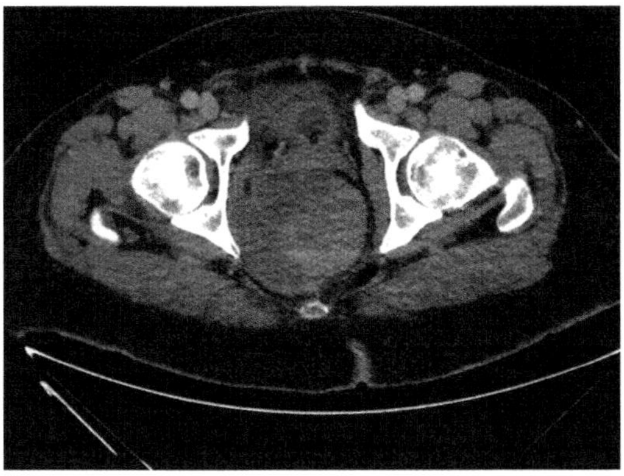

Fig. 20.3 Rectal adenocarcinoma with extraperitoneal perforation

eration, including the competence of the ileocecal valve and the level of obstruction. If the patient is slated for chemotherapy and radiation before formal resection, an ileostomy may be necessary. In cases of an incompetent ileocecal valve, a loop ileostomy is often the optimal choice. Conversely, if there's complete obstruction with a competent ileocecal valve, a loop colostomy is typically favored. If the cecum is nonviable or proximal perforation due to distal obstruction exists, a resection with an end stoma and mucous fistula is indicated. In distal obstruction cases, an end colostomy alone could lead to distal segment blowout. While self-expandable stents are reasonable for proximal lesions, rectal stenting is usually avoided due to potential complications like pain, tenesmus, incontinence, and stent migration. Placing a stent near the dentate line in distal rectal lesions could irritate the squamous columnar junction and should be avoided [22].

A bleeding locally advanced rectal tumor may pose challenges for excision compared to a similar lesion located more proximally. Therefore, alternative treatment avenues need to be explored. Given that distal lesions are more accessible via colonoscopic methods, endoscopic interventions like clipping and tumor fulguration become viable options. Additionally, radiofrequency ablation, utilizing a transanal endoscopic approach, has been noted as an alternative method for achieving hemostasis in cases of bleeding rectal malignancies [23]. Moreover, the extensive collateralization in the rectum enables the identification of bleeding sites for angioembolization. Furthermore, due to its fixed location within the pelvis, the tumor can serve as a stable target for therapeutic, and sometimes palliative, radiation. Systematic reviews have indicated pooled response rates of 81% in managing bleeding and discharge with the use of palliative external beam radiotherapy [24].

The most challenging scenario undoubtedly arises in the case of a perforated rectal cancer. While an extraperitoneal perforation can be managed through diversion followed by chemoradiotherapy, leading to definitive resection, a mid-rectal cancer with proximal extension and intraperitoneal perforation often necessitates swift action. In such cases, diversion alone insufficiently controls contamination, making resection the only viable option. Oncologic resection of the rectal malignancy entails ligating the superior rectal artery and dissecting in the total mesorectal excision (TME) plane. The objective is to achieve a margin of 5 cm for proximal rectal lesions, though margins of 2 cm or even down to 1 cm are acceptable for more distal lesions. Every effort should be made to achieve an R0 resection, which may involve multivisceral resection and could be unattainable without compromising oncologic outcomes. Given the hostile setting, anastomosis should be avoided in these circumstances.

Colonic Stenting

For managing obstructive colon lesions, the use of a self-expanding colonic stent may be considered for suitable patients. However, colonic stenting is not recommended for patients exhibiting signs of perforation, septic shock, hemodynamic instability, or peritonitis. This intervention can serve as a bridge to surgery or in a palliative context, allowing for a full bowel preparation and potentially enabling a primary anastomosis.

In a comparison of long-term outcomes, the patency rate at 18 months was 65.8% for patients undergoing colonic stenting, whereas it was 90.5% for those who underwent stoma creation [25]. A Dutch randomized controlled trial comparing stenting with resection for near-obstructing metastatic colon cancer was halted due to high perforation rates in the stenting group [26]. Unfortunately, the success rates in managing malignant extracolonic obstruction vary widely, and complication rates in such cases are significantly higher compared to primary colorectal cancer patients.

Several studies have highlighted the effectiveness of stenting as a temporary measure before definitive resection in patients with acute obstruction. It is generally advisable to wait for at least 10 days before proceeding with surgery, as this approach has been associated with lower laparoscopic conversion and leak rates, thus enhancing the feasibility of single-staged operations [27, 28].

Additionally, stenting facilitates a comprehensive evaluation of the remaining colon for synchronous lesions. Although experienced centers are increasingly employing colonic stents for more proximal cancers, caution is warranted, as this may pose technical challenges and increase the risk of perforation or stent failure in less experienced hands. Furthermore, stent placement should be avoided in patients who may require bevacizumab in the perioperative period, as it significantly elevates the risk of stent-related perforation compared to baseline populations.

Self-expanding colonic stents may be an option for managing obstructive colon lesions in some patients, providing a temporary remedy before surgery or in a palliative setting. Nonetheless, caution should be exercised as there is decreased utility in patients with extracolonic obstruction. Patients undergoing stenting should be monitored closely as insufflation in the setting of obstruction may lead to cecal perforation. Despite being effective in specific scenarios, meticulous patient selection and procedural proficiency are imperative to reduce risks and enhance outcomes.

While colonic stenting offers valuable benefits in certain cases of obstructive colon lesions, careful patient selection and procedural considerations are essential to minimize risks and optimize outcomes. Collaboration between multidisciplinary teams and adherence to established guidelines can aid in the safe and effective implementation of this intervention.

The effective management of acute complications of colon and rectal cancer often hinges upon multiple factors. It requires prompt action while ensuring that the patient's long-term oncologic prognosis is not compromised. Seeking assistance from consultants and experienced surgeons can greatly benefit the patient. Operative risk and surgical complications may ultimately result in delays in anticancer therapies and impact the overall prognosis.

References

1. Colorectal Cancer Statistics. How common is colorectal cancer? Retrieved March 18, 2024, from https://www.cancer.org/cancer/types/colon-rectal-cancer/about/key-statistics.html. Sung H, Ferlay J, Siegel RL, et al. Global cancer statistics 2020: globocan estimates of incidence and mortality worldwide for 36 cancers in 185 countries. CA Cancer J Clin. 2021;71(3):209–249.
2. Lin JS, Perdue LA, Henrikson NB, Bean SI, Blasi PR. Screening for colorectal cancer: updated evidence report and systematic review for the US preventive services task force. JAMA. 2021;325(19):1978.
3. Golder AM, McMillan DC, Horgan PG, Roxburgh CSD. Determinants of emergency presentation in patients with colorectal cancer: a systematic review and meta-analysis. Sci Rep. 2022;12(1):4366.
4. Smothers L, Hynan L, Fleming J, Turnage R, Simmang C, Anthony T. Emergency surgery for colon carcinoma. Dis Colon Rectum. 2003;46(1):24–30.
5. McArdle CS, Hole DJ. Emergency presentation of colorectal cancer is associated with poor 5-year survival. Br J Surg. 2004;91(5):605–9.
6. Lam AKY, Chan SSY, Leung M. Synchronous colorectal cancer: clinical, pathological and molecular implications. World J Gastroenterol. 2014;20(22):6815–20.
7. NCCN Clinical Practice Guidelines in Oncology – Colon Cancer; National Comprehensive Cancer Network. Retrieved March 21, 2024, from https://www.nccn.org/professionals/physician_gls/pdf/colon.pdf
8. Phang PT, MacFarlane JK, Taylor RH, et al. Effect of emergent presentation on outcome from rectal cancer management. Am J Surg. 2003;185(5):450–4.
9. Li Y, Wang J, Ma X, et al. A review of neoadjuvant chemoradiotherapy for locally advanced rectal cancer. Int J Biol Sci. 2016;12(8):1022–31.

10. Krarup PM, Nordholm-Carstensen A, Jorgensen LN, Harling H. Anastomotic leak increases distant recurrence and long-term mortality after curative resection for colonic cancer: a nationwide cohort study. Ann Surg. 2014;259(5):930–8.
11. Ellis CT, Maykel JA. Defining anastomotic leak and the clinical relevance of leaks. Clin Colon Rectal Surg. 2021;34(6):359–65.
12. Hsu MY, Lin JP, Hsu HH, Lai HL, Wu YL. Preoperative stoma site marking decreases stoma and peristomal complications: a meta-analysis. J Wound Ostomy Continence Nurs. 2020;47(3):249–56.
13. Wocn society, aua, and ascrs position statement on preoperative stoma site marking for patients undergoing ostomy surgery. J Wound Ostomy Continence Nurs. 2021;48(6):533–6.
14. Whitehead A, Cataldo PA. Technical considerations in stoma creation. Clin Colon Rectal Surg. 2017;30(3):162–71.
15. Horwood J, Hay D. The "glove cuff" technique for difficult stomas. Ann R Coll Surg Engl. 2009;91(5):438.
16. Meagher AP, Owen G, Gett R. Multimedia article. An improved technique for end stoma creation in obese patients. Dis Colon Rectum. 2009;52(3):531–3.
17. Du R, Zhou J, Wang F, et al. Whether stoma support rods have application value in loop enterostomy: a systematic review and meta-analysis. World J Surg Oncol. 2020;18(1):269.
18. Davis BR, Valente MA, Goldberg JE, et al. The American society of colon and rectal surgeons clinical practice guidelines for ostomy surgery. Dis Colon Rectum. 2022;65(10):1173–90.
19. Rørvig S, Schlesinger N, Mårtensson NL, Engel S, Engel U, Holck S. Is the longitudinal margin of carcinoma-bearing colon resections a neglected parameter? Clin Colorectal Cancer. 2014;13(1):68–72.
20. Steele SR, Hull TL, Hyman N, Maykel JA, Read TE, Whitlow CB. The ASCRS textbook of colon and rectal surgery. Springer Nature; 2021.
21. Cheynel N, Cortet M, Lepage C, Ortega-Debalon P, Faivre J, Bouvier AM. Incidence, patterns of failure, and prognosis of perforated colorectal cancers in a well-defined population. Dis Colon Rectum. 2009;52(3):406–11.
22. Ribeiro IB, de Moura DTH, Thompson CC, de Moura EGH. Acute abdominal obstruction: colon stent or emergency surgery? An evidence-based review. World J Gastrointest Endosc. 2019;11(3):193–208.
23. Vavra P, Dostalik J, Zacharoulis D, Khorsandi SE, Khan SA, Habib NA. Endoscopic radiofrequency ablation in colorectal cancer: initial clinical results of a new bipolar radiofrequency ablation device. Dis Colon Rectum. 2009;52(2):355–8.
24. Cameron MG, Kersten C, Vistad I, Fosså S, Guren MG. Palliative pelvic radiotherapy of symptomatic incurable rectal cancer – a systematic review. Acta Oncol. 2014;53(2):164–73.
25. Pattarajierapan S, Manomayangoon C, Tipsuwannakul P, Khomvilai S. Comparison of colonic stenting and stoma creation as palliative treatment for incurable malignant colonic obstruction. JGH Open. 2022;6(9):630–6.
26. Van Hooft JE, Bemelman WA, Oldenburg B, et al. Colonic stenting versus emergency surgery for acute left-sided malignant colonic obstruction: a multicenter randomized trial. Lancet Oncol. 2011;12:344–52.
27. Cui J, Zhang JL, Wang S, Sun ZQ, Jiang XL. A preliminary study of stenting followed by laparoscopic surgery for obstructing left-sided colon cancer. Zhonghua Wei Chang Wai Ke Za Zhi. 2011;14(1):40–3.
28. Lee GJ, Kim HJ, Baek JH, Lee WS, Kwon KA. Comparison of short-term outcomes after elective surgery following endoscopic stent insertion and emergency surgery for obstructive colorectal cancer. Int J Surg. 2013;11(6):442–6.

21 Surgical Decision-Making in Vascular Surgery: Practical Approaches to New Innovative Techniques and Revisiting Old Ones

Igor A. Laskowski, Sateesh Babu, Daniel Ventarola, Heepeel Chang, Arun Goyal, Joseph Fulton, and Rifat Latifi

Introduction

The art and the science development of surgery and the surgical decision-making have changed drastically and radically from many points of view, but most noticeably in vascular surgery from training of vascular surgeons, technical approaches to the same diseases that we have been looking after for decades, their overall management, and the surgical decision-making requiring into navigating the complexities of treating a diverse array of vascular conditions. There has been a considerable progress in the treatment of vascular pathology and thus major changes in decision-making in carotid disease [1–3], non-traumatic aortic dissection that expands with time [4–6], and traumatic aortic injuries previously deadly or with very high morbidity have been seem [7–11].

In addition, major progress has been made in the management of peripheral vascular disease as well [12–14]. The evaluation of patients requiring access for arteriovenous hemodialysis is one of the most common vascular procedures performed [15–17]. The management of venous disease management [18–20] will not be discussed in this chapter. However, we will discuss a rare but an important clinical entity that is the May-Thurner syndrome.

By exploring these specific clinical scenarios, we aim to illuminate the nuanced considerations, diagnostic challenges, and treatment options that vascular surgeons must navigate to deliver optimal care and achieve favorable outcomes for their patients.

The decision-making process in carotid surgery involves assessing the risk-benefit profile of carotid endarterectomy versus carotid artery stenting for the management of carotid artery disease. Factors such as patient comorbidities, lesion characteristics, and individualized risk assessment, and finally surgeon's and institutional

I. A. Laskowski (✉) · S. Babu · D. Ventarola · A. Goyal · J. Fulton
Vascular Section of the Department of Surgery, Westchester Medical Center, Valhalla, NY, USA

New York Medical College, Valhalla, NY, USA
e-mail: Igor.Laskowski@wmchealth.org; Sateesh.Babu@wmchealth.org; Daniel.Ventarola@wmchealth.org; Arun.Goyal@wmchealth.org; Joseph.Fulton@wmchealth.org

H. Chang
Westchester Medical Center, Valhalla, NY, USA
e-mail: Heepeel.Chang@wmchealth.org

R. Latifi
Department of Surgery, The University of Arizona, Tucson, AZ, USA

Tucson Medical Center, Department of Surgery, Tucson, AZ, USA
e-mail: Latifi@surgery.arizona.edu

R. Latifi (ed.), *Surgical Decision-Making*, https://doi.org/10.1007/978-3-031-67391-7_21

expertise play a pivotal role in determining the most appropriate treatment strategy to reduce the risk of stroke and improve long-term vascular health.

In aortic surgery, the decision-making process has changed dramatically from open surgery to minimally invasive -endovascular surgical approaches. This includes the evaluation of aortic aneurysms, dissections, and other complex aortic pathologies. In these conditions the surgical decision-making depends on the size, location, and morphology of the aortic lesion, as well as the patient's overall health status, to determine the most optimal timing and type of intervention, whether it be open surgical, endovascular, or hybrid procedures.

Peripheral vascular surgery presents unique challenges in decision-making, particularly in the context of peripheral arterial disease, critical limb ischemia, and venous insufficiency. The surgical decision-making must balance the goals of revascularization, limb salvage opportunity, and pain relief. All these require a comprehensive assessment of the patient's vascular anatomy, functional status, and quality of life considerations to tailor the most appropriate treatment approach for each individual. Furthermore, the evaluation of patients requiring access for hemodialysis as one of the most common vascular accesses in patients with kidney failure requires a very focused, individualized and patient centered surgical decision-making.

Modern Management of Acute Aortic Dissection

Acute aortic dissection (AAD) is an uncommon but potentially catastrophic condition that requires prompt intervention to assure patient survival. The AAD is defined as separation of the aortic wall due to a degenerative process of the media layer that results in formation of two separate lumens that may span the entire length of the aorta and beyond Fig. 21.1.

Two different clinical presentations that follow clinically distinct management pathways are known.

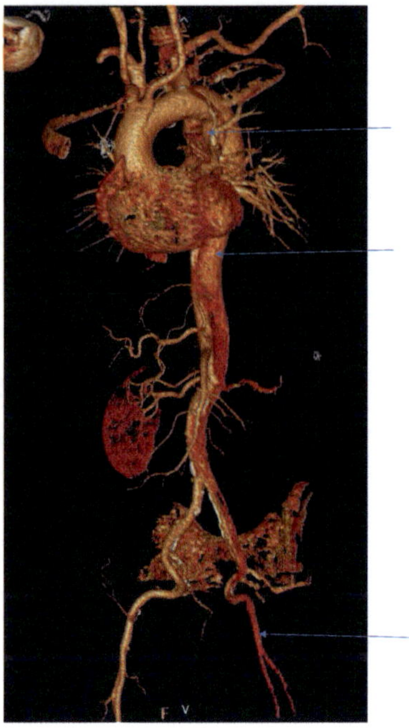

Fig. 21.1 Aortic dissection can extent from aortic arch and into femoral vessel

*Acute Stanford Type A dissection (DeBakey type 1 and 2 and Stanford Type A **)* (Figs. 21.2 and 21.3) involves the ascending part of the aorta with or without distal extension and is considered a surgical emergency. If untreated, patient mortality may be as high as 50% in 24 h from presentation. In addition, the involvement of aortic arch in dissection adds to the complexity of the management especially with regard to the need for and timing of the arch repair.

Acute Type B aortic dissection (aTBAD) (Figs. 21.2 and 21.4) involves descending part of the aorta and can be either an isolated occurrence without ascending aortic inclusion or as a residual dissection remaining after previous Type A repair. TBAD rarely presents as a true surgical emergency however in cases of malperfusion or frank aortic rupture emergent intervention should be considered.

Historically, main therapy for uncomplicated aTBAD without aortic rupture or end-organ malperfusion was medically aimed at blood pressure optimization with impulse control and close observation. However, medical management was shown to have up to 10% 30-day mortality and was asso-

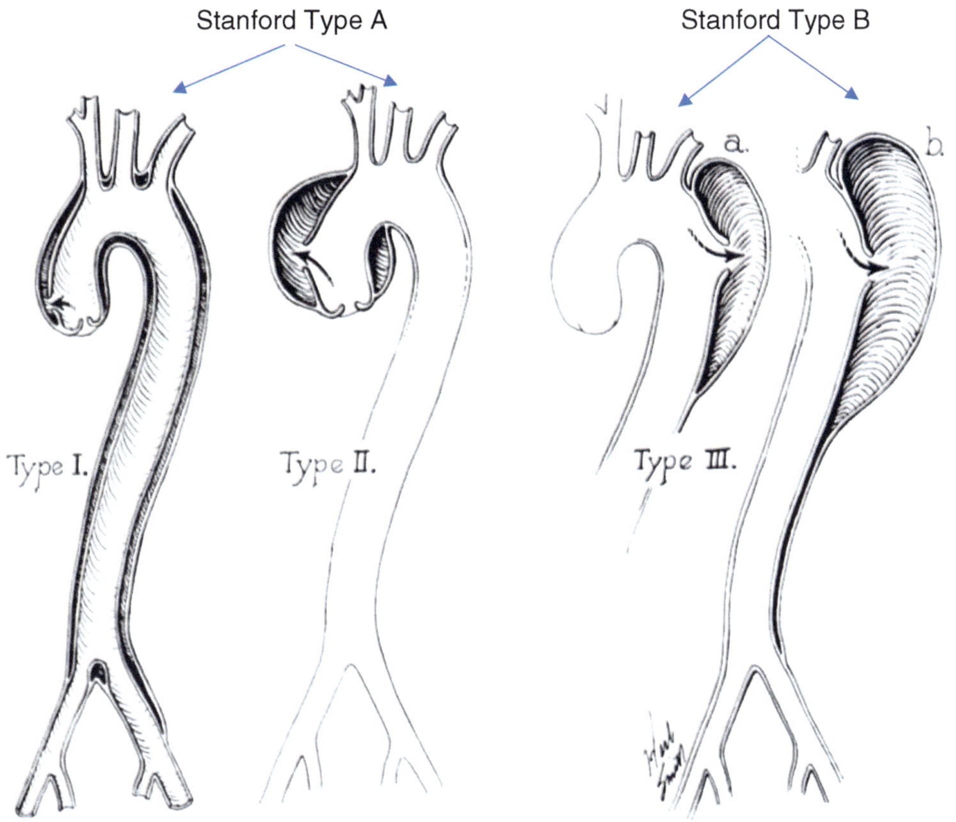

Fig. 21.2 DeBakey and Stanford aortic dissection classification**

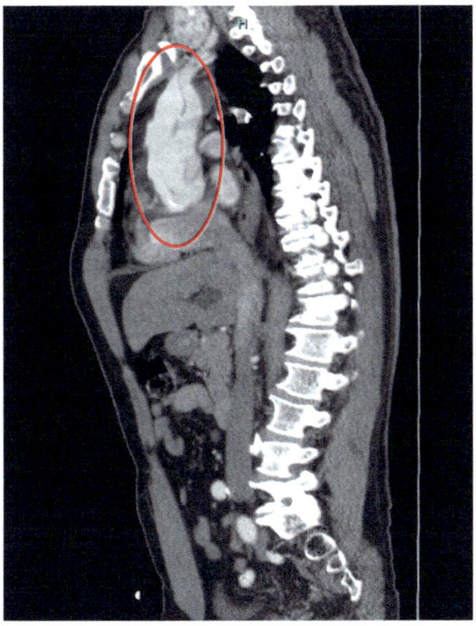

Fig. 21.3 Type A aortic dissection

ciated with a need for surgical interventions for aortic-related morbidity. In turn, any future aortic interventions following episode of TBAD were related to worse patient survival [21, 22].

With wide adaptation of endovascular therapies, thoracic endovascular aortic repair (TEVAR) for complicated and subsequently TBAD with high-risk anatomic features has been proposed and used with some success. The initial approach to dissection stenting was to cover the primary entry tear usually located in the very proximal descending thoracic aorta. The idea and hope behind this approach were to induce false lumen thrombosis once the entry tears were excluded. Because of the fact that more distal aortic reentry tears usually exist, this technique was found to be quite ineffective and persistent false lumen flow was present in up to 80% of patients [23]. In turn ongoing false lumen patency and pressurization can be directly related to the enlargement of aortic diameter in up to 50% of cases and may result in late aneurysmal aortic degeneration and rupture [24]. Additionally, it has been shown that presence of patent and partially thrombosed false lumens almost always leads to aortic diameter enlargement that at times may be very rapid specifically putting this patient population at even greater risk of failure after proximal TEVAR for TBAD [25]. Secondary tears have been frequently found in the paravisceral aortic segment where limitations of stent technology disallowed successful false lumen exclusion because of possibility of gut ischemia.

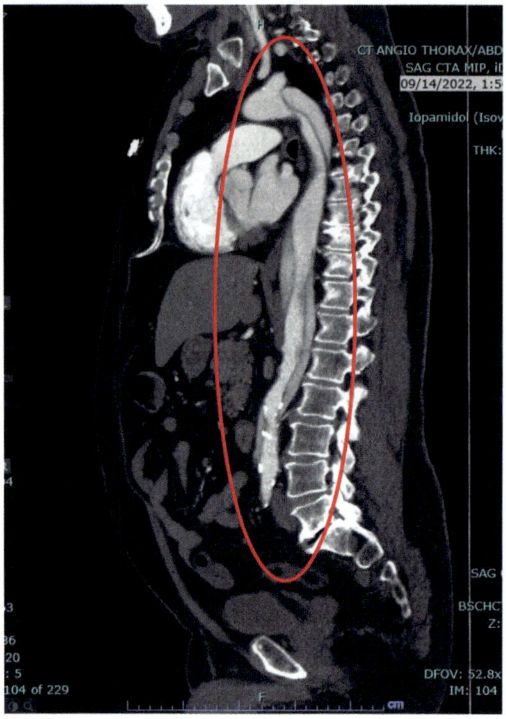

Fig. 21.4 Type B aortic dissection

Considering these obvious disadvantages of proximal tear only coverage an aortic dissection bare stent system graft (Cook Medical, Bloomington, IN) was introduced with the idea that it can be deployed in the paravisceral segment of the dissected aorta (Fig. 21.5). The combination with covered stent is known as dissection stent system and has been used in the attempt to increase true lumen of dissected aorta in the technique known as PETICOAT (provisional extension to induce complete attachment) [26, 27]. Unfortunately, the results of such repairs, again, showed high rate of false lumen flow, negative aortic remodeling, and presence of aneurysmal aortic degeneration in up to 63% of treated subjects in late period. This in turn lead to a significant number of secondary interventions including late open conversions when thoracoabdominal aneurysmal degeneration occurred (Fig. 21.6) [28, 29].

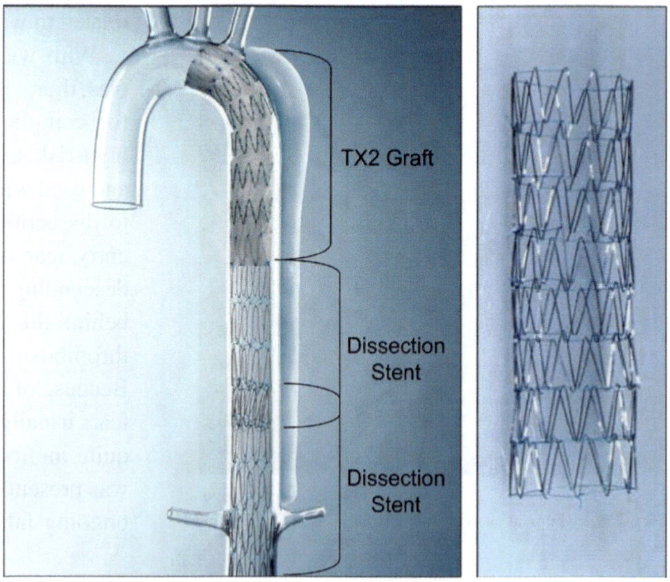

Fig. 21.5 Aortic dissection stent system

In order to address false lumen (FL) flow still present in patients with PETTICOAT, another step was added to the treatment algorithm. It involves angioplasty of the stented aortic segment with a large volume-low pressure balloon appropriately sized to the diameter of the aorta at the given segment. This approach if performed successfully allows for immediate re-lamination of the dissection flap in the position of outer aortic wall that is held in place by previously deployed stent. The procedure is known as STABILISE-stent-assisted balloon-induced intimal disruption and re-lamination in aortic dissection repair and was first described by Hofferberth [30] (Fig. 21.7).

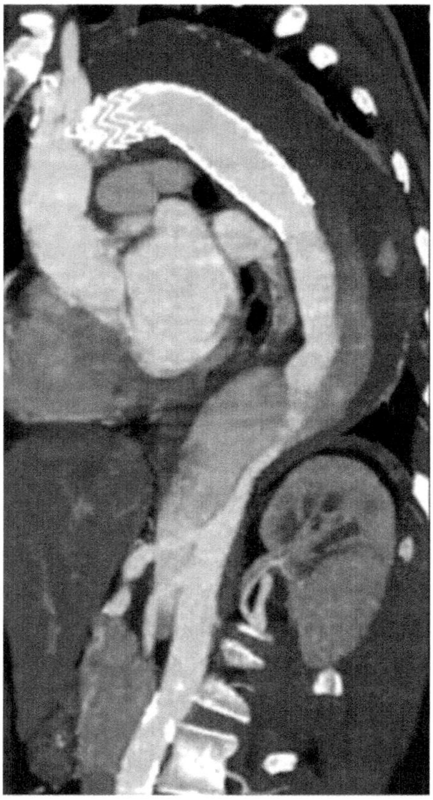

Fig. 21.6 Chronic postdissection TAAA following TEVAR for acute TBAD

Although this technique creates an immediate single aortic channel, concerns for aortic rupture and catastrophic failure exist. In the next part of this chapter, we will describe our institutional application of STABILISE technique in patients with acute and subacute TBAD that we feel provide save and durable outcome for this patient population.

Surgical Technique:

First step of evaluation and diagnosis of TBAD is based on imaging that is usually available before patient's arrival given the regional referral center role that our institution serves. If type A dissection is confirmed, an emergent open repair by the cardiothoracic part of our team is performed and decision for treatment of residual TBAD is made in the postoperative period during the same admission. Aortic measurements of true, false, and total aortic lumen and all aortic levels are obtained (Fig. 21.8).

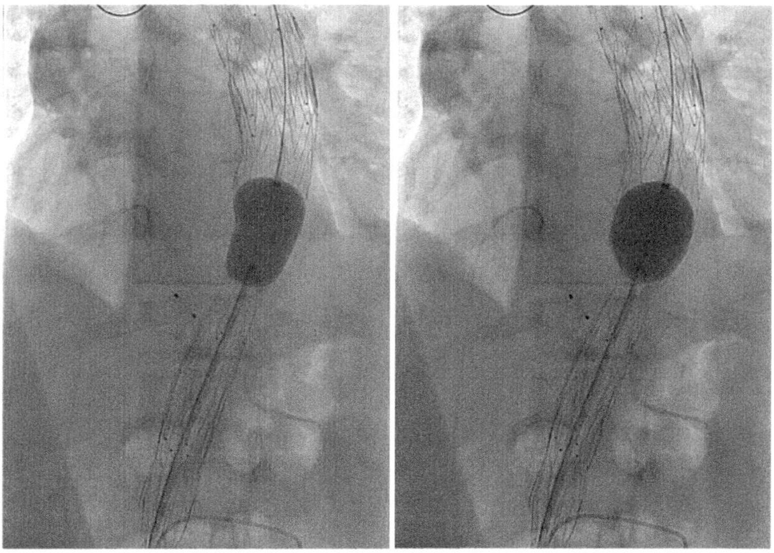

Fig. 21.7 Aortic angioplasty for immediate aortic remodeling in STABLIZE technique

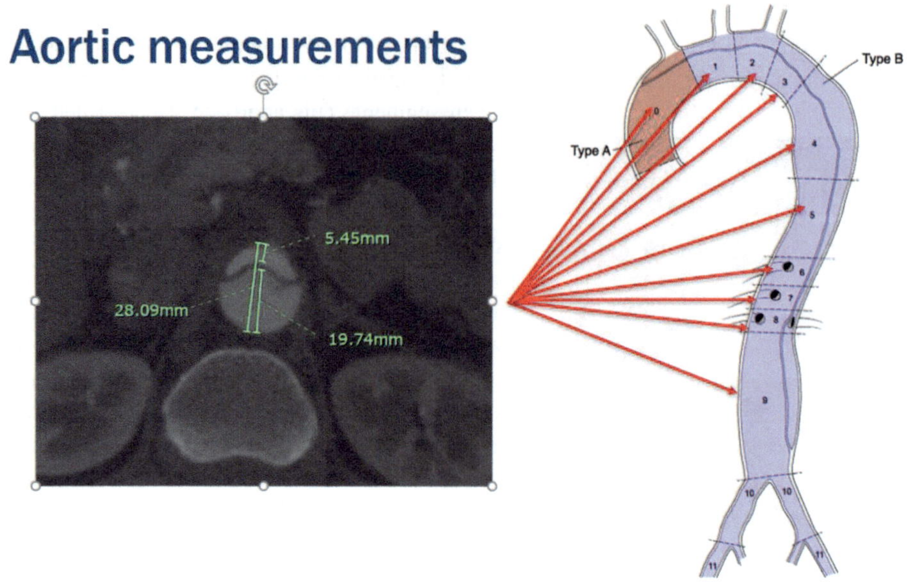

Fig. 21.8 Example of aortic measurement of TL and FL in the dissected aortic segment

All TBAD patients are admitted to the intensive care unit for initial management and necessary evaluation. If additional better-quality imaging is required prompt thin cut contrast enhanced computed tomography of the thorax, abdomen and pelvis (CTA) is performed. If absolute contraindications to iodinated contrast exist, Magnetic Resonance Angiography (MRA)may be utilized for further anatomic evaluation.

When isolated TBAD with organ malperfusion is present, an emergent repair using endovascular options is considered as the first line of therapy. In cases of frank aortic rupture, patients either undergo emergent open repair or multidisciplinary approach by vascular and cardiothoracic senior team members used to evaluate endovascular options and formulate treatment plan.

For patients with non-complicated, high risk features dissection with presence of two lumens, immediate medical management with blood pressure and impulse control is implemented. High risks feature TBAD is defined in cases when total aortic lumen is >40 mm, false lumen >22 mm, proximal aortic tear >10 mm, there is presence of ongoing chest pain regardless of blood pressure control, history of poor compliance with medical management of hypertension, and evidence of organ malperfusion on imaging [31]. Following qualification for surgical intervention timing of repair is defined as hyperacute when treated within first 24 h of presentation, acute-days 1–14 and subacute for those treated between day 15 and 90th day of presentation. Majority of our patients undergo repair during acute phase for isolated TBAD, and subacute for the residual dissection following TAD repair.

Imaging: CTA, MRI, TEE

All patients undergo baseline imaging evaluation that consisted of computed tomography angiography (CTA) with multiplanar reconstruction or gadolinium-enhanced magnetic resonance angiography when needed. Interprocedurally, all patients undergo transesophageal echocardiography for baseline assessment of aortic arch and ascending and proximal descending aorta for evaluation of a possibility of retrograde Type A dissection, new pericardial effusion, or any other acute changes.

Morphologic Aortic Assessment

Preoperative imaging was used for morphologic assessment of the entire aorta with assessment of aortic false lumen patency status, aortic arch involvement, and proximity to left subclavian artery, patency of aortic branch vessels with determination of the take-off from true or false lumen, and degree and symmetry of end-organ perfusion. Femoral access is evaluated in detail with particular attention to the extent of dissection and patency and diameter of iliac arteries, quality and diameter of femoral arteries with potential involvement in dissection, presence of atherosclerotic disease, and the level of femoral bifurcations bilaterally. This is especially important since we routinely use preclose technique with Perclose, Proglide devices (Abbott Cardiovascular Systems, IL, USA).

Preoperative Planning and Aortic Dissection

As a first step of preoperative planning of aortic dissection, we assess proximal extent of the dissection based on Ishimaru Zones. We always want to select aortic segment free of pathology as close to 2 cm in length for the proximal landing zone of the aortic stent graft. For elective cases, we attempt to preserve flow into left subclavian artery that is achieved by either revascularization with carotid to subclavian bypass grafting or with the use of Thoracic Branch Endograft (Gore and Ass, Flagstaff, AZ, USA). In all cases of FL visceral branch origin, we protect the branch vessels with a Glide Wire or end lumen catheter during distal aortic stenting with subsequent branch vessel patency and adjunct branch vessel stenting as needed (Fig. 21.8).

Technique

We perform all aortic dissection cases under general anesthesia in the hybrid operating room with the use of digital subtraction angiography. All patients undergo neuromonitoring with somatosensory evoked potential (SSEP) and motor evoked potential (MEP) throughout the case. We do not use cerebrospinal fluid drainage on routine basis. Bilateral ultrasound-guided percutaneous access with use of preclose Perclose ProGlide system technique is applied for the main device delivery. If ilio-femoral dissection is present, preferentially the non-dissected side is used for the device deployment. For initial vascular access, a Bentson wire (Boston Scientific, Marlborough, MA, USA) with 100 cm Pig tail catheter (Cook Medical) support is advance to ascending aorta with subsequent exchange for a 300 cm double curve Lunderquist® extra-stiff wire (Cook Medical). Contralateral diagnostic Pigtail catheter is advanced in a similar fashion and positioned in the ascending aorta. Femoral venous access is routinely established for temporary percutaneous pacing wires that are placed in the right ventricle. They are used for rapid cardiac pacing during stent deployment and during aortic angioplasty with rate set to 180 to 200 bpm. In the next step, aortic arch angiogram is performed and using information from the preoperative CTA, intraoperative confirmation of the position of arch vessels is made and final level of the proximal deployment of the first stent is selected. In cases where L SCA is involved and when GORE Thoracic Branch Endograft (TBE) is used, we obtain additional through and through wire access from the left wrist and out of the large sheath of the main device delivery as per Gore device IFU. In all other cases, our to go to device is Zenith TX2 when deployed into the native aorta or Zenith Alpha (Cook Medical) covered stents when deployment is into preexisting Dacron graft of either ascending aortic repair or an elephant trunk repair. For all cases requiring left SCA coverage that do not meet anatomic criteria for TBE, we perform carotid -to-subclavian bypass usually a day or two prior to the aortic stenting procedure.

Once proximal stent graft is in place, we continue to deploy covered stents to the level just proximal to celiac trunk. We do that to assure that all secondary tears of the aortic dissection flap are excluded as distally as possible. In our experience, this prevents ongoing false lumen flow that may lead to early repair failure. Once all covered stents are in place, we proceed with Zenith Dissection uncovered stents deployment in the remaining abdominal aorta all the way to the level of iliac bifurcation. At this point for those patients that Petticoat approach is intended, this completes the procedure.

Since in our experience, STABILISE technique has excellent outcomes we attempt it in all patients with TBAD that meet anatomic criteria of aortic diameters. We use modified criteria first established by Melissano and his group [32].

That part of the procedure is performed with a 46 mm Coda molding balloon (Cook), and the entire stented segment of the aorta to the infrarenal segment is angioplastied while rapid cardiac pacing is employed (Fig. 21.7). The goal is to dilate true aortic lumen to the total aortic diameter as per measurements from the preoperative imaging. In the next step, we perform confirmatory intravascular ultrasound of the entire aorta to determine presence of residual false lumen and we repeat aortic angioplasty at these levels until false lumen obliteration was achieved.

We routinely employ wire protection of all aortic branch vessels that come off the false lumen during aortic angioplasty (Fig. 21.9).

After intervention patients are observed in the intensive care unit with routine neurovascular checks and to maintain mean arterial pressures in the 90–100 mmHg range for first 72 h. Patients are on standard DVT prophylaxis, and antiplatelet regimen with aspiring 81 mg daily is implemented in those cases where TBED or adjunct branch vessel stenting was performed.

Patient undergo repeat CTA chest abdomen and pelvis evaluation before discharge to assess aortic remodeling results with particular attention to false, true and total lumen diameters, false lumen flow, and presence of endoleaks, type A retrograde dissection, and all organ perfusion.

To date, over 30 patients were treated using this approach with no intraoperative mortality and no aortic rupture in the course of aortic molding balloon. When compared to Petticoat, STABILISE technique achieved significantly smaller false lumen diameter and resultant abrogation of false lumen flow on follow-up imaging (Fig. 21.10). In addition, we did not observe retrograde type A dissection, open conversion, and new aortic branch vessel compromise or occlusion. We also did not observe neurologic complications both during the intervention and in the postoperative period. Realizing that more studies are needed to fully evaluate this approach, we feel that our treatment algorithm allows therapeutic options for patients with this challenging condition.

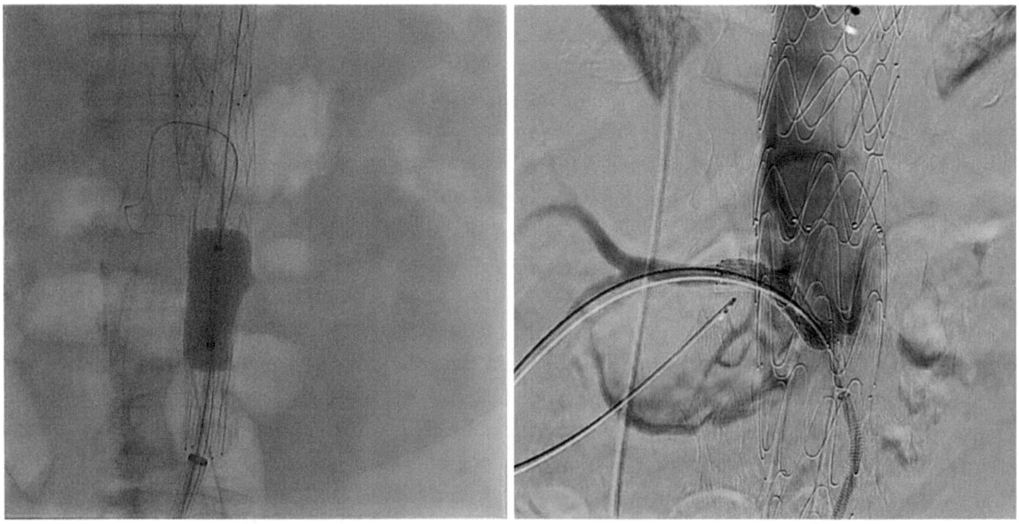

Fig. 21.9 Branch vessel wire protection and stenting after completion of aortic remodeling

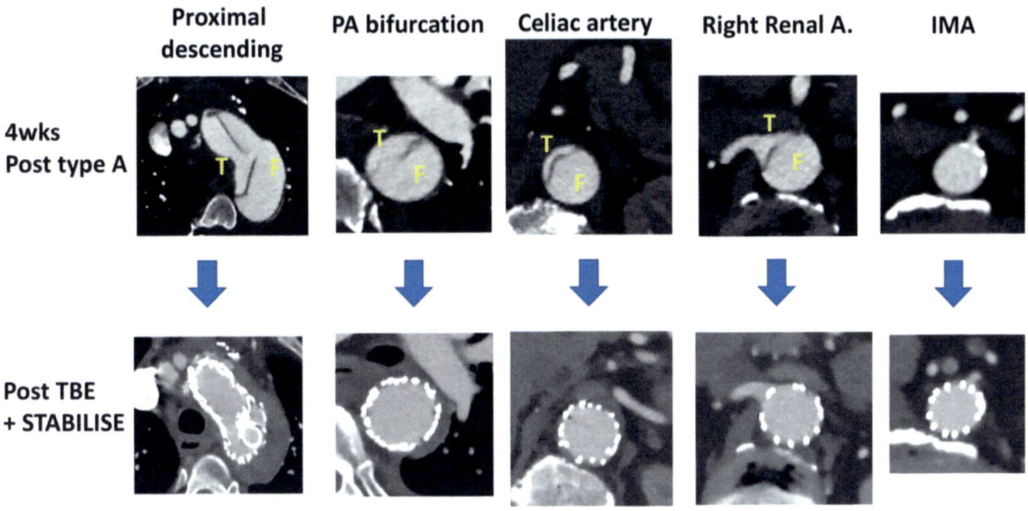

Fig. 21.10 Aortic remodeling after STABILISE technique on pre- and postoperative CTA imaging

Carotid Endarterectomy—Can We Make a Good Operation Better? Technical Considerations

Introduction

In the year 1913, James Ramsey Hunt, a young neurology attending from Columbia University presented a paper at the New York Academy of Medicine highlighting the role of carotid arteries in the causation of stroke [33]. Till that time, it was believed that stroke was essentially an intracranial pathology—hemorrhage, thrombosis, or tumor. Based on autopsy studies of brain and neck, Ramsey Hunt linked extracranial carotid artery disease to intracranial pathology. Miller Fisher, a Canadian neuropathologist who later headed the department in Harvard coined the term TIA (Transient Ischemic Attack) and furthered our understanding of stroke disorders. He postulated that one day, surgeons may be able to remove the "offending plaque." He also explained the mechanism of stroke in atrial fibrillation (cardioembolic). Egas Moniz from Portugal developed cerebral angiography making it possible to visualize the extracranial arteries and the intracranial vascular system. By late 1940s and early 1950s, the medical community became aware of the significance of carotid disease, there was angiography to confirm and visualize the disease, but there was uncertainty about how to treat this. Historically, Eastcott, Pickering, and Rob are credited to have done the first published carotid surgery in Saint Mary's Hospital in London in 1954 on a woman with carotid stenosis and TIA [34]. It is now confirmed that a surgeon in Argentina Raul Carrea performed in 1951 [35]. (Technically, the procedure was carotid artery reconstruction. Michael DeBakey performed carotid endarterectomy (CEA) in 1953, but did not publish it till much later) (Fig. 21.11) [37].

By 1980s, CEA became one of the most common procedures done in United States reaching 180,000 operations per year. Like so many other procedures in history of medicine, the results varied greatly from less than 3% stroke rate in some institutions to greater than 20% in some. This got the attention of media, causing public uproar. That was the force behind two large NIH sponsored studies here in US (NASCET—North American Symptomatic Carotid Endarterectomy Trial and ACAS—Atherosclerosis Carotid Artery Study) and almost similar study in Europe [38]. The conclusion of all three trials indicated

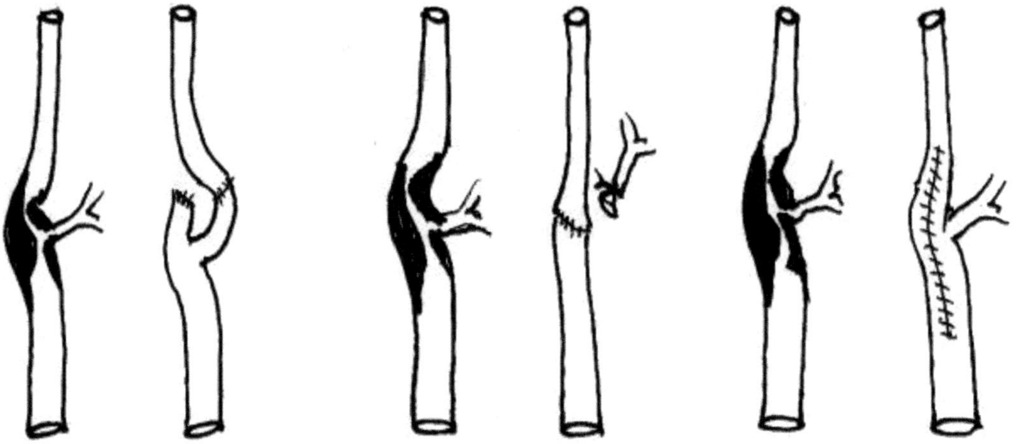

Fig. 21.11 Carotid endarterectomy techniques—historical perspective

that CEA is indicated in symptomatic patients a with hemodynamically significant carotid stenosis, provided the operation is performed with combined stroke and mortality rates of 3–5%. The neurologic community and surgeons were now held to a high standard of care, very much similar to cardiac surgeons doing CABG and transplant surgeons doing kidney transplantation. This was the beginning of accountability and a sort of code of conduct for the surgeons which also standardized the management of carotid disease—screening, diagnosis, indications, and expected outcomes.

The Operation

Carotid endarterectomy is a procedure which requires high technical skill as well as an understanding of brain physiology. This is an operation that has to be done technically perfect and physiologically right. The surgical team concept where every individual has the assigned role including the anesthesiologist, neuromonitoring personnel, circulating and the scrub nurse, the surgeon and his assistant—all doing work in synchrony. The postoperative care is as important as the surgery itself. Creation of clinical pathway (Carotid pathway) further streamlines the postoperative care by the PACU nurses who are knowledgeable about certain unique features of carotid surgery. For instance, hypotension calls for starting a pressor and not fluid bolus (as required in almost all other surgery cases). Similarly, the nursing staff should be aware of the significance of neck hematoma or hoarseness, laryngeal stridor, or new neurologic deficit, all of which require escalation of care and urgent intervention.

Regarding the conduct of surgery itself, some pointers are worth noting. Regarding type of anesthesia, whether regional or general has been looked at, extensively. There is no difference in outcome between those who use general anesthesia and those who use regional cervical block. It comes down to individual surgeon's preference, and the capability of anesthesia team to give a good regional block. Irrespective of the type of anesthesia, the conduct of operation requires, that in addition to doing a complete endarterectomy, a) there is adequate brain perfusion at all times and b) attention to technical steps to prevent embolization of atheromatous debris during surgery.

Assessment of Cerebral Tolerance to Internal Carotid Artery Clamping.

Brain is a remarkable organ, weighing 2% of the body weight, receives 15% of the cardiac output. Blood flow is 750-1000mls/minute. The normal resting flow is 50mls/100 g of tissue/minute. When brain blood flow drops to 30mls/100 g/min., there is ischemia and reduction of flow to 20mls/100 g/min or lower, thus results in cerebral infarction. It is important to maintain adequate flow when the internal carotid is clamped. There are ways of assessing the safety of internal carotid artery clamping:

1. Preoperative imaging studies—Helps to assess contralateral carotid, vertebral arteries, and circle of Willis. If contralateral carotid is occluded or if there is incomplete circle of Willis, shunting will be needed.
2. Operating on a wake patient (regional anesthesia)—Assessment of motor and cognitive function with clamping (not possible if general anesthesia is used).
3. Continuous EEG monitoring, evoke potentials monitoring (wave amplitude and pattern).
4. Measurement of cerebral blood flow (very cumbersome, not practical).
5. Measurement of stump pressure (50 mmHg acceptable, shunt required if lower).

The procedure begins with positioning, preparation, and draping of the fields. Head should be extended and turned away from the side of operation. It is important not to hyperextend the neck. Elderly patient may have degenerative disease of the spine. Hyperextension in these situations may cause vascular (vertebral artery) and nerve compression. It is important to seal the operative area with impervious barrier to prevent any escape of oxygen into the field from nasal cannula which if occurs can be a serious fire hazard. The field should be dried. Incision is oblique along the anterior border of sternomastoid. The external jugular vein coursing superficial to the muscle is ligated and divided. The muscle is retracted with retractors. Too aggressive retraction and placing the retractor blades too deep may by itself cause stretch injury to recurrent laryngeal nerve. The common carotid artery is exposed first. Some of the tributaries of IJV will need ligation. Middle thyroid vein in the lower part of the neck and facial vein is generally at the level of carotid bifurcation. If nerves are seen coursing anterior to the carotid artery, the most common being Ansa cervicalis, gentle dissection, and retraction are preferable to transection. Occasionally, the recurrent laryngeal nerve may course across the common carotid (nonrecurrent recurrent laryngeal nerve). The common carotid artery (CCA) is dissected first and controlled with vessel loop. Keeping close to CCA, the dissection proceeds cephalad, external carotid artery (ECA), and the very first branch of it, superior thyroid is controlled with vessel loops. Care should be taken to avoid dissection or rough manipulation of the carotid bulb, since this is the area of disease and rough handling, can cause embolization of atheromatous debris. The internal carotid artery (ICA) beyond the plaque should be dissected and controlled. Enough length of internal carotid should be dissected in case shunt is needed. It is important to identify the hypoglossal nerve which runs obliquely from lateral to medial about two inches cephalad to carotid bifurcation, however it can be lower. Once CCA, ECA, and ICA controlled, the patient is heparinized, adequacy of heparinization monitored with activated clotting time (ACT) which should be between 230 and 270 sec. ICA is clamped first followed by ECA and CCA. Arteriotomy begins in healthy CCA below the diseased area and is extended into the bulb on a slightly lateral location (arteriotomy too medial on the bulb may result in distortion of the bulb when closed and extended anteriorly in ICA beyond the plaque). Endarterectomy is begun after developing an appropriate plane (ideally between the inner and outer media). The entire plaque is removed. The arteriotomy should extend beyond the ending of endarterectomy. No part of the plaque should be left behind (complete endarterectomy), particularly on the internal carotid. If there is an intimal ledge, anchoring sutures may be used to tack the area to avoid dissection when flow is restored. Endarterectomy from ECA is done by eversion technique. All the debris, shards, and fibers are removed until the surface is smooth. The arteriotomy is closed with either a Dacron patch or bovine pericardial patch.

Unclamping Sequence (see diagram).

In order to prevent any embolization of particulate matter and/or air, proper unclamping sequence should be followed. This has five steps [36]

STEP 1. Unclamp the ICA and allow back bleeding (last few stiches are kept loose to allow this)
STEP 2. Re-clamp the ICA at its origin
STEP 3. Unclamp the ECA and let it bleed out
STEP 4. Unclamp the CCA directing the blood to ECA with ICA still clamped. Sutures are tied
STEP 5. Unclamp the ICA

Heparin is neutralized with protamine sulfate. After assuring complete hemostasis, incision is closed in layers (Fig. 21.12).

Eversion Endarterectomy

This is another technique popularized by the Albany group. In this technique, after dissection and clamping CCA, ECA, and ICA, the internal is transected obliquely from the carotid bulb.

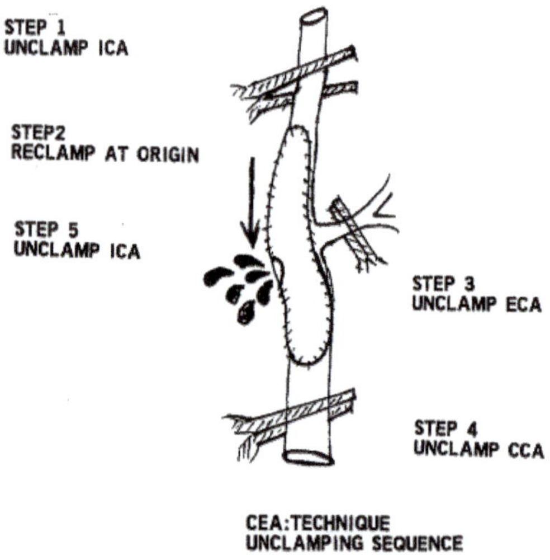

Fig. 21.12 Carotid endarterectomy unclamping sequence

After creating proper endarterectomy plane, the ICA wall is gently rolled back (everted) to sufficient length till the endpoint of the disease and plaque is removed. Similar maneuver is done on the common and external carotid. After completion, the ICA is anastomosed to the bulb. The advantages of this procedure being, no patch is required. Disadvantage is that if the disease is extensive, eversion is technically difficult or inadequate. It is also harder to use a shunt if required. Eversion endarterectomy requires experience and appropriate patient selection.

Complications

Every surgical procedure has complications, but hazards can be disastrous and thus safeguards during carotid endarterectomy are a must [39]. The goal is to minimize the incidence and under ideal situation, it should reach near zero. Some of the complications unique and specific to carotid endarterectomy are as follows:

1. Bleeding: Bleeding can happen after any operative procedure. When happens after CEA, it can have catastrophic consequences. Even moderate hematoma in the neck can cause venous compression, which results in laryngeal edema manifested initially by hoarseness and stridor soon after. This is a surgical emergency. It is important to remove the neck staples/sutures and sutures of the underlying layer to decompress the hematoma by bedside in PACU while preparations are made to return to OR. As soon as the hematoma is evacuated and the neck decompressed, patient will immediately feel better. The grave mistake is to attempt intubation of a patient in respiratory distress and stridor. Because of the laryngeal edema, the entrance to trachea will be pinhole, the anesthesiologist will not be able to intubate and aggressive attempts to intubate without first decompressing the neck will result in increasing anxiety on part of the patient, further anoxia and cardiac arrest.
2. Hypotension: Hypotension is seen in more than half of patients soon after the operation.

This is explained on the basis of irritability and alteration of the carotid baroreceptors which are a group of highly specialized cells located at the carotid bifurcation when stimulated baroreceptors cause hypotension and bradycardia. This is seen immediately or soon after the patient goes to Post Anesthesia Care Unit (PACU). It is important for the PACU nurse and other staff to be aware of this phenomenon. Unlike all other surgical procedures, where post-operative hypotension may indicate hypovolemia and calls for fluid bolus or blood, post-carotid endarterectomy hypotension needs pressor agents. The most commonly used agent is phenylephrine (Neosynephrine) given as a drip with dose titrated to keep systolic blood pressure around 110–129 mmHg. Hypotension generally lasts for about 4–6 hours as the body's autoregulation sets in by that time. If hypotension is not recognized or acted upon immediately, there is potential for the endarterectomized segment to thrombose with disastrous consequences. Hence the need for all CEA patients to be monitored for 6–8 hours in PACU.

3. Hypertension and Cerebral Hyper-perfusion Syndrome: Patients who have history of hypertension should be monitored in PACU and also afterwards to assure good control of blood pressure to normal range. Hypertension may facilitate bleeding at fresh surgical site. If that happens, measures described above should be followed in addition to controlling the blood pressure. In patients who had significantly compromised blood flow before operation (high grade stenosis of one carotid with total occlusion of contralateral carotid), intraoperative, peri-operative, and postoperative hypertension can lead to cerebral hyperperfusion syndrome. This is analogous to swelling of the limb and development of compartment syndrome which occurs after restoration of blood flow in situations of acute and profound limb ischemia. There is vasodilatation of the cerebral vascular bed in response to severely reduced flow. After CEA, there is sudden flooding of the brain with increased flow and if there is element of hypertension, this can lead to trans-vascular escape of fluid, cerebral edema, microhemorrhages and even intracerebral hemorrhage This is a serious complication with an incidence of about 0.5% of carotid endarterectomy cases, resulting in high morbidity and mortality [37]. Cerebral hyper-perfusion syndrome can happen within a few hours after surgery to a week or 10 days if patient has uncontrolled hypertension. Typically, patient complains of severe headache on the side of operation may have seizures or neurologic deficits similar to stroke [40]. Emergent CT scan, strict control of hypertension, barbiturates, and antiseizure drugs form the treatment strategy. Elective CEA should be postponed in patients with uncontrolled hypertension until their blood pressure is appropriately treated.
4. Nerve injury: Both cranial and other nerve injuries can happen in carotid operations[4]. The hypoglossal, vagus, and glossopharyngeal nerves are in close proximity to the artery. The recurrent laryngeal nerve is the most common to be injured. This can happen by excessive stretch by self-retaining retractors, or direct injury can occur by electrocautery, or transection during dissection CCA and ECA. Hoarseness and difficulty swallowing saliva can occur if there is paralysis of ipsilateral vocal cord. This is very disabling in addition to medicolegal implications. Otolaryngology consult should be sought early for proper evaluation of extent of disability and for intervention. Minor recurrent laryngeal nerve trauma will recover in a few weeks. The other nerve prone to injury is hypoglossal nerve which crosses from lateral to medial side. In most cases, it is about an inch or two higher cephalad to the carotid bifurcation. In some, it can cross lower, closer to carotid bifurcation. Transection can result in tongue deviated to the side of injury and affects the movement of tongue and ability to chew the food. Bilateral hypoglossal nerve injury results in paralysis of the tongue, causing obstruction of oropharyngeal area. Patient will require tracheostomy. Careful history should be taken in any patient who has had

CEA in the past who requires endarterectomy on the opposite side. In cases where hypoglossal or recurrent laryngeal nerve injury appears to have occurred, preoperative ENT evaluation is important. Injury to glossopharyngeal is rare, since it is not generally seen during carotid endarterectomy. However, in those situations where the bifurcation is high, or the disease is extensive that longer segment of ICA needs to be exposed, care should be taken to avoid injury to this nerve that courses anterior to ICA. Even clamp trauma to this nerve can cause significant pharyngeal dysfunction causing difficulty on swallowing. The recovery also is slow and some patients may require feeding tube or even PEG for feeding for 3–5 weeks which is the time it takes for the muscles of deglutition to recover. The other nerve prone for injury is the cervical and mandibular branch of the facial nerve. These can be injured when the neck incision extends higher than usual or from vigorous retraction by self-retaining retractors when the nerve gets compressed between the retractor blade and the mandible causes deviation of the angle of the mouth on the ipsilateral side. This is a significant complication because of cosmetic deformity. Injury to ansa cervicalis generally does not result in any sequalae. Very rarely, the spinal accessory nerve can be injured (it courses across sternocleidomastoid muscle high) resulting in difficulty in raising the shoulder. Hence it is important for the operating surgeon to be knowledgeable of relation of carotid artery to all the nerves and possible anatomic variations (Fig. 21.13).

5. Neurologic deficit after CEA: This is perhaps the most devastating to the patient and the surgeon. Neurologic deficit immediately after CEA is most likely due to technical factors and warrants immediate action. If the patient wakes up in the operating room with a neurologic deficit, the incision should be opened for direct inspection of the carotid artery. The arteriotomy should be reopened to directly inspect if there is an intimal flap, residual plaque, clamp trauma or platelet thrombi, etc., all of which should be addressed. Intraoperative duplex scan of the artery will be helpful. If no technical problems noted, then embolization of the plaque material/atheromatous debris to the brain is the most probable cause. This calls for urgent CT to rule out a bleed and consultation with neuro-

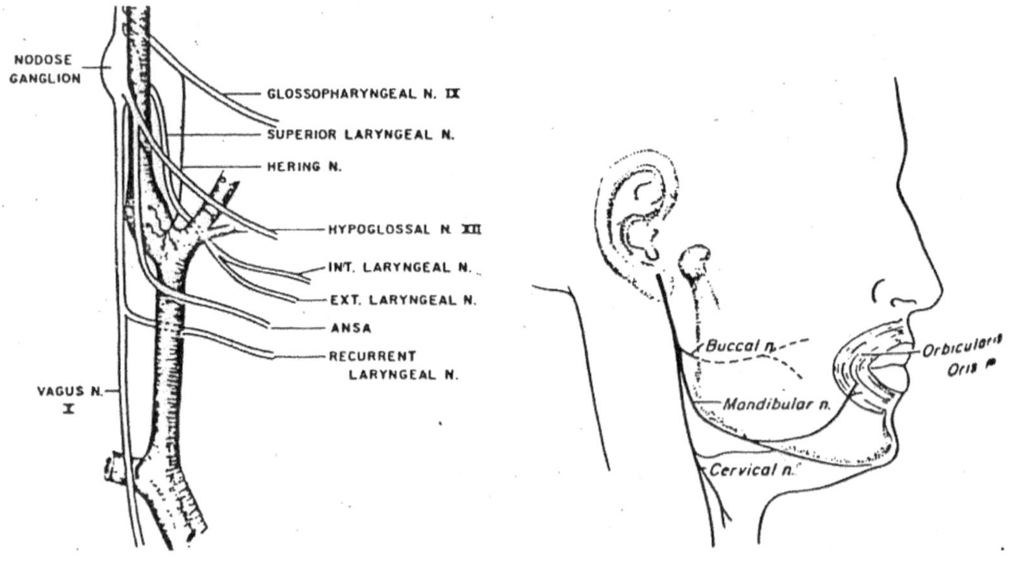

Fig. 21.13 Relation of nerves of the face and neck to carotid artery-surgical considerations

interventional experts. They have the ability to intervene and retrieve clot and debris from intracranial branches of ICA. All stroke centers have neuro-intervention specialists.

Conclusion

Carotid endarterectomy has been a time-tested operation for symptomatic carotid disease and in select asymptomatic patients. With meticulous attention to every detail like proper patient selection, appropriate indication, tailoring the type of anesthesia to patient's medical status, neuromonitoring, good surgical technique, and postoperative care by trained team guided by clinical pathway protocols, this procedure can be performed with stroke and death rates of 1% or lower. Acknowledging the vital importance of teamwork and practicing it as a habit has benefited patients enormously. This indeed is testament to modern surgery.

Advanced Peripheral Arterial Techniques for Limb Salvage: Role of Intravascular Lithotripsy

Introduction

Peripheral artery disease (PAD) is an important cause of cardiovascular morbidity and mortality, affecting over 230 million people worldwide [41–46]. Vascular calcification is a common feature in patients with PAD, especially in the setting of diabetes mellitus and/or end-stage renal disease, leading to poor prognosis and increased risk of major amputation. To date, limited therapeutic options are available to address severely calcified PAD including atherectomy and cutting balloons [42–46]. However, these devices have not been effective in plaque modification and vessel expansion as the presence of vascular calcification can interfere with the delivery of endovascular therapies, where it is responsible for suboptimal vessel expansion and increased risk of vascular complications including dissection and perforation. Consequently, there are higher use of provisional stents and increased risk of suboptimal stent-related restenosis. Moreover, although atherectomy has been shown to improve luminal diameter and reduce the need for bailout stenting, vascular complications such as distal atheroembolization remain a significant challenge [47–49].

Derived from renal lithotripsy, intravascular lithotripsy (IVL) is a novel technique that uses high-energy ultrasound waves to improve plaque modification and vessel compliance (Fig. 21.14) [50]. It uses pulsatile sonic pressure waves that pass through soft tissue and selectively interact strongly with high-density calcium, producing significant shear stresses that have the ability to fracture the calcium. Furthermore, it is designed to modify both intimal and medial calcium across a wide range of vascular applications to increase vessel compliance, restore vessel mobility, and provide new versatile treatment options for patients.

The Shockwave Medical Peripheral IVL System (Shockwave Medical, Fremont, CA)

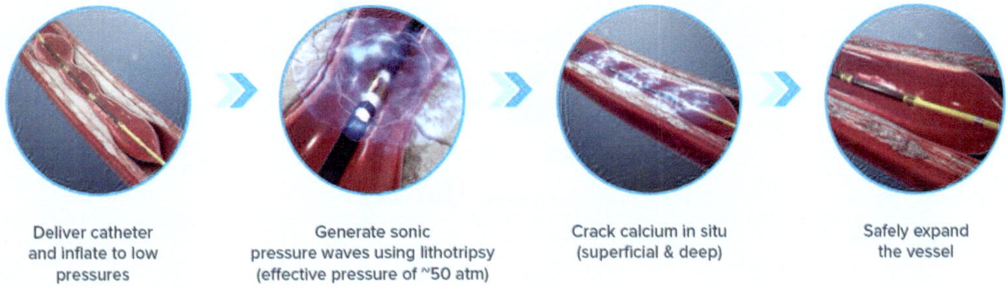

Fig. 21.14 Mechanism of action of the peripheral intravascular lithotripsy. *Reproduced with permission from Shockwave Medical*

received U.S. Food and Drug Administration (FDA) approval in 2016. This system consists of an IVL generator, a connector cable, and a catheter (Fig. 21.15a). The IVL catheter comprises an array of integrated lithotripsy emitters for the localized delivery of pulsatile mechanical energy and an integrated balloon (Fig. 21.15b). The IVL catheter is available in multiple sizes ranging from 2.5 mm to 12 mm and compatible with a 5 French to 8 French sheath and has working lengths of 110 cm and 135 cm to treat aorta to tibial and peroneal vessels (Fig. 21.16).

The IVL catheter contains an inflation lumen, a guidewire lumen, and the lithotripsy emitters (Fig. 21.16). The inflation lumen is used for inflation and deflation of the balloon with a 50:50 saline: contrast medium mixture. The guidewire lumen enables the use of a 0.014-inch guidewire to facilitate the advancement of the catheter to and through the target stenosis. The system is designed as "over-the-wire" (OTW) with a 110 cm or 135 cm shaft working length, and a minimum of a 5 French sheath is required at the access site. The balloon is located near the distal tip of the catheter. Two radiopaque marker bands within the balloon denote the length of the balloon to aid in the positioning of the balloon during treatment. The balloon is designed to provide an expandable segment of a known length and diameter at a specific pressure. The proximal hub has three ports: one for inflation/deflation of the balloon, one for the guidewire lumen, and one for connection to the IVL connector cable. The IVL catheter will deliver a maximum of 300 pulses or 10 cycles of 30 pulses per cycle for L6 and M5+ catheters and 160 pulses or 8 cycles of 20 pulses per cycle for S^4. It is recommended not to exceed 180 pulses in the same treatment segment.

Procedural Steps

The insertion site is accessed in a standard fashion using a micro-puncture system under ultra-

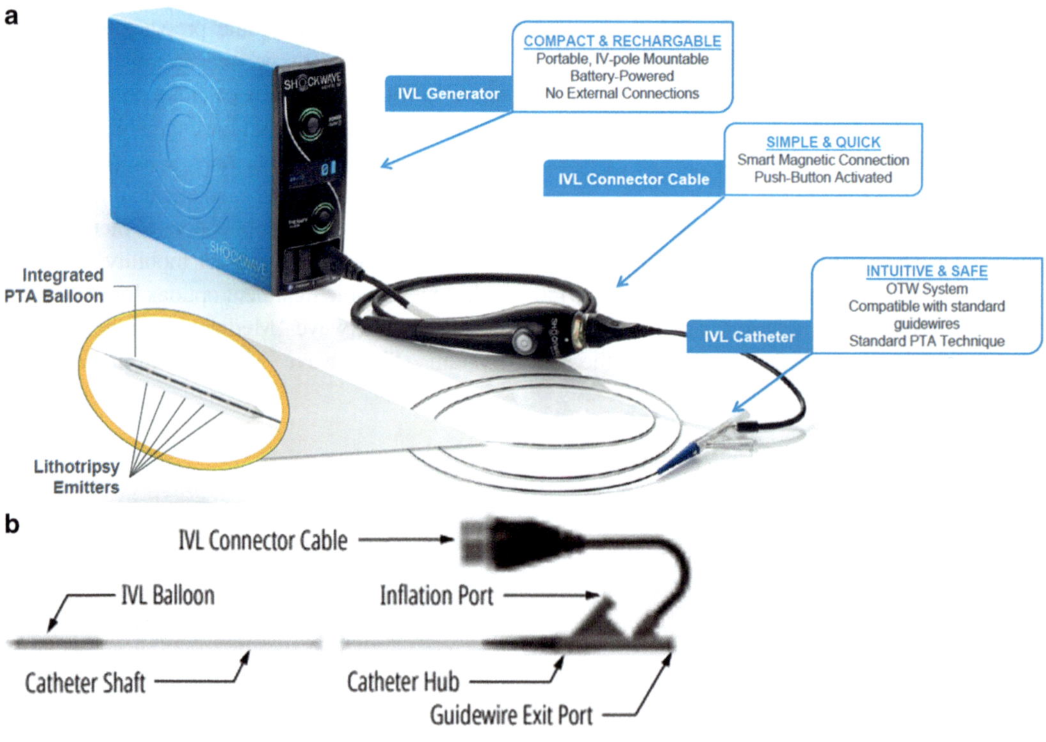

Fig. 21.15 Shockwave medical peripheral IVL system (**a**) with IVL catheter (**b**). (Reproduced with permission from Shockwave Medical)

SHOCKWAVE | L^6

Balloon Diameter (mm)	Balloon Length (mm)	Guidewire Compatibility (in)	Sheath Compatibility	Catheter Working Length (cm)	Max Pulse Count
10.0 & 12.0	30	0.018	8F	110	300
8.0 & 9.0	30	0.018	7F	110	300

SHOCKWAVE | M^{5+}

Balloon Diameter (mm)	Balloon Length (mm)	Guidewire Compatibility (in)	Sheath Compatibility	Catheter Working Length (cm)	Max Pulse Count
8.0	60	0.014	7F	135	300
6.5-7.0	60	0.014	6F*	135	300
3.5-6.0	60	0.014	6F	135	300

SHOCKWAVE | S^4

Balloon Diameter (mm)	Balloon Length (mm)	Guidewire Compatibility (in)	Sheath Compatibility	Catheter Working Length (cm)	Max Pulse Count	Pulses Per Second
2.5-4.0	40	0.014	5F	135	160	1

Fig. 21.16 Shockwave peripheral IVL catheter balloons. (Reproduced with permission from Shockwave Medical)

sound guidance, followed by upsizing to an appropriately sized sheath. Angiography is performed to localize and delineate the arterial lesion (Figs. 21.17a and 21.18a). Appropriate anticoagulation is initiated. A balloon catheter size is then selected in a 1:1 ratio with the reference vessel diameter. The IVL catheter is prepared by filling a 20 mL syringe with 5 mL of half-strength contrast medium and attaching the syringe to the inflation port on the catheter hub. The syringe is pulled back at least 3 times to release vacuum and allow the fluid to replace the air in the catheter. The guidewire port of the IVL catheter is then flushed with saline, and the protective sheath from the catheter is removed, and the IVL connector cable is inserted into a sterile sleeve and attached to the IVL generator. The 0.014-inch guidewire is used to traverse the treatment site under fluoroscopic guidance. The IVL catheter is then loaded over the guidewire and advanced through the sheath to the treatment site using the marker bands to aid in positioning. Once the IVL catheter is positioned and confirmed with fluoroscopy, the IVL balloon is inflated up to 4 atm, and IVL is activated for up to 20 pulses for S^4 and 30 pulses for M^{5+} and L^4 by pressing the activation button (Figs. 21.17b-c and 21.18b). The balloon is then inflated up to 6 atm under fluoroscopy. Then, the balloon is deflated, and additional treatments can be performed as needed by repositioning the IVL and repeating the sequence as necessary. If multiple inflations are required due to a lesion length greater than the IVL balloon length, the recommended balloon overlap is at least 1 cm. After treatment, completion angiography is performed to assess post-intervention results (Figs. 21.17d and 21.18c).

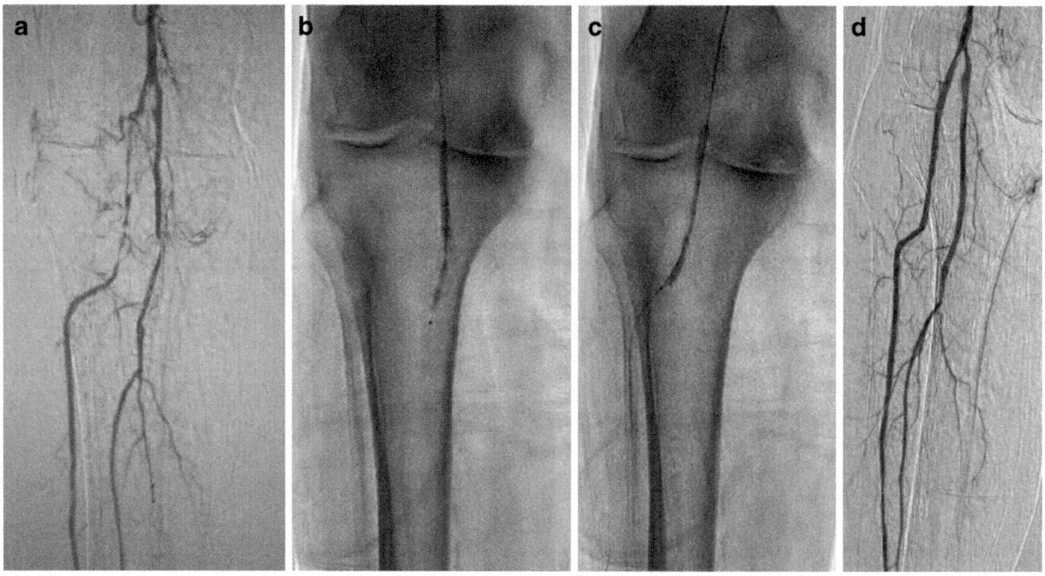

Fig. 21.17 Right lower extremity angiography demonstrating severe long segment calcified stenoses of the anterior tibial artery and tibioperoneal trunk (**a**) treated with 4 mm × 60 mm IVL catheter with a total of 300 pulses (**b**-**c**). Completion angiography illustrating significant luminal expansion of the treated vessels with no residual stenoses (**d**)

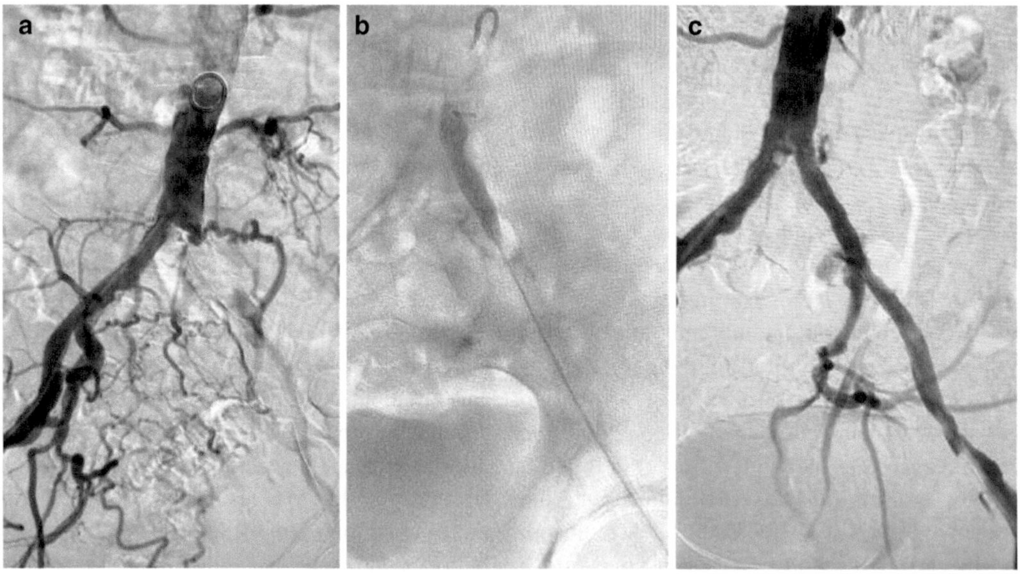

Fig. 21.18 Angiography illustrating severely calcified left iliac arterial system (**a**) treated with the IVL (**b**) alone. Completion angiography demonstrates significantly improved flow to the left iliac arterial system (**c**)

Clinical Evidence of Intravascular Lithotripsy in Peripheral Artery Disease

The DISRUPT PAD I and II were multi-center retrospective studies of prospectively collected data to investigate the short-term safety and efficacy of the IVL for treating calcified, occlusive femoropopliteal lesions [51, 52]. The results showed 100% procedural success with a dramatic reduction in stenosis severity, high acute gain, and minimal vessel injury. There were no major adverse events or revascularizations after the index procedure, and vessel patency was durable out to 6 months, with primary patency rates of 82.1%. The DISRUPT PAD III RCT trial was the first randomized controlled study comparing the outcomes of IVL and percutaneous transluminal angioplasty (PTA) to prepare the lesions before drug-coated balloon (DCB) or stenting for occlusive femoropopliteal lesions [53]. Compared to the PTA group, the IVL group had higher procedural success and balloon/stent expansion with significantly lower residual stenosis and flow-limiting dissection rates (Table 21.1 and Fig. 21.19). Two-year follow-up results revealed significantly higher primary patency in the IVL group versus PTA group (70.3% vs. 51.3%; $P = 0.003$) [54]. DISRUPT PAD III observational study (OS) was a prospective, non-randomized, multi-center, single-arm study conducted to assess the real-world acute performance of IVL in the treatment of calcified, stenotic peripheral arteries that may not qualify for inclusion in the RCT [55]. Of the 1531 lesions treated in the iliac, common femoral, superficial femoral, popliteal, and infrapopliteal arteries, 90% presented with moderate or severe calcification, with an average calcified length of 115 mm. The use of IVL resulted in a final residual diameter stenosis of 24% with only 0.7% and 0.2% experiencing final dissections (Type D–F) and perforations, respectively (Table 21.1 and Fig. 21.19). Notably, there were no instances of embolization, thrombus formation, no-reflow or abrupt closure.

Table 21.1 Summary of DISRUPT PAD III RCT and OS trials

	DISRUPT PAD III RCT	DISRUPT PAD III OS
No.	306 (153 IVL)	1367
Vessel	SFA/popliteal	Iliac, CFA, SFA/popliteal, Infrapopliteal
Dissection (type D-F)	0%	0.7%
Perforation	0%	0.2%
Embolization	0%	0%
Slow flow/no-reflow	0%	0%
Abrupt closure	0%	0%
Thrombus	0%	0%

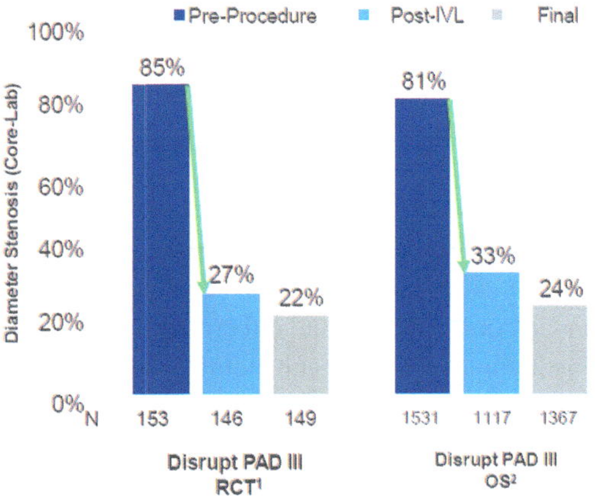

Fig. 21.19 Efficacy of IVL in reducing the residual diameter stenosis in Disrupt PAD III RCT and OS studies

The sub-analysis of the DISRUPT PAD III OS study showed promising results in the use of IVL in calcific infrapopliteal lesions, with 100% successful IVL catheter delivery and no flow-limiting dissection, perforation, distal embolization, slow flow, no-reflow, or abrupt closure [56]. The Disrupt BTK study was a prospective, non-randomized, multi-center feasibility, and safety trial composed of 20 patients (mean age 79.0 ± 9.6 years; 14 men) with Rutherford category 1 to 5 ischemia with moderate to severe calcified infrapopliteal stenosis treated with IVL and followed for 30 days [57]. IVL catheter delivery was successful in 95%, with a 46.5% acute reduction in percent diameter stenosis of target lesions, one dissection, and 2 stents placed. None of the subjects experienced thrombus formation, abrupt closure, distal embolization, or perforation, with no composite of major adverse events at 30 days. There were no device-related complications. The results of this pilot study demonstrated that calcified, stenotic infrapopliteal arteries can be safely and successfully treated with intravascular lithotripsy. The effect of IVL on calcific plaque under the stent strut has also been reported in the carotid, mesenteric, and lower extremity arterial systems. While IVL can modify the calcific plaque under a peripheral stent, improving stent expansion, the long-term impact of this approach will need to be examined in larger clinical studies.

Conclusion

IVL represents a promising endovascular technique for limb salvage and improved outcomes in patients with calcified PAD. Clinical evidence underscores its safety and effectiveness in achieving luminal gain and enhancing vessel patency with minimal risk of complications. However, further research is warranted to elucidate its long-term benefits and applicability in specific patient populations.

The May–Thurner Syndrome

The May–Thurner Syndrome (MTS) is compression of the left common iliac vein from the right iliac artery and vertebral body. This condition was first described by an autopsy study performed by May and Thurner in 1957 [58]. The clinical condition of left iliac vein stenosis was described by Cockett [59].

Anatomy

The left iliac vein is present between the body of the lumber vertebra and the right iliac artery (Fig. 21.20). This causes a physiologic stenosis

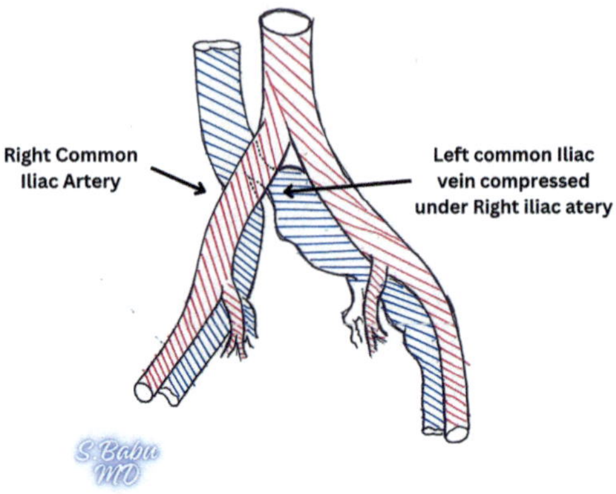

Fig. 21.20 Left common iliac vein compression by right common iliac artery

which is very common. A CT scan study shows that 25% of asymptomatic patients have 50% stenosis and two-thirds of asymptomatic patients have 25% stenosis [60]. When this stenosis becomes exaggerated and causes clinical symptoms, it is diagnosed as MTS.

Clinical Presentation

MTS is present two times more commonly in women as compared to men. MTS has two distinct clinical presentations which include thrombotic vs non-thrombotic.

Patients with non-thrombotic MTS have chronic left lower extremity symptoms of venous insufficiency. Nonspecific symptoms of chronic venous disease include heaviness, achiness, swelling, throbbing, and itching (HASTI Symptoms). A significant number of patients have venous claudication which is defined as pain and stiffness of the leg with exercise and improvement with rest and elevation.

Swelling of the lower extremity is a common condition with differential diagnosis of venous insufficiency, deep venous thrombosis, lymphedema, heart failure, medications, leg injury, morbid obesity, and prolonged inactivity in a sitting position.

Chronic venous disease is a common disorder that has manifestations ranging from varicose veins to venous ulcerations. Chronic venous disease is best classified by CEAP classification which includes clinical, etiological, anatomic, and pathophysiological categories. Non-thrombotic MTS patients can have concomitant lower extremity varicose veins due to primary superficial venous reflux along with left iliac vein obstruction.

Thrombotic MTS occurs due to deep venous obstruction of the left iliac vein from left iliac vein stenosis. Deep venous thrombosis can occur due to a history of thrombophilia or transient risk factors such as pregnancy, surgery, prolonged immobilization, or oral contraceptive pills. Thrombotic MTS is often diagnosed with acute ileo-femoral DVT. These patients present with acute pain and swelling of the left lower extremity. In more severe cases, patients can present with phlegmasia cerulea dolens. Some patients with thrombotic MTS present with chronic left ileo-femoral DVT. These patients have a history of DVT which was treated with anticoagulation in the past and have chronic post-phlebitic syndrome. These patients have venous claudication with severe venous stasis changes in the left leg.

Multiple other conditions cause iliac vein and IVC stenosis and thrombosis. These conditions include iliac vein and IVC thrombosis due to thrombophilia; iliac vein and IVC stenosis due to congenital webs and atresia; external compression due to malignancy; a catheter or IVC filter-associated stenosis and thrombosis. These conditions necessitate the same diagnostic studies and often similar treatment approaches as MTS.

Imaging Studies

1. Duplex scan is the most important initial diagnostic study. Duplex scan for suspected patients in the vascular lab involves lower extremity duplex and iliac vein and inferior vena cava scan. A lower extremity duplex scan is useful for the diagnosis of deep venous thrombosis and deep and superficial venous reflux. An inferior vena cava and iliac vein study is useful to determine any deep venous thrombosis in this segment. The extent of left iliac vein stenosis is harder to determine by duplex scan.
2. Contrast CT scan with venography has higher sensitivity and specificity to detect left iliac vein stenosis and deep venous thrombosis. CT scan is also useful to determine external causes of compression of the iliac vein by malignancy, uterine fibroid, lymphadenopathy, or hematoma.
3. Magnetic resonance venography is an alternative to CT venography. This study is rarely used due to the length of time it takes to do the test as compared to a contrast CT scan.
4. Venography: Venogram of iliac veins and inferior vena cava can be done by femoral vein, popliteal vein, and jugular vein based on the treatment plan. A venogram will show severe iliac vein stenosis and occlusion; however, it will miss moderate iliac vein stenosis even in multiple projections.
5. Intravascular Ultrasound (IVUS): IVUS is the gold standard for diagnosis of MTS. IVUS provides information regarding the degree and length of stenosis. This information is useful for accurate deployment of stents. It should be noted that physiologic stenosis of 50% is present in many asymptomatic patients. Treatment with iliac vein stents should be done in patients with severe symptoms that interfere with the patient's activities.

Treatment of MTS

Non-thrombotic MTS often presents with lower extremity chronic venous disease. These patients are initially treated with compression stockings, leg elevation, exercise involving ambulation, and weight loss if needed. Patients are evaluated with a lower extremity venous duplex scan. Patients who have significant saphenous venous reflux and fail conservative treatment are first treated with radiofrequency ablation of the saphenous vein. Patients who continue to have swelling of the left lower extremity undergo a duplex scan of iliac veins and IVC. These patients who have severe symptoms undergo venogram and IVUS procedures. We do a venogram for non-thrombotic patients by accessing the common femoral vein by ultrasound guidance. A 6 Fr

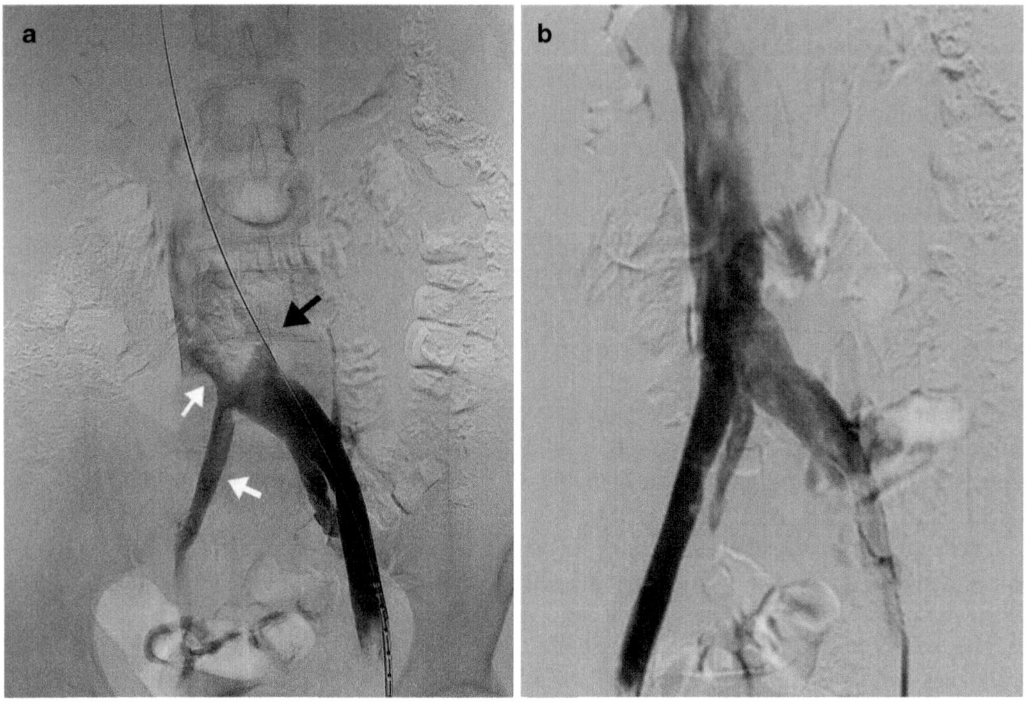

Fig. 21.21 (**a**) Venogram showing severe common iliac vein stenosis (black arrow), White arrows showing filling of collateral veins. (**b**) Venogram after left common iliac vein stent placement

sheath is placed in the femoral vein, and venogram is performed in AP and oblique projections. Venogram generally shows patent left iliac vein and IVC with no significant stenosis. Stenosis on venogram is only seen if it is severe (Fig. 21.21a). Next 6 Fr sheath is exchanged over wire for 9 Fr sheath. IVUS is performed over 0.035 guide wire (Fig. 21.22a). In patients with severe symptoms and with the presence of over 50% stenosis on IVUS, a left common iliac vein stent is placed. IVUS is useful to determine the extent of the iliac vein stent. Generally, Wallstent, Zilver Vena, or Abre stent are deployed. The diameter of the stents is 14–16 mm, and the length of stents ranges from 60 to 100 mm. Extending the stent beyond the stenosis into IVC is desirable (Fig. 21.21b). Angioplasty of the iliac vein is done using a 14 to 16-mm balloon. A completion IVUS is done (Fig. 21.22b). Patients are on bed rest for 2 hours and then discharged home. Post-procedure patients are placed on anticoagulation for 4 weeks. They are then placed on antiplatelet for 6 months. Patients undergo duplex scans at 1 month and 6 months to confirm the patency of the stent. This procedure has been shown to improve patient symptoms with a 4-year patency of 93% [61].

Thrombotic MTS presents with either acute ileo-femoral vein DVT or chronic ileo-femoral vein DVT. Clinical presentation and management of these two conditions differ.

Patients with acute thrombotic MTS present with severe acute pain and swelling of the left lower extremity. These patients are often unable to ambulate due to the extent of pain. Duplex scan is done which will confirm ileo-femoral vein acute DVT. The initial treatment of acute thrombotic MTS is leg elevation in the Trendelenburg position and high-dose intravenous heparin protocol if the patient has no contraindication for anticoagulation. For patients who have respiratory distress or hypoxia, a contrast CT scan of the chest is done to check for pulmonary embolism. Some patients also undergo CT venography to determine the extent of thrombosis. The patient is then booked in the angio-suite for mechanical

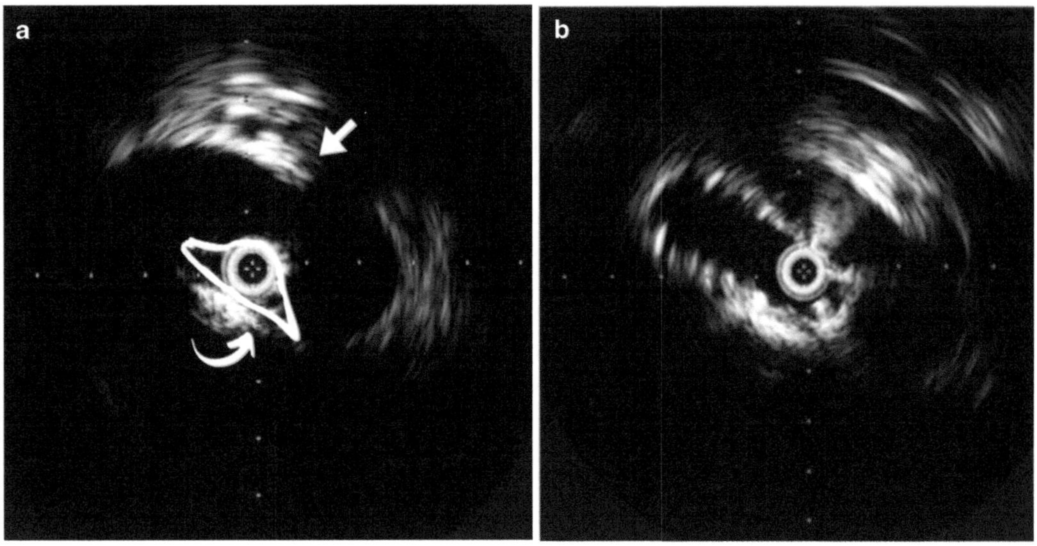

Fig. 21.22 (**a**) IVUS shows the left common iliac vein (curved arrow) and right common iliac artery (top arrow). (**b**) IVUS of left common iliac vein after stent

thrombectomy, thrombolysis, angioplasty, and stenting. Placement of temporary or removable IVC filters is considered in patients who have limited lung reserve due to pulmonary embolism or free-floating thrombus. Most patients do not require IVC filter placement.

In the angio-suite, patients are placed in the supine position and a duplex scan is done for patency of femoral and popliteal veins. The procedure is most commonly performed under conscious sedation; however, some patients require monitored anesthesia care or general anesthesia. We can access the left popliteal vein percutaneously with ultrasound guidance with the patient in a supine position with the leg bent. Initially, a 6 Fr sheath is placed, and a venogram is done to a patent segment of the femoral vein. A glide wire along with a glide catheter is used to go through the thrombosed femoral and iliac vein up to IVC. Next 6 Fr sheath is exchanged over a wire for a 9 Fr sheath. We use 8 Fr Angiojet-Zelante catheters for thrombolysis and mechanical thrombectomy of femoral and iliac vein thrombosis. Initially, a power pulse is used for thrombolysis with up to 10 mg of tissue plasminogen activator (TPA). TPA is allowed to dwell in the thrombus for 20 minutes. Next mechanical thrombectomy is done with multiple passes through the thrombus. A repeat venogram is done to assess the extent of clearance. In some cases, clot maceration is done with repeat mechanical thrombectomy. IVUS is done to access the extent of left iliac vein stenosis, and stenting of the iliac vein is done from IVC to the distal extent of stenosis [64, 65].

After the procedure anticoagulation with heparin is continued. This is later switched to Lovenox, DOAC, or Coumadin for 6 months. The patient is also evaluated for thrombophilia and if present will need lifelong anticoagulation. This procedure has replaced catheter-directed thrombolysis in our institution which takes 1 to 2 days of treatment in the intensive care and multiple visits to the angio-suite.

Patients with acute thrombotic MTS can also be treated with an indigo penumbra 8 Fr suction device and an Inari 13-F ClotTriever device. ClotTriever device has the advantage that it can be used for chronic thrombotic MTS.

Chronic thrombotic MTS presents with post-phlebitic syndrome with leg pain, swelling, advanced chronic venous stasis, and venous claudication. These patients undergo diagnostic studies including venous duplex and CT venography. Patients are initially seen in an outpatient setting and are brought to the angio-suite electively.

ClotTriever procedure involves percutaneous access of the patent distal femoral or popliteal vein under ultrasound guidance. Initially, a 6 Fr sheath is placed and a venogram is done to access the thrombosed segment. Using a glide wire and catheter thrombosed segment of the femoral and iliac vein is crossed up to IVC. Next 13 Fr ClotTriever sheath is placed, and the funnel is deployed. Next ClotTriever catheter is placed into IVC over the guide wire proximal to the thrombus. The coring element and collection bag are opened, and the coring element is pulled back to remove the clot from the vessel wall. If resistance is met during thrombectomy, coring element is disengaged and re-engaged beyond the stenosis. The area of iliac vein stenosis is treated with angioplasty. After the thrombectomy, iliac stenosis is stented. The main advantage of this system is that it can treat both acute and chronic deep venous thrombosis. This system also does not require thrombolytic treatment. The results of the ClotTriever device have been outlined in the Cloud Registry which shows 91% of patients have near complete thrombectomy (determined by Marder score) with an adverse event rate of 0.2%. Patients had immediate improvement of symptoms as shown by the Villalta scale before and after the procedure [62, 63].

Patients with thrombotic MTS who are treated with iliac stents have 2-year primary assisted and secondary patency of 88 and 96% [66].

Conservative Treatment

Many patients with isolated left leg swelling and non-thrombotic MTS elect not to have interventional treatment. These patients are treated with compression stockings, leg elevation, and exercise as tolerated. Some of these patients with chronic swelling have components of lymphedema, and they can be managed by manual lymphatic drainage and/or venous and lymphatic pumps.

In our clinical practice, we have also treated patients with acute thrombotic MTS with long-term anticoagulation and conservative treatment. We have seen some of these patients recover with minimal sequelae. CAVENT trial [67] showed a lower incidence of postphlebitic syndrome in patients with ileo-femoral DVT treated with catheter-directed thrombolysis (CDT) as compared to anticoagulation alone. ATTRACT [68] trial showed no improvement with CDT as compared to anticoagulation. Both of these trials were not specific for MTS and did not employ newer technology.

Patients with chronic thrombotic MTS can also be treated conservatively. These patients require anticoagulation if they have thrombophilia or recurrent DVTs. Some patients without thrombophilia can be treated with a 6-month course of anticoagulation and then it can be stopped.

Conclusions

MTS presents with left lower extremity swelling with venous claudication symptoms. Imaging studies including venous duplex, venogram, and IVUS are useful for the diagnosis of MTS. Physiologic stenosis of the left iliac vein is common and therefore accurate diagnosis requires a combination of clinical criteria and imaging study. Patients with non-thrombotic MTS are treated with left common iliac vein angioplasty and stent placement. Patients with acute and chronic thrombotic MTS are treated with thrombectomy of the ileo-femoral segment along with iliac vein angioplasty and stent. These patients require long-term anticoagulation. Some patients with less severe symptoms can be treated conservatively.

Evaluation of a Patient for Hemodialysis Access

Hemodialysis is the most prevalent form of renal replacement therapy (RRT), with the others being peritoneal dialysis and kidney transplant. For patients receiving hemodialysis, their longevity is proportional to the quality of their dialysis, which in turn is proportional to the quality of access to their vasculature. It is important that the vascular access for hemodialysis be reliable, adequate to deliver prescribed dialysis, suitable to patient's given needs, and with low complication rates. The options for vascular access include:

1. Arteriovenous fistula: a surgical connection between an artery and a vein. This is usually in the upper extremity, but can be performed in the lower extremity.
2. Arteriovenous graft: a conduit is connected between an artery and a vein. The conduit is directly accessed for dialysis.
3. Central venous catheter: a flexible, double lumen tube inserted into a large, central vein.

The National Kidney Foundation's Kidney Disease Outcomes Quality Initiative (KDOQI) has provided evidence-based guidelines for hemodialysis vascular access since 1996, with the most recent update being in 2019 [69].

These are commonly referred to as the "KDOQI guidelines" and form the basis for much of the decision-making regarding the care of chronic kidney disease (CKD) patients and their vascular access. The Work Group which wrote the guidelines was multidisciplinary and included nephrologists, radiologists, vascular surgeons, and vascular access nurses. While the emphasis of the previous guidelines published in 2006 was "fistula first," an important new concept introduced in the most recent update is that of the End-Stage Kidney Disease (ESKD) Life-Plan.

The ESKD Life-Plan is an individualized roadmap of the patient's vascular access needs over their lifetime. It helps prepare for, create, and preserve access for dialysis, as well as for the next vascular access before the current one fails. This considers the patient's current and anticipated medical, functional, and psychosocial status to determine the optimal dialysis modalities and access options. Important factors to assess include:

1. Patient goals, preferences, and life expectancy.
2. Comorbidities and functional status.
3. Vascular anatomy and suitability for different access types.
4. Prior access history and complications.
5. Social support and logistics.

Keeping this ESKD Life-Plan in mind, the access surgeon's goal should be to provide the right access, in the right patient, at the right time, for the right reasons. This involves a collaborative process between the patient, their care partners, and the multidisciplinary care team. This shared decision-making approach ensures the Life-Plan aligns with the patient's goals, preferences, and values. The Life-Plan requires regular review and updates as the patient's condition, needs, and desires can change over time.

Pre-Access Evaluation by the Surgeon

Initial evaluation of a patient for new hemodialysis access emphasizes physical exam.

1. Arterial.
   (a) Character of peripheral pulses, including brachial, radial, and ulnar arteries.
   (b) Allen test, assess adequacy of palmar arch collateralization.
2. Venous.
   (a) Assess for edema, arm size, and collateral veins which could indicate central venous obstruction.
   (b) Visible, palpable veins such as cephalic and basilic veins.
   (c) Look for older, failed, previous fistulas or grafts.
3. Pump.
   (a) Assess for signs of heart failure.

Vein mapping should routinely be obtained. This could be performed in the office by the surgeon or can be done in a peripheral vascular lab. Mapping includes vessel diameter, depths, and quality. While there is not a strict minimum vein or artery diameter on vessel mapping, arteries and veins <2 mm in diameter should undergo careful evaluation for quality and feasibility to create a functioning access. There are emerging studies that can be done to be more inclusive for traditionally excluded vessels.

KDOQI Guidelines for Access Selection

1. Central venous catheters are least preferred. They are associated with higher rates of bacteremia, interventions, and central vein stenosis.
2. AVF are preferred over AVG but not always.
   (a) In some populations, AVF have longer secondary patency rates and less interventions.
   (b) In older adults >60 years.
      (i) AVG may have higher secondary patency rates in first 18 months.
      (ii) AVG have shorter time to cannulation, less adjuvant procedures.
3. In patients with >1 year life expectancy.
   (a) Distal AVF, such as radiocephalic or snuffbox.
   (b) Forearm loop AVG or proximal forearm fistula, such as Gracz fistula.
4. In patients with <1 year life expectancy.
   (a) Brachiocephalic AVF with high likelihood of unassisted maturation.
   (b) Upper arm AVG.

Management After Access Is Created

Once the access has been created, the patient should be seen within 2 weeks to assess for early complications, such as thrombosis, immaturity, infection, pain, ischemia, weakness, numbness, or edema. Grafts can typically be accessed at this time with adequate graft incorporation. For AVF, the next visit should be at 4–6 weeks to assess maturation by physical exam or duplex. With current guidelines, the "Rule of 6's" is no longer sacrosanct (6 mm in diameter, 600 cc/min, <6 mm depth). Duplex exam criteria for maturation include a vessel diameter of >4 mm, >400 ml/min, straight length > 10 cm, and a depth of <6 mm. Typically, if after 6 weeks from creation, the fistula has not adequately matured, further waiting will not help. At this point, fistulagram with possible angioplasty is warranted.

Once the access is being used, the patient should undergo regular physical exams to detect clinical indicators of flow dysfunction or late complications such as steal, aneurysms, or infection. Surveillance imaging is not recommended for either AVF or AVG. Similarly, pre-emptive angioplasty of AVF or AVG with stenosis not associated with clinical indicators is not recommended. Clinical indicators suggesting a clinically significant stenosis of access include:

1. Physical examination.
   (a) Ipsilateral extremity edema and/or prominent collaterals.
   (b) Aneurysmal degeneration of the fistula.
   (c) Abnormal thrill or bruit.
   (d) Failure of the fistula to collapse with arm elevation.
2. Dialysis.
   (a) New issues with cannulation.
   (b) Prolonged bleeding after decannulation.
   (c) Aspiration of clots during dialysis.
   (d) Inadequate flow rates or elevated venous pressures.
   (e) Inadequate clearance with dialysis.

Patients with suspected clinically significant stenosis should proceed to fistulagram.

Summary and the Future of Surgical Decision-Making in Vascular Surgery

Vascular surgery has evolved significantly over the years, probably beyond anyone imagination, and it is a result of advancements in technology [70], surgical techniques, and medical knowledge leading to improved outcomes for patients with vascular conditions, and modernization of new hospital [71]. In the past, vascular surgery primarily focused on open surgical procedures, such as bypass grafts and endarterectomies, to treat ischemia and other vascular problems. However, with the advent of minimally invasive techniques, such as angioplasty and stenting, vascular surgeons are now able to treat many conditions with less risk, shorter recovery times, and improved patient comfort.

The use of imaging technologies, such as ultrasound, CT scans, and MRIs, has also revolutionized the field of vascular surgery by allowing for more accurate diagnosis and treatment planning. Additionally, the development of advanced endovascular devices and materials has expanded the range of conditions that can be treated through minimally invasive approaches. Furthermore, the field of vascular surgery continues to evolve with ongoing research and advancements in areas such as vascular biology, genetics, and regenerative medicine. These advancements hold promise for personalized treatment approaches and improved outcomes for patients with vascular conditions.

Overall, the evolution of vascular surgery has been marked by a shift toward less invasive procedures, greater precision in diagnosis and treatment, and a focus on improving patient outcomes and quality of life. As technology and medical knowledge continue to advance, the future of vascular surgery looks promising, with continued improvements in patient care and treatment options on the horizon [72–74].

In the future, vascular surgery is likely to continue to evolve in several key areas, driven by advancements in technology, research, and medical knowledge. Some potential directions in which vascular surgery may be heading include:

1. *Personalized Medicine:* With the growing understanding of genetics and molecular biology, vascular surgeons may be able to tailor treatment plans based on the individual patient's genetic profile, optimizing outcomes and reducing the risk of complications. Arrest and regression of atherosclerosis will become more prevalent based on previous pioneering studies [75–78].
2. *Minimally Invasive Techniques:* The trend toward less-invasive procedures is likely to continue, with further advances in endovascular devices, robotics, and imaging technologies allowing for even more precise and effective treatment of vascular conditions with reduced risks and quicker recovery times.
3. *Regenerative Therapies:* Research in regenerative medicine holds promise for developing new therapies that can repair damaged blood vessels and improve blood flow, potentially offering novel treatment options for patients with vascular diseases [78–81].
4. *Telemedicine and Remote Monitoring:* The use of telemedicine and remote monitoring technologies may become more prevalent in vascular surgery, allowing for more efficient follow-up care, remote consultations, and monitoring of patients' conditions without the need for frequent in-person visits [82–84].
5. *Artificial Intelligence (AI):* AI algorithms may play an increasingly important role in helping vascular surgeons analyze complex imaging data, predict outcomes, and optimize treatment plans, leading to more precise and personalized care for patients [85–89].

Overall, the future of vascular surgery is likely to be characterized by continued innovation, personalized approaches to treatment, and the integration of advanced technologies to further improve outcomes and patient care. Collaboration between vascular surgeons, researchers, and technology developers will be key to driving these advancements and shaping the future of vascular surgery.

References

Sect. 1: Introduction

1. AbuRahma A. An analysis of the recommendations of the 2022 Society for Vascular Surgery clinical practice guidelines for patients with asymptomatic carotid stenosis. J Vasc Surg. 2024;79(5):1235–9. https://doi.org/10.1016/j.jvs.2023.12.041. Epub 2023 Dec 27
2. Zohourian T, Hines G. The evolution of current Management for Carotid Artery Bifurcation Disease. Cardiol Rev. 2024;32(3):257–62. https://doi.org/10.1097/CRD.0000000000000497. Epub 2022 Dec 20
3. Brott TG, Calvet D, Howard G, Gregson J, Algra A, Becquemin JP, de Borst GJ, Bulbulia R, Eckstein HH, Fraedrich G, Greving JP, Halliday A, Hendrikse J, Jansen O, Voeks JH, Ringleb PA, Mas JL, Brown MM, Bonati LH. Carotid stenosis Trialists' collaboration. Long-term outcomes of stenting and endarterectomy for symptomatic carotid stenosis: a preplanned pooled analysis of individual patient data. Lancet Neurol. 2019;18(4):348–56. https://doi.org/10.1016/S1474-4422(19)30028-6. Epub 2019 Feb 6. PMID: 30738706; PMCID: PMC6773606

4. Applefeld WN, Jentzer JC. Initial triage and Management of Patients with acute aortic syndromes. Cardiol Clin. 2024;42(2):195–213. https://doi.org/10.1016/j.ccl.2024.02.007. Epub 2024 Mar 15
5. Naito N, Takagi H. Optimal timing of pre-emptive thoracic endovascular aortic repair in uncomplicated type B aortic dissection: a network meta-analysis. J Endovasc Ther. 2024;9:15266028241245282. https://doi.org/10.1177/15266028241245282. Epub ahead of print
6. Bozso SJ, Nagendran J, Chu MWA, Kiaii B, El-Hamamsy I, Ouzounian M, Forcillo J, Kempfert J, Starck C, Moon MC. Three-year outcomes of the dissected aorta repair through stent implantation trial. J Thorac Cardiovasc Surg. 2024;167(5):1661–1669.e3. https://doi.org/10.1016/j.jtcvs.2022.08.040. Epub 2022 Sep 11. PMID: 36220703
7. Gogna S, Gachabayov M, Goyal P, Latifi R. Does endovascular repair for blunt traumatic aortic injuries provide better outcomes compared to its open technique? A systematic review and meta-analysis. Surg Technol Int. 2021;39:283–96. https://doi.org/10.52198/21.STI.39.CV1489. PMID: 34736285
8. Al Tannir AH, Biesboer EA, Pokrzywa C, Golestani S, Kukushliev V, Jean X, Harding E, de Moya MA, Morris R, Kugler N, Schellenberg M, Murphy PB. Open versus endovascular repair of penetrating non-aortic arterial injuries: a systematic review and meta analysis. Injury. 2024;55(3):111368. https://doi.org/10.1016/j.injury.2024.111368. Epub 2024 Jan 19
9. Harky A, Bleetman D, Chan JSK, Eriksen P, Chaplin G, MacCarthy-Ofosu B, Theologou T, Ambekar S, Roberts N, Oo A. A systematic review and meta-analysis of endovascular versus open surgical repair for the traumatic ruptured thoracic aorta. J Vasc Surg. 2020;71(1):270–82. https://doi.org/10.1016/j.jvs.2019.05.011. Epub 2019 Jul 18. PMID: 31327611
10. Alremeithi R, Tran QK, Quintana MT, Shahamatdar S, Pourmand A. Approach to traumatic cardiac arrest in the emergency department: a narrative literature review for emergency providers. World J Emerg Med. 2024;15(1):3–9. https://doi.org/10.5847/wjem.j.1920-8642.2023.085. PMID: 38188559; PMCID: PMC10765073
11. Al-Thani H, Hakim S, Asim M, Basharat K, El-Menyar A. Patterns, management options and outcome of blunt thoracic aortic injuries: a 20-year experience from a tertiary care hospital. Eur J Trauma Emerg Surg. 2022;48(5):4079–91. https://doi.org/10.1007/s00068-022-01930-1. Epub 2022 Mar 14. PMID: 35286404; PMCID: PMC9532277
12. Menard MT, Farber A, Powell RJ, Rosenfield K, Conte MS, Hamza TH, Kaufman JA, Cziraky MJ, Creager MA, Dake MD, Jaff MR, Reid D, Sopko G, White CJ, Strong MB, van Over M, Chisci E, Goodney PP, Gray B, Kayssi A, Siracuse JJ, Choudhry NK, BEST-CLI Investigators. Quality of life in patients with chronic limb-threatening ischemia treated with revascularization. Circulation. 2024;149(16):1241–53. https://doi.org/10.1161/CIRCULATIONAHA.123.065277. Epub 2024 Apr 10. PMID: 38597097
13. Zhou Y, Wang T, He H, Li Q, Wan Z, Lu P, Shu C. Comparative effectiveness of endovascular treatment modalities for de novo femoropopliteal lesions at long-term follow-up: a network meta-analysis of randomized controlled trials. Int J Cardiol 2024 Jun 1;404:131977. doi: https://doi.org/10.1016/j.ijcard.2024.131977.. Epub 2024 Mar 18.
14. Yuan Z, Levitan B, Deng H, Szarek M, Bauersachs RM, Berkowitz SD, Haskell L, Barnathan ES, Bonaca MP. Quantitative benefit-risk evaluation of rivaroxaban in patients after peripheral arterial revascularization: the VOYAGER PAD trial. J Am Heart Assoc. 2024;13(8):e032782. https://doi.org/10.1161/JAHA.123.032782. Epub 2024 Apr 2. PMID: 38563380
15. Lok CE, Huber TS, Orchanian-Cheff A, Rajan DK. Arteriovenous access for hemodialysis: a review. JAMA. 2024;331(15):1307–17. https://doi.org/10.1001/jama.2024.0535.
16. Kingsmore DB, Edgar B, Aitken E, Calder F, Franchin M, Geddes C, Inston N, Jackson A, Jones RG, Karydis N, Kasthuri R, Mestres G, Papadakis G, Sivaprakasam R, Stephens M, Stevenson K, Stove C, Szabo L, Thomson PC, Tozzi M, White RD. Quality assurance in surgical trials of arteriovenous grafts for haemodialysis: a systematic review, a narrative exploration and expert recommendations. J Vasc Access. 2024:11297298241236521. https://doi.org/10.1177/11297298241236521. Epub ahead of print
17. Milders J, Ramspek CL, Janse RJ, Bos WJW, Rotmans JI, Dekker FW, van Diepen M. Prognostic models in nephrology: where Do we stand and where Do we go from here? Mapping out the evidence in a scoping review. J Am Soc Nephrol. 2024;35(3):367–80. https://doi.org/10.1681/ASN.0000000000000285. Epub 2023 Dec 12. PMID: 38082484; PMCID: PMC10914213.
18. Fayyaz F, Vaghani V, Ekhator C, Abdullah M, Alsubari RA, Daher OA, Bakht D, Batat H, Arif H, Bellegarde SB, Bisharat P, Faizullah M. Advancements in varicose vein treatment: anatomy, pathophysiology, minimally invasive techniques, sclerotherapy, patient satisfaction, and future directions. Cureus. 2024;16(1):e51990. https://doi.org/10.7759/cureus.51990. PMID: 38344644; PMCID: PMC10853729.
19. Cai PL, Hitchman LH, Mohamed AH, Smith GE, Chetter I, Carradice D. Endovenous ablation for venous leg ulcers. Cochrane Database Syst Rev. 2023;7(7):CD009494. https://doi.org/10.1002/14651858.CD009494.pub3. PMID: 37497816; PMCID: PMC10373122
20. Huang Y, Zhang D, Zhou C, Zhang Y, Shi C, Chen Q. The first meta-analysis research on the effects of endovenous laser ablation combined with saphenofemoral junction high ligation of the great saphenous vein. Lasers Med Sci. 2023;38(1):175. https://doi.org/10.1007/s10103-023-03833-y.

Sect. 2: Modern Management of Acute Aortic Dissection

21. Durham CA, Cambria RP, Wang LJ, Ergul EA, Aranson NJ, Patel VI, Conrad MF. The natural history of medically managed acute type B aortic dissection. J Vasc Surg. 2015;61(5):1192–8.
22. Brunkwall J, Kasprzak P, Verhoeven E, Heijmen R, Taylor P, ADSORB Trialists, Alric P, Canaud L, Janotta M, Raithel D, Malina W, Resch T, Eckstein HH, Ockert S, Larzon T, Carlsson F, Schumacher H, Classen S, Schaub P, Lammer J, Lönn L, Clough RE, Rampoldi V, Trimarchi S, Fabiani JN, Böckler D, Kotelis D, Böckler D, Kotelis D, von Tenng-Kobligk H, Mangialardi N, Ronchey S, Dialetto G, Matoussevitch V. Endovascular repair of acute uncomplicated aortic type B dissection promotes aortic remodelling: 1 year results of the ADSORB trial. Eur J Vasc Endovasc Surg. 2014;48(3):285–91. https://doi.org/10.1016/j.ejvs.2014.05.012. Epub 2014 Jun 22. Erratum in: Eur J Vasc Endovasc Surg. 2015 Jul;50(1):130. Böckler, D [removed]; von Tenng-Kobligk, H [corrected to von Tengg-Kobligk, H].
23. Eggebrecht H, Nienaber CA, Neuhäuser M, Baumgart D, Kische S, Schmermund A, Herold U, Rehders TC, Jakob HG, Erbel R. Endovascular stent–graft placement in aortic dissection: a meta-analysis. Eur Heart J. 2006;27(4):489–98.
24. Brunkwall J, Kasprzak P, Verhoeven E, Heijmen R, Taylor P, ADSORB Trialists, Alric P, Canaud L, Janotta M, Raithel D, Malina W, Resch T, Eckstein HH, Ockert S, Larzon T, Carlsson F, Schumacher H, Classen S, Schaub P, Lammer J, Lönn L, Clough RE, Rampoldi V, Trimarchi S, Fabiani JN, Böckler D, Kotelis D, Böckler D, Kotelis D, von Tenng-Kobligk H, Mangialardi N, Ronchey S, Dialetto G, Matoussevitch V. Endovascular repair of acute uncomplicated aortic type B dissection promotes aortic remodelling: 1 year results of the ADSORB trial. Eur J Vasc Endovasc Surg. 2014;48(3):285–91. https://doi.org/10.1016/j.ejvs.2014.05.012. Epub 2014 Jun 22. Erratum in: Eur J Vasc Endovasc Surg. 2015 Jul;50(1):130
25. Miyahara S, Mukohara N, Fukuzumi M, Morimoto N, Murakami H, Nakagiri K, Yoshida M. Long-term follow-up of acute type B aortic dissection: ulcer-like projections in thrombosed false lumen play a role in late aortic events. J Thorac Cardiovasc Surg. 2011;142(2) Tolenaar JL, van Herwaarden JA, Verhagen H, Moll FL, Muhs BE, Trimarchi S. Importance of entry tears in Type B aortic dissection prognosis. Ann Cardiothorac Surg. 2013 Sep;2(5):631
26. Rong D, Ge Y, Liu J, Liu X, Guo W. Combined proximal descending aortic endografting plus distal bare metal stenting (PETTICOAT technique) versus conventional proximal descending aortic stent graft repair for complicated type B aortic dissections. Cochrane Database Syst Rev. 2019;2019(10):CD013149. https://doi.org/10.1002/14651858.CD013149.pub2. PMID: 31684692; PMCID: PMC682012;
27. Niklas N, Królikowska K, Zdrodowska K, Gutowski P, Kazimierczak A, Rynio P. The rate of postoperative complications in complicated acute, and subacute type B aortic dissections after TEVAR vs. PETTICOAT procedures: systematic review and meta-analysis. Medicina (Kaunas). 2023;59(12):2150. https://doi.org/10.3390/medicina59122150. PMID: 38138253; PMCID: PMC10744781
28. Lombardi JV, Gleason TG, Panneton JM, Starnes BW, Dake MD, Haulon S, Mossop PJ, Segbefia E, Bharadwaj P, STABLE II investigators. Five-year results of the STABLE II study for the endovascular treatment of complicated, acute type B aortic dissection with a composite device design. J Vasc Surg. 2022;76(5):1189–97.
29. Mascia D, Rinaldi E, Salvati S, et al. Thoracic endovascular aortic repair with additional distal bare stents in type B aortic dissection does not prevent long-term aneurysmal degeneration. J Endovasc Ther. 2021;28:425–33. STABLE I and II long term trial
30. Hofferberth SC, Nixon IK, Boston RC, et al. Stent-assisted balloon-induced intimal disruption and relamination in aortic dissection repair: the STABILISE concept. J Thorac Cardiovasc Surg. 2014;147:1240–5. https://doi.org/10.1016/j.jtcvs.2013.03.036.
31. Herajärvi J, Mustonen C, Kesävuori R, Raivio P, Biancari F, Jermaine M. Juvonen T impact of high-risk features on outcome of acute type B aortic dissection. JTCVS Open. 2023;13:20–31.
32. Melissano G, Bertoglio L, Rinaldi E, Mascia D, Kahlberg A, Loschi D, De Luca M, Monaco F, Chiesa R. Satisfactory short-term outcomes of the STABILISE technique for type B aortic dissection. J Vasc Surg 2018 Oct;68(4):966–975. doi: https://doi.org/10.1016/j.jvs.2018.01.029.. Epub 2018 Mar 30.

Sect. 3. Carotid Endarterectomy—Can We Make a Good Operation Better? Technical Considereations

33. Hunt JR. The role of the carotid arteries in the causation of vascular lesions of the brain, with remarks on certain special features of the symptomatology. Am J Med Sci. 1914;147:704–13.
34. Eastcott HHG, Pickering GW, Rob CG. Reconstruction of internal carotid artery in a patient with intermittent attacks of hemiplegia. Lancet. 1954;2:994–6.
35. Carrea RMM, Murphy G. Surgical treatment of spontaneous thrombosis of the internal carotid artery in the neck: carotid-carotidal anastomosis: report of a case. Acta Neurol Latinoam. 1955;1:71–8.
36. Moniz E, Moniz E. L'encephalographie arterielle, son importance dans la localization des tumeurs cerebrales. Rev Neurol (Paris). 1927;2:72–90.
37. DeBakey ME. Successful carotid endarterectomy for cerebrovascular insufficiency. Nineteen-year follow-up. JAMA. 1975;233(10):1083–5.

38. North American Symptomatic Carotid Endarterectomy Trial Collaborators. Beneficial effect of carotid endarterectomy in symptomatic patients with high-grade carotid stenosis. N Engl J Med. 1991;325:445–53.
39. Matsumoto GH, Cossman D, Callow AD. Hazards and safeguards during carotid endarterectomy. Technical considerations. Am J Surg. 1977;133(4):458–62.
40. Delgado MG, Bogousslavsky J. Cerebral Hyperperfusion syndrome and related conditions. Eur Neurol. 2020;83(5):453–7.

Sect. 4: Use of Advanced Peripheral Arterial Techniques for Limb Salvage: Role of Intravascular Lithotripsy

41. Aday AW, Matsushita K. Epidemiology of peripheral artery disease and Polyvascular disease. Circ Res. 2021;128(12):1818–32.
42. Kawaguchi R, Tsurugaya H, Hoshizaki H, Toyama T, Oshima S, Taniguchi K. Impact of lesion calcification on clinical and angiographic outcome after sirolimus-eluting stent implantation in real-world patients. Cardiovasc Revasc Med. 2008;9(1):2–8. https://doi.org/10.1016/j.carrev.2007.07.004.
43. Lee MS, Canan T, Rha SW, Mustapha J, Adams GL. Pooled analysis of the CONFIRM registries: impact of gender on procedure and angiographic outcomes in patients undergoing orbital atherectomy for peripheral artery disease. J Endovasc Ther. 2015;22(1):57–62.
44. Babaev A, Zavlunova S, Attubato MJ, Martinsen BJ, Mintz GS, Maehara A. Orbital atherectomy plaque modification assessment of the femoropopliteal artery via intravascular ultrasound (TRUTH study). Vasc Endovasc Surg. 2015;49(7):188–94.
45. Fanelli F, Cannavale A, Gazzetti M, et al. Calcium burden assessment and impact on drug-eluting balloons in peripheral arterial disease. Cardiovasc Intervent Radiol. 2014;37(4):898–907.
46. Wardle BG, Ambler GK, Radwan RW, Hinchliffe RJ, Twine CP. Atherectomy for peripheral arterial disease. Cochrane Database Syst Rev. 2020;9(9):CD006680.
47. Roberts D, Niazi K, Miller W, Krishnan P, Gammon R, Schreiber T, Shammas NW, Clair D, DEFINITIVE Ca++ Investigators. Effective endovascular treatment of calcified femoropopliteal disease with directional atherectomy and distal embolic protection: final results of the DEFINITIVE Ca^{++} trial. Catheter Cardiovasc Interv. 2014;84(2):236–44.
48. McKinsey JF, Zeller T, Rocha-Singh KJ, Jaff MR, Garcia LA, DEFINITIVE LE Investigators. Lower extremity revascularization using directional atherectomy: 12-month prospective results of the DEFINITIVE LE study. JACC Cardiovasc Interv. 2014;7(8):923–33.
49. Banerjee A, Sarode K, Mohammad A, Brilakis ES, Banerjee S, Shammas GA, Shammas NW. Safety and effectiveness of the Nav-6 filter in preventing distal embolization during Jetstream Atherectomy of Infrainguinal peripheral artery lesions. J Invasive Cardiol. 2016;28(8):330–3.
50. Cleveland RO, McAteer JA. Physics of shock-wave lithotripsy. In: Smith's textbook of Endourology. Hoboken: Wiley-Blackwell; 2012. p. 527–58.
51. Brodmann M, Werner M, Brinton T, et al. Safety and performance of Lithoplasty for treatment of calcified peripheral artery lesions. J Am Coll Cardiol. 2017;70(7):908–10.
52. Brodmann M, Werner M, Holden A, Tepe G, Scheinert D, Schwindt A, Wolf F, Jaff M, Lansky A, Zeller T. Primary outcomes and mechanism of action of intravascular lithotripsy in calcified, femoropopliteal lesions: results of Disrupt PAD II. Catheter Cardiovasc Interv. 2019;93(2):335–42.
53. Tepe G, Brodmann M, Werner M, Bachinsky W, Holden A, Zeller T, Mangalmurti S, Nolte-Ernsting C, Bertolet B, Scheinert D, Gray WA, Disrupt PAD III, Investigators. Intravascular lithotripsy for peripheral artery calcification: 30-day outcomes from the randomized Disrupt PAD III trial. JACC Cardiovasc Interv. 2021;14(12):1352–61.
54. Tepe G, Brodmann M, Werner M, Bachinsky W, Holden A, Zeller T, Mangalmurti S, Nolte-Ernsting C, Virmani R, Parikh SA, Gray WA, Disrupt PAD III Investigators. Intravascular lithotripsy for peripheral artery calcification: mid-term outcomes from the randomized Disrupt PAD III trial. JSCAI. 2022;1(4):1–8.
55. Armstrong E. Late breaking clinical trial and shockwave-sponsored symposium. VIVA; 2022.
56. Adams G, Soukas PA, Mehrle A, Bertolet B, Armstrong EJ. Intravascular lithotripsy for treatment of calcified Infrapopliteal lesions: results from the Disrupt PAD III observational study. J Endovasc Ther. 2022;29(1):76–83.
57. Brodmann M, Holden A, Zeller T. Safety and feasibility of intravascular lithotripsy for treatment of below-the-knee arterial Stenoses. J Endovasc Ther. 2018;25(4):499–503.

Sect. 5. The May–Thurner Syndrome

58. May R, Thurner J. The cause of the predominantly sinistral occurrence of thrombosis of the pelvic veins. Angiology. 1957;8(5):419–27. https://doi.org/10.1177/000331975700800505.
59. Cockett FB, Thomas ML, Negus D. Iliac vein compression. Its relation to iliofemoral thrombosis and the post-thrombotic syndrome. Br Med J. 1967;2(5543):14–9. https://doi.org/10.1136/bmj.2.5543.14. PMID: 6020994; PMCID: PMC1841147
60. Kibbe MR, Ujiki M, Goodwin AL, Eskandari M, Yao J, Matsumura J. Iliac vein compression in

an asymptomatic patient population. J Vasc Surg. 2004;39(5):937–43. https://doi.org/10.1016/j.jvs.2003.12.032.
61. Yin M, Huang X, Cui C, Ye K, Li W, Lu X, Lu M, Jiang M. The effect of stent placement for May-Thurner syndrome combined with symptomatic superficial venous reflux disease. J Vasc Surg Venous Lymphat Disord. 2015;3(2):168–72. https://doi.org/10.1016/j.jvsv.2014.11.006. Epub 2015 Jan 17
62. Abramowitz S, Shaikh A, Mojibian H, Mouawad NJ, Bunte MC, Skripochnik E, Lindquist J, Elmasri F, Khalsa B, Bhat A, Nguyen J, Shah N, Noor SS, Murrey D, Gandhi S, Raskin A, Schor J, Dexter DJ. Comparison of anticoagulation vs mechanical thrombectomy for the treatment of iliofemoral deep vein thrombosis. J Vasc Surg Venous Lymphat Disord. 2024;24:101825. https://doi.org/10.1016/j.jvsv.2024.101825. Epub ahead of print
63. Dexter DJ, Kado H, Shaikh A, at. Safety and effectiveness of mechanical Thrombectomy from the fully enrolled Multicenter, prospective CLOUT registry. JSCAI. 2023:100585. https://doi.org/10.1016/j.jscai.2023.100585.
64. Murali N, Gupta R, Desai KR. The role of iliac vein stent placement in pelvic venous disorder management. J Vasc Surg Venous Lymphat Disord. 2024;12(2):101696. https://doi.org/10.1016/j.jvsv.2023.101696. Epub 2023 Nov 15
65. Villalba LM, Bayat I, Dubenec S, Puckridge P, Thomas S, Varcoe R, Vasudevan T, Tripathi R. Review of the literature supporting international clinical practice guidelines on iliac venous stenting and their applicability to Australia and New Zealand practice. J Vasc Surg Venous Lymphat Disord. 2024:101843. https://doi.org/10.1016/j.jvsv.2024.101843. Epub ahead of print
66. Raju S, Ward M Jr, Davis M. Relative importance of iliac vein obstruction in patients with post-thrombotic femoral vein occlusion. J Vasc Surg Venous Lymphat Disord. 2015;3(2):161–7. https://doi.org/10.1016/j.jvsv.2014.10.004. Epub 2014 Dec 12
67. Haig Y, Enden T, Grøtta O, Kløw NE, Slagsvold CE, Ghanima W, Sandvik L, Hafsahl G, Holme PA, Holmen LO, Njaaastad AM, Sandbæk G, Sandset PM, CaVenT Study Group. Post-thrombotic syndrome after catheter-directed thrombolysis for deep vein thrombosis (CaVenT): 5-year follow-up results of an open-label, randomized controlled trial. Lancet Haematol. 2016;3(2):e64–71. https://doi.org/10.1016/S2352-3026(15)00248-3. Epub 2016 Jan 6
68. Vedantham S, Goldhaber SZ, Julian JA, Kahn SR, Jaff MR, Cohen DJ, Magnuson E, Razavi MK, Comerota AJ, Gornik HL, Murphy TP, Lewis L, Duncan JR, Nieters P, Derfler MC, Filion M, Gu CS, Kee S, Schneider J, Saad N, Blinder M, Moll S, Sacks D, Lin J, Rundback J, Garcia M, Razdan R, VanderWoude E, Marques V, Kearon C. ATTRACT trial Investigators. Pharmacomechanical catheter-directed thrombolysis for deep-vein thrombosis. N Engl J Med. 2017;377(23):2240–52. https://doi.org/10.1056/NEJMoa1615066. PMID: 29211671; PMCID: PMC5763501

Sect. 6: Evaluation of a Patient for Hemodialysis Access

69. Lok CE, et al. KDOQI vascular access guideline work group. KDOQI clinical practice guideline for vascular access: 2019 update. Am J Kidney Dis. 2020;75(4/suppl 2):S1–S164.

Sect. 7: Summary and Future of Vascular Surgery

70. Latifi R, Rhee P, Gruessner R, editors. Technological advances in surgery, trauma, and critical care. Springer; 2015.
71. Latifi R, editor. The modern hospital. Patient Centered, disease based, research oriented, technology driven. Switzerland AG: Springer Nature; 2019.
72. Sinha K, Berczeli M, Lumsden AB, Roy TL. Imaging: new frontiers in vascular training. Methodist Debakey Cardiovasc J. 2022;18(3):39–48. https://doi.org/10.14797/mdcvj.1093. PMID: 35734160; PMCID: PMC9165676
73. Kwak SH, Hernandez-Cancela RB, DiCorpo DA, Condon DE, Merino J, Wu P, Brody JA, Yao J, Guo X, Ahmadizar F, Meyer M, Sincan M, Mercader JM, Lee S, Haessler J, Vy HMT, Lin Z, Armstrong ND, Gu S, Tsao NL, Lange LA, Wang N, Wiggins KL, Trompet S, Liu S, RJF L, Judy R, Schroeder PH, Hasbani NR, Bos MM, Morrison AC, Jackson RD, Reiner AP, Manson JE, Chaudhary NS, Carmichael LK, Chen YI, Taylor KD, Ghanbari M, van Meurs J, Pitsillides AN, Psaty BM, Noordam R, Do R, Park KS, Jukema JW, Kavousi M, Correa A, Rich SS, Damrauer SM, Hajek C, Cho NH, Irvin MR, Pankow JS, Nadkarni GN, Sladek R, Goodarzi MO, Florez JC, Chasman DI, Heckbert SR, Kooperberg C, Dupuis J, Malhotra R, de Vries PS, Liu CT, Rotter JI, Meigs JB, Cohorts for Heart and Aging Research in Genomic Epidemiology (CHARGE) Consortium. Time-to-event genome-wide association study for incident cardiovascular disease in people with type 2 diabetes. Diabetes Care. 2024:dc232274. https://doi.org/10.2337/dc23-2274. Epub ahead of print
74. Jockisch RD, Davey CR, Keller SMP, Lahoti S, Bramlet MT. Pioneering patient-specific approaches for precision surgery using imaging and virtual reality. J Vis Exp. 2024;(206) https://doi.org/10.3791/66227.
75. Dudrick SJ. Regression of atherosclerosis by the intravenous infusion of specific biochemical nutrient substrates in animals and humans. Ann Surg. 1987;206(3):296–315. https://doi.

org/10.1097/00000658-198709000-00008. PMID: 3115205; PMCID: PMC1493195.

76. Gould KL, Martucci JP, Goldberg DI, Hess MJ, Edens RP, Latifi R, Dudrick SJ. Short-term cholesterol lowering decreases size and severity of perfusion abnormalities by positron emission tomography after dipyridamole in patients with coronary artery disease. A potential noninvasive marker of healing coronary endothelium. Circulation. 1994;89(4):1530–8. https://doi.org/10.1161/01.cir.89.4.1530.
77. Trounson A, McDonald C. Stem cell therapies in clinical trials: progress and challenges. Cell Stem Cell. 2015;17(1):11–22. https://doi.org/10.1016/j.stem.2015.06.007.
78. Zhang J, Bolli R, Garry DJ, Marbán E, Menasché P, Zimmermann WH, Kamp TJ, Wu JC, Dzau VJ. Basic and translational research in cardiac repair and regeneration: JACC state-of-the-art review. J Am Coll Cardiol. 2021;78(21):2092–105. https://doi.org/10.1016/j.jacc.2021.09.019. PMID: 34794691; PMCID: PMC9116459.
79. Kir D, Patel MJ, Munagala MR. What is the status of regenerative therapy in heart failure? Curr Cardiol Rep. 2021;23(10):146. https://doi.org/10.1007/s11886-021-01575-3.
80. Ogay V, Sekenova A, Li Y, Issabekova A, Saparov A. The therapeutic potential of mesenchymal stem cells in the treatment of atherosclerosis. Curr Stem Cell Res Ther. 2021;16(7):897–913. https://doi.org/10.2174/1574888X16999210128193549.
81. Latifi R, Doarn C, Merrell R, editors. Telemedicine, telehealth, and telepresence: principles, strategies, applications, and new directions. Switzerland: Springer Nature; 2020.
82. Gachabayov M, Latifi LA, Parsikia A, Latifi R. Current state and future perspectives of telemedicine use in surgery during the COVID-19 pandemic: a scoping review protocol. Int J Surg Protoc. 2020;24:17–20. https://doi.org/10.1016/j.isjp.2020.10.002. Epub 2020 Oct 24. PMID: 33140036; PMCID: PMC7584517
83. Lareyre F, Chaptoukaev H, Kiang SC, Chaudhuri A, Behrendt CA, Zuluaga MA, Raffort J. Telemedicine and digital health applications in vascular surgery. J Clin Med. 2022;11(20):6047. https://doi.org/10.3390/jcm11206047. PMID: 36294368; PMCID: PMC9604656.
84. Chen AJ, Yeh SL, Delfin D, Hoal G, Barron N, Riedinger T, Kashanijou N, Lieland J, Bickel K, O'Connell JB, Ulloa JG. Telemedicine and vascular surgery: expanding access and providing care through the COVID-19 pandemic. Am Surg. 2022;88(10):2561–4. https://doi.org/10.1177/00031348221109464. Epub 2022 Jun 19. PMID: 35722888; PMCID: PMC9209855.
85. Yew SN, Khor BY, Wong E, Gwilym BL, Bosanquet DC. Telemedicine in vascular surgery during COVID-19 pandemic: a systematic review and narrative synthesis. Ann Vasc Surg. 2023;93:166–73. https://doi.org/10.1016/j.avsg.2023.03.023. Epub 2023 Apr 1. PMID: 37011724; PMCID: PMC10065869
86. Tran Z, Byun J, Lee HY, Boggs H, Tomihama EY, Kiang SC. Bias in artificial intelligence in vascular surgery. Semin Vasc Surg 2023 Sep;36(3):430–434. doi: https://doi.org/10.1053/j.semvascsurg.2023.07.003.. Epub 2023 Aug 1.
87. Zarkowsky DS, Stonko DP. Artificial intelligence's role in vascular surgery decision-making. Semin Vasc Surg. 2021;34(4):260–7. https://doi.org/10.1053/j.semvascsurg.2021.10.005. Epub 2021 Oct 27
88. Dossabhoy SS, Ho VT, Ross EG, Rodriguez F, Arya S. Artificial intelligence in clinical workflow processes in vascular surgery and beyond. Semin Vasc Surg. 2023;36(3):401–12. https://doi.org/10.1053/j.semvascsurg.2023.07.002. Epub 2023 Jul 22. PMID: 37863612; PMCID: PMC10956485
89. Thaxton C, Dardik A. Computer science meets vascular surgery: keeping a pulse on artificial intelligence. Semin Vasc Surg. 2023;36(3):419–25. https://doi.org/10.1053/j.semvascsurg.2023.05.003. Epub 2023 May 27. PMID: 37863614; PMCID: PMC10589450.

Surgical Decision-Making in the Management of Polytrauma Patients

22

Anthony Duncan, Ergest Isak, Mentor Ahmeti,
and Anthony Duncan

Abbreviations

AIS	Abbreviated Injury Score
ATLS	Advanced Trauma Life Support
DCR	Damage Control Resuscitation
DCL	Damage Control Laparotomy
DCO	Damage Control Orthopedics
TBI	Traumatic Brain Injury

Introduction

Polytrauma is not a novel term within the medical field, originally described by Border et al. as encompassing any patient who has sustained two or more significant injuries [1]. Its most recent iteration, established by the Berlin definition, is evidence-based and encompasses all patients with an Abbreviated Injury Score (AIS) of greater than or equal to 3 in two or more bodily systems [2]. Despite continuous research and advances in polytrauma management, it remains a significant global cause of mortality, despite notable improvements in medical care and trauma management [3, 4]. Managing polytrauma patients necessitates a multidisciplinary approach, swift assessment, and well-coordinated care to optimize outcomes. This chapter delineates the fundamental principles and steps essential to the effective management of polytrauma patients.

A. Duncan

A. Duncan · E. Isak
Department of Surgery, University of North Dakota School of Medicine and Health Science, Grand Forks, ND, USA
e-mail: Anthony.Duncan@und.edu; ergest.isak@und.edu

M. Ahmeti (✉)
Department of Surgery, University of North Dakota School of Medicine and Health Science, Grand Forks, ND, USA

Department of Trauma and Acute Care Surgery, Sanford Medical Center Fargo, Fargo, ND, USA

Initial Assessment and Stabilization

Primary Survey

Upon the patient's arrival at the hospital, a meticulously organized approach to their management becomes imperative. The foundations of this initial management can be discovered in the Advanced Trauma Life Support (ATLS) guidelines, which serve to enhance the quality and efficiency of care for polytrauma cases. The primary survey in ATLS adheres to the ABCDE approach, addressing the following key aspects: Airway, Breathing, Circulation, Disability, and Exposure [5].

R. Latifi (ed.), *Surgical Decision-Making*, https://doi.org/10.1007/978-3-031-67391-7_22

Airway

Airway management takes precedence in ATLS and should be addressed before proceeding with the rest of the algorithm [5]. Additionally, in these patients, the mechanism of injury should be carefully considered, and cervical spine stabilization should be maintained if necessary. Assessing the patient's response is crucial, as it enables the determination of airway patency and the sufficiency of cerebral oxygen supply for cognitive function. If issues arise with the patient's oxygenation, simple interventions can be attempted to improve the situation, such as oral suctioning or the use of a chin lift/jaw thrust to enhance airway patency.

In most clinical scenarios involving patients with a Glasgow Coma Scale (GCS) score of less than 8, securing a definitive airway becomes imperative. This is typically achieved through the insertion of an endotracheal tube, a method widely recommended. In the context of polytrauma, many clinicians advocate for the use of video laryngoscopy, as it reduces strain on the neck in patients with potential cervical spine injuries and has shown to increase first-attempt intubation success rates [6, 7].

If endotracheal intubation is unsuccessful or not feasible, the next step involves establishing a surgical airway. This can be accomplished through either cricothyroidotomy or tracheostomy. Cricothyroidotomy is often preferred as it is less technically challenging and can be performed more expeditiously. Both percutaneous and open techniques have been described, with animal models demonstrating that an open scalpel technique is superior in terms of achieving a timely airway [8, 9].

Breathing

Breathing is the vital process responsible for oxygenating the blood, primarily reliant on lung parenchyma. The initial assessment entails several key steps: auscultating for bilateral breath sounds, monitoring pulse oximetry readings, and observing respiratory rate and effort. Absence of breath sounds warrants immediate consideration of conditions that could compromise respiration, such as tension pneumothorax or hemothorax. Left untreated, these conditions can swiftly escalate into life-threatening emergencies. Depending on the clinical setting and availability of supplies, the choice between needle thoracentesis, finger thoracostomy, or tube thoracotomy should be made. When opting for needle thoracentesis, it should be executed at the fifth intercostal space, just anterior to the mid-axillary line, with a prompt transition to tube thoracostomy as soon as practical [10]. Tube thoracostomy placement is ideally positioned at the fifth intercostal space along the mid-axillary line.

Circulation

In the Advanced Trauma Life Support (ATLS) protocol, the "C" signifies "Circulation," highlighting its pivotal role in managing a patient's cardiovascular system during trauma care [5]. Swift and precise assessment of circulatory status is paramount, as inadequate perfusion can lead to life-threatening complications. Healthcare providers concentrate on evaluating critical parameters, including blood pressure, heart rate, capillary refill time, and overall hemodynamic stability. Identifying and controlling sources of blood loss are of paramount importance during this phase. External blood loss can be readily detected through observation and physical examination, with common external bleeding sites including long-bone fractures and scalp lacerations. On the other hand, internal blood loss can be more challenging to pinpoint. To aid in diagnosis, chest X-rays can be used to assess intrathoracic hemorrhage, and a focused assessment with sonography (FAST) examination can provide valuable information, although it may not entirely rule out internal bleeding. In cases where significant blood loss is suspected, initiating a balanced transfusion of packed red cells, fresh frozen plasma, and platelets at a 1:1:1 ratio as soon as possible has been shown to improve outcomes compared to crystalloid resuscitation [11, 12]. Hemostatic resuscitation studies reported the ratio for platelets in pooled packs. It is important to note that platelet volume nomenclature has changed to platelet units which are equivalent to 6 platelet packs, as to reduce confusion, the actual transfusion ratio should be 6:1:6. More recently, there has been a shift toward using whole blood, where available, for cases involving significant blood loss [13, 14]. Tranexamic acid (TXA) has also demonstrated promise in trauma patients, as it effectively reduces the rate of fibrinolysis, preserving clot integrity. Administration should begin with a 1-gram bolus within 3 hours of the initial injury, followed by an additional 1-gram infusion over the subsequent 8 hours [15–17].

Disability

The assessment of a patient's disability status necessitates a comprehensive evaluation of their entire neurological condition. This encompasses obtaining the Glasgow Coma Scale (GCS) score, conducting a thorough examination of pupils, and assessing motor and sensory functions in the extremities to detect any deficits. It is of utmost importance to meticulously document and record these findings, as this documentation serves as a baseline to monitor for any potential deterioration in the patient's condition. In cases where a patient presents with a diminished level of consciousness, traumatic brain injury should always be a primary consideration.

Exposure/Environment

During this phase of the evaluation, it is essential to remove all of the patient's clothing to facilitate a comprehensive head-to-toe examination, which includes the back, to uncover any potential concealed injuries. Additionally, meticulous care must be exercised to prevent the onset of hypothermia by providing warm blankets to shield the patient from temperature loss and maintain their body heat.

Management priorities

While the linear sequence of airway-breathing-circulation has been a long-standing principle taught for decades and adopted by the ATLS course for ease of didactic teaching, management of polytrauma patients should focus on addressing immediately life-threatening injuries. While a principle of Tactical Combat Casualty Care for decades, recently this concept has been gaining acceptance in civilian trauma management, supported by civilian evidence as described by Ferrada that hypotensive patients who underwent intubation before blood transfusion exhibited a significantly higher mortality rate compared to those who underwent transfusion first [18]. Conversely, other studies indicate no disparity in mortality when comparing CAB (Circulation-Airway-Breathing) and ABC sequences [19]. We maintain the belief that there is no one-size-fits-all approach for polytrauma patients, given the unique patterns of injury each individual presents with. Particularly, in real-time situations where multiple issues demand simultaneous attention, patients should be assessed and treated for the most immediate concern—whether it be hypovolemic shock or critical hypoxia. Authors are excited to learn that new ATLS formats will shift from the historic ABCDE to xABCDE priority, where **x** stands for e-**x**-anguination and/or e-**x**-tremity, in recognition of evidence available.

Management of injuries based on system

Damage Control Resuscitation (DCR)

DCR was initially developed by the military after witnessing the benefit of giving whole blood to patients. As polytrauma patients undergo continued blood loss, there is a shift toward the trauma patient lethal triad including metabolic acidosis, hypothermia, and coagulopathy. DCR focuses on prevention of the coagulopathy aspect of the lethal triad but must occur in conjunction with immediate control of bleeding, either by direct pressure, tourniquets, or damage control laparotomy (DCL) depending on the scenario. DCR does not substitute bleeding control. There continues to be a growing amount of evidence for use of balanced transfusion or whole blood in trauma patients with limiting the amount of crystalloid products given [12]. Despite lack of controlled randomized trials, benefits of whole blood continue to be described; including a decreased amount of excess volume given compared to component therapy, better coagulation profile, improved function of product, decreased 24-hour and in-hospital mortality, and decreased complication rates [12, 20, 21].

Traumatic Brain Injury (TBI)

The initial evaluation of polytrauma patients with suspected TBI should prioritize the assessment of neurological status. The Glasgow Coma Scale (GCS) remains a valuable tool for quantifying the severity of TBI. The goal of preventing secondary injury in traumatic brain injury (TBI) is a crucial focus of evidence-based management. It is one of the major effects clinicians can have to prevent worsening of patient outcomes. The two major and preventable causes that are seen to cause secondary injury are hypoxia and hypotension.

Maintaining adequate cerebral perfusion pressure (CPP) by optimizing blood pressure and oxygen delivery to the brain is essential. Cerebral perfusion pressure = mean arterial pressure-ICP. Current guidelines support the use of advanced monitoring techniques to guide the management of TBI in polytrauma patients [22]. Intracranial pressure (ICP) monitoring is crucial for early detection and management of intracranial hypertension, which can lead to secondary brain injury. Classical recommendations per the Brain Trauma Foundation recommend maintaining an ICP of ≤22. However, more recent studies suggest that a patient specific ICP goal is more correlated with improved outcomes [23, 24]. There has recently been questioning if agents like hypertonic saline or mannitol are beneficial. While they have been shown to decrease ICP, there appears to be no benefit in mortality or neurological outcome with them [25–27].

Two recent randomized control trials evaluated the utility of using prophylactic hypothermia in severe TBI. They differed slightly with one using hypothermia in patients with elevated ICP and the other study performed this in patients without elevated ICP [28, 29]. While prophylactic hypothermia was successful at decreasing ICP, but at the cost of increased mortality and worst neurological outcomes [28, 29]. Further, patients with TBI that present with accidental hypothermia are found to have significantly higher rates of mortality [30].

Surgical Interventions: In select cases of severe TBI, surgical interventions like decompressive craniectomy have gained prominence as a means to reduce intracranial pressure and prevent herniation. Some data suggests that use of decompressive craniectomy can improve outcomes, particularly in patients with refractory intracranial hypertension [31, 32]. In contrast, the DECRA study showed while early decompressive craniectomy decreased intracranial pressure, it was associated with worst 6-month mortality [33]. However, the correct patients that would benefit most from decompressive craniectomy and have meaningful quality of life are still being investigated.

Hypoxia and hypotension are associated with poorer outcomes in TBI patients, emphasizing the importance of oxygenation and hemodynamic stability. Addressing injuries that cause hemodynamic instability becomes a priority in patients with TBI. Additionally, avoiding hypercapnia and maintaining normocapnia, as well as managing temperature to prevent hyperthermia, have been shown to reduce secondary injury. Close neurological monitoring, the use of advanced neuromonitoring techniques, and a multidisciplinary approach are integral to the evidence-based prevention of secondary brain injury in TBI patients.

Abdominal Injuries

Damage Control Laparotomy

Damage Control Laparotomy (DCL) continues to be a fundamental part of trauma surgery. DCL focuses on controlling hemorrhage and contamination while minimizing operative time to save the physiologic reserve of the patient. Typical indications for DCL are as follows: metabolic acidosis (pH < 7.2), hypothermia (<35 °C), coagulopathy, patients who are unstable and operation will last longer than 2 hours, or patients that will require further intra-abdominal surgical evaluation at a later time [34].

Combination of improvements in temporary abdominal closures and hemostatic resuscitation over the past decade have made the DCL more efficient and decreased the rate of complications we see. As stated above the focus of DCL is first controlling hemorrhage and second, contamination. Hemorrhage should be controlled with timely repair, packing, simple ligation, or temporary shunts. Hollow viscus injuries should be resected and anastomosis left for the time of definitive repair. Multiple different methods of temporary negative pressure systems exist commercially or can be fashioned with equipment readily available in the operating room, to serve as an optimal method of temporary abdominal closure. The initial portion consists of a porous plastic covering that allows extraction of fluid while preventing the formation of adhesions. In authors' experience, a sterile X-ray film cover with perforations works very well, is inexpensive and readily available. Foam or operating room sterile towels are then placed with an eventual occlusive dressing overtop with airtight drains being laid in bilateral gutters. Negative pressure is then typically applied between 100 and 150 mmHg. There are also readily available commercial products that include all parts in a single package. Once the patient has been removed from the operating room, focus should be placed on further resuscitation, hemodynamic stability, correction of acid/base, electrolyte abnormalities and rewarming.

After the patient has been stabilized and physiologically optimized in the ICU setting, they should be considered for return to the operating room either for repeat exploration or definitive repair. While multiple centers and surgeons will opt for an arbitrary 48-hour period, we recommend returning to the operating room once the patient is physiologically optimized.

With the evolution of and utilization of the open abdomen strategy, it is important to keep in mind closure of the abdomen. Delay in closure is associated with increase in ventral hernias, enterocutaneous or entero-atmospheric fistulas, and loss of abdominal domain. One recent study showed that closure of the abdomen within 8 days can minimize complications [35].

Non-operative management

High quality data shows the benefit of non-operative management (NOM) within abdominal trauma in certain clinical situations [36, 37]. The current standard of care for the majority of patients with blunt abdominal trauma who are hemodynamically stable without peritonitis is to pursue further radiological work up with computed tomography. However, patients who are hemodynamically unstable or exhibit peritonitis on examination should undergo surgical intervention, as stated above.

The management of transient responders involves institutional resources (availability of interventional radiology or surgical capabilities) to address the cause of hemodynamic instability. In facilities with quick access to interventional radiology, stable patients with solid organ injuries of advanced grading will often be effectively treated with angioembolization or other interventional radiologic interventions. Our institution uses the American Association for Surgery of Trauma grading of solid organ injuries.

Patients with known injuries who are being managed with NOM require hospital admittance with close monitoring for changes in the patient's clinical status. There are no current recommendations on the frequency of monitoring; however, it typically consists of serial laboratory values, NPO status, initial short-term limitations of activity, and repeat abdominal examinations. Clinicians also need to maintain a high index of suspicion for injuries that are often missed on the patient's initial CT scan, including hollow viscus injuries and diaphragmatic injuries. Furthermore, patients who experience deterioration in their clinical status should undergo operative intervention as quickly as possible.

Thoracic Injuries

Injuries resulting from trauma stand as the primary global cause of mortality. In the United States, thoracic trauma contributes to as much as 35% of trauma-related fatalities, involving a diverse array of injuries resulting in significant morbidity and mortality [38, 39]. Thoracic trauma is seen in approximately two-thirds of trauma patients and with varying degrees of severity, often ranging from simple rib fractures to more complex penetrating injuries. Thoracic trauma is broadly categorized as blunt or penetrating trauma. Blunt chest trauma is the most common, accounting for 80% of incidents, with less than 10% needing any form of surgical intervention vs. 15 to 30% in patients that sustained penetrating chest injuries [38]. However, blunt chest trauma directly contributes to 20 to 25% of trauma deaths [38]. Mortality rates, second only to head injuries, emphasize the critical significance of prompt and effective initial management. Timely diagnosis and treatment can prevent a significant number of these fatalities [38].

The management of chest trauma can be categorized into three specific tiers of care: prehospital trauma support, in-hospital or emergency room trauma support, and surgical trauma support [36]. Recognizing thoracic injuries at each care level is pivotal for subsequent outcomes. The initial resuscitation and management of a patient with chest trauma adhere to protocols outlined in Advanced Trauma Life Support (ATLS) [5]. Following a primary survey, the focus is on promptly excluding or addressing immediately life-threatening injuries, such as tension pneumothorax, massive hemothorax, flail chest, cardiac tamponade, aortic injury, and tracheobronchial disruption.

Prehospital support: The initial evaluation of the trauma patient begins with the primary survey, which is an essential step in recognizing immediately life-threatening conditions such as tension pneumothorax, pulmonary contusion, massive hemothorax, and cardiac tamponade. General inspection of the thorax for asymmetry; palpation for tenderness, crepitus, and flail segments; percussion; and auscultation [sensitivity of 90% and specificity of 98% will aid in identifying life-threatening conditions such as tension pneumothorax, which may necessitate immediate intervention such as needle decompression or tube thoracostomy [40, 41]. Given that tension pneumothorax stands as the most frequently reversible cause of death in trauma patients experiencing cardiac arrest, prompt and accurate assessment is crucial [42–44].

In-hospital support: The assessment of patients with thoracic trauma commences with Advanced Trauma Life Support (ATLS) and subsequently utilizes diverse imaging methods contingent on the initial symptoms observed. Swift intervention is imperative for life-threatening injuries identified during the initial trauma assessment.

Ever since its initial formal description nearly five decades ago, the emergency department thoracotomy (EDT) has remained a subject of debate for many years [45]. Research indicates that outcomes depend on the mechanism of injury, anatomic location of injury, and the presence of signs of life on arrival [39]. Defined by the American College of Surgeons Committee on Trauma in 2001, signs of life are considered present with any of the following: pupillary response, spontaneous ventilation, presence of carotid pulse, measurable or palpable blood pressure, extremity movement, or cardiac electrical activity [45]. In penetrating chest trauma, the survival rate after resuscitative thoracotomy is 8.8%, contrasting with 1.4% in blunt chest trauma. Notably, patients with penetrating chest trauma and signs of life upon arrival have an overall survival rate of 19.4% in contrast to 4.6% overall survival in blunt chest trauma with signs of life present upon arrival [46]. There have recently been some suggestions as to different indications in pediatric patients compared to adult patients [47, 48]. Adult and pediatric patient indications/contraindications for resuscitative thoracotomy include [49–51]:

Adult Indications:

Salvageable postinjury cardiac arrest:

- Patients sustaining witnessed penetrating trauma with <15 minutes of prehospital CPR.
- Patients sustaining witnessed blunt trauma with <5 minutes of prehospital CPR.

Persistent severe postinjury hypotension (SBP $\leq$ 60 mmHg) due to:

- Cardiac tamponade.
- Hemorrhage—intrathoracic, intra-abdominal, extremity, cervical.
- Air embolism.

Adult Contraindications:

- Penetrating trauma: CPR > 15 minutes and no signs of life (pupillary response, respiratory effort, or motor activity).
- Blunt trauma: CPR > 5 minutes and no signs of life or asystole.

Pediatric Indications:

- Pediatric patients with penetrating thoracic or abdominopelvic injury and signs of life on presentation.
- Pediatric patients with blunt injury and signs of life on presentation.

Pediatric Contraindications:

- Pediatric patients with penetrating thoracic or abdominopelvic injury without signs of life on presentation.
- Pediatric patients with blunt injury without signs of life on presentation.

Hemothorax and pneumothorax are the most common injuries frequently encountered in thoracic trauma. These can be definitively managed through the use of a chest tube in 80% of cases [39]. Approximately 10% of all trauma patients and 30% of those with chest trauma exhibit rib fractures [43]. Initial management in patients with three or more rib fractures entails ensuring adequate analgesia, thoracostomy drainage if required, and pulmonary hygiene. Effective pain control is paramount and involves a multimodal approach beginning with acetaminophen and NSAIDs, with opioids administered on an as-needed basis. Regional anesthesia, such as epidural anesthesia can be used as a step-up approach for patients with multiple or displaced rib fractures, and for those with pain unresponsive to pharmacologic management [45]. Surgical rib fixation is typically performed within 48 to 72 hours of the injury and is reserved for cases where adequate pain control cannot be achieved and for patients facing impending respiratory failure or unable to wean off ventilatory support [39]. Certain patients require urgent or emergent operative intervention. Thoracotomy performed in the operating room is indicated for various conditions in thoracic trauma including massive hemothorax with blood loss ≥1500 mL initially or > 200 mL/hour of chest tube output over 2–4 hours, cardiac tamponade, great vessel injury, significant air leak persisting after thoracostomy placement, confirmed tracheobronchial injury, and open pneumothorax [34]. As minimally invasive techniques have become more popular, video-assisted thoracoscopic surgery (VATS) has been increasingly used in favor of thoracotomy in hemodynamically stable trauma patients, leading to faster recovery, reduced postoperative pain, and greater visualization of the entire pleural place for diagnosing and treating commonly missed injuries such as retained hemothoraces and diaphragmatic lesions [38, 52, 53].

Orthopedic Management

Orthopedic injuries are a significant source of hemorrhagic shock and blood loss for polytrauma patients and must be considered and addressed in the acute setting. It has been estimated that a significant amount of musculoskeletal injuries are missed during the primary survey [54].

Pelvic fractures can cause a significant amount of blood loss without external physical signs other than vital changes. Open long-bone fractures also must be recognized and addressed as they have major vascular supply and will have no means of self-tamponade. Orthopedic trauma surgery has also taken a similar paradigm shift from what was previously known as “Early Total Care” (ETC) to what is now standard of care as “Damage Control Orthopedics” (DCO). The notion that the polytrauma patients with significant musculoskeletal injuries were considered too physiologically unstable to undergo any major orthopedic surgery was questioned by the Bone et al. study in 1989 [55]. This landmark study found that early fixation of all long-bone fractures within 24 hours of initial injury led to reduced morbidity among patients, including reduced pulmonary complications and length of ICU and hospital stay [55]. The term "Early Total Care" was shortly established following this study, and it referred to definitive fracture surgery within 24–48 hours for all long-bone fractures in a polytrauma patient. The practice of ETC was challenged as studies that followed found a rise in pulmonary complications and multiorgan dysfunction observed in polytraumatized and physiologically unstable patients that were managed using this approach. The studies described these complications as arising from the "second hit" or inflammatory response associated with fracture surgery [56]. This led to the emergence of "DCO." Modeled after the concept of "damage control surgery," "DCO" emphasizes that a certain subgroup of patients require further resuscitation and medical optimization prior to undergoing definitive fracture surgery and thus, temporizing measures such as external fixation of fractures can lead to more favorable outcomes in such patient groups [57]. Current recommendations though are for open fractures to be taken to the OR within 24 hours for initially debridement and possible early closure [55].

Infection Prevention and Antibiotics

Prophylactic Antibiotics

Prompt antibiotic use is important in indicated clinical settings, while not overusing to create antibiotic resistance is also essential. The usage of antibiotics must still be driven by the etiology of disease process that the patient is experiencing. Patients who have open fractures, lacerations, or concern for viscus injuries justify the usage of antibiotics. The majority of trauma centers will have intuitional protocols for recommended antibiotic and dosages given their area specific microbiome. Those who are being taken to the operating room for intervention also justify the use of prophylactic antibiotics given within one hour prior to incision. In regard to doing open abdomen, evidence shows that there is a benefit in prompt prophylactic administration of antibiotics and early discontinuation in appropriate patients [58].

Multidisciplinary Care

Team Collaboration

The polytrauma patient often presents with injuries spanning various medical specialties, necessitating a comprehensive, multidisciplinary treatment approach. The optimal approach to caring for multiply injured patients requires a multidisciplinary team, including but not limited to trauma surgeons, orthopedic surgeons, anesthesiologists, intensivists, neurosurgeons, maxillofacial surgeons, ophthalmologists, diagnostic/interventional radiologists, and various other specialists [59]. Vertical integration of various teams within the healthcare system is essential in the delivery of care and management of the polytrauma patient. This includes integration of nursing, advanced practice providers, pharmacists, blood bank, case managers, social workers, clinical psychiatry, and physical and occupational therapists to name a few.

This comprehensive approach to managing polytraumatized patients spans across various disciplines, commencing in the prehospital phase with the involvement of early responders and emergency medical service (EMS) personnel. It is these highly specialized prehospital teams who are tasked with the initial assessment, stabilization, and transportation of the polytrauma patient to the nearest trauma center equipped to address their needs [60]. Given the substantial volume of trauma patients, accurate triage is crucial, with over 90% best served in local community hospitals [60]. The remaining 10%, comprising severely injured individuals necessitating higher level of care at Level I and II trauma centers, demands a multidisciplinary approach to enhance overall clinical outcomes [60]. When in the trauma bay, effective, closed-loop communication and level-appropriate division of tasks among members of the team is of crucial importance in effectively managing a polytrauma patient [61]. Team members such as anesthesiologists play a major role in both the peri-operative and intraoperative care of the polytrauma patient. Ensuring that recommended large bore peripheral IV access (or when not possible adequate vascular access, intraosseous needle, central venous line, or arterial line for hemodynamic monitoring) has been obtained for resuscitation and infusion of intravenous fluids, blood products, and medications is a task that can be accomplished by trained emergency room providers while the trauma surgeon can focus on the operative management aspect of the patient. Once the patient has been stabilized, the intensivists not only provide additional critical care to trauma patients but are also intimately involved in consulting and coordinating care between different members of the healthcare team. Thus, successful integration of a collaborative, multidisciplinary team approach in managing the polytrauma patient is crucial for minimizing complications, lowering mortality rates, and expediting recovery following injury [59].

Sugested Readings

1. Border JR, LaDuca J, Seibel R. Priorities in the management of the patient with polytrauma. Prog Surg. 1975;14:84–120.
2. Rau CS, Wu SC, Kuo PJ, Chen YC, Chien PC, Hsieh HY, et al. Polytrauma defined by the new berlin definition: a validation test based on propensity-score matching approach. Int J Environ Res Public Health. 2017;14(9)
3. Iyengar KP, Venkatesan AS, Jain VK, Shashidhara MK, Elbana H, Botchu R. Risks in the management of polytrauma patients: clinical insights. Orthop Res Rev. 2023;15:27–38.
4. van Breugel JMM, Niemeyer MJS, Houwert RM, Groenwold RHH, Leenen LPH, van Wessem KJP. Global changes in mortality rates in polytrauma patients admitted to the ICU-a systematic review. World J Emerg Surg. 2020;15(1):55.
5. American College of Surgeons. Committee on T. Advanced trauma life support: ATLS: student course manual. 10th ed. Chicago: American College of Surgeons; 2018. 1, 391 pages: illustrations (chiefly colour) p.
6. Goutcher CM, Lochhead V. Reduction in mouth opening with semi-rigid cervical collars. Br J Anaesth. 2005;95(3):344–8.
7. Li T, Jafari D, Meyer C, Voroba A, Haddad G, Abecassis S, et al. Video laryngoscopy is associated with improved first-pass intubation success compared with direct laryngoscopy in emergency department trauma patients. J Am Coll Emerg Physicians Open. 2021;2(1):e12373.
8. Andresen AEL, Kramer-Johansen J, Kristiansen T. Percutaneous vs surgical emergency cricothyroidotomy: An experimental randomized crossover study on an animal-larynx model. Acta Anaesthesiol Scand. 2019;63(10):1306–12.
9. Karlsson T, Brannstrom A, Gellerfors M, Gustavsson J, Gunther M. Comparison of emergency surgical cricothyroidotomy and percutaneous cricothyroidotomy by experienced airway providers in an obese, in vivo porcine hemorrhage airway model. Mil Med Res. 2022;9(1):57.
10. Inaba K, Branco BC, Eckstein M, Shatz DV, Martin MJ, Green DJ, et al. Optimal positioning for emergent needle thoracostomy: a cadaver-based study. J Trauma. 2011;71(5):1099–103; discussion 103.
11. Borgman MA, Spinella PC, Perkins JG, Grathwohl KW, Repine T, Beekley AC, et al. The ratio of blood products transfused affects mortality in patients receiving massive transfusions at a combat support hospital. J Trauma. 2007;63(4):805–13.
12. Kornblith LZ, Howard BM, Cheung CK, Dayter Y, Pandey S, Busch MP, et al. The whole is greater than the sum of its parts: hemostatic profiles of whole blood variants. J Trauma Acute Care Surg. 2014;77(6):818–27.
13. Gerard J, Mueck K, Lubkin D, Hatton G, Wade C, Cotton B, et al. An assessment of the safety, hemostatic efficacy, and clinical impact of low-titer group O whole blood in children and adolescents. J Trauma Acute Care Surg. 2023;95:497.
14. Kemp Bohan PM, McCarthy PM, Wall ME, Adams AM, Chick RC, Forcum JE, et al. Safety and efficacy of low-titer O whole blood resuscitation in a civilian level I trauma center. J Trauma Acute Care Surg. 2021;91(2S Suppl 2):S162–S8.
15. Collaborators C-t. Effects of tranexamic acid on death, disability, vascular occlusive events and other morbidities in patients with acute traumatic brain injury (CRASH-3): a randomised, placebo-controlled trial. Lancet. 2019;394(10210):1713–23.
16. Davis S, Nawab A, van Nispen C, Pourmand A. The role of tranexamic acid in the management of an acutely hemorrhaging patient. Hosp Pharm. 2021;56(4):350–8.
17. Fischer K, Awudi E, Varon J, Surani S. Role of tranexamic acid in the clinical setting. Cureus. 2020;12(5):e8221.
18. Ferrada P. Shifting priorities from intubation to circulation first in hypotensive trauma patients. Am Surg. 2018;84(2):e75–e6.
19. Ferrada P, Callcut RA, Skarupa DJ, Duane TM, Garcia A, Inaba K, et al. Circulation first—the time has come to question the sequencing of care in the ABCs of trauma; an American Association for the Surgery of Trauma multicenter trial. World J Emerg Surg. 2018;13:8.
20. Hanna K, Bible L, Chehab M, Asmar S, Douglas M, Ditillo M, et al. Nationwide analysis of whole blood hemostatic resuscitation in civilian trauma. J Trauma Acute Care Surg. 2020;89(2):329–35.
21. Sivertsen J, Braathen H, Lunde THF, Kristoffersen EK, Hervig T, Strandenes G, et al. Cold-stored

leukoreduced CPDA-1 whole blood: in vitro quality and hemostatic properties. Transfusion. 2020;60(5):1042–9.

22. Carney N, Totten AM, O'Reilly C, Ullman JS, Hawryluk GW, Bell MJ, et al. Guidelines for the management of severe traumatic brain injury. Fourth Edition Neurosurgery. 2017;80(1):6–15.
23. Maas AIR, Menon DK, Adelson PD, Andelic N, Bell MJ, Belli A, et al. Traumatic brain injury: integrated approaches to improve prevention, clinical care, and research. Lancet Neurol. 2017;16(12):987–1048.
24. Zeiler FA, Ercole A, Cabeleira M, Beqiri E, Zoerle T, Carbonara M, et al. Patient-specific ICP epidemiologic thresholds in adult traumatic brain injury: a CENTER-TBI validation study. J Neurosurg Anesthesiol. 2021;33(1):28–38.
25. Roquilly A, Moyer JD, Huet O, Lasocki S, Cohen B, Dahyot-Fizelier C, et al. Effect of continuous infusion of hypertonic saline vs standard care on 6-month neurological outcomes in patients with traumatic brain injury: the cobi randomized clinical trial. JAMA. 2021;325(20):2056–66.
26. Schwimmbeck F, Voellger B, Chappell D, Eberhart L. Hypertonic saline versus mannitol for traumatic brain injury: a systematic review and meta-analysis with trial sequential analysis. J Neurosurg Anesthesiol. 2021;33(1):10–20.
27. van Veen E, Nieboer D, Kompanje EJO, Citerio G, Stocchetti N, Gommers D, et al. Comparative effectiveness of mannitol versus hypertonic saline in patients with traumatic brain injury: a CENTER-TBI study. J Neurotrauma. 2023;40(13–14):1352–65.
28. Andrews PJ, Sinclair HL, Rodriguez A, Harris B, Rhodes J, Watson H, et al. Therapeutic hypothermia to reduce intracranial pressure after traumatic brain injury: the Eurotherm3235 RCT. Health Technol Assess. 2018;22(45):1–134.
29. Cooper DJ, Nichol AD, Bailey M, Bernard S, Cameron PA, Pili-Floury S, et al. Effect of early sustained prophylactic hypothermia on neurologic outcomes among patients with severe traumatic brain injury: the POLAR randomized clinical trial. JAMA. 2018;320(21):2211–20.
30. Rosli D, Schnuriger B, Candinas D, Haltmeier T. The impact of accidental hypothermia on mortality in trauma patients overall and patients with traumatic brain injury specifically: a systematic review and meta-analysis. World J Surg. 2020;44(12):4106–17.
31. Lan Z, Richard SA, Li Q, Wu C, Zhang Q, Chen R, et al. Outcomes of patients undergoing craniotomy and decompressive craniectomy for severe traumatic brain injury with brain herniation: a retrospective study. Medicine (Baltimore). 2020;99(43):e22742.
32. Sahuquillo J, Dennis JA. Decompressive craniectomy for the treatment of high intracranial pressure in closed traumatic brain injury. Cochrane Database Syst Rev. 2019;12(12):CD003983.
33. Cooper DJ, Rosenfeld JV, Murray L, Arabi YM, Davies AR, D'Urso P, et al. Decompressive craniectomy in diffuse traumatic brain injury. N Engl J Med. 2011;364(16):1493–502.
34. Lock JF, Anger F, Germer CT. Management of traumatic intestinal injury of mass casualties. Chirurg. 2017;88(10):848–55.
35. Mahoney EJ, Bugaev N, Appelbaum R, Goldenberg-Sandau A, Baltazar GA, Posluszny J, et al. Management of the open abdomen: a systematic review with meta-analysis and practice management guideline from the Eastern Association for the Surgery of Trauma. J Trauma Acute Care Surg. 2022;93(3):e110–e8.
36. Leppaniemi AK, Haapiainen RK. Selective non-operative management of abdominal stab wounds: prospective, randomized study. World J Surg. 1996;20(8):1101–5; discussion 5–6.
37. Stawicki SP. Trends in nonoperative management of traumatic injuries—a synopsis. Int J Crit Illn Inj Sci. 2017;7(1):38–57.
38. Ludwig C, Koryllos A. Management of chest trauma. J Thorac Dis. 2017;9(Suppl 3):S172–S7.
39. Edgecombe L, Sigmon DF, Galuska MA, Angus LD. Thoracic trauma. Treasure Island: StatPearls; 2023.
40. Waydhas C, Sauerland S. Pre-hospital pleural decompression and chest tube placement after blunt trauma: a systematic review. Resuscitation. 2007;72(1):11–25.
41. Barton ED, Epperson M, Hoyt DB, Fortlage D, Rosen P. Prehospital needle aspiration and tube thoracostomy in trauma victims: a six-year experience with aeromedical crews. J Emerg Med. 1995;13(2):155–63.
42. McPherson JJ, Feigin DS, Bellamy RF. Prevalence of tension pneumothorax in fatally wounded combat casualties. J Trauma. 2006;60(3):573–8.
43. Bushby N, Fitzgerald M, Cameron P, Marasco S, Bystrzycki A, Rosenfeld JV, et al. Prehospital intubation and chest decompression is associated with unexpected survival in major thoracic blunt trauma. Emerg Med Australas. 2005;17(5–6):443–9.
44. Mistry N, Bleetman A, Roberts KJ. Chest decompression during the resuscitation of patients in prehospital traumatic cardiac arrest. Emerg Med J. 2009;26(10):738–40.
45. Galvagno SM Jr, Smith CE, Varon AJ, Hasenboehler EA, Sultan S, Shaefer G, et al. Pain management for blunt thoracic trauma: a joint practice management guideline from the eastern association for the surgery of trauma and trauma anesthesiology society. J Trauma Acute Care Surg. 2016;81(5):936–51.
46. Rhee PM, Acosta J, Bridgeman A, Wang D, Jordan M, Rich N. Survival after emergency department thoracotomy: review of published data from the past 25 years. J Am Coll Surg. 2000;190(3):288–98.
47. Prieto JM, Van Gent JM, Calvo RY, Rooney AS, Martin MJ, Sise MJ, et al. Nationwide analysis of resuscitative thoracotomy in pediatric trauma: Time to differentiate from adult guidelines? J Trauma Acute Care Surg. 2020;89(4):686–90.
48. Selesner L, Yorkgitis B, Martin M, Ng G, Mukherjee K, Ignacio R, et al. Emergency department thoracot-

omy in children: a pediatric trauma society, western trauma association, and eastern association for the surgery of trauma systematic review and practice management guideline. J Trauma Acute Care Surg. 2023;95(3):432–41.
49. Burlew CC, Moore EE, Moore FA, Coimbra R, McIntyre RC Jr, Davis JW, et al. Western Trauma Association critical decisions in trauma: resuscitative thoracotomy. J Trauma Acute Care Surg. 2012;73(6):1359–63.
50. Yamamoto R, Suzuki M, Nakama R, Kase K, Sekine K, Kurihara T, et al. Impact of cardiopulmonary resuscitation time on the effectiveness of emergency department thoracotomy after blunt trauma. Eur J Trauma Emerg Surg. 2019;45(4):697–704.
51. Seamon MJ, Haut ER, Van Arendonk K, Barbosa RR, Chiu WC, Dente CJ, et al. An evidence-based approach to patient selection for emergency department thoracotomy: a practice management guideline from the Eastern Association for the Surgery of Trauma. J Trauma Acute Care Surg. 2015;79(1):159–73.
52. Zhao L, Han Z, Liu H, Zhang Z, Li S. Delayed traumatic diaphragmatic rupture: diagnosis and surgical treatment. J Thorac Dis. 2019;11(7):2774–7.
53. Goodman M, Lewis J, Guitron J, Reed M, Pritts T, Starnes S. Video-assisted thoracoscopic surgery for acute thoracic trauma. J Emerg Trauma Shock. 2013;6(2):106–9.
54. Stevens NM, Tejwani N. Commonly missed injuries in the patient with polytrauma and the orthopaedist's role in the tertiary survey. JBJS Rev. 2018;6(12):e2.
55. Bone LB, Johnson KD, Weigelt J, Scheinberg R. Early versus delayed stabilization of femoral fractures. A prospective randomized study. J Bone Joint Surg Am. 1989;71(3):336–40.
56. Pape HC, Hildebrand F, Pertschy S, Zelle B, Garapati R, Grimme K, et al. Changes in the management of femoral shaft fractures in polytrauma patients: from early total care to damage control orthopedic surgery. J Trauma. 2002;53(3):452–61; discussion 61–2.
57. Obertacke U, Kleinschmidt C, Dresing K, Bardenheuer M, Bruch J. Repeated routine determination of pulmonary microvascular permeability after polytrauma. Unfallchirurg. 1993;96(3):142–9.
58. Goldberg SR, Henning J, Wolfe LG, Duane TM. Practice patterns for the use of antibiotic agents in damage control laparotomy and its impact on outcomes. Surg Infect. 2017;18(3):282–6.
59. Bach JA, Leskovan JJ, Scharschmidt T, Boulger C, Papadimos TJ, Russell S, et al. The right team at the right time—multidisciplinary approach to multitrauma patient with orthopedic injuries. Int J Crit Illn Inj Sci. 2017;7(1):32–7.
60. McSwain N, Rotondo M, Meade P, Duchesne J. A model for rural trauma care. Br J Surg. 2012;99(3):309–14.
61. Ruchholtz S, Waydhas C, Lewan U, Piepenbrink K, Stolke D, Debatin J, et al. A multidisciplinary quality management system for the early treatment of severely injured patients: implementation and results in two trauma centers. Intensive Care Med. 2002;28(10):1395–404.

Decision-Making in Complex Dento-Alveolar Trauma in the Maxillofacial Region

23

Lumnije Kqiku and Kurt Alois Ebeleseder

Introduction

General Remarks

Maxillofacial trauma, skull fractures, and dento-alveolar injuries are frequently found in blunt and penetrating trauma patients.

About 50% of isolated cases of traumatic dental injuries occur in children and teenagers, 19% in girls, and 33% of all boys are affected.

Dento-alveolar trauma has multiple etiologies including traffic collisions, sports injuries and falls, assaults, or industrial mishaps [1–3].

Proper decision-making on the treatment of dento-alveolar injuries is necessary to avoid serious long-term morphologic, functional, and aesthetic consequences. In addition to soft tissue injuries, dental trauma is the most common facial trauma in the maxillofacial region and primarily affects the anterior region of the teeth [4–7].

In clinical situations with polytraumatized patients showing multiple facial, orbital, and skull fractures, bleeding, dental avulsions, fractures of the alveolar process, intrusions, and severe intraoral soft tissue injuries, surgical decision-making is very important. The decision to perform definitive treatment during emergency or subsequently, once the major and high-risk injuries have been taken care and swelling has subsided, is a matter of intuition, patient's physiology, and overall clinical status. Tooth avulsion, on the other hand, needs to be treated properly and immediately [8].

In fractures of the alveolar process, a quick decision should be made between manual reposition/splinting and open surgery (Figs. 23.1 and 23.2).

This means that for complex trauma, early recognition of all injuries is necessary for the decision between closed treatment (nasal tampons, intermaxillary fixation, rigid and flexible splints for dental injuries) and open treatment (surgical intervention).

Facial fractures such as nasal bone fractures, naso-orbito-ethmoid complex fractures, orbital fractures, zygomaticomaxillary complex fractures, Le Fort fractures (Le Fort type 1,2,3), and mandibular fractures (body, symphysis mentalis, ramus, condyle, coronoid process, alveolar crest) are the most common injuries in maxillofacial emergencies. Dento-alveolar injuries are associated with all types of facial trauma, and surgical decision-making should be guided by clinical scenario.

L. Kqiku (✉) · K. A. Ebeleseder
Department of Dental Medicine and Oral Health, Division of Restorative Dentistry, Periodontology and Prosthodontics, Medical University of Graz, Graz, Austria
e-mail: lumnije.kqiku@medunigraz.at; kurt.ebeleseder@medunigraz.at

R. Latifi (ed.), *Surgical Decision-Making*, https://doi.org/10.1007/978-3-031-67391-7_23

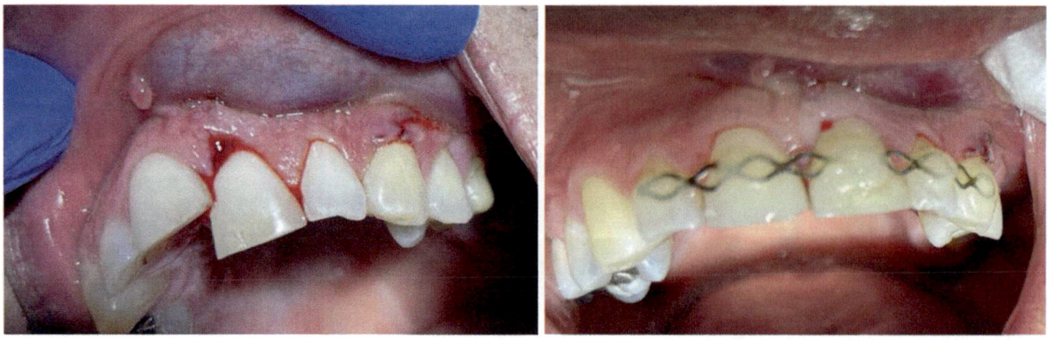

Figs. 23.1 and 23.2 Alveolar process fracture/manual reposition and splinting immediately after trauma

Classification of Dento-Alveolar Injuries

The most commonly used classification system for dental trauma is Andreasen's classification (accepted by the WHO in 1972 and propagated by the International Association of Dental Traumatology, IADT) which is applied to both primary and permanent teeth [9]. It distinguishes between 4 types of fractures (crown fracture, crown root fracture, root fracture, and fracture of the alveolar process) and 6 types of luxations, respectively, dislocations (concussion, subluxation, lateral luxation, extrusion, intrusion, and avulsion).

This means that dento-alveolar injuries are described as syndromes. A more analytic classification describes the tooth as composed of five tissues that can also be injured independently from each other [10, 11]. Thus, any injured tooth is described in five aspects: Dental *H*ard tissue, *E*ndodontium, *P*eriodontal ligament, *A*lveolar bone, and *G*ingiva.

By this method, also uninjured aspects are described automatically (Table 23.1 depicts this classification).

Fracture injuries of the dental hard tissues comprise crown fracture, crown root fracture, and root fracture (Fig. 23.3), while *the Endodontium (dental pulp)* can be affected together with all forms of dento-alveolar injuries. It can be injured in the form of an indirect exposure (dentin fracture), a direct exposure to the oral cavity, an internal exposure to the injured periodontal ligament (in root fractures), a strain, a contusion, or a separation (Fig. 23.4). On the other hand, *the Periodontium* is affected in so-called *Luxation injuries.*

Six injury types with different healing patterns can be distinguished:

Concussion

A slight injury to the periodontal ligament with edema and partial bleeding but without mobility of the affected tooth.

Subluxation

An injury with partial rupture of the periodontium structures accompanied by lip swelling and gingival sulcus bleeding.

Extrusion

An injury to the tooth characterized by a subtotal rupture of the *periodontal ligament* resulting in partial displacement of the tooth out of its socket.

The affected tooth is elongated with high mobility to axial direction, accompanied by strong gingival sulcus bleeding and possible rupture of the papillae. The resulting hematoma pushes the tooth far out of the alveolus (Fig. 23.5).

Table 23.1 The HEPAG classification[a]

Teeth	H	E	P	A	G
22	Uninjured	Uninjured	Uninjured	Uninjured	Uninjured
21	Small crown fracture	Necrotic	Avulsion/dry (hopeless)	Uninjured	Laceration of the mesial papilla
11	Root fracture	Partially necrotic	Extrusion	Uninjured	Laceration of the mesial papilla
12	Uninjured	Uninjured	Uninjured	Uninjured	Uninjured

H hard tissues (injury of dental-alveolar hard tissues),
E endodontium (injury of endodontics /dental pulp),
P periodontium (injury of periodontium),
A alveolar bone (injury of alveolar process) and
G gingiva (injury of gingiva) (HEPAG)
[a]HEPAG classification [10, 11]

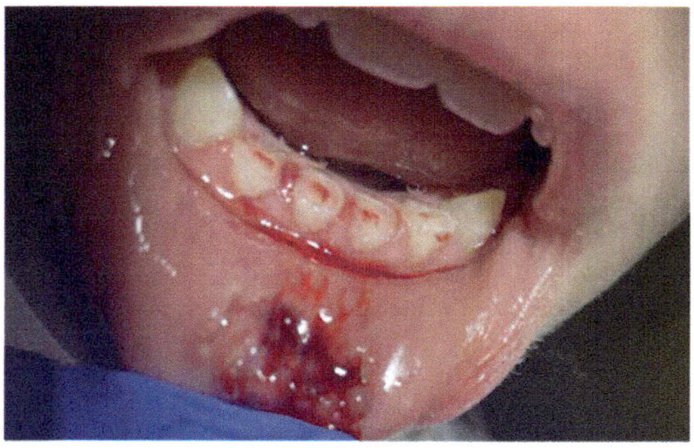

Fig. 23.3 Clinical examination immediately after injuries: crown fractures of four adjacent lower incisor teeth with exposed dental pulps and concomitant lip laceration which could bear tooth fragments

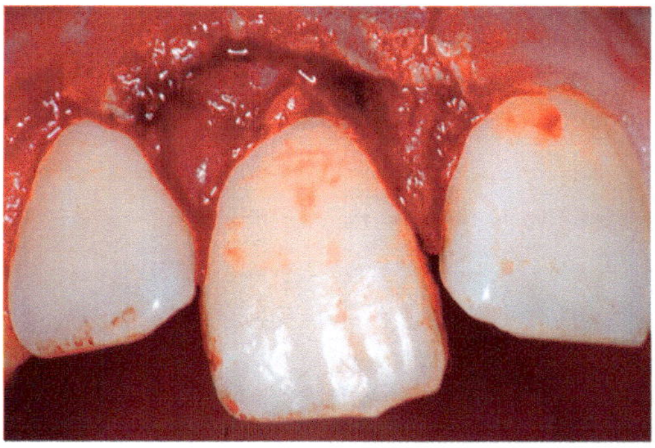

Fig. 23.4 Internal exposure of dental pulp to the injured periodontal ligament (in root fractures). Initial presentation after the injuries. Pulpal rupture was visible intraorally in the fractured root tooth

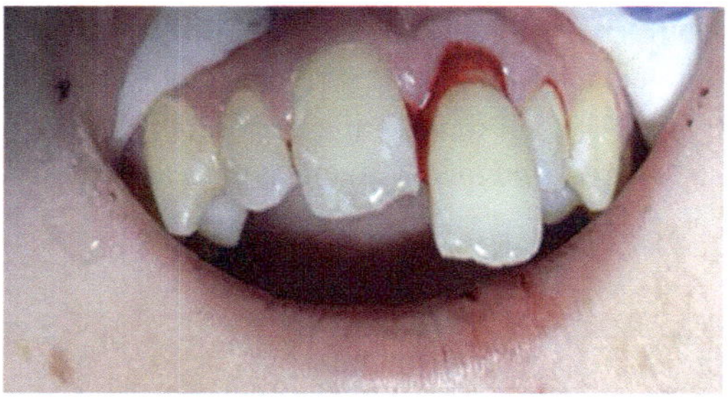

Fig. 23.5 Extrusion of the left maxillary central incisor. The affected tooth is elongated with high mobility in the axial direction, accompanied by bleeding in the gingival sulcus

Lateral luxation

Displacement of the tooth in labial or palatal direction. Lateral luxation injury is accompanied by partial separation of the periodontal ligament, fracture of the buccal lamella with the fragment remaining fixed to the root, and pinching of the root apex into the bone. The tooth is immobile. Accompanying injuries can be a contusion of the labial and bruising of the palatal gingiva and a laceration of papillae (Fig. 23.6).

Intrusion

Traumatic intrusion of a permanent tooth is a rare but serious injury [12–15].

The tooth is displaced axially into the alveolar bone and frequently penetrating the labial bone plate, may disappear completely in the tissues, or is penetrating the nasal cavity. This injury is most accompanied by moderate bleeding from the nose, total rupture, and crushing of the periodontium, contusion of the dental socket without alveolar bleeding, fracture of the buccal lamella of the root apex, rupture of the gingival papillae, and rupture of the gingiva (Fig. 23.7).

Avulsion

Avulsion is a complete displacement of the tooth out of its socket and is one of the most serious dental injuries to the permanent tooth, seen in 0.5–16% of all dental injuries [16, 17]. Prompt and correct emergency management and a long-term treatment plan are important for a good prognosis (Figs. 23.8 and 23.9).

The alveolar bone can be fractured or comminuted. A special injury is the fracture of the alveolar process, a rare but complex dental injury. It may be associated with injured jaws and joints. Not only is the alveolar bone involved, but also the alveolar sockets, the pulps, and the periodontal ligament of several teeth, the free and attached gingiva, and in some cases the alveolar mucosa. Clinically, one or more teeth are displaced in the same direction and can be moved as a unit. Concomitant injuries such as laceration of the gingiva, root fractures, crown fractures, extrusion, or avulsion can frequently be found (Fig. 23.10).

Concomitant injuries of the gingiva or oral mucosa can be found in the form of laceration, contusion, or abrasion of gingiva or oral mucosa.

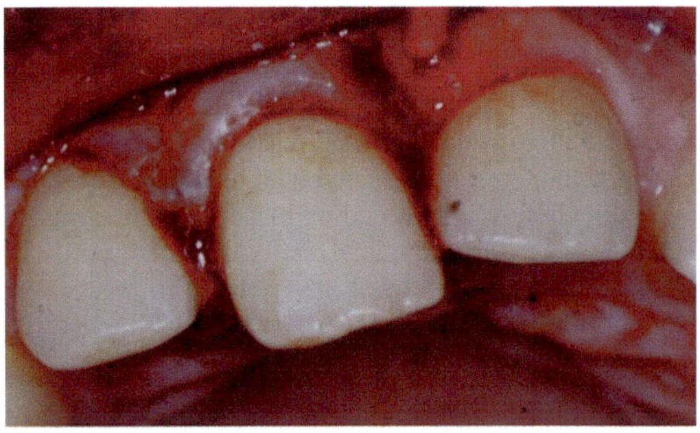

Fig. 23.6 Lateral dislocation. Displacement of the teeth in the palatal direction

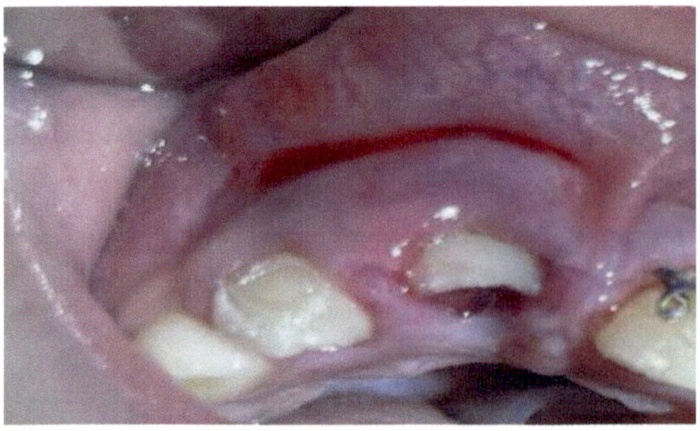

Fig. 23.7 Intrusion. The tooth is axially displaced into the alveolar bone

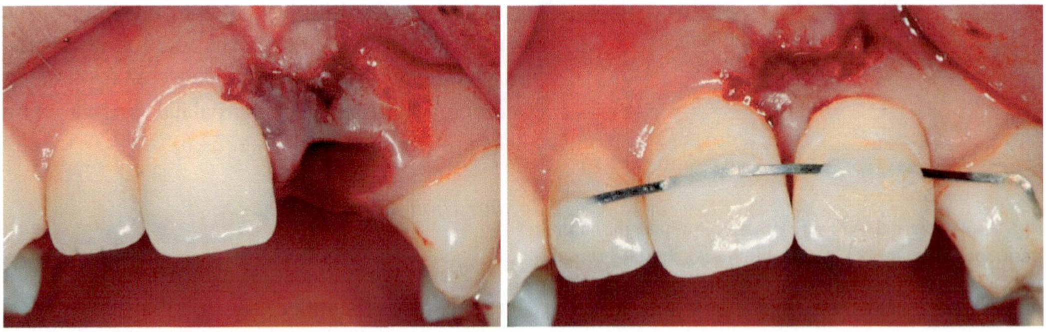

Figs. 23.8 and 23.9 Avulsion, clinical situation after complete displacement of the tooth from its socket. Emergency management/prompt replantation of the avulsed tooth

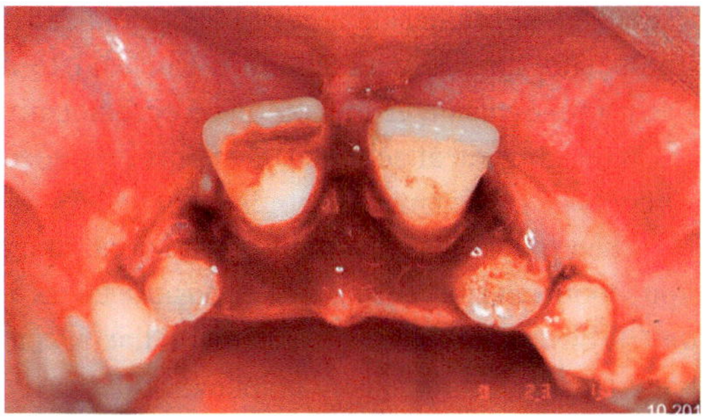

Fig. 23.10 Fracture of the alveolar process. Bucal lamelle fracture of the alveolar process

Emergency Management

Evaluation

Generally, examination of a patient with a traumatic dental injury is very important for the correct diagnosis and treatment of soft and hard tissue injuries.

Clinical examination includes complete medical and surgical history, particularly the history of any bleeding disorder, followed by the inspection, palpation, percussion, sensitivity test, occlusion testing, and radiographic examination.

Detailed mechanism of injury, including suspicion of mistreatment/child or elderly abuse required very important information that needs to be documented in medical records. Photographs and detailed documentation according to HEPAG (Table 23.1) play a key role for an exact diagnosis, treatment, prognosis, and follow-up of dento-alveolar trauma. Cleaning of the face and the oral cavity with water or saline and the application of local anesthesia are frequently necessary but not in every case.

The HEPAG classification describes the tooth as composed of five tissues that can also be injured independently from each other [10, 11]. Arranging the findings in the form of a table is depicted below. Example with 4 teeth being described, two of them injured (Table 23.1):

Management

To improve prognosis and minimize complications, a prompt and correct emergency management is necessary as long as life-threatening injuries are taken care of first. A delay in treatment of more than 12 hours can re-effect prognosis of the involved structures [18].

The dento-alveolar trauma management should be based on five principles:

1. Reducing microbial burden measures.
2. Minimally invasive initial treatment.
3. Early functionality.
4. Substance-saving restorations (especially for young patents) and.
5. Multidisciplinary approach.

Antimicrobial Therapy

Microbially induced healing disorders following dento-alveolar trauma include multiple root resorption, endodontic and periodontal/gingival healing disorders, and healing disorders of the alveolar bone. Most of these possibilities can be prevented by reducing microbial burden with measures such as splinting of mobile teeth, avoidance of mushy food, active oral hygiene, disinfection of mucous membranes with chlorhexidine, systemic administration of antibiotics, and treatment/coverage of all wounds.

Opinions on the use of systemic antibiotics in dento-alveolar injuries are divergent.

The International Association of Dental Traumatology/IADT guidelines recommend systemic use of antibiotics in specific situations, such as open wounds or fractures that extend into the oral cavity.

In general, short courses of antibiotics are recommended to minimize the development of antibiotic resistance.

Minimally Invasive Initial Treatment (Table 23.2)

Dental Hard Tissues

Extractions and other non-essential surgical interventions as part of initials care should be avoided. If an avulsed tooth is brought in, replantation must be attempted without delay, even if the extraoral tolerance time (less than 60 minutes) has been exceeded. This requirement arises from the fact that many circumstances are not known at the time of the initial treatment that

Table 23.2 Minimally invasive initial treatment—summary

1. Avoid extractions
2. Replantation of teeth, no interventions on the periodontal membrane
3. Leaving and covering mobile parts of the alveolar bone
4. Gentle reduction of teeth and alveolar bone, splinting
5. No gingival excision
6. Search for tooth fragments in perforated lip wounds
7. Atraumatic, not self-dissolving, monofilament sutures
8. Preservation of original fragments in physiological solution
9. Pulpotomy instead of pulpectomy

allows a planned, detailed decision on further treatment. A superfluous replantation is easier to reverse than an erroneous non-replantation.

If teeth or parts of teeth are missing, a reasonable search should be made at the site of the accident. In many cases, the reattachment of an original fragment can save the patient a costly restoration, although there is a refracture rate of approx. 30% mostly due to new trauma of which the patient should be made aware [19]. Often, however, lost teeth are swallowed or aspirated and can be seen in the chest X-ray (CXR) and need to be removed. If they are swallowed and seen in the stomach, they should be removed endoscopically.

Teeth with fractured roots should be properly reduced and splinted rigidly.

Endodontium

In the case of violations of endodontic tissue, the following vitality-preserving measures are preferred: direct capping which should be performed within 2 hours after pulp exposure, pulpotomy, or pulpectomy.

Periodontium

Repositioning of dislocated teeth is desirable and should be performed, when possible. Proper repositioning of bone and teeth not only reduces wound gaps and re-arranges the cellular architecture of the periodontal ligament, but it also facilitates gingival adaption and thus protects the periodontal wound from superinfection. Intrusion trauma should rather be reduced orthodontically. Immediate surgical repositioning can lead to a short-term avulsion of the tooth and occasionally to loss of gingival attachment due to the expanded alveolus.

When repositioning a tooth from lateral luxation, tooth and bone must be repositioned as a unit. The accompanying fracture of the buccal bone lamella can be easily palpated in the vestibule as a bone edge behind which the root is wedged. Subluxations and extrusions require gentle reduction. The first important step in the treatment of an avulsed tooth is to decide on immediate treatment, known as immediate replantation at the site of the injury.

It is important to hold the tooth by the crown and not to touch the root so as not to damage the root cement layer. After replantation, the tooth should be held in place, if possible, by lightly biting on a clean cloth.

If immediate replantation is not possible, the avulsed tooth can be stored in a suitable transport medium such as DENTOSAFE (Dental Rescue Box for Storing Tooth or Tooth Fragments), milk, egg-white, saliva, or saline solution. Anything else is not recommended because of possible damage to the periodontal ligament cells.

During replantation, with the exception of a brief removal of visible particles under flowing saline solution, interventions on the periodontal membrane should be avoided [20]. A reliably necrotic periodontal membrane does not need to be removed and can be used as a drug carrier (20-minute bath in antibiotic solution) [21, 22]. Periodontal ligament can help maintaining the alveolar anatomy and symmetry in adults only (in juveniles, ankylosis can cause a local alveolar growth inhibition). After replantation, the extracted tooth must be stabilized. All these decision-making steps for the treatment of an avulsed tooth are crucial to increase the chances of long-term preservation of an avulsed tooth.

Alveolar Bone

Hasty removal of fractured pieces should be avoided. Comminuted fractures often heal surprisingly well under prolonged antibiotic cover (14 days). Septa that have remained in place need not to be removed if they are covered with gingiva. Removal of the entire mobile section together with the traumatized teeth has catastrophic consequences for further prosthetic and functional restoration because the entire alveolar ridge must first be reconstructed by osteoplasty before it can be restored prosthetically [23]. When deciding whether to operate on an alveolar process fracture, several factors must be considered before a final decision can be made. An important factor that may influence the decision is the severity of the fracture.

Simple, non-displaced fractures may heal on their own with conservative treatment such as manual reduction and systemic antibiotics.

In the case of a complex and displaced fracture of the alveolar process, the decision for surgery is always made. Failure to properly stabilize the alveolar process fracture may compromise jaw function and lead to other complications. The general health of the patient also plays an important role in the decision-making process, for example, patients with a weakened immune system are not optimal cases for surgical intervention.

Gingiva and Facial Soft Tissue

Traumatic gingival flaps should first be repositioned to their original position and fixed with a few atraumatic sutures as possible, even if they do not appear to be particularly well supplied with blood. Once the alveolar bone and all teeth have been properly repositioned, the gingiva can be repositioned easily. To avoid pressure of the sutures on the papillae, the splint can be used as an abutment for the knot. For this reason, it is more favorable to suture the gingiva *after* tooth splinting. Repositioned teeth, splint, and sutures then act as a biologic unit.

Absorbable sutures are less suitable for gingival adaptation than non-absorbable, synthetic monofilament material due to their tendency to bacterial colonization and their sometimes-prolonged dwelling time.

If parts of the gingiva are missing, immediate coverage with the aid of a small sliding flap is indicated, especially if marginal bone would otherwise be exposed.

Facial soft tissue lacerations should be sutured *after* the treatment of the dento-alveolar structures. Perforating lacerations in combination with tooth crown fractures should make the operator aware of a possible impaction of tooth fragments in the lip wound (Figs. 23.11 and 23.12). The sutures should be removed 4–6 days after surgery.

Splinting and Immobilization (Table 23.3)

It has been a long matter of debate whether traumatically loosened teeth should be splinted or not. The first authors to question the benefits of splinting around 50 years ago were Andreasen et al. in 1975 [24]. They assumed different premises at

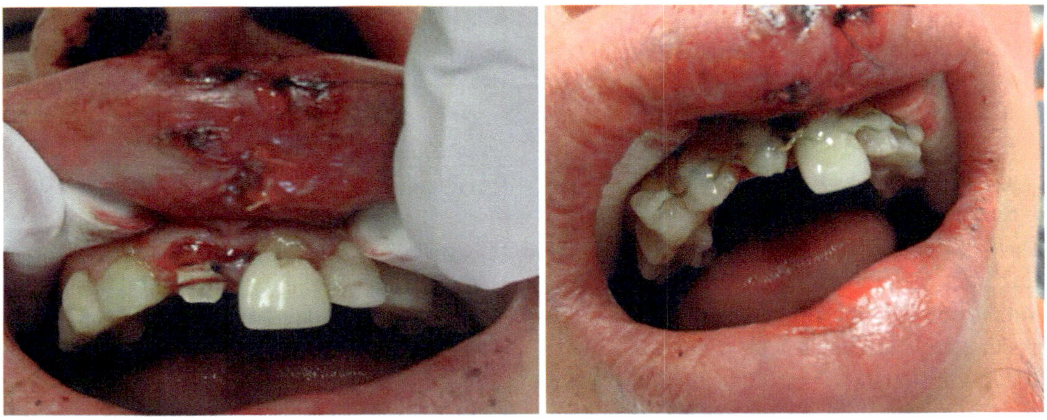

Figs. 23.11 and 23.12 Facial soft tissue injuries combined with dental alveolar injuries

Table 23.3 Splinting

General splinting duration 3–6 weeks
Purpose of the splint:
Restoration of hygiene and chewing function
Fixation of the tooth in the repositioned position
Immobilization in case of alveolar bone fracture and root fractures (splinting duration up to 2 months)
Possible disadvantages of the splint:
Gingivitis due to lack of hygiene
Ankylosis after replantation

that time: firstly, the term "splinting" usually meant surgical wire ligature fixation, and secondly they based their view on experimental studies, most of which were carried out on monkey teeth after artificially induced avulsions.

There is no longer any question that wire ligation splinting has a destructive effect on the gingiva and periodontium [25] and that even previously untraumatized teeth can be loosened as a side effect. Today's post-traumatic splints must be flexible and able to support mastication and cleaning. It is important to note that the patient needs the masticatory load necessarily for healing. Additionally, traumatized teeth often have a tendency to sink back into the luxation position after repositioning (extrusion, lateral luxation, intrusion) and cause permanent malocclusion. Regarding this aspect, it is therefore desirable to fix the tooth at least for 1–2 weeks in the position in which it should heal.

The benefit of splinting lies in the resumption of physiological masticatory loading. Thus, it provides functional input for healing of the periodontal ligament and hard substance (in alveolar fractures and root fractures) and an easier adaptation of the gingiva during first-aid treatment. An adverse effect of a splint may be the accumulation of plaque in cases of bad oral hygiene. In case of alveolar bone fracture 6 weeks and in case of root fracture 3–6 months, splinting is required. IADT guidelines for dental trauma treatment have shorter splinting periods. Splints made of composite resin and a metallic, orthodontically inactive arch bar are the most suitable splints. Today, the Titanium Trauma Splint (TTS) is estimated to be the gold standard of splinting traumatically mobile teeth.

Substance-Saving Restorations

In crown fractures, sealing of exposed dentin with dentin bonding helps avoiding pulp necroses especially in children. As up to 60% of fracture area are covered by dentin tubules, untreated dentinal wounds after crown fractures are a threat to the vitality of the dental pulp.

Reattachment of the original fragment is present. If the fragment is lost, an immediate build-up of the fractured crown with composite is recommended. In case of single tooth loss: implant, autotransplant, or orthodontic gap closure should be planned.

Interdisciplinary coNcept

Maxillofacial and dental traumata are practically always interdisciplinary cases. They often begin as oral-surgical emergency treatments and continue as cases for the specialized endodontist. If the patient is a child, also special knowledge on pedodontics is to be applied including orthodontic or prosthetic aspects. If a child has special needs, a continuous cooperation with pediatric surgery is advocated.

Post-initial Treatment

Further measures during first month of treatment are suture removal, mobility testing (the Periotest® device can be recommended), post-primary restoration, endo monitoring or intervention, spontaneous re-eruption, and surgical or orthodontic measures.

Clinical and radiographic follow-ups should be made after 2–8 weeks, 4 months, 6 months, 1 year, and yearly for 5 years.

Conclusions

Maxillofacial and dental-alveolar trauma often creates a chaotic situation, especially when children and adolescents are involved. Such situations can affect important decisions. In fact, correct decisions should be made regardless of whether the treatment is performed by surgeons, general dentists, or specialists.

The goals of the decision-making process for maxillofacial and dental trauma include increased treatment efficiency, increased comfort for the emergency physician (pediatric dentist or maxillofacial surgeon), decreased waiting time, and improved prognosis.

All dislocation injuries should be treated promptly. Replantation is the treatment of choice for avulsed teeth and must be performed immediately. The decision to replant a tooth is almost always the right one, even if the extraoral time is more than 60 minutes. The tooth can still be extracted later if extracted at an appropriate time after a rapid interdisciplinary assessment. Repositioning and splinting minimize gaps and facilitate healing. Splinting is considered the best method to maintain the repositioned tooth or alveolar attachment fracture in the correct position and to promote initial healing and function. The duration of splinting varies and depends on the type of injury.

All wound openings must be closed, and gingival adherent or torn mucosa must be sutured. Direct capping or pulpotomy of the exposed pulp should be performed in the first session.

Measures to reduce the microbial burden should be applied and close follow-ups play an important role in improving the prognosis of dento-alveolar trauma. Overall, complex cases of maxillofacial and dental trauma require careful and thorough decision-making, a balance of clinical expertise, and collaboration with other specialists to prevent further damage and ensure the best possible outcome for the patient.

*Finally, the following are key step*s in the management of complex maxillofacial and dento-alveolar trauma:

1. *Communication with the patient:* In complex maxillofacial and dental trauma, effective communication with the patient throughout the decision-making process is essential to explain all treatment options and steps, potential risks, and benefits, and to ensure appropriate follow-up care.
2. *Stabilization of patients* as necessary before initiating treatment.
3. *Immediate evaluation of injuries:*
   Assess the extent and severity of the injury, including imaging studies to determine the nature of the injury.
4. *Prioritization of treatment:* Treat serious injuries that are considered a risk to the patient's overall health before performing cosmetic or functional treatments, and.
5. *Multidisciplinary approach*
   The need for a multidisciplinary approach to the management of acute complex maxillofacial and dental trauma should not be underestimated, especially with pediatric, otolaryngology, plastic reconstructive surgery, and other. This multidisciplinary team approach is essential to ensure comprehensive patient. Knowledge on treatment options taking into account the long-term implications of the severity of the injuries is necessary from the beginning.

References

1. Noffze MJ, Tubbs RS. Rene le fort 1869-1951. Clin Anat. 2011;24(3):278–81.
2. Kaul RP, Sagar S, Singhal M, Kumar A, Jaipuria J, Misra M. Burden of maxillofacial trauma at level 1 trauma center. Craniomaxillofac Trauma Reconstr. 2014;7(2):126–30.
3. Andreasen JO. Etiology and pathogenesis of traumatic dental injuries. A clinical study of 1298 cases. Scand J Dent Res. 2014;78:329–42.
4. Borssen E, Holm AK. Traumatic dental injuries in a cohort of 16-year-olds in northern Sweden. Endod Dent Traumatol. 1997;13:276–80.
5. Bastone EB, Freer TJ, McNamara JR. Epidemiology of dental trauma: a review of the literature. Aust J Dent. 2000;1:2–9.
6. Glendor U. Epidemiology of traumatic dental injuries – a 12 year review of the literature. Dent Traumatol. 2008;24:603–11.
7. Andreasen JO, Andreasen FM. Classification, etiology and epidemiology. In: Andreasen JO, Andreasen FM, editors. Textbook and color atlas of traumatic injuries to the teeth. Copenhagen: Munksgaard; 1996. p. 151–80.
8. Andreasen JO. Delayed replantation after submucosal storage in order to prevent root resorption after replantation. An experimental study in monkeys. Int J Oral Surg. 1980;9(5):394–403.
9. WHO – World Health Organization. Application of the international classification of diseases and stomatology. Geneva: IDCDA; 1992.

10. Ebeleseder K. A suggestion of a new classification system of traumatic dental injuries. Endod Dent Traumatol. 1994;10:39.
11. Filippi A, Tschan J, Pohl Y, Berthold H, Ebeleseder K. A retrospective classification of tooth injuries using a new scoring system. Clin Oral Investig. 2000;4(3):173–5.
12. Kirschner H. Atlas der chirurgischen Zahnerhaltung. Band I. 1st ed. Munich: Hanser; 1996. p. 11.
13. Andreasen JO, Bakland LK, Matras R, Andreasen FM. Traumatic intrusion of permanent teeth. Part 1. An epidemiological study of 216 intruded permanent teeth. Dent Traumatol. 2006;22:83–9.
14. Andreasen JO, Bakland LK, Matras R, Andreasen FM. Traumatic intrusion of permanent teeth. Part 2. A clinical study of the effect of preinjury and injury factors (such as sex, age, stage of root development, tooth location and extent of injury including number of intruded teeth) on 140 intruded permanent teeth. Dent Traumatol. 2006;22:90–8.
15. Andreasen JO, Bakland LK, Matras R, Andreasen FM. Traumatic intrusion of permanent teeth. Part 3. A clinical study of the effect of treatment variables such as treatment delay, method of repositioning, type of splint, length of splinting and antibiotics in 140 teeth. Dent Traumatol. 2006;22:99–111.
16. Glendor U, Halling A, Andersson L, Eilert-Petersson E. Incidence of traumatic tooth injuries in children and adolescents in the county of Vastmanland, Sweden. Swed Dent J. 1996;20:15–28.
17. Andreasen JO, Andreasen FM, Andersson L. Textbookand color atlas of traumatic injuries to the teeth. 5th ed. Oxford: Wiley Blackwell; 2018.
18. Andreasen JO, Andreasen FM. Avulsions. In: Andreasen JO, Andreasen FM, Andersson L, editors. Textbook and color atlas of traumatic injuries to the teeth. 4th ed. Oxford: Wiley-Blackwell; 2007. p. 444–88.
19. Andreasen JO, Andreasen FM, Skeie A, Hjørting-Hansen E, Schwartz O. Effect of treatment delay upon pulp and periodontal healing of traumatic dental injuries – a review article. Dent Traumatol. 2002;18(3):116–28.
20. Andreasen FM, Andreasen JO. Crown fractures. In: Andreasen JO, Andreasen FM, editors. Textbook and color atlas of traumatic injuries to the teeth. St. Louis: Mosby; 1994.
21. Cvek M, Cleaton-Jones P, Austin J, Lownie J, King M, Fatti P. Effect of topical application of doxycycline on pulp revascularization and periodontal healing in reimplanted monkey incisors. Endod Dent Traumatol. 1990;6:170–6.
22. Cvek M, Cleaton-Jones P, Austin J, et al. Pulp revascularization in reimplanted immature monkey incisors–predictability and the effect of antibiotic systemic prophylaxis. Endod Dent Traumatol. 1990;6(4):157–69.
23. Andreasen JO, Borum MK, Jacobsen HL, Andreasen FM. Replantation of 400 avulsed permanent incisors. 4. Factors related to periodontal ligament healing. Endod Dent Traumatol. 1995;11(2):76–89.
24. Andreasen J. The effect of splinting upon periodontal healing after replantation of permanent incisors in monkeys. Acta Odontol Scand. 1975;6(33):313–23.
25. Oikarinen K, Gundlach KK, Pfeifer G. Late complications of luxation injuries to teeth. Endod Dent Traumatol. 1987;3(6):296–303.

Part IV

Special Issues in Surgical Decision Making

The Surgeon's Response to a Patient Death

24

Erin Switzer and Terence O'Keeffe

Why Is this Different for Surgeons?

Although a patient's death is something that is going to affect any doctor who provides direct patient care, we would argue that proceduralists in general and surgeons specifically are at increased risk of directly contributing to a patient's death and therefore the anguish and stress associated with this. Taking a patient to the operating room and performing a complex operation which can have an uncertain result can make the surgeon feel directly responsible for the outcome even if the best result is intended, which is particularly true for emergency operations. However, even in the best of hands, the mortality rate for surgery is NOT zero, and it behooves us to ensure during our conversations with the patient about consent for surgery, that we provide realistic expectations for the patient and their family. Many of us have been faced with desperate patients and/or families who wish to have "everything done," regardless of the actual chances of success or the possible consequences. One of our roles needs to be in taking counsel with the other caregivers of these patients to make sure that we are of course "doing no harm," but additionally that we are able to provide realistic expectations of the outcomes of surgery, so that hopes are not unduly raised, only to be dashed again if complications occur. The American College of Surgeon's NSQIP risk calculator (accessible at https://riskcalculator.facs.org/RiskCalculator/) is an invaluable tool that can help inform a conversation with patients' and their families and may actually help surgery be avoided in cases where the outcome is unlikely to be successful.

Expected vs. Unexpected Deaths

Again, although surgeons are not the only doctors that run up against unexpected patient deaths, many practitioners are operating on patients at the extremes of life, on patients who have very disordered physiology, e.g., trauma patients or patients with sepsis, have severe chronic conditions, e.g., vascular patients, or have a disease that is literally trying to kill them and the surgeon is trying to fight that e.g., patients with cancer. Under any of these circumstances, surgeons will be exposed to unexpected deaths more frequently than other physicians, and thus surgical decision-making is significantly more difficult.

A patient dying of metastatic cancer may often have a different impact on their surgeon that a patient who had been recovering well from their operation, and then suddenly passes away from an unexpected complication. In the former case, the death might be considered a relief for the patient, their family, and even the surgeon,

E. Switzer · T. O'Keeffe (✉)
Division of Trauma/Surgical Critical Care/General Surgery, Department of Surgery, Augusta University, Augusta, GA, USA
e-mail: eswitzer@augusta.edu; tokeeffe@augusta.edu

R. Latifi (ed.), *Surgical Decision-Making*, https://doi.org/10.1007/978-3-031-67391-7_24

who may wish for a merciful release for their patient if recovery is not possible. Nevertheless, many surgical oncologists and/or surgeons who perform palliative surgery may still form strong bonds with their patients. To a certain extent, this may depend on how the surgeon identifies with their patient as well as with their family, their social circumstances, and the specific disease.

In another example, many trauma surgeons will be all too familiar with the change in epidemiology of gun violence that has occurred over the last few years, with many more children and adolescents suffering injuries [5]. These patients are infinitely more stressful to operate on, and the challenge of then talking to the family of a child who has passed away from gun violence is one we would not wish on anyone.

Most of us will still remember the first patient that we cared for that died—the authors certainly still have a strong recollection of that event. Over time physicians who deal with death on a regular basis develop coping mechanisms to at least partially insulate themselves from the emotional distress that they may feel from this. That doesn't mean that we forget, but this ability to be at least somewhat dispassionate can help to prevent burnout and keep the surgeon functioning to the best of their ability.

Second Victim Syndrome

The death of a patient is clearly traumatic for the patient's family and loved ones, and is something all doctors try to avoid to the best of their abilities, but there is increasing evidence that surgeons can also suffer emotional angst and suffering in a constellation of symptoms that has been referred to as second victim syndrome [10]. In a paper from 2017 by Han et al., up to 84% of surgeons reported feelings of anxiety, guilt, sadness, shame, and anger [6]. These feelings were pronounced in some cases, with a surgeon writing "We all hide our grief, suffer in silence. The pain can be close to debilitating." In the world of surgery, resilience and stoicism are thought highly of, and this can make it harder to acknowledge our feelings after a poor patient outcome.

Guilt

Guilt can be a powerful emotion that the surgeon has to deal with after the death of a patient, particularly if the surgeon ascribes some blame to themselves for the cause of the death. In his book "Complications. A surgeons note on an imperfect science," Dr. Gawande describes his emotions "I felt a sense of shame like a burning ulcer. This was not guilt: guilt is what you feel when you have done something wrong. What I felt was shame: I was what was wrong." [4] These emotions can be especially damaging to surgeons early in their career, such as residents, who may not have yet dealt with a patient's death. In one recent study, 88% of residents reported being part of a medical error, with 86% of these surgery residents experiencing emotional sequelae. A good peer support system in the residency, in addition to a sympathetic program director can make sure that the resident is able to move through this trauma effectively. Unfortunately, in this study, only 24% of the respondents stated that they had received emotional support [7].

Acceptance

As surgeons, we need to accept that death is unfortunately an integral part of our lives; on many occasions we are merely trying to slow the inexorable march of a disease, or trying to bring comfort to a patient. End of life care may be a larger or smaller part of a surgeon's practice, depending on their exact specialty. Burnout appears to be highest amongst intensivists and is also very high in general surgeons, which is not surprising considering the number of life and death circumstances that are encountered by these specialists. In addition, much has been written on compassion fatigue amongst nurses, oncologists, and intensivists, but less data exists in the literature regarding the incidence and the difficulties surgeons experience with it. Unless the surgeon is careful, this can be an unfortunate consequence of over-exposure to the seriously ill and dying. The COVID-19 pandemic in 2020 and 2021 was a once in a lifetime event for many of us, who often provided ICU care as we were unable to operate, and saw death on a scale that was highly unusual. For some doctors, there were tragic consequences, and more than a few suicides in doctors have been reported as an aftermath of the chaotic breakdown of our medical systems during that time.

Burnout

Surgeon burnout is increasingly being recognized as a serious entity, with up to 35% of general surgeons reporting symptoms of burnout, with an incidence of up to 70% in trainees. Burnout is covered eloquently elsewhere, so will not be covered exhaustively here, but it is clear that there are many forces at play. The emotional distress associated with caring for dying patients can certainly predispose to burnout, but it can also be a consequence of systemic organizational problems, which may be more relevant as more and more surgeons become employees of large heath care systems, as opposed to group or academic practice [3, 8].

Performance Issues and Resilience

After caring for a patient who dies, a surgeon will likely need to emotionally and mentally pivot and refocus so they can effectively perform their other immediate clinical demands. This may be extremely difficult. In general, in the case of an unexpected intra-operative death on an elective list, the surgeon would be wise to postpone or reschedule other non-urgent cases to give them time to regain their equilibrium and to be able to devote the necessary physical and mental energy to a new operation. Acute care surgeons find themselves in the situation of operating on high-risk cases with greater frequency, and so are likely to experience this event more often, and may not have this option to step "away" from call commitments in this event. Nevertheless, experiencing a patient death in the middle of a busy 24-hour call can be a significant drain, and if at all possible, at least a few minutes of time away from patient care to compose oneself is advisable and very necessary. Having a debrief with the rest of the surgical team is very important to ensure that all members can continue to function at their best, as it is easy to suffer from compassion fatigue in the aftermath of a patient's death.

The challenge of continuing to perform at one's best for each new consult or subsequent operation cannot be understated, and although surgeons are proud of their "grit," we must be mindful of our own vulnerabilities and respond appropriately for the safety of all our patients [1]. In another quote from his book "Complications" Dr. Gawande writes about a colleague who had made an error: "Afterward, he could barely bring himself to operate. When he did operate, he became tentative and indecisive. The case affected his performance for months." Seeking guidance from a senior colleague may be helpful in these circumstances to help the surgeon find their equilibrium anew [4]. This may be particularly important if the surgeon has to operate on another patient with a similar condition, where fear of the outcome can impact the surgeons' performance—asking for assistance may help the physician overcome this hurdle.

Patient and Hospital Factors

Some of the fear and stress that comes from dealing with a patient's death are related to the interaction with the patient's family, particularly if the death has been in any way unexpected. Grief manifests in different ways in people, and both aggressive verbal and physical outbursts are not uncommon, and can be directed at the physician, even if they have done their utmost to avoid a bad outcome. Unfortunately, there have even been instances in which patients or their family have targeted and killed physicians for real or perceived dereliction of care. In our increasingly multicultural society, there are also additional factors that come into play, depending on the ethnicity and/or belief systems of the patient and their family. Most surveys show that between 70% and 80% of people in the United States believe in God in some form, and up to 80%

believe in miracles [9]. This can make the process of death harder for some families to accept, especially if this has been an unexpected event. Dealing with a patient's family members who do not accept their death can certainly increase the physician's stress and discomfort, which can be especially problematic with brain death, as the patient's body remains warm and vital, despite their lack of brain function and clinical diagnosis of death.

It is also relatively common to face legal repercussions in cases with a patient death, especially if it is felt to be related to the care provided. This may cause the surgeon to be less forthcoming about the circumstances of the death, in an attempt to avoid litigation, which may in turn make the patient's family feel that there is something to hide, and actually make litigation MORE likely. Most of the studies around medical litigation seem to favor full disclosure and a timely honest conversation about the complication as the best way to avoid a medical malpractice suit, although this will likely be very uncomfortable in the moment.

Although surgeons have by tradition always had some form of oversight of their performance in our weekly mortality and morbidity conferences, most hospital organizations have a parallel but different process known as peer review. In the case of the hospital peer review committee, the peers are usually NOT surgeons, and the process unfolds very differently and can be a source of additional stress and concern for the surgeon. Having experience on these committees, and having experienced how surgeons respond to them, it is clear that this kind of oversight, while well-intended and necessary to identify issues, is not well liked by the average physician, who nearly always regards the review as punitive in nature.

While many surgeons are their "own worst enemy" in terms of how they review their own cases in terms of the patient's death, fear of retribution from the patient's family, the hospital or even the State medical board may compound the stress from the event and contribute to the "second victim syndrome."

How Can Surgeons Find Effective Coping Mechanisms?

Although things do seem to be changing, we are often taught in medical training to maintain a certain degree of emotional detachment. The predominant surgical culture in US medical establishments would regard a physician's emotional response to death as a sign of weakness and unprofessionalism. Nevertheless, it is important to acknowledge the death of a patient in whose care we were involved, and also to acknowledge the feelings that are evoked within us. This will help us to become more aware of the needs of our patients and also to recognize our own needs. Physicians who deal with death on a regular basis must develop coping mechanisms to at least partially insulate themselves from the emotional distress that they may feel from this. These coping strategies can be healthy or unhealthy. The later tend to provide only temporary relief and are generally maladaptive and serve to suppress the emotion or response rather than process and acknowledge it. Table 24.1 lists some "good" and "bad" coping mechanisms.

At the outset it may be helpful to some degree, to share feelings of loss with members of the family of the deceased. The grief of the family must of necessity take precedence, but sometimes family members, too, can gain a great deal of comfort from sharing experiences with someone who has been involved with the care of their relative. All too often in medicine we do not acknowledge events such as this, and our own feelings get lost because we then become involved with new cases and new situations. As surgeon intensivists, we were very busy early in the COVID-19 pandemic, caring for patients both surgically and in the intensive care units. Due to the quarantining and restrictions set in place, there was limited personal interaction and connection with patients' families. We felt the negative impact when this component of the coping strategy broke down.

The support of our peers is another avenue from which we can draw assistance. This includes our partners, senior colleagues, mentors, or others in positions of authority. This may be more

Table 24.1 Coping strategies

Negative	Positive
Alcohol or substance misuse	Talking openly with the patient's family
Suppression of your emotions	Attending the patient's funeral
Feeling guilty and blaming yourself	Supporting the surgical team
Brooding over events	Guidance/support from colleagues
Obsessing how things could have been different	Support from your family
Blaming others—anesthesia, nurses, colleagues, patient, family	Seeking professional help

difficult if the surgeon is a solo practitioner, and especially in the case of the rural surgeon who may not have professional colleagues in close vicinity. Academic or group practice will afford more local opportunities for peer-to-peer counseling and support, however, with the explosion of Information Technology over the last decade, peer support is much more accessible independent of geographic location or practice size. For instance, numerous applications and mobile Apps have been developed as resources and to provide various surgeon and non-surgeon physician specific support network for its users. Likewise, social media can provide another way for surgeons to interrelate and commiserate.

The importance of personal family connections obviously cannot be over-emphasized here, whether it is a spouse, siblings, or other family members in the medical profession, who may be sources of support, sounding boards, or even able to provide advice from their own real-life experiences. Having good family relationships that allow the surgeon to decompress, relax with, and discuss the issue in an unguarded fashion is absolutely essential for their emotional well-being. The unconditional love that we receive from our families at times like these allows us to remain grounded and get through what can be very difficult times.

Many surgeons find solace in their pastimes, whether these consist of physical activities or more cerebral pursuits. Having a sport, hobby, or social outlet outside of work may also be a good way to find work-life balance, and enable the surgeon to move through the emotional turmoil of the death of a patient. Personal strategies, such as practicing meditation and mindfulness, can regulate stress and anxiety, and help a surgeon refocus by observing and acknowledging thoughts and emotions and allowing them to pass. Physical exercise with its endorphin-promoting effects may be a particularly effective way to mitigate against the multiple types of stress associated with such an event.

Professional organizations are starting to recognize the emotional strain modern medical practice puts upon the practitioner. There are an increasing number of resources available to help surgeons deal with these stressors [2].

Conclusions

How we deal with a patient's death can define us; whether we wall ourselves off, become emotionally over attached and vulnerable, or in those cases where it leads to consequences in terms of anger, depression, or even substance abuse. The pressures of modern surgical practice and the increasing expectations of patients can make what is a highly rewarding career increasingly fraught with difficulties. Surgeon burnout is real, and we need to come up with ways to openly discuss it, and provide support to those surgeons in their time of need. The individual physician needs to have insight into their own feelings and either have robust coping strategies of their own, or seek appropriate help when it is needed. Although the notion of "second victim syndrome" may not be fashionable amongst our profession, where we pride ourselves on our resilience, we must not fool ourselves that our junior colleagues and trainees wish to continue to suffer in silence, and we must remove the stigma. Personally we would rather be cared for by a surgeon who is affected by a patient's death, than one who has become stone-hearted to the suffering of his patients. This is what we entered the sacred profession of surgery for, to alleviate suffering, and we should keep that foremost in our minds.

Conflicts of Interests There are no identifiable conflicts of interests to report.

The authors have no financial or proprietary interest in the subject matter or materials discussed in the manuscript.

References

1. Burkhart RA, et al. Grit: a marker of residents at risk for attrition? Surgery. 2014;155(6):1014–22.
2. El Hechi MW, et al. Design and impact of a novel surgery-specific second victim peer support program. J Am Coll Surg. 2020;230(6):926–33.
3. Ferguson CM. Addressing the source of surgeon burnout. Bull Am Coll Surg. 2015;100(7):73–4.
4. Gawande A. Complications: a surgeon's notes on an imperfect science. New York: Metropolitan Books; 2002.
5. Goldstick JE, et al. Current causes of death in children and adolescents in the United States. N Engl J Med. 2022;386(20):1955–6.
6. Han K, et al. The surgeon as the second victim? Results of the Boston intraoperative adverse events surgeons' attitude (BISA) study. J Am Coll Surg. 2017;224(6):1048–56.
7. Khansa I, Pearson GD. Coping and recovery in surgical residents after adverse events: the second victim phenomenon. Plast Reconstr Surg Glob Open. 2022;10(3):e4203.
8. Maslach C, Leiter MP. The truth about burnout: how organizations cause personal stress and what to do about it. San Francisco: Jossey-Bass; 1997.
9. The Harris poll. Americans' belief in god, miracles and heaven declines. From http://www.theharrispoll.com/health-and-life/Americans__Belief_in_God__Miracles_and_Heaven_Declines.html.
10. Wu AW. Medical error: the second victim. The doctor who makes the mistake needs help too. BMJ. 2000;320(7237):726–7.

The Surgeon's Burnout: How to Deal with It

25

Christina Colosimo, Sai Krishna Bhogadi, and Bellal Joseph

Irrespective of seniority, most of us in the world of medicine in general, and surgery in particular, go through situations where we feel helpless, lose interest, and feel unappreciated; everything looks bleak, and it's difficult to muster up the energy to care. There comes a time when dragging ourselves out of bed requires the strength of Hercules, problems look overwhelming and even breathing becomes a task. The impact of such feelings forces individuals to reconsider their self-worth, and this cascade of events eventually leads to helplessness. Experiencing these feelings most of the time may lead them to suffer burnout, which can threaten one's career, relationships, and health.

What Is Burnout?

It is not surprising that the term "burnout" was coined by American psychologist Herbert Freudenberger in 1974 to describe, "the consequences of severe or prolonged stress and anxiety experienced by people working in the healing professions" [1]. Maslach and Jackson later defined burnout as "a syndrome of emotional exhaustion and cynicism that occurs frequently among individuals who do people work of some kind" [2]. In simple terms, burnout refers to a mental or physical collapse caused by overwork or stress. It has been described in the literature as a syndrome of emotional, mental, and physical exhaustion, high depersonalization, and a feeling of low personal accomplishment caused by excessive and prolonged stress [3].

It is well established that emotional exhaustion lies at the center of the problem and excessive psychological and emotional demands result in emotional exhaustion. Depersonalization is a tendency to view others in a markedly detached manner and represents the individual's attempt to protect against further emotional exhaustion. All these components are self-perpetuating and ultimately lead to a mixed matrix propagating the other components. Burnout is a continuous variable ranging from emotional exhaustion to low personal accomplishment.

Burnout syndrome is an endless list of problems including physical illness, emotional lability, increased turnover, absenteeism, poor job performance, drug abuse, and negative attitudes that have been associated with burnout. These problems present as a part of a "generalized psychological distress" which is variable in each individual [4]. Burnout leading to burnout syndrome ultimately occurs in individuals who require spending time and intensive involvement with other people. Given the severity and impact an individual has, it is important to deal with burnout in a defined stepwise approach.

C. Colosimo · S. K. Bhogadi · B. Joseph (✉)
Division of Trauma, Critical Care, Burns, and Emergency Surgery, Department of Surgery, University of Arizona, Tucson, AZ, USA
e-mail: ccolosim@arizona.edu; saikbhogadi@arizona.edu; bjoseph@arizona.edu

R. Latifi (ed.), *Surgical Decision-Making*, https://doi.org/10.1007/978-3-031-67391-7_25

At Risk Population

The phenomenon of burnout has been investigated in a wide variety of occupations, including physicians and surgeons. In the published literature, up to 40% of practicing surgeons suffer from considerable stress and subsequent burnout during their career that may affect their personal and professional performance. Campbell et al. reviewed burnout among 582 American surgeons and found that one-third (32%) of them had high levels of emotional exhaustion, whereas 13% had higher depersonalization, and 4% indicated a low level of personal accomplishment [5]. In a systematic review and meta-analysis including 27 articles with 8617 surgeons, the prevalence of burnout was found to be 47%, with rates per specialty ranging between 15% and 77% [6]. In a recent systematic review and meta-analysis on trends in surgeon burnout in the US and Canada including 103 studies representing 63,587 individuals, 41% of the surgeons met criteria for burnout [7].

Burnout more likely occurs in young female surgeons who have younger children or delay childrearing and assume greater parental responsibility while they have similar clinical duties as male surgeons [8]. Younger surgeons experience more emotional stress as a result of different social expectations regarding the balance of career, family, and personal growth and development. The implication is that we continue to fail to prepare our young trainees to survive in their personal and professional lives while maintaining good mental health. The impact of this failure is substantial as literature demonstrates that many of these young burned out practitioners leave surgical specialties to retrain in other specialties or begin retiring earlier [9].

Although some evidence demonstrated that physicians in private practice might be at a greater risk for burnout, there is no difference in burnout among surgeons based on practice setting. However, some limited evidence suggests that there may be some differences in burnout among different surgical subspecialties [10]. The surgical specialties involved with the care of emergencies and acute adverse events are usually at higher risk of burnout due to their longer work hours and stressful nature of the field. In a survey conducted on the members of the Eastern Association for the Surgery of Trauma and American Association for the Surgery of trauma, 40% of the trauma surgeons reported symptoms of post-traumatic stress disorder (PTSD) and 15% had a diagnosis of PTSD [11].

Burnout is not limited to practicing physicians or surgeons, and there are other vulnerable groups including medical students and residents who suffer from burnout. More than half of the medical students in the US manifest burnout while in medical school. Nearly 38% of orthopedic surgery residents and 45% of vascular surgery trainees reported symptoms of burnout in surveys, with sizeable amount of trainees reporting mistreatment, duty hour violations, thoughts of attrition, specialty change, and suicide [12, 13]. High levels of stress and burnout have also been reported in nurses. Burnout is higher in acute pediatric nurses compared to non-acute care nurses. Similar results have been reported in nurses working night shifts and those involved in the intensive care setting [14].

Burnout vs. Stress

Often burnout and stress are words that are used interchangeably however they are not the same. Constant stress causes an individual to initiate losing interest that may have been a motivator to take on a certain role in the first place. Like burnout, stress can also affect the quality of family relationships and the nature of the doctor–patient relationship. The difference is that stressed people can imagine and visualize rationally. Often the condition is reversible and once the stress is managed or dealt with, people are often able to successfully manage their professional performance and feel better. On the other hand, burnout deters one's ability to rationalize or imagine and ultimately the ability to reverse the condition is complex, requiring management of more than one condition.

Burnout is often associated with a devoid of motivation. It can result in feeling as though one "has nothing left to do," negative attitudes toward patients, and a reduced feeling of competence. People with high levels of burnout are hopeless and cannot see the positive changes in their situation. In contrast to stress, burnout is characterized by disengagement. It produces blunted feelings and causes helplessness, hopelessness, loss of motivation, and ideals. It may lead to detachment and depression. Primary damage in burnout is emotional and may make life seem not worth living. However, burnout is a psychological construct to investigate the stress.

Measuring Tools

The Maslach Burnout Inventory is a reliable measurement instrument to sample large populations for stress [8]. This measuring tool has separate subscales to evaluate each domain of burnout [15]. There are some standard categorical thresholds to classify each domain score as high, moderate, or low. According to this classification scoring system, surgeons are considered as high scores in depersonalization and emotional exhaustion [8]. However, burnout in the surgical environment is sparsely reviewed and the quantitative assessment of surgical burnout is limited.

Burnout in Surgeons

As mentioned in the previous sections, the prevalence of burnout in surgeons is very high. This indicates that there is a concern in the personal and professional life of the surgeons. Surgeons work long for irregular hours, deal repeatedly with their patients, and make considerable sacrifices to practice in their field. They have an unwritten but understood code of rules and expectations. This code includes coming in early and staying late, working nights and weekends, performing a high volume of procedures, meeting multiple simultaneous deadlines, never complaining, and keeping personal problems away from work.

Ultimately all of these qualities are both defined and rendered by the surgeons; however, when there is no fine line between dedication and hard work it can lead to unhealthy and self-destructive behavior, which can affect patient care as well.

COVID-19 Pandemic and Burnout

The COVID-19 pandemic has led to unprecedented impact on people, healthcare workers, and the healthcare system alike. Healthcare systems all over the world had to deal with patients beyond their capacities, often with limited staff. Many surgeons significantly curtailed elective surgeries and were deployed on the teams providing frontline treatment. In addition to being in the frontline teams, surgeons also provided acute care surgery support whenever necessary. Similar to professionals from other specialties, surgeons faced extreme levels of burnout during the pandemic. In a systematic review including 19 articles with 3866 surgical trainees, the prevalence of burnout in surgical trainees during the pandemic was reported between 9.1% and 95.2%, with general surgery having the highest burnout rates (33.1–95.2%) compared to other surgical specialties. Another systematic review by Shaikh et al. assessing burnout among surgeons and surgical trainees during the COVID-19 pandemic also found high rates of burnout ranging from 6% to 86% [16].

There are several theories behind increased burnout in surgeons and surgical trainees during the pandemic. Limited prior working experience with this patient population and sudden increase in the COVID-19 patient clinical load, redeployment to COVID-19 wards, reduction in the regular operative cases, decreased hands-on experience, and not being able to complete case requirements are some factors that have been proposed as the possible reasons. In addition, repeated episodes of quarantine and self-isolation, violence and harassment, lack of psychological support, stigmatization and discrimination, and concerns of care for family members have placed surgeons and health care workers at higher risk for burnout during the pandemic.

Causes

There are several causes for burnout. Originally, it stems from the occupation, however anyone who is overworked is at risk of burnout. Additionally, lifestyle and personality traits contribute to burnout. Being younger and having a spouse employed outside the home is associated with a higher risk of burnout. It means that lack of balance among career, family, and personal growth in the younger surgeons is directly associated with burnout. On the other hand, having children is associated with a lower risk of burnout [10]. Causes of burnout are presented in Table 25.1 [10, 17, 18].

One or combination of these factors can predispose a professional to burnout. Excess workload, inefficiency, loss of self-sufficiency, and a lack of meaning in work seem to be central factors to cause burnout among surgeons [19]. There is a probability that gender differences may be another cause of burnout. Female physicians have a higher level of burnout in comparison to their male counterparts. However, among surgeons, gender disparity does not have a robust impact on burnout [14]. In a survey including 291 trauma surgeons, poor work-life balance, being midcareer, having more work hours, fewer awake hours at home, and feeling that there is a better job were identified as predictors of burnout [20].

Table 25.1 Causes of burnout [10, 17, 18]

Work related
Lack of control over the work
Lack of appreciation for decent work
Uncertain job expectations
Doing unchallenging work
Working in a high-pressure situation
Lifestyle related
Uneven distribution of time between work and personal life making a safe training environment
Lack of relaxation and socializing time
Lack of enough sleep
Taking on too many duties without enough help
Research and educational situation
Lack of supportive relationships
Personality traits
Type A personality
Perfectionistic feeling
Negative view of oneself and world

Surgeons and Sleep Deprivation

Surgeons often work for long hours with erratic schedules with constant on-call duties and emergencies which create a perfect storm where adequate restful sleep becomes a rare commodity. Sleep deprivation among professionals working in high-risk industries has been shown to be a proven factor in the loss of civilian life. Constant sleep deprivation affects cognitive function, the very bedrock on which surgeons build their precision and decision-making prowess. Since surgery is a field where split-second decisions can be life-altering, sleep deprivation in surgeons is a major issue that needs attention. In a systematic review of 33 studies assessing sleep deprivation in surgery, sleep deprivation was found to negatively impact technical performance with a 12–32% decrement in performance [21]. This issue of sleep deprivation is even more significant in acute care surgeons as their clinical activities include surgical critical care, emergency general surgery, and trauma, all of which require around-the-clock clinical coverage. In a 6-month prospective study of 224 acute care surgeons by Coleman et al., surgeons reported feelings of moderate, very, or extreme burnout for 25.7% of days during the study period, and feelings of being moderately, slightly, or not at all rested occurred 75.91% of days. Decreased amount of time between the inhouse calls, reduced sleep duration, and having a bad patient outcome have been linked to greater feelings of daily burnout [22].

Signs and Symptoms

Burnout occurs gradually over a period of time. Signs and symptoms of burnout are subtle at first, but they get worse over time. It is associated with depression and anxiety. In a study, evaluating members of the American College of Surgeons, approximately 30% of study participants screened positive for depression [10]. Some reports also suggest that the exhaustion component of the burnout syndrome may be related to depression.

Burnout and depression among practicing surgeons are independent predictors of medical errors. The inherent stressful nature of the surgery along with excessive and erratic work hours put surgeons at a much higher risk for burnout and may also affect personal relationships. The increasing incidence of divorce after 30 years of marriage is the highest among surgeons, regardless of the amount of work resources or hours worked. Moreover patients with chronic burnout have specific cognitive impairments in nonverbal memory and attention [23].

Symptoms of Surgeon's Burnout

Signs and symptoms of surgeons' burnout can be broadly classified into three groups: physical, behavioral, and emotional. Physical signs and symptoms include feeling tired most of the time, change in appetite or sleep habits, frequent headache and body pain, and reduced immunity. Among the emotional symptoms; loss of motivation, negative attitude, feeling failure, decreased satisfaction, feeling hopeless and helpless, and detachment are remarkable. Furthermore, isolation, careless attitude, generalizing frustration toward others, and procrastination are among the emotional factors associated with burnout.

Surgeons, with high levels of burnout, are more likely to report increasing intake of alcohol, keeping things to themselves, engaging in less sports or recreation and mixing less with friends in response to work-related stress [14].

Consequences of Burnout

In the demanding world of surgery, where precision is paramount and split-second decisions can be a matter of life and death, burnout emerges as a silent but pervasive threat. Beyond the immediate toll it takes on an individual, burnout casts a long shadow, influencing not only the surgeon but also the entire healthcare ecosystem.

(a) *Effects at the Individual Level:*

Previous reports have identified burnout to be associated with numerous detrimental personal consequences, including a higher risk of mental health disorders and poorer physical quality of life [24]. Among surgical trainees, burnout has been linked with higher levels of depression, anxiety, PTSD, and suicidality [25]. Burnout has also been associated with unhealthy behaviors in surgical trainees such as alcohol misuse and engaging less frequently in exercise.

(b) *Impact on Patient Care:*

Burnout poses a threat to patient-centered care, a principle which is the cornerstone of medicine. As surgeons battle with their own emotional and physical exhaustion, the ability to connect empathetically with patients diminishes. The downstream effect is a potential decline in patient satisfaction and trust [26]. The manifestation of burnout has been associated with challenges in cognitive task performance, posing a concern for surgeons and their professional aptitude [27]. Higher levels of emotional exhaustion and burnout have been linked with greater number of perceived medical errors [28, 29]. In a systematic review and meta-analysis by Al-Ghunaim et al., burnout was found to be associated with 2.5-fold increased risk of involvement in medical error [30].

Burnout Prevention

Considering the early symptoms of burnout as warning signs is important. By having insight to these warning signs and recognizing them early, we can prevent a major breakdown and the development of burn out. Taking steps to get life back into balance can prevent burnout from becoming a full-scale failure. Individual efforts to develop a balance between personal and professional life may help reduce burnout rate in surgeons. Overall, enhanced institutional support and increased opportunities for professional progression can decrease burnout rate among surgeons [31]. One effective method to prevent burnout among surgeons is to actively protect their personal and professional well-being at physical, emotional, psychological, and spiritual levels. These efforts need to occur from medical school through retirement.

Burnout Prevention in Surgeons

Even though the prevalence of burnout is higher among surgeons compared to other specialties, surgeons are less likely to seek help compared to other medical professionals [32]. This is highly concerning as surgeons have higher rates of suicide compared to other physicians and individuals in other occupations [33]. We need to encourage discussions on this topic and create a culture where trainees and surgeons feel supported to express their struggles. Measures to prevent burnout must be taken at the individual and institutional level. There are several tips which will help in burnout prevention among surgeons. *Starting the day with a relaxing protocol and meditation will help inspire the individual. Surgeons should adopt healthy eating, exercising, and sleeping habits. By getting* plenty of rest, they will have enough energy and flexibility to deal with the environmental irritations. They should halt overextending themselves and set their limitations. Additionally, it is exceedingly imperative that a surgeon knows how to manage stress. All these elements can have a crucial role in preventing burnout.

Moreover, co-worker and spouse support, as well as positive patient interactions, can buffer work overload and emotional demands, thereby positively influencing surgeon's well-being. In order to decrease unnecessary tension and fortify support mechanisms for surgeons, Wallace et al. believe that a categorized group can strengthen functional teams by providing team construction and social events, enabling feedback and working for common aims. This will help alleviate tension and its consequences [34].

Other personal strategies that may help increase well-being of individual surgeons include participating in research, following educational activities outside work environment, paying particular attention to important personal relationships, performing spiritual practices, recognizing the importance of one's work, promoting personal interests outside work, engaging in mentorship, and creating a balance between personal and professional life [31]. Surgeons who can determine what is important in their life and put energy for their goals may have a lower risk for developing burnout. Additional coping factors to decrease burnout include getting regular sleep, obtaining personal medical care, and exercise. There are several organizational strategies for coping with burnout that are represented in Table 25.2 [35–38].

Table 25.2 Preventing strategies [35–38]

Personal
Identify stress and emotional burnout and approve adaptive coping strategies
Cultivate a healthy personal relationship and spiritual practices
Find medical and/or mental health care when needed or directed
Preserve appropriate nutrition and physical fitness
Attempt to create and sustain a work-life balance
Organizational
Developing administrative leadership to identify at risk surgical residents
Making a safe training situation
Providing stress controlling training
Create relationship-building opportunities for residents and their spouses and families
Identify the critical contributors to burnout among female and young residents
Providing research and educational situation
Making a constructive mentorships and relation between residents and faculty

Coping with all predisposing factors will help prevent burnout. Surgeons must be proactive about any work issue which exists in the work environment and try to approach and elucidate them. The individual should be completely aware of their responsibilities at the workplace and ask their mentor about all of the dimensions of their duty. Doing a constant duty for a long time may result in impatience and tiredness. Therefore, it is helpful to ask for a new task or role.

Recovering

While burnout happens with its warning signs, it is crucial to take it seriously and try to recover from it. The first step of recovery is to slow down and take a break. It is equal to time for healing. Ultimately if burnout is inevitable, the best solution is to ask for a complete break from work to recover and recharge one's mood and perspective. Sharing feelings with others and trusting them can relieve tension and burnout criteria. Finally, surgeons should reevaluate and set goals and priorities that they define as reachable and important contributors to their overall happiness.

Conclusion

Both symptoms and diagnosis of burnout are common among medical field personnel, especially in surgeons. Further understanding of the factors that predispose surgeons to burnout may benefit the patients and the profession. It lays responsibility on national organizations to help set new standards of identification and treatment of burnout. Advocating active surveillance and development of targeted interventions by national organizations may promote wellness among surgeons.

Conflicts of Interests There are no identifiable conflicts of interests to report.

The authors have no financial or proprietary interest in the subject matter or materials discussed in the manuscript.

References

1. Freudenberger HJ. Staff burn-out. J Soc Issues. 1974;30(1):159–65.
2. Maslach C, Jackson SE. The measurement of experienced burnout. J Organ Behav. 1981;2(2):99–113.
3. Melnitchouk N, Dimou F, Eckelbarger D, Riall T, Elmore L, Jeffe D, Jin L, Awad M, Turnbull I, Brandt M. Surgeon burnout: defining, identifying, and addressing the new reality. Clin Colon Rectal Surg. 2019;32(06):407–14.
4. Serenari M, Cucchetti A, Russo PM, Fallani G, Mattarozzi K, Pinna AD, Colonnello V, Poggioli G, Cescon M. Burnout and psychological distress between surgical and non-surgical residents. Updat Surg. 2019;71:323–30.
5. Campbell DA Jr, Sonnad SS, Eckhauser FE, Campbell KK, Greenfield LJ. Burnout among American surgeons. Surgery. 2001;130(4):696–702.; discussion 702-695. https://doi.org/10.1067/msy.2001.116676.
6. Jesuyajolu D, Nicholas A, Okeke C, Obi C, Aremu G, Obiekwe K, Obinna I. Burnout among surgeons and surgical trainees: a systematic review and meta-analysis of the prevalence and associated factors. Surg Pract Sci. 2022;10:100094.
7. Etheridge JC, Evans D, Zhao L, Ibrahim N, Wick EC, Freischlag JA, Brownstein MR. Trends in surgeon burnout in the US and Canada: systematic review and meta-regression analysis. J Am Coll Surg. 2023;236(1):253–65.
8. Dyrbye LN, Shanafelt TD, Balch CM, Satele D, Sloan J, Freischlag J. Relationship between work-home conflicts and burnout among American surgeons: a comparison by sex. Arch Surg. 2011;146(2):211–7. https://doi.org/10.1001/archsurg.2010.310.
9. Cimbak N, Stolarski A, Moseley J, O'Neal P, Whang E, Kristo G. Burnout leads to premature surgeon retirement: a nationwide survey. J Surg Res. 2019;2(3):159–69.
10. Shanafelt TD, Balch CM, Bechamps GJ, Russell T, Dyrbye L, Satele D, Collicott P, Novotny PJ, Sloan J, Freischlag JA. Burnout and career satisfaction among American surgeons. Ann Surg. 2009;250(3):463–71.
11. Joseph B, Pandit V, Hadeed G, Kulvatunyou N, Zangbar B, Tang A, O'Keeffe T, Wynne J, Green DJ, Friese RS, Rhee P. Unveiling posttraumatic stress disorder in trauma surgeons: a national survey. J Trauma Acute Care Surg. 2014;77(1):148–54.; discussion 154. https://doi.org/10.1097/ta.0000000000000271.
12. Chia MC, Hu Y-Y, Li RD, Cheung EO, Eng JS, Zhan T, Sheahan MG III, Bilimoria KY, Coleman DM. Prevalence and risk factors for burnout in US vascular surgery trainees. J Vasc Surg. 2022;75(1):308–15. e304
13. Somerson JS, Patton A, Ahmed AA, Ramey S, Holliday EB. Burnout among United States orthopaedic surgery residents. J Surg Educ. 2020;77(4):961–8.
14. Sharma A, Sharp DM, Walker LG, Monson JR. Stress and burnout among colorectal surgeons and colorectal nurse specialists working in the National Health Service. Color Dis. 2008;10(4):397–406. https://doi.org/10.1111/j.1463-1318.2007.01338.x.
15. West CP, Huschka MM, Novotny PJ, Sloan JA, Kolars JC, Habermann TM, Shanafelt TD. Association of perceived medical errors with resident distress and empathy: a prospective longitudinal study. JAMA. 2006;296(9):1071–8. https://doi.org/10.1001/jama.296.9.1071.
16. Shaikh CF, Kelly EP, Paro A, Cloyd J, Ejaz A, Beal EW, Pawlik TM. Burnout assessment among surgeons and surgical trainees during the COVID-19 pandemic: a systematic review. J Surg Educ. 2022;79(5):1206–20.
17. Galaiya R, Kinross J, Arulampalam T. Factors associated with burnout syndrome in surgeons: a systematic review. Ann R Coll Surg Engl. 2020;102(6):401–7.
18. Robinson DBT, Luton O, Mellor K, James OP, Hopkins L, Powell AG, Hemington-Gorse S, Harries RL, Egan RJ, Lewis WG. Trainee perspective of the causes of stress and burnout in surgical training: a qualitative study from Wales. BMJ Open. 2021;11(8):e045150.
19. Shanafelt T, Dyrbye L. Oncologist burnout: causes, consequences, and responses. J Clin Oncol. 2012;30(11):1235–41. https://doi.org/10.1200/jco.2011.39.7380.

20. Brown CV, Joseph BA, Davis K, Jurkovich GJ. Modifiable factors to improve work-life balance for trauma surgeons. J Trauma Acute Care Surg. 2021;90(1):122–8.
21. Whelehan DF, McCarrick CA, Ridgway PF. A systematic review of sleep deprivation and technical skill in surgery. Surgeon. 2020;18(6):375–84.
22. Coleman JJ, Robinson CK, von Hippel W, Holmes KE, Kim J, Pearson S, Lawless RA, Hubbard AE, Cohen MJ. What happens on call doesn't stay on call. The effects of in-house call on acute care surgeons' sleep and burnout: results of the surgeon performance (SuPer) trial. Ann Surg. 2023;278(4):497–505.
23. Peterson U, Demerouti E, Bergstrom G, Samuelsson M, Asberg M, Nygren A. Burnout and physical and mental health among Swedish healthcare workers. J Adv Nurs. 2008;62(1):84–95. https://doi.org/10.1111/j.1365-2648.2007.04580.x.
24. Jennings JM, Gold PA, Nellans K, Boraiah S. Orthopaedic surgeons have a high prevalence of burnout, depression, and suicide: review of factors which contribute or reduce further harm. J Am Acad Orthop Surg. 2022;30(5):e528–35.
25. Williford ML, Scarlet S, Meyers MO, Luckett DJ, Fine JP, Goettler CE, Green JM, Clancy TV, Hildreth AN, Meltzer-Brody SE. Multiple-institution comparison of resident and faculty perceptions of burnout and depression during surgical training. JAMA Surg. 2018;153(8):705–11.
26. Byrd J, Knowles H, Moore S, Acker V, Bell S, Alanis N, Zhou Y, d'Etienne JP, Kline JA, Wang H. Synergistic effects of emergency physician empathy and burnout on patient satisfaction: a prospective observational study. Emerg Med J. 2021;38(4):290–6.
27. Österberg K, Skogsliden S, Karlson B. Neuropsychological sequelae of work-stress-related exhaustion. Stress. 2014;17(1):59–69.
28. Crijns TJ, Kortlever JT, Guitton TG, Ring D, Barron GC. Symptoms of burnout among surgeons are correlated with a higher incidence of perceived medical errors. HSS J. 2020;16(2_suppl):305–10.
29. Joseph B, Tseng ES, Zielinski MD, Ramirez CL, Lynde J, Galey KM, Bhogadi SK, El-Qawaqzeh K, Hosseinpour H. Feeling like an imposter: are surgeons holding themselves back? BMJ Special J. 2023;8:e001021.
30. Al-Ghunaim TA, Johnson J, Biyani CS, Alshahrani KM, Dunning A, O'Connor DB. Surgeon burnout, impact on patient safety and professionalism: a systematic review and meta-analysis. Am J Surg. 2022;224(1):228–38.
31. Bertges Yost W, Eshelman A, Raoufi M, Abouljoud MS. A national study of burnout among American transplant surgeons. Transplant Proc. 2005;37(2):1399–401. https://doi.org/10.1016/j.transproceed.2005.01.055.
32. Gerada C, Jones R. Surgeons and mental illness: a hidden problem? BMJ. 2014;348
33. Harvey SB, Epstein RM, Glozier N, Petrie K, Strudwick J, Gayed A, Dean K, Henderson M. Mental illness and suicide among physicians. Lancet. 2021;398(10303):920–30.
34. Wallace JE, Lemaire J. On physician well being-you'll get by with a little help from your friends. Soc Sci Med. 2007;64(12):2565–77. https://doi.org/10.1016/j.socscimed.2007.03.016.
35. EbrAHIMI S. Burned-out surgeons–a review of risk factors and intervention types. Maastricht Stud J Psychol Neurosci. 2015;4
36. Espeland KE. Overcoming burnout: how to revitalize your career. J Contin Educ Nurs. 2006;37(4):178–84.
37. Shanafelt, T. D., Gorringe, G., Menaker, R., Storz, K. A., Reeves, D., Buskirk, S. J., Sloan, J. A., & Swensen, S. J. (2015). Impact of organizational leadership on physician burnout and satisfaction. Mayo Clin Proc, https://doi.org/10.1016/j.mayocp.2015.01.012.
38. Shanafelt TD, Kaups KL, Nelson H, Satele DV, Sloan JA, Oreskovich MR, Dyrbye LN. An interactive individualized intervention to promote behavioral change to increase personal well-being in US surgeons. Ann Surg. 2014;259(1):82.

When Should We Quit Operating?

26

Stanley J. Dudrick, Edward S. Anderson,
and Rifat Latifi

"However, difficult and demanding many of these decisions have been, often accompanied by lingering anxiety, self-doubt, and other manifestations of emotional and psychological distress, no more formidable and personal challenge must be faced and confronted by the practicing, operating surgeons than the decision as to when it is time for them to stop operating. Yet, this is both in their best interests, and in the best interests of their patients, especially from the standpoints of trust, safety, efficacy, optimal outcomes, and personal and professional responsibility, duty, honor, and character". Stanely J. Dudrick, MD, FACS

During their professional lifetimes, surgeons must make many decisions, virtually daily, often continually, mostly "on the spot," sometimes "life or death," and almost always critically important to the optimal care, outcomes, and well-being of their patients. During their professional lifetimes, surgeons must make many decisions, virtually daily, often continually, mostly "on the spot," sometimes "life or death," and almost always critically important to the optimal care, outcomes, and well-being of their patients. These decisions are based primarily on the cumulative knowledge, experience, judgment, and wisdom gained throughout years of education, training, mentoring, conferences, consultations, study, and introspection; coupled with dedication, motivation, persistence, resilience, integrity, equanimity, core values, ethics, and courage; along with a wide variety of additional, often unique, virtues which comprise the individual essence and character of each of the multitude of surgeons throughout the world. However difficult and demanding many of these decisions have been, often accompanied by lingering anxiety, self-doubt, and other manifestations of emotional and psychological distress, no more formidable and personal challenge must be faced and confronted by the practicing, operating surgeons than the decision as to when it is time for them to stop operating. Yet, this is both in their best inter-

Dr. Stanely Dudrick, MD, FACS passed away on January 18, 2020, at age almost 75. The editor and the published decided to republish this chapter the way it was published on the first edition. Correspondence about this chapter send to the editor of this tome, Rifat Latifi, MD.

S. J. Dudrick (Deceased)
Surgery, The Commonwealth Medical College, Scranton, PA, USA

E. S. Anderson
Physician Assistant Studies, Misericordia University, Dallas, PA, USA

Emeritus of Surgery, Yale University Medical School, New Haven, CT, USA

R. Latifi (✉)
Department of Surgery, The University of Arizona, Tucson, AZ, USA

Tucson Medical Center, Department of Surgery, Tucson, AZ, USA
e-mail: Latifi@surgery.arizona.edu

R. Latifi (ed.), *Surgical Decision-Making*, https://doi.org/10.1007/978-3-031-67391-7_26

ests, and in the best interests of their patients, especially from the standpoints of trust, safety, efficacy, optimal outcomes, and personal and professional responsibility, duty, honor, and character.

It would be uncommon for all surgeons to agree completely to follow an identical pathway or algorithm in the decision-making process related to the management of any surgical problem. Although the mechanisms and principles of obtaining a comprehensive history and physical examination, together with appropriate indicated hematologic, biochemical, nutritional, immunologic, genetic, and imaging (ultrasonic, radiologic, magnetic resonance) studies have been well established, the decisions to use them judiciously, and in a specific order of priority vary quite a lot among surgeons, as does the subsequent use of more complicated, sophisticated, and expensive techniques and technologies in establishing a provisional or definitive diagnosis, proposing a therapeutic plan, and informing and educating the patient regarding the risks, potential complications, and prognosis, together with the preoperative preparations and measures, and the essentials of postoperative care, recovery, convalescence, and rehabilitation requisite for optimal outcomes. Many other general and specific patient-centered aspects must be incorporated into wise decision-making, including personal, family, financial, health-care insurance, employment, social, spiritual, religious considerations, et cetera. There are myriad other compounding and/or confounding factors which can significantly complicate the process, particularly in patients with multiple complex problems, patients with various kinds and degrees of organ and/or system failures, undernutrition, trauma, infections, old age, frailty, et cetera. Thus, it is obvious that making the same series of decisions in all patients with the same apparent problem is promulgated by the myth of "routine care for routine patients." There are no uniformly routine situations in real life, and it is this type of "one size fits all" thinking and rote decision-making that can result in surgical management, operative errors, and misadventures that can lead to undue complications, morbidity, and mortality, which continue to exist at unacceptable, recalcitrant levels despite current measures to avoid or minimize them. The apparently untoward, unanticipated, unavoidable occurrence or result can almost always be traced back to a conscious or subconscious decision on the part of the surgeon not to follow his or her own established principles and practices proficiently, meticulously, and conscientiously. Why do these unfortunate, preventable, quixotic consequences continue to occur arguably to the most intelligent, educated, experienced, disciplined, hard-working, motivated, accomplished, respected surgeons on earth? If the answer to this question were obvious and readily discernable, the situation would have been arrested, reversed, diminished, or prevented years ago; but it persists today virtually unabated, tragically, and stubbornly, despite apparent national, institutional, societal, professional, and personal efforts to solve, correct, and obviate the problems. Perhaps it has continued to exist because we have only nibbled at the edges of the problems and have been treating symptoms or modulating untoward consequences rather than identifying and attacking all of the root causes of poor outcomes. In accordance with the wisdom and pronouncement of Pogo, "We have met the enemy, and he is us" [1]. As surgeons, we have all experienced a less than optimal result of even our best efforts to alleviate or correct a serious patient condition ordinarily amendable to judicious surgical treatment. Why has the patient not responded as predicted, planned, and expected, based on our previous experience or historical expectations? Was the failure to achieve the ideal or "perfect" result predetermined by a combination, or set of confounding circumstances, which would interdict our usual efforts or attempts, despite our strict observance of, and adherence to, the highest standards of care? Were we naively expecting that this commonly straightforward patient could have the "routine" problem "slam-dunked" by the surgeons' skill, expertise, and experience? I teach students, residents, and others that there are no "routine surgical patients," but there are some "routine surgeons." Most of the time they can play the poker game well and comfortably, but when they are dealt an unusual, weak, or strange hand, they will lose their money or chips if they think that they can win the pot every time because they are such superior poker players. As recorded in the Country Western ballad, "The Gambler:" "If you're gonna play the game boy, you gotta learn to play it right. You've got to know when to hold'em, know when to fold'em, know when to walk away, know when to run. You never count your money, when your sittin' at the table; there'll be time enough for countin', when the dealin's done. Every gambler knows that the secret to survivin' is knowin' what to throw away and knowin' what to keep. 'Cause every hand's a winner and every hand's a loser, and the best that you can hope for is to die in your sleep" [2]. Even the world's best poker player cannot win the pot if he or she is dealt an extremely poor hand of cards, and even the best of surgeons cannot cure all of their patients, because not only are they compelled to work with the patient that they are dealt, but also, despite their exceptional efforts, skills, and talents, the desired outcome may elude them when the odds are so greatly against success. Although ethical surgeons are not gamblers, they must know and cope with similar sets of probability, percentages, and unknown other inherent factors such as risks, luck, and chance, that influence the results of their decisions and "bluffing" is never allowed or acceptable in surgery.

My first Professor of Surgery, Dr. Isadore S. Ravdin, frequently pointed out to the medical students, surgical residents, and others that, "one cannot make a silk purse out of a sow's ear," especially when the operative goals could not be achieved as planned, secondary to an impossible pathologic situation, and/or untoward or unintended consequences. Indeed, the wisdom that he and my other mentors imparted to me, starting as a medical student and then throughout my surgical residency training and research fellowship, has influenced me greatly throughout my surgical career. In those days, it was either conventional or the rule, that a surgeon relinquish a leadership role as a Chairman or Chief of a Surgical Service at 65 years of age. This also applied to operative surgery, or at least to major operative surgery, and most surgeons would plan their projected length of time practicing operative surgery from the completion of their training and board certification on that basis. However, this "mandatory retirement" was not uniformly accepted or applied throughout the country, and subsequently, after the legislation dealing with age discrimination in 1986 came into play, many surgeons have continued to operate well beyond the year of their 65th birthday.

When I was a student and intern at the bottom of the surgical food chain, I witnessed more than a few conversations among the older residents regarding the quality of the attending surgeons' decisions in patient management and the operative procedures. After a case which might not have had an ideal intraoperative experience or result, a resident would comment negatively about the surgeon thusly, "Did you see how the old man ripped out the gallbladder and caused all that bleeding?" Or, "Can you believe how roughly he tore through the adhesions and into the intestine?" Or, "He was in such a hurry that the patient lost at least two units of blood because he wouldn't stop to clamp all the vessels he cut across." Or, "Why does he keep doing these big cases when they all seem to get complications secondary to his roughness or impatience?" These were very disturbing, often whispered, conversations among the house staff, which obviously frustrated and frightened them and me. I was in no position to judge them or the staff surgeons involved, but I was indelibly impressed that I would never want to find myself in a comparable position as a surgeon who was judged to be "over the hill" by his assistants, subordinates, or colleagues. Even worse, not to be informed, counseled, or advised by colleagues as to their concerns, but rather to be allowed to continue to perform below standards and, perhaps, thereby not to be aware of secondary adverse consequences to the patient and to the reputation of the surgeon.

By the time that I had completed my Chief Residency year in General Surgery, I had made the prospective decision that I would stop operating at age 65 in order not to embarrass myself, not to compromise the ideal standards of operative care, and not to cause any untoward complications or outcomes in my patients related to my diminishing competencies and skills secondary to my aging.

In his Presidential Address to the Forty-first Scientific Meeting of the North American Chapter of the International Society for Cardiovascular Surgery in Washington, DC, in June, 1993, Lazar Greenfield chose to address the end of mandatory retirement as the broader question of the performance of aging surgeons [3]. He stated that, "This is a touchy issue because most of us feel that we are constantly getting better at what we do, when, in fact, we are aging….Although very little is known about the behavior of aging surgeons, there is a great deal of interest in the older worker in general, particularly with reference to job safety and productivity. In fact, it is surprising to learn that in the science of applied ergonomics, which addresses the interaction between the worker and job demands, the older worker is defined as anyone over 40 years of age. You will be delighted to learn that this is believed to be the time of the *onset of slowed performance, decreased ability to learn new skills, increased accidents, rigidity, poor health, irritability, and resistance to supervision* [4]. Other studies suggest a *decline in motivation, creativity, and ability to cope with stress* [5]. Is this stereotype accurate and is there any relevance to the field of surgery? It may be helpful to review the known physiology of aging, depressing as it is. Although *joint mobility decreases only slightly* between the ages of 20 and 60 years of age, *the incidence of arthritis increases markedly* beyond age 45 years and there is *reduced motion of the lumbar spine* [6]. The *decrease in overall elasticity can limit leg and arm movements*, with *more rapid shoulder muscle fatigue* [6]. Maximal strength is achieved between the ages of 20 and 30 years, with a slow decline into the 40s and then an accelerated decline, more prominent in the legs and trunk than in the arms. For women, muscle strength remains at about two thirds that of men. For both sexes, finger and arm strength decrease after age 40 years, and maximum grip strength falls by 50% between age 25 and 79 years [7]. Overall there is a 25% loss of strength by age 65 years. This is generally the result of muscle wasting and weakness, fewer functioning motor units, and reduced nerve conduction impulse velocity. Similarly, maximum oxygen capacity peaks at about 20 years and then declines so that at age 65 years, it is 70% of that for a 25-year-old person [8]. Part of this change in performance is likely caused by the effects of progressive inactivity. However, there is an age-related reduction in the ability to diffuse lactate after maximal exercise beginning at age 30 years, which decreases endurance [9]. Heart rate during maximal exercise also decreases with age from values of 195 beats/min at age 24 years to 175 beats/min at 50 years and 165 beats/min at 65 years of age [8]. This increases the perceived effort for the older cohort and decreases workload capacity. For surgeons, however, the issue is performance rather than workload. In the workplace, performance is defined as the ratio of allowed time for a specific task to the actual time taken for the job. Engineering studies show a consistent decline in mean performance ratings with increased age [10]. This appears to be caused by a reduced signal/noise ratio from sensory organs to the brain and within the brain. This is why the older person asks you to speak louder. To compensate for this, there is a spontaneous tendency to adopt strategies to optimize performance [11]. These are more successful in preserving timing and action sequence for familiar tasks than actual reaction times and complex decisions. This is because of difficulty in switching attention from one task to another in older cohorts. With aging, it takes longer to retrieve information from memory and make decisions that require use of specific short-term memory. Perhaps the most common physiologic age-related change is in our vision, which is caused by pupil shrinkage, hardening and yellowing of the lens, loss of accommodation, and greater light scattering in the ocular media. Better lighting, visual aids, and minimal glare will improve performance. Studies show that optimal performance requires 50% more illumination for workers aged 40–55 years and 100% more for workers over age 55 years [12]. Older workers are also less tolerant of heat stress, which may explain why I find myself complaining more about the temperature in the operating room.

These effects have led to recommendations in industry to use ergonomic job design to sustain productivity and to retain the skills and knowledge of the older worker in supervisory positions. However, more longitudinal studies of performance are needed to increase the validity of these age-related changes [13]. Because aging is a complex phenomenon involving many organs and systems, it would be advantageous to have a model system to investigate the mechanisms" [3].

Greenfield [3] states further, "Because we are not likely to be able to influence the rate of physiologic aging any time soon, what are the problems related to aging that surgery must face? One is the end of mandatory retirement. Federal legislation enacted in 1986 now prohibits employers from requiring their employees to retire when they reach a specific age. An exception to this law allows colleges and universities to require tenured faculty to retire at age 70 years but only until Dec. 31, 1993. However, in 1991 Michigan passed its own legislation barring any age-related mandatory retirement. At the University of Michigan the number of faculty who are age 60 years or older has increased 37% in the past 12 years, whereas the overall size of the faculty has increased only 2%. With the option to continue after age 70 years for the past 3 years, 60% have chosen to stay and one study predicts a future 1-year retention rate of 85% for faculty reaching 70 years of age. In the United States today only 11.5% of medical faculty are 60–69 years old and only 2% are over 70 years of age" [3].

"In the absence of mandatory retirement, both academic departments and private practices will have to face medicolegal and economic challenges. The economic challenge includes not only the cost of compensation, but also the restricted ability to bring in younger surgeons. The medicolegal issue has surfaced as a matter of disclosure of the surgeon's health, beyond the nature and risks of the procedure. As more data on outcomes become available, hospitals and patients will make comparisons and expect reassurance that the aging surgeon is not declining in performance. These comparisons are difficult and obviously heavily dependent on the level of patient risk that the surgeon is willing to accept. We are having difficulty just deciding who should drive. The number of U.S. motorists 65 years of age or older has doubled since the 1980s to a total of about 22 million, and the numbers continue to increase. The data show that drivers over age 65 years as a group do not represent a hazard to the public because their crash rate per mile is increased only slightly until they reach age 75 years. However, these older drivers are more vulnerable to injury once a crash has occurred. Compared with drivers under 20 years of age, drivers over age 64 years were five times more likely to die in a survey of 15,336 two-car fatal crashes" [14].

"In addition to crashes, older drivers are overrepresented in the frequency of traffic violations such as failure to yield, failure to stop, inattention, and safe-movement violations. However, they are underrepresented in recklessness, following too closely, and alcohol violations. The federal highway safety standard for driver licensing requires that reexamination occur at least every four years and tests of knowledge and visual acuity are done. It also calls for driver deficiencies and limitations to be identified and that remedial measures or termination of licensure occur for individuals failing to meet the standards. There is great variation in how the states handle this responsibility, but most require vision testing at some age threshold, whereas only a few require knowledge or road testing. Authorities in the field suggest that vision testing be expanded to include both acuity under reduced illumination and dynamic visual acuity [15]. The data also suggest that the frequency of examination be increased to every 2 years when the driver reaches age 70–75 years and consideration be given to issuance of restricted licenses to avoid high-risk traffic areas" [3].

Greenfield [3] then points out that, "There is obvious sensitivity to any suggestion of discrimination against the elderly, and this has kept some states from enacting any age-driven reforms. However, it is interesting that we use age-based criteria in many other public policies such as eligibility for Social Security, Medicare, housing programs, and tax benefits. At the other end of the spectrum, individuals are not permitted to drive until age 16 years and are not legally able to purchase or consume alcoholic beverages until 21 years of age. These choices are obviously based on administrative expediency because it would be much more costly to make individual assessments. However, state administrators find themselves subject to liability for failing to identify the disabilities of drivers who subsequently cause death or damages. So we can begin to see some similarities here to the responsibilities we face in the credentialing of older surgeons. The public can quite legitimately ask why it is that the older person must take an examination to drive but not to be an operating surgeon. If we respond that we monitor for adverse outcomes, the question becomes why it is necessary for an adverse outcome to occur before something is done. Acting on a single adverse outcome would surely be challenged in court, but to wait for multiple adverse outcomes invites the plaintiff's attorney to include the Chief of Surgery in the suit. The concept of calculated risk would certainly not be acceptable when there is a group at risk, such as in a commercial airplane. In fact, the Federal Aviation Administration has been able to withstand a number of legal challenges to its requirement that commercial pilots flying larger planes retire at age 60 years. It is less comforting to realize that the rule does not apply to smaller commuter flights and private pilots. However, there are no data to suggest that older commercial pilots have more accidents. Indeed, the defense to the rule has been the legal technicality that the older pilot challenging the rule must show that his performance is as good as that of any other older pilot and because there are no other older pilots, it is a catch 22. The Office of Aviation Medicine within the Federal Aviation Administration has initiated a research project to look at the relationship between aging and accidents and develop a battery of tests to select individuals capable of flying beyond age 60 years. That may be difficult, however, because pilots as a group have a much higher death rate than the general population, peaking at the 55–59 year age group for reasons that are unclear. However, pilots who retire early have a longer life expectancy" [3].

"To return to our primary concern, there is recent information on the changes in cognitive functions of older physicians. The data come from a new computerized neuropsychologic screening battery entitled the Assessment of Cognitive Functions [16]. Rather than test expert knowledge, this instrument assesses mental functions that use the limbic system to learn, store, and retrieve information. Damage to the limbic system produces gross memory deficits characteristic of dementia of the Alzheimer type. This battery also tests attention, language, calculations, visuospatial operations, and reasoning by 21 subtests sampling 16 cognitive domains. The Assessment of Cognitive Functions, was administered to 1002 physicians in Florida, Texas, and Massachusetts, ranging from 25 to over 75 years of age. The tests were validated by concurrent testing of normal and mildly impaired control persons, and the confounding factors of emotional state, medication, sleep deprivation, and intellectual ability were found not to influence the results. …There is a gentle downward slope for both physicians and normal subjects for the first three decades and a more rapid decline after age 65 years. … Obviously, there is great variability among individuals at advanced ages and a substantial number will continue to function at levels comparable to those of younger people. In fact, four out of five physicians in the age range of 70–74 years function as well intellectually as those in the prime decades of 45–64 years. However, because these are cross-sectional rather than longitudinal studies, they are particularly vulnerable to the law of the jungle, because only the fit survive to be tested. Interestingly, when 445 physicians were asked, 'Have you noticed any signs of diminished personal cognition?' the admission of cognitive problems was also proportional to age" [3, 16].

"Word-name blockage was reported by 33% of physicians over 65 years, whereas only 10–20% under 55 years of age had this problem. Problems with short-term recall were reported by 40% of physicians 65 years or older, whereas only 22% under age 55 years were affected. Most physicians also reported using compensatory mechanisms to cope with perceived losses such as keeping notes and lists. So if we assume that most physicians will or should recognize the signs of mental and physical aging, it should follow that they will adjust their work load and realize that retirement is better than the loss of one's professional reputation. In the sports' world, a good example is Ted Williams, who hit a home run his final time at bat for the Red Sox: a much better conclusion than watching the 42-year-old Willie Mays waving at fastballs he once hit into the stands. Of course, the penalty is much higher if you are a boxer who makes one too many trips into the ring, as Muhammed Ali found out, only to have his former sparring partner, Larry Holmes, demolish him. However, it is not unusual for some surgeons to ignore the signs and keep operating well beyond the loss of their skills. All of us have known such situations and usually been unable or unwilling to do much about them. Perhaps the most famous is the story of the last years of Ferdinand Sauerbruch, as described in the book The Dismissal by Thorwald" [3, 17].

Why and how is it that otherwise gifted surgeons have little or no insight into their deterioration or can be so unwilling to give up operating? Deckert [18] has identified three physician traits that can account for this behavior [18]. "The first trait is poor self-esteem. This is surprising at first glance, but it refers to the tendency for physicians to identify themselves with what they do rather than who they are as a person. As an example, he relates the comment of a 70-year-old surgeon who said, 'I know I have no business doing surgery anymore, but what good is a surgeon who doesn't operate?' The second trait is ignorance or rejection of death, which seems even more unusual because physicians deal with death every day. He points out that physicians deal with other peoples' death and as a group are extremely afraid of disease and death. Studies show that most people come to the realization that life is finite and death is real in their 40s, whereas physicians do not adjust until their 60s. The third trait is resistance to change, which characterizes physicians reluctant to accept the need to adjust to advancing age and who boast, 'I'll never retire!' This is easy to understand because it requires facing the previous issue of loss of self-worth and confronting one's own death" [3].

Greenfield [3] concluded his address with: "It is clear that we need better data on the performance of aging surgeons from the standpoint of longitudinal rather than cross-sectional studies. Both cognitive and functional test results should be evaluated under controlled circumstances so that objective as opposed to subjective criteria for performance can be established. Above all, we need to remove the stigma associated with retirement and construct ways for productive members of our society to continue to retain their self-esteem as they enter the final chapters of their career" [3].

Specific problems, examples, and studies related to aging surgeons including their proficiency, operative mortality, cognitive changes, neuropsychologic tests, decay of skills, surgical risk factors, surgeon fatigue, time to leave active practice, and other less specific estimates of competence and safety, have not been yielding uniformly unequivocal data or information which is as conclusive as had been anticipated regarding definitive resolution of some of the study objectives originally hypothesized [19–26].

More recently, Whitehead [27], in a short communication on the internet entitled, "When Should Surgeons Stop Operating" highlighted a two-day series of assessments for older surgeons to evaluate physical and cognitive function, a program offered at Sinai Hospital in Baltimore. She noted that some of the declines that accompany aging include increasing fatigue, forgetfulness, and reduced eyesight. She then pointed out that other professions maintain a close watch for such changes in order to protect the public, and some even have a firm age cut-off. For example, airline pilots are required to retire at age 65, and some firefighters must step down by age 57, however, no nationwide age-related cut-offs, required assessments, or guidelines currently exist to ensure that physicians provide their services safely and competently. She added that we all know octogenarians who can play a respectable game of tennis, and others in the same age group who cannot even walk to the mailbox. The same can be said for surgeons; many still do great work in their 70s, but others should not even be allowed in the operating room [27].

Recently, the American Medical Association took the initiative in this situation, convening a group of physician members to recommend guidelines for assessing the skills and the abilities of physicians late in their careers. However, no definitive action has been announced by July, 2015, nor has any indication been made as to who would be charged with conducting such assessments of competency. In the United States, one of every four licensed physicians is older than 65 years, with 40% of them actively practicing according to the AMA statistics. Their goal in creating guidelines is to head-off calls for a mandatory retirement age, especially for surgeons, while still safeguarding patients. Mark R. Katlic, MD [28], a thoracic surgeon at Sinai Hospital in Baltimore, in his seventh decade of age, was not involved in generating the AMA report, but has been a strong proponent of guidelines tied to competency, particularly for surgeons [28]. He published his work on "The Aging Surgeon" in the Annals of Surgery in 2014 and reported several disquieting anecdotes that he had heard regarding excellent surgeons with exemplary reputations and respect, who ran into trouble as they got older. One requested a colleague to lead him back to his office after an operation because he wasn't sure that he could find it. Another ordinarily meticulous surgeon began to show up to work appearing sloppy and unclean. Yet another surgeon actually fell asleep while performing a surgical procedure in the operating room! To dramatize his message, he abstracted the tragic and heartbreaking late years of Ferdinand Sauerbruch (1875–1951), one of the world's greatest surgeons, who for years was a brilliant diagnostician and exquisite technician in his clinic and operating theaters in Berlin. However, in his late 60s, his colleagues noted that Sauerbruch, "had sudden changes in mood and periods of forgetfulness." He "struck assistants with instruments during operations, which were performed with growing clumsiness, dragging tissues and tearing blood vessels." In part because of the success related to his international fame and generation of financial resources, the Faculty and Administration failed to intervene, and individual efforts by his friends suggesting retirement were flatly rejected. After a prominent actor succumbed to bleeding during a simple herniorrhaphy and a child died after a stomach resection because Sauerbruch failed to restore gastrointestinal continuity, he finally acceded to demands to retire in 1949 at age 74 when threatened with a humiliating public dismissal. Despite this, he had little insight and continued to operate in his home with disastrous results. His 1953 autobiography is entitled, "Master Surgeon." Sixty years since then, there are overwhelming anecdotes and some published evidence that the aging surgeon remains a problem, which has piqued Katlic's interest and efforts [28].

Katlic [28] says, "I think the general public would be very interested to know that surgeons don't police themselves well as a profession. It often takes a bad complication that hurts a patient before something serious is done. Surgery requires solid mental and physical capabilities that some older surgeons may be lacking. Fine motor skills are needed to wield sharp scalpels; endurance is essential for long procedures, and quick reaction times are a must too. If a problem arises in the operating room, surgeons need to analyze the situation swiftly and make decisions on the fly" [28]. A surgical oncologist at Eastern Virginia Medical School, Roger Perry, MD [29], says "this key problem solving ability, known as fluid intelligence, can decline with age. No operation is ever the same as any other. You need to be able to figure out things as you go, and when problems arise, recognize an alternative" [27–29].

How can we determine whether and when a surgeon can no longer be trusted wielding a scalpel during a major operative procedure? Katlic [28] and Perry [29] say, "The key is creating a series of tests and guidelines that check capabilities instead of chronological age. The Aging Surgeon Program at Sinai Hospital is one example of this initiative" [27]. "Created by Katlic in 2014, the program invites surgeons from around the world to come to Baltimore to take a two-day test that rates their physical and cognitive abilities. Among the many skills and attributes examined, the tests evaluate hearing, vision, and hand-eye coordination. Surgeons who are concerned about their health can opt to take the tests, but hospitals can also request evaluations of their surgeons. The results and recommendations –

good or bad – are entirely confidential and are supplied solely to the individual who requested the evaluation" [27].

While it may sound like a good option for senior surgeons, the program has had its difficulties. For one, not a single doctor has stepped forward to date to take the test as of July, 2015 [27]. "However, we've learned that a number of physicians have opted to retire when threatened to be put through our program," Katlic says [27, 28].

"Stanford Health took a similar approach in 2012 when it created the Late Career Practitioner Policy requiring physicians over the age of 75 years to be screened every two years. The policy has faced opposition among Stanford Faculty members with some arguing that there is research proving that older physicians are more likely to make mistakes than younger physicians. Some critics of these sorts of tests and guidelines say that they are needlessly discriminatory and should focus on competency, not age. Others point out that physicians, of all people, have the training and experience to evaluate their own health and shouldn't need outside oversight. But that's not good enough, Katlic [28] and Perry [29] say. Doctors, are human too" [27]. "Most people, regardless of the field they fall into, fail to recognize that they are not doing as well as they used to," Perry [29] said. "We all know people in our families who are driving that shouldn't be – but if you speak to them, they think that they are perfectly fine." Perry [29] thinks that, "with time, the need for competency tests will become accepted by doctors. And with that acceptance, participation in the Aging Surgeon Program will increase, too" [27]. Katlic [28] concludes with, "such an assessment would balance the dignity of a committed practitioner and his or her value to society with patient safety and liability risk...a comprehensive, multidisciplinary, objective, and confidential evaluation. Both the surgeon and society deserve no less" [28].

"When should we quit operating?" has been a difficult question to answer for surgeons throughout the centuries; and it has become ever more trying, demanding, formidable, and controversial as our patients and surgeon population age and live longer; and as our society becomes more complex and demanding. No uniformly recognized, accepted, enforced laws, rules, regulations, standards, practices, or guidelines have been established, and little progress has been made in defining and managing this onerous problem. Prior to the Age Discrimination in Employment Act (ADEA) in 1986 in the United States, the mandatory retirement age of 65 years served as a generally, though not entirely, accepted landmark or milestone for surgeons to relinquish their leadership positions of authority, and concurrently to surrender their major operative privileges and complex patient management activities and responsibilities. This was somewhat helpful in avoiding and ameliorating the problem of the aging surgeon. However, the mandate against age discrimination has had a significant impact on surgical practice, both positive and negative, and many of the resulting consequences have been noted, described and/or discussed throughout this chapter, together with what relatively little relevant or representative literature has been published to date. Moreover, in addition to the studies and presentations of some of our most intellectual, philosophical, responsible, and concerned individual surgeon colleagues, some of our most respected and honorable professional societies and governing bodies have undertaken the challenges to elucidate and resolve this "Gordian knot" problem, including the American College of Surgeons, the American Board of Surgery, the American Medical Association, and others. To date, no definitive conclusions or recommendations have been forthcoming, although it is inevitable that the greater health care community and the patient population will demand and expect the resolution of this problem in the near future. It is highly unlikely that any resolution will be acceptable to everyone, but such is the nature of human behavior, and rational, logical, moral, and ethical decisions must prevail. Until the definitive adjudication of the time for surgeons to quit operating occurs, we will continue to be dependent upon the innate insight, judgment, wisdom, integrity, character, competence, strength, skills, ethics, health, finances, and other personal factors of the individual surgeons to make this often distressing decision and to "do the right thing."

On a personal note, at the time of this writing, the author is 80 years old and has refrained completely from operative surgery and acute patient management for five years since his 75th birthday in 2010. It was not easy or pleasing to do, and there has not been a day since then that I have not missed doing what I loved most, but I have maintained my long-standing modified, prospective decision, and I have only returned to the operating theater on a few occasions since then to provide requested consultations to my younger staff colleagues or trainees who sought the benefits of my more extensive experience. To be candid and honest, I have greatly enjoyed those occasional sojourns to the operating suite, and I cherished the gratifying opportunity to continue to be useful in sharing my accrued experience, judgment, and wisdom.

On the other hand, I have not really retired from life or from the microcosm of academic medicine and surgery. I have been occupied 40–80 hours a week (sometimes more) lecturing, teaching, and mentoring medical students, PA students, residents, fellows, other members of the health care community; supervising history-taking, physical examinations, surgical skills sessions, simulation exercises; advising, counseling, writing reference letters, making personal telephone, and cyber contacts to advocate for students, residents, and fellows; presenting lectures, conferences, seminars throughout the country; writing papers, chapters, books, usually with younger co-authors at all levels; giving mock oral examinations; traveling throughout the world lecturing at major professional meetings and learning; spending more time with my wife of 57 years and family of six children, 16 grandchildren, and one great grandchild; and enjoying more time with them in our beloved New Hampshire lake house. There are so many other wonderful, challenging, and exciting things for me to do and enjoy that I don't have time or desire to reflect upon the past "glory days" of surgery, because I am trying to help promote the future greatness of surgery via the brightest generation of young aspirants to our specialty that I have ever known.

To conclude my tale, I had made the decision when I was completing my Chief Residency in surgery in 1967, that if I lived and enjoyed good, functional mental, emotional, and physical health, that I would quit operating at age 65 years, not really expecting to reach that age. I did not want to be the failing "old man" who was "losing it" in the operating room and thereby endangering the patient, distressing the nurses and house staff, and compromising a reputation which I would have worked hard to achieve and maintain as a safe, competent, and perhaps even an exceptional, surgeon. I wanted to quit surgery while I still could play an acceptable, safe, efficacious, non-embarrassing, no fumbles surgical game and walk away with my head held high in the knowledge that I had had a gratifying, effective, distinguished surgical career.

As I approached my 65th year, it became apparent to me that I still had the strength, energy, endurance, cognitive ability, eye-hand coordination, competence, and other skills, together with a rich experience and successful record of complex surgical management of countless critically ill patients, that I might extend my original planned operative exit to age 70, while spending more time sharing my patient load with my younger surgical colleagues and residents in order to reduce my workload and to increase theirs, to the benefit of their experience and expertise and to my extended operative longevity. I enjoyed that period, and when I talked of quitting operating at age 70, my colleagues at all levels assured me that I still could "handle the toughest cases" with ease, safety, and competence, and they convinced me to continue on a bit longer. I persuaded my closest professional and personal surgical friends to swear that they would not allow me to embarrass myself or to perform below my own high standards, and that they would discretely inform me when it was "time to hang up the cleats," and "turn in the uniform." Indeed, I regularly checked with them as to whether I was still doing "OK."

As I approached age 75, became an Emeritus Professor, Emeritus Chairman of Surgery, and Emeritus Program Director of Surgery, I reasoned that it was time to become an emeritus operative and practicing surgeon. All of the wind socks were blowing in the same direction.

Moreover, at age 74, I underwent a successful triple coronary artery bypass procedure which took a little wind out of my sails, and although I returned to the operating room a few months, postoperatively; I knew deep within my body and soul that it was time to close the curtain, and I did so without histrionics, fanfare, or regrets, definitively and without recourse at age 75, which was 10 years longer than I had originally planned. I am greatly blessed to have had the opportunity to help my fellow human beings with my surgical efforts for 43 years as a board certified surgeon, and a total of 49 years, including my internship, surgical residency, and fellowship. Since then, I have been enjoying life as a surgical educator, scientist, mentor, writer, lecturer, husband, and parent; and cherishing the opportunities to continue to be as useful as I can be for as long as I am able. Who could want, or ask for anything more?

References

1. Pogo KW. Daily comic strip. Earth day, Post-Hall Syndicate. Simon & Schuster; 1971.
2. Bradley R, Nehra M, Nehra A, Folkes J. The gambler. Sony/ATV Music Publishing, LLC; 1978.
3. Greenfield LJ. "Farewell to surgery," presented as the presidential address at the forty-first scientific meeting of the International Society for Cardiovascular Surgery, North American Chapter, Washington, DC, June 7–8, 1993. J Vasc Surg. 1994;19:6–14.
4. Stauger R. Boredom on the assembly line: age and personality variables. Indust Gerontol. 1975;30:23–43.
5. Benson R. Management perceptions of older employees. Mon Labor Rev. 1978;101:33–5.
6. Hauon engineering guide to equipment design... McGraw Hill, New York; 1963.
7. Garg A, Funke S, Janisch D. One-handed dynamic pulling strength with special applications to lawn mowers. Ergonomics. 1988;31:1139–53.
8. Astrand PO, Rodahl K. Textbook of work physiology. New York: McGraw Hill; 1977.
9. Tzankoff SP. Age-related differences in lactase distribution kinetics following maximal exercise. Eur J Appl Physiol. 1979;42:35–40.
10. Karnes EW, Freeman A, Whalen J. Engineering work standards for warehouse operations: effects of performance ratings, age, gender and neglected variables. In: Trends in ergonomics/human factors III (part A). New York: Elsevier Science; 1986. p. 535–43.
11. Welford AT. Changes of performance with age: an overview. In: Aging and human performance. New York: Wiley; 1985. p. 333–65.
12. Required Quantity and Quality of Light Committee. Selection of illuminance values for interior lighting design (RQQ report 6). J Illuminat Eng Soc. 1980;9:188–90.
13. Garg A. Ergonomics and the older worker: an overview. Exp Aging Res. 1971;17:143–55.
14. Partyka S. Comparison by age of drivers in two-car fatal crashes. Washington, DC: National Highway Traffic Safety Administration. U.S. Department of Transportation; 1983.
15. Waller PF. Renew licensing of older drivers... transportation in an aging society, Special report No. 218 72-100, vol. 2. Washington, DC: Transportation Research Board, National Research Council; 1988.
16. Powell DH, Whitla D. Profiles in cognitive aging. Cambridge: Harvard Press; 1994.
17. Thorwald J. The dismissal: the last days of Ferdinand Sauerbruch. New York: Pantheon; 1962.
18. Deckert GH. How to retire happy. Med Econ. 1992;69:73–80.
19. Neumayer LA, Gawande AA, Wang J, Giobbie-Hurder MS, Itani KMF, Fitzgibbons RJ Jr. Proficiency of surgeons in inguinal hernia repair: effect of experience and age. Ann Surg. 2005;242:344–8. discussion 348–352
20. Waljee JF, Greenfield LJ, Dimick JB, Birkmeyer JD. Surgeon age and operative mortality in the United States. Ann Surg. 2006;244:353–62.
21. Bieliauskas LA, Langenecker S, Graver C, Jin Lee H, O'Neill J, Greenfield LJ. Cognitive changes and retirement among senior surgeons (CCRASS): results from the CCRASS study. J Am Coll Surg. 2008;207:69–78. discussion 78–79
22. Boom-Saad Z, Langenecker SA, Bieliauskas LA, Graver CJ, O'Neill J, Caveney AF. Surgeons outperform normative controls on neuropsychologic tests, but age-related decay of skills persist. Am J Surg. 2008;195:205–9.
23. Blasier RB. The problem of the aging surgeon. Clin Orthop Relat Res. 2009;467:402–11.
24. Tuwairqi K, Selter JH, Sikder S. Assessment of surgeon fatigue by surgical simulators. Open Access Surg. 2015;8:43–50.
25. Garrett K, Kaups KL. The aging surgeon: when is it time to leave active practice? Bull Am Coll Surg. 2014;99:32–5.
26. Drag LL, Bieliauskas LA, Langenecker SA, Greenfield LJ. Cognitive functioning, retirement status, and age: results from the cognitive changes and retirement among senior surgeons study. J Am Coll Surg. 2010;211:303–7.
27. Whitehead N. http://www.npr.org/sections/health-shots/2015/06/18/414912417/when-should-surgeons-stop-operating
28. Katlic MR, Coleman J. The aging surgeon. Ann Surg. 2014;260(2):199–201.
29. Perry PR. Governors' committee on physician competency and health. Bull Am Coll Surg. 2013;

27 Stanley J Dudrick: A Life of a Giant in Surgery and Surgical Decision to Transition to a New Role or No Role At All

Rifat Latifi

Introduction

As discussed eloquently and comprehensively in the previous chapter (Chap. 26) of this book written by professor Dr Stanley J Dudrick, MD, FACS, (Fig. 27.1), we surgeons make many important decisions that continuously affect the lives and our patients throughout our career, but there is no bigger decision, and more important one that we make in our own lives than that to decision to stop operating and transition into a different pace of life. But the transition from active practice to retirement is a necessary phase in the career of every surgeon. The questions, when, how, and why are well addressed in this chapter, and I will not delve on them, but it is clear (although some of us do not like it) that as we surgeons age, we may experience physical and cognitive changes that can affect our ability to perform surgery safely and effectively. All of these natural changes are often time very difficult to be self-recognized by many. We all have seen surgeons who struggle to even walk, who look really sick, and yet, come to participate in national and international meetings. I have often asked myself; would I want to look like that and still be present in the public? Do not know what is the right answer. But when I have seen some of the giants of surgery whom I have revere for years in a state that they could not even keep the coffee or drink in their hand, could not remember any one around them, and nodding to everything they hear, I had mixed feelings. Just wanted to remember them as the giant of surgical history that they were.

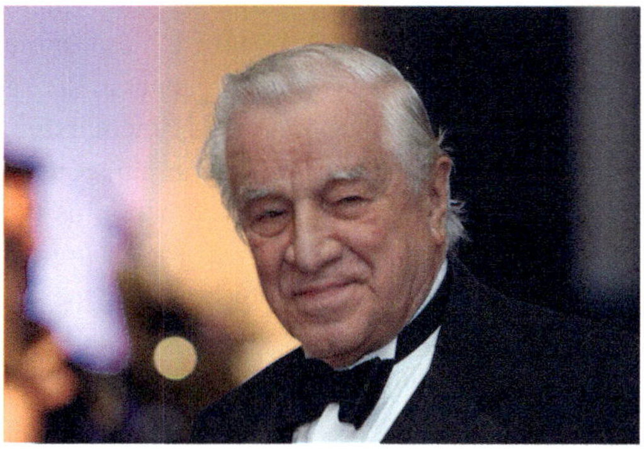

Fig. 27.1 Dr. Stanley J Dudrick, MD, FACS

These changes are normal part of aging, and some of use will have more and some of us will have less, but the fact is that can include decreased dexterity, visual acuity, and reaction time, as well as memory decline. Retiring at the appropriate time allows us to maintain high standards of patient care and safety. And, if possible, to transition from active surgical practice on the educational and teaching only position, and participating in teaching and quality conferences, will be an amazing opportunity to continue to

R. Latifi (✉)
Department of Surgery, The University of Arizona, Tucson, AZ, USA

Tucson Medical Center, Department of Surgery, Tucson, AZ, USA
e-mail: Latifi@surgery.arizona.edu

R. Latifi (ed.), *Surgical Decision-Making*, https://doi.org/10.1007/978-3-031-67391-7_27

further contribute. While at the University of Arizona, the weekly Morbidity and Mortality conferences and surgical grand rounds were often attended by great names of surgery, particularly during the fall, winter, and spring seasons such as Professors Robert M Zollinger, Lazar Greenfield, and many other retired local surgeons. Their presence represented an extraordinary opportunity for the young and not so young surgeons to hear some incredible comments that she light of major experience in a thoughtful way. They were all retired, but the department of surgery leadership, invited them to be part of the department faculty, and allowed an academic platform to pass on the knowledge, expertise, and more importantly wisdom to younger generations of surgeons through teaching and mentorship. Transitioning to retirement allows us surgeons to focus on our own health and well-being, as the demanding and high-stress nature of surgical practice can take a toll on physical and mental health over time.

For the first edition of this book, I have asked my mentor and a true friend to write the chapter on when should we quit. In this editorial special chapter, I wanted the reader to know a bit more about the author, professor Dr. Stanley Dudrick a renowned surgeon and pioneer in the field of parenteral nutrition. He has revolutionized the treatment of patients with gastrointestinal failure "who should not, cannot eat or will not eat" by developing the total parenteral nutrition (TPN), a life-saving technique for millions of patients over the year. This breakthrough method involved providing all essential nutrients directly into the central veins, bypassing the digestive system, and allowing the intestinal problem to heal.

Dr. Dudrick's work in TPN has significantly improved the outcomes for patients with conditions such as gastrointestinal disorders, cancer, and severe malnutrition. His research and innovations have saved countless lives and have become a standard practice in the medical field. In addition to his contributions to parenteral nutrition, Dr. Dudrick has also made significant advancements in the field of surgery, particularly in the areas of trauma and critical care. He has published numerous papers and authored several books on these topics, further solidifying his reputation as a leading expert in the field. Overall, Dr. Stanley Dudrick's work has had a profound impact on the field of medicine, and his dedication to improving patient care has earned him recognition and respect from colleagues and patients alike.

The Phone Call that Changed My Life

When April 8, 1985 I left Kosova and arrived at JFK to join Drita and our two daughters, Kalterina and Qendresa (54 days old), born in New York city, and whom I have not seen her yet, I had no idea where I was going, what will I do with my life in the USA. All I knew, somehow one day, I will write a book or two, train in the USA and achieve whatever potential I could that possibly had. First year and half was not easy. As I am writing this personal essay, I opened a book "America's Art" by Smithsonian American Art Museum, and on chapter two, "This other Eden" describing the early live of immigrants in the new world, it says: "*Immigrants endured hardship on their journeys and in their first years in America.*" So, struggling in a new world it was nothing new. Except I traveled by plane to JFK, and not by ship. Following a stint of being unemployed at all, while I was studying English language and preparing for the famous ECFMG exam, later converted to USLME, I was lucky to work with another luminary in the field of nutrition, Professor Hussein Ghadimi, in New York, where I delved into the intricacies of the biochemistry of amino acids, a subject that I loved during medical school with similar passion as surgery, physiology, and anatomy. But this was non-operative practice and not a surgical discipline. I wanted to continue my surgical career and was determined to carve a path in the surgical world of the USA. This led to make one of the first "surgical decision" and decided to make a bold leap and leave New York to go to Houston drawn by the allure of the Texas Medical Center, despite lacking any "surgical" connections in Texas. It turned out that Texas was very good to me, and I loved Houston, and Texas. Leaving amongst cowboys and science was exactly what I was missing.

The serendipitous encounter that led me to meet Dr. Stanley J. Dudrick, MD, FACS in Houston, Texas in December 1987 was nothing short of a stroke of luck that altered the course of not just my life and my career but also the lives of my family. It was the decision to leave New York, and go to Texas this leap of faith that brought me into the orbit of Dr. Thomas Klima, a pathologist at the Texas Heart Institute, after being introduced to him by a private practice pathologist in South Houston, who said to me: "*I cannot give you the job, because if do I will ruin your prospect of becoming an academic surgeon, but go and meet dr. Klima.*" After short introduction with him, he took phone roster and meticulously made 29 phone calls in a single afternoon trying to secure me a paying research position at the Texas Medical Center. The first 28 inquiries that Friday afternoon yielded no fruitful outcomes, it was the 29th call that reverberated with fate. On a Saturday morning in December 1987, a phone call from Dr. Dudrick not only altered the trajectory of my life and career but also laid the foundations for a profound partnership that spanned over three remarkable decades. While awaiting to meet him 2 day later in his office, I read a paper that he has just published 3 months earlier in the Annals of Surgery that month on regression of atherosclerosis by the intravenous infusion of specific biochemical nutrient substrates in animals and humans [1] and thought that was fascinating study that in a sense it was a continuation of TPN. The meeting went very well, and December 14, 1987, I became a member of Dr. Dudrick' team and was back in the operating room after year and half of hiatus, joined the man who has changed the practice of medicine and surgery for ever by inventing the total parenteral nutrition [2–5] (Fig. 27.2).

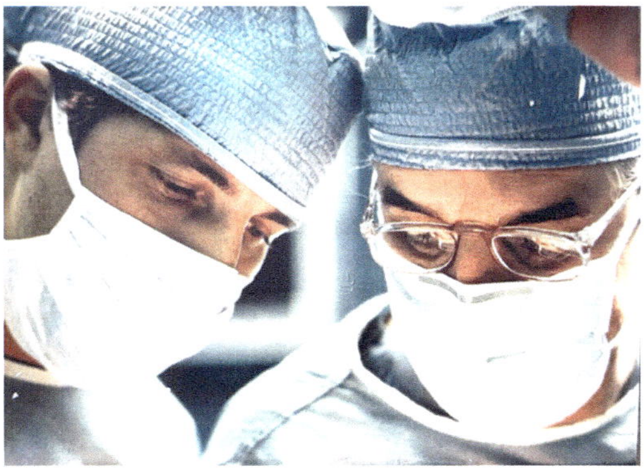

Fig. 27.2 Drs. Dudrick and Latifi, circa spring 1988, Hermann Memorial Hospital, Texas Medical Center

Under Dr. Dudrick's revered mentorship, I left the orthopedics and became eventually trauma and general surgeon, and was fortunate to learn insights and knowledge from one of the luminaries of world surgery. Our collaboration not only resulted in the co-creation and refinement of various publications and books but also marked my debut in the esteemed journal, Surgical Clinics of North America in 1991, a volume that Dr. Dudrick edited [6–11]. Beyond our professional endeavors, Dr. Dudrick transcended the role of mentor to become a cherished friend, guiding me through the intricacies of reoperative surgery and offering steadfast support during challenging moments.

The indelible mark left by Dr. Dudrick was not solely confined to his pioneering work in total parenteral nutrition (TPN) [2–5], which earned him the well-deserved moniker of the "father of intravenous feeding." His legacy extended beyond his groundbreaking innovations, elevating him to the echelons of medical and surgical luminaries like Joseph Lister and Alexander Fleming and others. As a founding member of the American Society for Parenteral and Enteral Nutrition and a pivotal figure in the establishment of the Oley Foundation, his dedication to advancing patient care and championing the field of nutrition set a standard of excellence that reverberates throughout the medical community. Over the span of 30 years, we continued to work closely and publish together [12–48] books, book chapters, and other papers.

As I reflect on the remarkable career and enduring legacy of Dr. Stanley J. Dudrick, I am reminded of his boundless impact on the field of medicine, his unparalleled contributions to patient care, teaching and education, and his unwavering dedication to excellence. From his foundational work in TPN to his pivotal role in shaping surgical education and patient advocacy, Dr. Dudrick's influence resonates far and wide, touching the lives of countless individuals across the globe.

My journey alongside Dr. Dudrick was not just a professional partnership, but a transformative experience that shaped my career and instilled in me a deep sense of purpose and dedication to patient care, practicing it to this day. His belief in me, from offering me my first job in the United States to guiding me through the intricacies of reoperative surgery and beyond, will forever remain etched in my DNA make up, that constantly I pass on to students of surgery. The lessons I learned from him, the wisdom he imparted, and the unwavering support he provided continue to inspire me in my practice every day.

As we remind ourselves of and celebrate the life to Dr. Dudrick, we honor his remarkable achievements, his pioneering spirit, and his profound commitment to advancing the field of surgery. His legacy lives on in the countless lives he touched, the innovations he brought to the forefront, and the indelible mark he left on the hearts of all who had the privilege of knowing him. Dr. Dudrick's, legacy will continue to shine brightly in the world of medicine, and his spirit will forever guide us in our pursuit of excellence and compassion in patient care.

Now, When Should We Really Quit or Transition to a New Role or No Role At All?

When I asked him to write this chapter for the first edition of this book, shortly after he retired, he was very happy to do it. I have read this chapter many times, and I urge everyone to read it, times and times again. I decided to publish Dr. Dudrick's chapter without any changes as remarkable contribution to the field, that is very much in the minds of many surgeons around the world. Knowing when to call it not a quit, but an end is probably as important as when we started. His personal anecdote shared in the last few paragraphs provides a poignant reflection on the journey of a seasoned surgeon who meticulously planned his retirement from the operating room based on a commitment to maintain his professional integrity and safeguarding patient well-being. The narrative captures the ethos of excellence and humility that defined the surgeon's ethos, showcasing a deep-seated dedication to upholding the highest standards of surgical practice and ensuring that his legacy remained untarnished.

The surgeon's decision to set a "retirement age of 65," rooted in a desire to exit the surgical arena while still at the peak of his/her capabilities, underscores the unwavering commitment to prioritizing patient safety and preserving the reputation the surgeon had diligently cultivated over the years. The self-awareness and foresight demonstrated in the decision-making process reveal a profound sense of responsibility and integrity, encapsulating a deep respect for the craft of surgery and the well-being of those under his care. Much has changed since he and many surgeons, if healthy, thought they will retire at that age or about (1–19 under references for retirement).

As the narrative unfolds, it chronicles Dr. Dudrick's and many others contemplation and eventual extension of planned retirement age to 70, guided by a desire to share their wealth of experience and knowledge with younger colleagues while continuing to deliver exceptional surgical care. The sense of camaraderie and mutual respect permeating his interactions with colleagues, who affirmed his continued competence and proficiency, speaks to the deep bonds of professional respect and trust that defined his surgical career.

The surgeon's transition to an emeritus status at age 75, prompted by a combination of physical health considerations and a profound recognition of timing and readiness, exemplifies a graceful and dignified exit from the operating room. His introspective reflections on undergoing a coronary artery bypass procedure and the subsequent realization of the need to gracefully conclude his surgical practice underscore a sense of acceptance and peace with his decision, devoid of regret, or hesitation.

The narrative culminates in a heartfelt expression of gratitude for the opportunity to serve humanity through surgical care, coupled with a poignant acknowledgment of the rich tapestry of roles and experiences that now define his post-operative life. The surgeon's embrace of the multifaceted aspects of his existence beyond the operating room—as an educator, mentor, writer, and family member—reflects a profound sense of fulfillment and contentment in a life lived with purpose and impact.

In conclusion, the narrative eloquently captures the essence of a surgical career marked by dedication, foresight, humility, and a deep-seated commitment to ethical practice and patient welfare. The surgeon's journey serves as a testament to the transformative power of self-awareness, integrity, and a steadfast dedication to excellence that transcends the surgical realm. The thoughtful consideration and deliberate planning that guided the surgeon's retirement decision reflect a profound sense of responsibility and foresight, underpinned by a steadfast commitment to upholding professional standards and ensuring optimal patient care.

Moreover, the surgeon's willingness to adapt his original retirement timeline and seek guidance from trusted colleagues and family underscore a spirit of collaboration, mentorship, and continuous self-assessment. The narrative showcases the importance of humility, self-reflection, and the cultivation of supportive professional relationships in navigating pivotal career transitions with grace and purpose.

The final chapters of the surgeon's career, marked by a graceful transition to emeritus status and a renewed focus on sharing knowledge, wisdom, and experiences with the next generation of medical professionals, highlight a legacy rooted in service, dedication, and a deep-seated passion for the art of surgery. The surgeon's ability to pivot from a distinguished surgical practice to a fulfilling role as an educator, scientist, and mentor speaks to a resilient spirit and an unwavering commitment to lifelong learning and growth.

Ultimately, the narrative encapsulates a life lived with purpose, integrity, and a profound dedication to the well-being of others. The surgeon's journey serves as a powerful reminder of the enduring impact of compassion, humility, and ethical practice in shaping a meaningful and fulfilling career in medicine. The legacy of dedication, excellence, and service that defines Dr. Dudrick story will continue to inspire and resonate with future generations of medical professionals, embodying the timeless values and principles that define the noble calling of healing and caregiving.

The Role of Leaders in Surgery in Navigating the Retirement Process for Senior Surgeons

Leaders in surgery must play a pivotal role in navigating the retirement process for senior surgeons with grace, respect, and sensitivity. When facilitating the transition for a revered surgeon nearing the end of their surgical career, it is essential for leaders to approach the situation with compassion, understanding, yet straight and to outline clear by flexible transition process, to be worked out. An effective way to initiate retirement discussions is through one-on-one conversations in a private and comfortable setting, allowing for candid dialogue and mutual respect.

During these conversations, leaders should acknowledge the surgeon's illustrious career, contributions to the field, and the impact they have had on patients, young surgeons and colleagues, and the institution itself. It is crucial to emphasize the surgeon's expertise, dedication, and lasting legacy while acknowledging the challenges that come with aging, including any physical limitations that may affect their ability to practice surgery safely and effectively.

By expressing genuine appreciation for the surgeon's lifelong commitment to patient care and surgical excellence, leaders can help create a supportive and dignified environment for the retirement transition. Openly discussing the surgeon's future plans, aspirations, and concerns allows for a collaborative approach to decision-making, where the surgeon feels empowered and respected throughout the process.

Leaders should offer guidance, resources, and support to assist the surgeon in transitioning to a new role or phase of their career or life, whether it involves reducing surgical responsibilities, focusing on patient care in a non-operative capacity, or engaging in mentorship and teaching. Providing options for professional development and continued involvement in the surgical community can help the retiring surgeon to maintain a sense of purpose and fulfillment beyond their active operating years.

Additionally, leaders should involve the surgeon in succession planning and mentorship opportunities, ensuring a smooth transition of patient care responsibilities and knowledge transfer to younger colleagues. Recognizing the retiring surgeon's expertise and experience by creating opportunities for them to share their insights, teach best practices, and often impart wisdom and dignity to the next generation of surgeons can be profoundly rewarding for both the retiree and the surgical team.

Above all, leaders should approach the retirement process of their elderly colleagues with empathy, sensitivity, and a deep appreciation for the surgeon's lifelong dedication to the field of surgery. And remember, one day you will come of age of retirement too. By fostering a culture of respect, support, and gratitude, leaders can honor the retiring surgeon's legacy and ensure a dignified and meaningful transition into the next chapter of their professional journey.

In my previous role as Chairman of Surgery at a leading university hospital, the Westchester Medical Center in Valhalla, NY, I had a meaningful discussion with a 76-year-old surgeon who was grappling with a significant hand tremor. Walking together in the serene hospital park, I gently placed my hand on his shoulder to broach the topic of his future plans for transition. I asked him directly has he considered retiring from the operating room while he was still at the pinnacle of his abilities, wanting to be remembered solely for his exceptional expertise. It was a conversation he had been waiting to have, and he expressed relief that finally discussing this pivotal decision with someone from the leadership. Subsequently, he made the decision to step away from surgery much easier but continued to care for patients on an outpatient's basis and taught medical students and residents finding immense fulfillment of joy in his new role.

Conclusion

While the decision to step away from active practice may have come with mixed emotions and uncertainties about leaving behind the familiar and the thrill of surgery, most surgeons find solace and fulfillment in the idea to continue making a lasting impact through teaching and mentorship. By sharing their knowledge, experiences, and insights with aspiring surgeons, the surgeons see an opportunity to influence the future of healthcare, inspire excellence, and leave a legacy that extended beyond the confines of the operating room. In embracing this new chapter of their career, the surgeon can renew purpose and a sense of fulfillment in knowing that he/she is passing on their expertise to shape the future of the surgical field.

The decision to transition from active surgical practice to teaching and mentorship (if there is such possibility, and majority of surgeons do not have that luxury) is not an easy one, but should be planned in advance. After years of honing our skills in the operating room and building a successful career, the surgeons must reflect on their journey and realized that they had reached a point where they wanted to give back and contribute in a different way. We have to recognize that our passion for surgery and patient care could be channeled into shaping the next generation of surgeons, helping them navigate the complexities of the field, and instilling in them the importance of empathy, ethics, and continuous learning. Above all we have to accept one day that our era has ended or is about to end, and only thing will be left is what we have taught other and what we wrote and publish in the process.

References

1. Dudrick SJ. Regression of atherosclerosis by the intravenous infusion of specific biochemical nutrient substrates in animals and humans. Ann Surg. 1987;206(3):296–315. https://doi.org/10.1097/00000658-198709000-00008. PMID: 3115205; PMCID: PMC1493195.
2. Dudrick SJ, Vars HM, Rawnsley HM, Rhoads JE. Total intravenous feeding and growth in puppies. Fed Proc. 1966;25(2):481.

3. Dudrick SJ, Drick S. Longterm total parenteral nutrition with growth in puppies and positive nitrogen balance in patient. Surg Forum. 1967;18:356–7.
4. Dudrick SJ. Rhoads Lecture: a 45-year obsession and passionate pursuit of optimal nutrition support: puppies, pediatrics, surgery, geriatrics, home TPN, A.S.P.E.N., et cetera. JPEN J Parenter Enteral Nutr. 2005;29(4):272–87. https://doi.org/10.1177/0148607105029004272.
5. Dudrick SJ. History of parenteral nutrition. J Am Coll Nutr. 2009;28(3):243–51. https://doi.org/10.1080/07315724.2009.10719778.
6. Dudrick SJ, Latifi R. Total parenteral nutrition in surgery current status. Contemp Surg. 1992;41:41–8.
7. Dudrick SJ, Latifi R, Adams PR. Arrest and reversal of atherosclerosis with parenteral nutrition. Surg Clin NA. 1991;71(3):665–75. PMID 1904650.
8. Dudrick SJ, Latifi R, Fosnocht D. Management of the short bowel syndrome. Surg Clin NA. 1991;71(3):625–43.
9. Dudrick SJ, Latifi R, Schrager R. Nutritional management of inflammatory bowel disease. Surg Clin NA. 1991;71(3):609–23.
10. Latifi R, McIntosh J, Dudrick SJ. Nutritional support in acute and chronic pancreatitis. Surg Clin NA. 1991;71(3):579–95. PMID 1904645.
11. Latifi R, Killam R, Dudrick SJ. Nutritional support in liver failure. Surg Clin NA. 1991;71(3):567–478.
12. Gould KL, Martucci JP, Goldberg DI, Hess MJ, Latifi R, Dudrick SJ. Short term cholesterol lowering decreases size and severity of perfusion abnormalities by positron emission tomography after dipyridamole in patients with coronary artery disease: a potential noninvasive marker of healing coronary endothelium. Circulation. 1994;89(4):1530–8. PMID 8149518.
13. Dudrick SJ, Latifi R. Total parenteral nutrition part II: administration, monitoring and complications. Pract Gastroenterol. 1992;16(7):29–38.
14. Dudrick SJ, Latifi R. Total parenteral nutrition part I: indications and techniques. Pract Gastroenterol. 1992;16(6):21–9.
15. Latifi R, Dudrick SJ, editors. The biology and practice of current nutrition support. 2nd ed. Landes Bioscience: Georgetown; 2003.
16. DeMaria EJ, Latifi R, Sugerman HJ, editors. Laparoscopic bariatric surgery: techniques and outcomes. Landes Bioscience: Georgetown; 2002.
17. Latifi R, Dudrick SJ, editors. Current surgical nutrition. Georgetown: R.G. Landes; 1996.
18. Dudrick SJ, Pimiento JM, Latifi R. Short bowel syndrome: a clinical update. In: Latifi R, editor. Surgery of complex abdominal wall defects: practical approaches. Cham: Springer International; 2017. p. 225–42.
19. Latifi R, Dudrick S, Merrell R. The new surgeon: patient-centered, disease-focused, technology-driven, and team-oriented. In: Technological advances in surgery, trauma, and critical care. New York: Springer; 2015.
20. Dudrick S, Pimiento J, Latifi R. Short bowel syndrome: a clinical update. In: Latifi R, editor. Surgery of complex abdominal wall defects. Springer Science+Business Media New York; 2013.
21. Latifi R, Dudrick SJ, Perch PG. Nutritional management of chronic pancreatitis: current concepts. In: Latifi R, Dudrick SJ, editors. The biology and practice of current nutritional support. 2nd ed. Georgetown: Landes Bioscience; 2003. p. 334–45.
22. Latifi R, SJ, Dudrick SJ. Nutrition support in acute pancreatitis. In: Latifi R, Dudrick SJ, editors. The biology and practice of current nutritional support. 2nd ed. Georgetown: Landes Bioscience; 2003. p. 320–33.
23. Dudrick SJ, Fizan A, Latifi R. Nutritional and metabolic management of short bowel syndrome. In: Latifi R, Dudrick SJ, editors. The biology and practice of current nutritional support. 2nd ed. Georgetown: Landes Bioscience; 2003. p. 261–74.
24. Latifi R, Dudrick SJ. Total parenteral nutrition: current concepts and practice. In: Latifi R, Dudrick SJ, editors. The biology and practice of current nutritional support. 2nd ed. Georgetown: Landes Bioscience; 2003. p. 208–18.
25. Horowitz D, Latifi R. Radiologic assessment of nutritional and metabolic status. In: Latifi R, Dudrick SJ, editors. The biology and practice of current nutritional support. 2nd ed. Georgetown: Landes Bioscience; 2003. p. 181–91.
26. Lanning DA, Latifi R. Wound healing: the role of nutrient substrates. In: Latifi R, Dudrick SJ, editors. The biology and practice of current nutritional support. 2nd ed. Georgetown: Landes Bioscience; 2003. p. 88–102.
27. Azimuddin K, Latifi R, Ivatury RR. Acute phase proteins: the utility in nutrition support of critically ill patients. In: Latifi R, Dudrick SJ, editors. The biology and practice of current nutritional support. 2nd ed. Georgetown: Landes Bioscience; 2003. p. 63–71.
28. Latifi R, Azimuddin K. Biochemistry of amino acids: clinical implications. In: Latifi R, Dudrick SJ, editors. The biology and practice of current nutritional support. 2nd ed. Georgetown: Landes Bioscience; 2003. p. 52–62.
29. Dudrick SJ, Latifi R, Castro GA. Digestion and absorption. In: O'Leary JP, editor. The physiologic basis of surgery. 2nd ed. Baltimore: Williams & Wilkins; 1996. p. 365–75.
30. Mason GR, Kahrilas PJ, Otterson MF, Lang IM, Telford GL, Telford SW, Sarna KS, Cowles VE, Koch TR, Debas HT, Gittes G, Jaffe M, Dudrick SJ, Latifi R, Castro GA. The digestive system. In: O'Leary JP, editor. The physiologic basis of surgery. 2nd ed. Baltimore: Williams & Wilkins; 1996. p. 406–40.
31. Dudrick SJ, Zarif A, Latifi R. Nutritional and metabolic Management of Short Bowel Syndrome. In: Latifi R, Dudrick SJ, editors. Current surgical nutrition. R.G. Landes and Chapman & Hall; 1996. p. 309–17.

32. Anain PM, Matarese LE, Latifi R, Steiger E. Home parenteral nutrition in patients with gastrointestinal tract failure. In: Latifi R, Dudrick SJ, editors. Current surgical nutrition. R.G. Landes and Chapman & Hall; 1996. p. 297–308.
33. Latifi R, Burns GA, Dudrick SJ. Nutritional support of chronic pancreatitis. In: Latifi R, Dudrick SJ, editors. Current surgical nutrition. R.G. Landes and Chapman & Hall; 1996. p. 243–54.
34. Latifi R, Dudrick SJ. Nutrition support of acute pancreatitis. In: Latifi R, Dudrick SJ, editors. Current surgical nutrition. R.G. Landes and Chapman & Hall; 1996. p. 229–42.
35. Latifi R, Dudrick SJ. Total parenteral nutrition: current concepts and indications. In: Latifi R, Dudrick SJ, editors. Current surgical nutrition. R.G. Landes and Chapman & Hall; 1996. p. 45–56.
36. Horowitz DR, Latifi R. Radiological assessment of nutritional and metabolic status. In: Latifi R, Dudrick SJ, editors. Current surgical nutrition. R.G. Landes and Chapman & Hall; 1996. p. 33–43.
37. Latifi R, Dudrick SJ. Effects of nutrients in acute pancreatitis. In: Latifi R, Dudrick SJ, editors. Surgical nutrition: strategies in critically ill patients. Springer-Verlag, R.G. Landes; 1995. p. 147–51.
38. Dudrick SJ, Latifi R. Amino acids in critically ill patients. In: Latifi R, Dudrick SJ, editors. Surgical nutrition: strategies in critically ill patients. Springer-Verlag, R.G. Landes; 1995. p. 31–43.
39. Dudrick SJ, Latifi R. Management of Patients with short bowel syndrome. In: Kirby DF, Dudrick SJ, editors. Practical handbook in clinical practice. CRC Press; 1994. p. 215–26.
40. Dudrick SJ, Latifi R. Total parenteral nutrition. In: Kirby DF, Dudrick SJ, editors. Practical handbook in clinical practice. CRC Press; 1994. p. 135–64.
41. Latifi R, Dudrick SJ. Nutrition in surgical patients. In: Kirby DF, Dudrick SJ, editors. Practical handbook in clinical practice. CRC Press; 1994. p. 165–82.
42. Latifi R, Dudrick SJ. Hepatic encephalopathy: nutrition and metabolic implications of amino acids. In: Latifi R, editor. Amino acids in critical care and cancer. Austin: R.G. Landes Publishing Company; 1994. p. 125–36.
43. Dudrick SJ, Latifi R. Nutritional support: general principles, indications, and techniques. In: Quigley EMM, Sorrell MF, editors. The gastrointestinal surgical patient: preoperative and postoperative care. Baltimore: William & Wilkins; 1994.
44. Dudrick SJ, Latifi R. Surgery and nutrition in the elderly. In: O'Donnell P, editor. Geriatric urology. St. Louis: Mosby; 1993. p. 105–13.
45. Dudrick SJ, Latifi R, Castro GA. Digestion and absorption. In: O'Leary JP, editor. The physiologic basis of surgery. Baltimore: Williams & Wilkins; 1993. p. 365–75.
46. Mason GR, Kahrilas PJ, Otterson MF, Lang IM, Telford GL, Telford SW, Sarna KS, Cowles VE, Koch TR, Debas HT, Gittes G, Jaffe M, Dudrick SJ, Latifi R, Castro GA. The digestive system. In: O'Leary JP, editor. The physiologic basis of surgery. Baltimore: Williams & Wilkins; 1993. p. 340–75.
47. Dudrick SJ, Latifi R. Total parenteral nutrition in the treatment of atherosclerosis. In: Van Way III CW, editor. Handbook of surgical nutrition. Philadelphia: JB Lippincott; 1992. p. 259–71.
48. Dudrick SJ, Adams PR, Englert DM, Latifi R, Feste A. Arrest and regression of atherosclerosis by intravenous infusion of specially formulated nutrient substrates. In: Takehiko T, Akira O, editors. Nutritional support in organ failure. Amsterdam/New York/Oxford: Elsevier; 1990.

Further Readings

Bhatt NR, Morris M, O'Neil A, Gillis A, Ridgway PF. When should surgeons retire? Br J Surg. 2016;103(1):35–42. https://doi.org/10.1002/bjs.9925. Epub 2015 Nov 18.

Gotlib Conn L, Wright FC. Retirement plans and perspectives among general surgeons: a qualitative assessment. Can J Surg. 2018;61(5):319–25. https://doi.org/10.1503/cjs.011217. PMID: 30246991; PMCID: PMC6153102.

Anteby R, Sinyard RD 3rd, Healy MG, Warshaw AL, Hodin R, Ellison EC, Phitayakorn R. Passing the scalpel: lessons on retirement planning from retired academic surgeons. Am J Surg. 2022;224(1 Pt A):166–71. https://doi.org/10.1016/j.amjsurg.2021.11.025. Epub 2021 Nov 29.

Flint L, Scott-Conner CE. What constitutes a successful retirement? Invited commentary on: Anteby and coauthors, passing the scalpel: lessons on retirement planning from retired academic surgeons. Am J Surg. 2022;224(1 Pt A):172–3. https://doi.org/10.1016/j.amjsurg.2022.01.001. Epub 2022 Jan 6.

Buckley R. How do trauma surgeons retire with grace? Injury. 2023;54(10):110999. https://doi.org/10.1016/j.injury.2023.110999. Epub 2023 Aug 9.

Buccimazza I. When should surgeons retire? S Afr J Surg. 2016;54(4):3–4.

Hewitt L, Ashford B. Career reflections of retired surgeons. ANZ J Surg. 2023;93(1–2):21–3. https://doi.org/10.1111/ans.18173. Epub 2022 Nov 24.

Stolarski A, Moseley JM, O'Neal P, Whang E, Kristo G. Retired surgeons' reflections on their careers. JAMA Surg. 2020;155(4):359–61. https://doi.org/10.1001/jamasurg.2019.5476. PMID: 31968054; PMCID: PMC6990937.

Kim NE, Moseley JM, O'Neal P, Whang E, Itani KMF, Kristo G. Retired surgeons as mentors for surgical training graduates entering practice: an underutilized resource. Ann Surg. 2021;273(3):613–7. https://doi.org/10.1097/SLA.0000000000003272.

Part V

The Final Word

Epilogue: Quo Vadis Surgical Decision-Making

28

Rifat Latifi

"In a surgeon (Foreword to: Marx Thorek. Surgical Errors and Safeguards, Fourth edition, Philadelphia: J.B. Lippincott Company; 1943.), there is no quality of mind more to be desired than that of judgment. It is judgment even more than skill that makes him truly a successful surgeon."

Hugh Devine, 1943[1].

Introduction

In this epilogue as the concluding chapter of this book on Surgical Decision-Making: Evidence and Beyond, Second Edition, I want to remind the reader one more time, the profound impact that these decisions have on the lives of our patients, and frankly in our own lives as surgeons as well. Each page of every chapter of this book, each case presented and analyzed, and each insight shared by the authors have deepened our understanding and brought us closer to the nuances and dynamic nature of surgical decision-making.

As we reflect on the myriad factors that influence surgical decision-making, it becomes clear that it is not merely a matter of following guidelines or protocols, or check list. It is a delicate dance between art and science, a harmonious blend of technical proficiency and human compassion. Moreover, it is a culmination of experience, intuition, education, and unwavering dedication to patient care that forms the foundation upon which these critical decisions are made. These decisions, however, in case of emergencies and when things are seemingly out of control, are not always understandable by the team, and only the surgeon may be able to explain the decision, although not all the time.

Through the exploration of real-life scenarios and review of the evidence in each chapter of this book, and often real-life practices described by authors, I am hoping that collectively as a group of surgeons, interested in surgical decision-making, we have advanced the understanding of this complex process and further uncovered the inherent complexities and challenges that surgeons face in the decision-making process. In doing so, this book reviews the role of and the evolution of surgical practices, through advancements in technology, and the shifting paradigms that shape our approach to patient care.

R. Latifi (✉)
Department of Surgery, The University of Arizona, Tucson, AZ, USA

Tucson Medical Center, Department of Surgery, Tucson, AZ, USA
e-mail: Latifi@surgery.arizona.edu

R. Latifi (ed.), *Surgical Decision-Making*, https://doi.org/10.1007/978-3-031-67391-7_28

But let me warn you the reader: if you were expecting to completely grasp how surgical-making decision by the conclusion of this book, you may find that you are not completely satisfied [1]. Although we have delved into various aspects of this intricate topic, there are still many unknowns that necessitate further research. This research should be conducted by surgeons working together with experts who specialize in understanding the mind, brain function, and methods for influencing or training the brain.

In his book "Modern Surgery" published as a second edition in late 1939, Professor Max Thorek, the founder of International College of Surgeons, quotes the renowned English surgeon Lord Moynihan in the first chapter titled "The Surgeon and his Art."

> Surgery is not only a matter of operating skillfully. It must engage in its service qualities of mind and heart that raise it to the very highest pinnacle of human endeavor. A patient can offer you no higher tribute than to entrust you with his life and his health, and by implication, with the happiness of all his family. To be worthy of this trust we must submit for a lifetime to the constant discipline of unwearied effort in the search of knowledge, and most reverent devotion to every detail in every operation that we perform [2–4].

Professor Thorek continues his chapter with:

> " There is no human calling which demands from those who follow it a greater endowment of the best human qualities and the highest developments of technical knowledge and skill than art of surgery." Further, he writes "On the other hand, the surgeon's judgment, knowledge and skill may save a life otherwise doomed; Erroneous or careless surgical procedures may and often do bring either death or life-long misery to a patient who has had a comparatively easily corrected condition" [2].

I should add to these beautifully written words, that should guide every surgeon, that avoiding carelessness and adventurous surgical behavior is a must for every surgeon, every student of surgery, every member of the surgical team, irrespective the stage of their surgical life. The only way to do so, it is for us surgeons to be prepared well, have utmost respect for every procedure, and know everything that is to know about the patient, including past surgical history, the anatomy (often distorted from previous procedures), physiology and patients state of mind, and patient's wishes and goals of end-of-life.

After thoroughly studying Thorek's comprehensive insights, I have come to appreciate more the complexity and significance of surgery, which has long been regarded as one of the noblest arts. While surgical decision-making has evolved over the years, maintaining respect for the patient, disease, and procedures, as well as a commitment to continuous improvement, remains constant. The inherent complexity of making surgical decisions is deeply ingrained in the hearts, minds, and their beings of surgeons.

The methods of surgical decision-making in the present day differ from those used in the past, with technological advancements revolutionizing the field of medicine and surgery. The convergence of surgeon intuition, creativity, and knowledge and comfort with cutting-edge medical technologies has led to a significant transformation in the practice of surgery. Innovations such as laparoscopy, robotics, nanotechnology, genetics, virtual reality, and bioengineering have reshaped the surgical landscape, empowering patients to actively engage in their own healthcare and achieve better outcomes. As a result, hospitals have adapted to support these advancements, and surgeons have embraced a patient-centered, disease-focused, technology-driven, and collaborative approach to healthcare [5, 6].

However, despite the various considerations discussed in this book, the ultimate decisions regarding whether to operate, when to operate, and which approach to take rely solely on the surgeon, and it is a complex interplay of experience of the surgeon, intuition, education, training, exposure, and the surgeon's commitment to providing the best possible care for the patient.

When evaluating the advancements in technology across the spectrum, it is evident that surgical outcomes have improved, leading to reduced morbidity and mortality rates and a higher quality of life for patients. However, at its essence, surgical decision-making transcends mere evidence-based explanations; it lies at the heart of being a surgeon. It involves blending technical expertise with a relentless drive to heal patients and a constant willingness to question and evaluate our own actions.

It is crucial for surgeons to recognize that not every decision made will be correct, and it is essential to acknowledge and learn from mistakes when they occur. True surgical competence involves an ongoing process of self-reflection and a willingness to continuously strive for improvement.

To quote again Professor Max Thorek: "*To fail to admit one's mistakes is to block progress; an honest declaration of error is the first step toward its correction. In this age of cooperation in the science of healing, the surgeon who fears loss of prestige through acknowledgment of fault violates not only faith to himself, but also unjust to his calling*" [7]. Acknowledging potential mistakes in decision-making can undoubtedly lead us to discover new approaches when caring for future patients. Most importantly, will teach the new generations of surgeons dealing with our own errors, and learn from such mistakes.

Ultimately, we aspire for this collaborative effort to motivate others to focus their research endeavors on this subject. Particularly, experienced surgeons should strive to elucidate their decision-making processes more effectively. Integrating discussions on decision-making into surgical planning and team debriefings could be a valuable practice for every surgeon, as advocated by the senior author of this chapter.

As I reflect on the conclusion of this journey that began several years ago, the decision to embark on the creation of the second edition of this book fills me with a sense of hope and renewed creativity. On a very personal note, among >20 book manuscripts I have been involved with over the years, this one stands out as the pinnacle of my satisfaction. Instead of experiencing fatigue, I found myself energized and genuinely delighted with the final result. I hope that this book has ignited a spark of curiosity and reflection in our readers, prompting them to delve deeper into the intricacies of surgical decision-making. May it serve as a catalyst for further research, dialogue, and collaboration among surgeons, educators, and healthcare professionals, driving us toward excellence and innovation in the field of surgery.

In closing, I extend my gratitude to all those who have contributed to this collective effort and to the patients who entrust us with their care. The journey of surgical decision-making is a continuous one, marked by challenges, triumphs, and opportunities for growth, an often with disappointments, that we never forget, but learn from. Let us embrace this journey with humility, compassion, and a steadfast commitment to providing the best possible care for those who place their trust in our hands.

References

1. Latifi R, Latifi F. Final thoughts on surgical decision-making. In: Latifi R, editor. Surgical decision making-beyond the evidence based surgery. Springer; 2016.
2. Thorek M. Modern surgery. Philadelphia: J. P. Lippincott; 1939. Groves EW. The life and work of Moynihan. Br Med J 1940;1(4136):601–606.
3. Groves EW. The life and work of Moynihan. Br Med J. 1940;1(4136):601–6.
4. Groves EW. The life and work of Moynihan: part II. Br Med J. 1940;1(4137):649–51.
5. Latifi R, editor. The modern hospital. Patient centered, disease based, research oriented, technology driven. Switzerland AG: Springer Nature; 2019.
6. Latifi R, Dudrick SJ, Merrell CR. The new surgeon: patient-centered, disease-focused, technology-driven, and team-oriented. In: Latifi R, et al., editors. Technological advances in surgery, trauma and critical care. New York: Springer Science+Business Media; 2015.
7. Thorek M. Surgical errors and safeguards. 4th ed. Philadelphia: J.B. Lippincott; 1943.

Index

R. Latifi (ed.), *Surgical Decision-Making*, https://doi.org/10.1007/978-3-031-67391-7

B

C

F

G

H

U

V

W

X

Y

Z